Paediatric Oncology

Paediatric Oncology
Clinical practice and controversies

Edited by

P.N. Plowman
The Hospital for Sick Children, Great Ormond Street, London

C.R. Pinkerton
The Royal Marsden Hospital, Surrey

CHAPMAN & HALL MEDICAL
London · New York · Tokyo · Melbourne · Madras

Published by Chapman & Hall, 2-6 Boundary Row, London SE1 8HN

Chapman & Hall, 2-6 Boundary Row, London SE1 8HN, UK

Blackie Academic & Professional, Wester Cleddens Road,
Bishopbriggs, Glasgow G64 2NZ, UK

Chapman & Hall, 29 West 35th Street, New York NY10001, USA

Chapman & Hall Japan, Thomson Publishing Japan, Hirakawacho
Nemoto Building, 6F, 1-7-11 Hirakawa-cho, Chiyoda-ku, Tokyo 102,
Japan

Chapman & Hall Australia, Thomas Nelson Australia, 102 Dodds
Street, South Melbourne, Victoria 3205, Australia

Chapman & Hall India, R. Seshadri, 32 Second Main Road, CIT East,
Madras 600 035, India

First edition 1992
Reprinted 1993

© 1992 Chapman & Hall

Typeset in 10/12 Palatino by Photoprint, Torquay, Devon
Printed in Great Britain at The University Press, Cambridge

ISBN 0 412 39780 3   0 442 31595 3(US)

A catalogue record for this book is available from the British Library
Library of Congress Cataloging-in-Publication Data available

Contents

Contents

Contents

Contributors

R.P. A'Hern
Statistician
The Royal Marsden Hospital
Fulham Rd
London

U. Bertram
Chief
Dept of Paediatrics
General Hospital
D-6450 Hanau
Germany

V. Broadbent
Consultant Paediatric Oncologist
Dept of Paediatrics
Addenbrooke's Hospital
Cambridge, and
The Hospital for Sick Children,
Great Ormond Street,
London

M. Carli
Associate Professor of Paediatrics
Division of Haematology and Oncology
Dept of Paediatrics
University of Padova
Italy

G. Cecchetto
Division of Paediatric Surgery
Dept of Paediatrics
University of Padova
Italy

A.C. Chu
Consultant Dermatologist
Dept of Experimental Dermatology and
    Immunology
Royal Postgraduate Medical School
Hammersmith Hospital
Du Cane Rd
London

J.K. Cowell
Head, Haematology and Oncology Research
    Unit
Oncology Group
Institute for Child Health
London

E. Douek
Research Fellow
Imperial Cancer Research Fund
Dept of Medical Oncology
St Bartholomew's Hospital
West Smithfield
London

H. Ekert
Director
Dept of Clinical Haematology and Oncology
Royal Children's Hospital
Melbourne
Victoria 3052
Australia

U. Göbel
Professor and Chairman
Dept of Haematology and Oncology
Kinderklinik der Heinrich-Heine-Universität
D-4000 Düsseldorf
Germany

A. Goldman
Senior Lecturer in Palliative Care
Dept of Haematology and Oncology
The Hospital for Sick Children
Great Ormond Street
London

M. Guglielmi
Professor of Paediatric Surgery
Dept of Paediatrics
University of Padova
Italy

I.M. Hann
Consultant Haematologist
Dept of Haematology and Oncology
The Hospital for Sick Children
Great Ormond Street
London

J.R. Hardy
Consultant Physician
Dept of Medical Oncology
The Royal Marsden Hospital
Fulham Rd
London

J.L. Hungerford
Consultant Ophthalmic Surgeon
Dept of Ophthalmology
St Bartholomew's Hospital
West Smithfield
London

H. Jürgens
Professor and Chairman
Dept of Haematology and Oncology
Universitäts Kinderklinik
D-4400 Münster
Germany

S.J. Kellie
Staff Oncologist
Dept of Paediatrics
Westmead Hospital
Westmead, NSW
Australia

J.T. Kemshead
Director
Imperial Cancer Research Fund Paediatric
    and Neuro-Oncology Group
Frenchay Hospital
Bristol

J.E. Kingston
Senior Lecturer and Honorary Consultant
Dept of Paediatric Oncology
St. Bartholomew's Hospital
West Smithfield
London

J. de Kraker
Paediatric Oncologist
Dept of Paediatric Oncology
Emma Kinderziekenhuis
Meibergdreef 9
1105 AZ Amsterdam
The Netherlands

R. Ladenstein
Research Associate
Centre Leon Berard
28 Rue Laennec
Lyon
France

F. Lampert
Chief
Dept of General Paediatrics, Haematology
    and Oncology
Universitaets Kinderpoliklinik
D-6300 Giessen
Germany

L.S. Lashford
ICRF Clinical Fellow
Dept of Paediatric Oncology
St James's University Hospital
Becket Street
Leeds

I. van Loo
Dept of Paediatrics
Academic Hospital
Wassenaarseweg 62
Leiden
The Netherlands

H.P. McDowell
Consultant Paediatrician
Royal Liverpool Children's Hospital
Alder Hey
Liverpool

C.D. Mitchell
Senior Lecturer
Dept of Haematology and Oncology
The Hospital for Sick Children
Great Ormond Street
London

P. Morris Jones
Reader in Child Health
Dept of Paediatric Oncology
Royal Manchester Children's Hospital
Pendlebury
Manchester

J. Ninane
Paediatric Oncologist
Service d'Hematologie Pediatrique
Universite Catholique de Louvain
Cliniques Universitaires Saint-Luc
Avenue Hippocrate 10
1200 Brussels
Belgium

V. Ninfo
Professor of Pathology
Dept of Pathology
University of Padova
Italy

D.R. Newell
Senior Lecturer
Division of Oncology
Cancer Research Unit
The Medical School
Framlington Place
The University
Newcastle upon Tyne

A. Oakhill
Consultant Paediatric Haematologist/
  Oncologist
Dept of Paediatric Oncology
Bristol Royal Hospital for Sick Children
St Michael's Hill
Bristol

O. Oberlin
Paediatric Oncologist
Paediatric Dept
Institute Gustave Roussy
94805 Villejuif Cedex
France

N. Patel
Community Liaison Sister
Children's Unit
The Royal Marsden Hospital
Downs Road
Sutton Surrey

C. Patte
Paediatric Oncologist
Paediatric Dept
Institut Gustave Roussy
94805 Villejuif Cedex
France

xvii

Contributors

T. Philip
Director
Centre Leon Berard
28 Rue Laennec
Lyon
France

C.R. Pinkerton
Consultant Paediatric Oncologist
Children's Dept
The Royal Marsden Hospital
Downs Road
Sutton
Surrey

P.N. Plowman
Consultant Radiotherapist
Dept of Radiotherapy
St Bartholomew's Hospital
West Smithfield London, and
Dept of Haematology and Oncology
The Hospital for Sick Children,
Great Ormond Street
London

H.G. Prentice
Consultant Physician
Dept of Haematology
Royal Free Hospital School of Medicine
Rowland Hill Street
London

J. Pritchard
Senior Lecturer and Consultant Paediatric
    Oncologist
The Institute for ChildHealth and
The Hospital for Sick Children
Great Ormond Street
London

H. Riehm
Chief
Dept of Paediatric Haematology/Oncology
Medical School
D-3000 Hannover
Germany

E.A. Shafford
Honorary Clinical Assistant
Dept of Paediatric Oncology
St Bartholomew's Hospital
West Smithfield
London

S.M. Shalet
Consultant Endocrinologist
Dept of Endocrinology
Christie Hospital
Wilmslow Rd
Withington
Manchester

G. Sotti
Division of Radiation Therapy
General Hospital of Padova
Padova
Italy

G.G. Steel
Section Head
Radiotherapy Research Unit
The Institute of Cancer Research: Royal
    Cancer Hospital
Belmont
Sutton
Surrey

C.A. Stiller
Statistician
Childhood Cancer Research Group
Dept of Paediatrics
University of Oxford
Oxford

D.M. Tait
Consultant in Radiotherapy and Oncology
Children's Dept
The Royal Marsden Hospital
Downs Road
Sutton
Surrey

T.J. Triche
Pathologist-in-Chief and Chairman
Dept of Pathology and Laboratory Medicine
Children's Hospital
Los Angeles
California 90027
USA

W.H.B. Wallace
Research Fellow in Endocrinology
Dept of Endocrinology
Christie Hospital
Wilmslow Rd
Withington
Manchester

T.E. Wheldon
Head of Laboratory Section
Dept of Radiation Oncology
Cancer Research Campaign Beatson
  Laboratories
Bearsden
Glasgow

K. Winkler
Professor and Chairman
Dept of Haematology and Oncology
Universitäts-Kinderklinik
D-2000 Hamburg 20
Germany

Preface

This book aims to present a succinct but detailed and up to date overview of the most important aspects of managing children with cancer. In contrast to the major American texts which present a treatment philosophy based on the CCG or POG protocols, this volume has a predominantly European slant.

The chapters on individual diseases contain details of clinical presentation, diagnostic work-up, new imaging techniques and current management with chemotherapy, radiotherapy and surgery. We have tried not to present treatment methods in a didactic fashion, but rather to discuss through these core chapters the 'pros' and 'cons' of different therapeutic philosophies.

There is a chapter on pathology which considers the application of modern techniques such as electron microscopy, immunocytochemistry and molecular biology. Similarly, there are chapters on innovative treatment approaches such as megatherapy with marrow rescue, tumour targetting and immunotherapy.

Furthermore, the important subject of avoiding, detecting and managing late sequelae is covered, together with issues such as children in the community and care of the dying child.

At the end of each chapter in Part Two, we have included sections presenting controversies as they relate to diagnosis and management, with references to contemporary work relevant to each controversy. In some cases, these have been compiled by the editors themselves.

Our book is aimed at practising paediatric oncologists seeking an overview of European and North American therapeutic strategies discussed in an objective manner. It should also appeal to general paediatricians, particularly those involved in shared care of children with cancer, who may require an accessible summary of clinical features and modern management.

P.N. Plowman, C.R. Pinkerton

Part One

Scientific and Diagnostic Principles

Chapter 1

Aetiology and epidemiology

C. A. STILLER

1.1 INCIDENCE

Cancer is predominantly a disease of ageing and it is very rare in childhood. In Western populations, only around 0.5% of all cancers occur in children aged under 15 years. The incidence rate is typically in the range 110–130 per million children per year, with the rate in the UK being towards the lower end of this range; this translates into a risk of 1 in 600 that a child will be affected during the first 15 years of life. Therefore, in the UK, which currently has a population of 11 million children, 1200 new cases of childhood cancer can be expected during a year. A general practitioner whose list includes 500 children could expect to see two newly diagnosed cases of childhood cancer during 35 years in practice; to have more than five such patients would be very unusual. The numbers of childhood cancers occurring in the combined lists of large group practices, however, would obviously be greater. In a typical health district containing 50 000 to 75 000 children, between five and ten new cases may be expected per year.

Childhood cancers exhibit a great diversity of histological type and anatomical site but the carcinomas most frequently seen in Western adults – those of lung, female breast, stomach and large bowel – are all extremely rare among children. Cancer incidence data for adults are nearly always grouped according to the International Classification of Diseases (ICD). In the ICD, however, cancers other than leukaemias, lymphomas and melanomas are classified by site of origin. While this is satisfactory for the great majority of neoplasms in adults, it is more appropriate for childhood tumours to be classified according to their histology. A classification scheme for childhood cancers has been developed (Birch and Marsden, 1987) with the groups defined according to codes for morphology as well as topography in the International Classification of Diseases for Oncology (ICD-O). The 12 major diagnostic groups are: leukaemias; lymphomas; brain and spinal tumours; sympathetic nervous system tumours; retinoblastoma; kidney tumours; liver tumours; bone tumours; soft tissue sarcomas; gonadal and germ cell tumours; epithelial tumours; other and unspecified malignant neoplasms. This scheme was used for a recent monograph on the international incidence of childhood cancer (Parkin et al., 1988a), and it is intended that it should become the standard classification for the presentation of childhood cancer incidence data.

The largest population-based series of childhood cancers in the world is the National Registry of Childhood Tumours, which covers

England, Scotland and Wales and is maintained at the Childhood Cancer Research Group in Oxford. Copies of all notifications to the national cancer registration schemes since 1962 for children aged under 15 have been sent to the Registry. The diagnoses on these registrations are verified against medical records and amended where necessary. Table 1.1 shows the registration rates for Great Britain during 1971–1980, a period when the child population was on average 12.4 million. The data are based on those published in the monograph on international incidence rates. As cancer registration is not quite complete, these registration rates are underestimates of the true incidence rates. Comparison with other sources of ascertainment, however, suggests that over 90% of childhood cancers are registered.

About one-third of all childhood cancers are leukaemias, and of these over three-quarters are of the acute lymphoblastic type (ALL). Between a quarter and a fifth are brain and spinal tumours, of which astrocytoma is the most common histological type. Neuroblastoma, retinoblastoma, Wilms' tumour and hepatoblastoma – the distinctive embryonal tumours of childhood – account for 15% of all registrations. Lymphomas account for a further 11%, with non-Hodgkin's lymphoma (NHL) somewhat more common than Hodgkin's disease. Two diagnostic groups have been omitted from Table 1.1. The first of these is Langerhans cell histiocytosis. Ascertainment of this group of disorders by general cancer registries is very incomplete, and some forms at least are not regarded as neoplasms. Data from the Manchester Children's Tumour

Table 1.1 Registration rates for childhood cancer in England, Scotland and Wales, 1971–80 (National Registry of Childhood Tumours data). Total rates are standardized to world population

| Diagnostic group | Total registrations | Annual rates per million for age group | | | | Total (age standardized) | Sex ratio (M/F) |
		0	1–4	5–9	10–14		
Total	12 557	127.3	148.0	85.8	80.4	106.7	1.3
I Leukaemias	4295	26.9	64.6	29.8	20.1	37.5	1.3
Acute lymphoblastic	3362	13.2	55.4	24.0	13.0	29.7	1.4
Acute non-lymphoblastic	722	8.7	6.8	4.8	5.7	6.0	1.2
Chronic myeloid	97	2.4	0.9	0.5	0.8	0.8	1.4
Other and unspecified	114	2.7	1.5	0.5	0.7	1.0	0.9
II Lymphomas	1390	3.8	6.9	11.5	15.2	10.6	2.3
Hodgkin's disease	571	–	1.3	4.1	8.2	4.1	2.5
Non-Hodgkin*	779	2.5	5.3	7.3	6.7	6.1	2.4
Other reticuloendothelial	40	1.3	0.3	0.2	0.3	0.3	0.9
III Brain and spinal	2948	18.8	27.3	25.4	20.7	24.1	1.2
Ependymoma	352	3.9	4.8	2.3	1.8	3.1	1.3
Astrocytoma	1103	5.3	9.5	9.4	8.6	8.9	1.1
Medulloblastoma	596	4.2	6.1	5.6	3.3	5.0	1.7
Other and unspecified	897	5.3	6.9	8.0	7.0	7.2	1.2
IV Sympathetic nervous	746	24.8	12.4	3.0	1.5	7.2	1.4
Neuroblastoma	730	24.4	12.1	3.0	1.4	7.0	1.4
Other	16	0.4	0.2	0.0	0.1	0.1	1.0

Table 1.1 *continued*

Diagnostic group	Total registrations	Annual rates per million for age group				Total (age standardized)	Sex ratio (M/F)
		0	1–4	5–9	10–14		
V Retinoblastoma	341	16.7	6.8	0.3	0.0	3.5	1.0
VI Kidney	769	14.0	15.6	3.7	0.9	7.4	1.0
Wilms' tumour	749	13.9	15.6	3.5	0.6	7.2	1.0
Renal carcinoma	16	–	–	0.1	0.3	0.1	1.7
Other and unspecified	4	0.1	0.1	0.0	–	0.0	–
VII Liver	103	4.2	1.5	0.3	0.3	1.0	0.9
Hepatoblastoma	79	3.8	1.4	0.2	0.1	0.8	0.8
Hepatic carcinoma	24	0.4	0.2	0.1	0.3	0.2	1.4
VIII Bone	631	0.3	1.0	3.9	9.9	4.5	1.2
Osteosarcoma	354	–	0.2	1.7	6.3	2.4	1.1
Ewing's sarcoma	237	0.3	0.5	1.9	3.1	1.7	1.2
Other and unspecified	40	–	0.2	0.3	0.5	0.3	1.5
IX Soft tissue sarcomas	753	11.1	7.6	5.2	5.1	6.4	1.4
Rhabdomyosarcoma	484	6.6	6.1	3.7	2.2	4.2	1.6
Fibrosarcoma†	106	1.4	0.3	0.6	1.4	0.8	1.0
Other and unspecified	163	3.1	1.3	0.8	1.6	1.3	1.2
X Gonadal and germ cell	293	4.9	3.2	1.1	2.5	2.5	0.8
Non-gonadal germ cell	99	2.1	1.2	0.5	0.6	0.9	0.7
Gonadal germ cell	178	2.7	2.0	0.6	1.7	1.5	1.0
Other and unspecified	16	0.1	0.1	0.1	0.2	0.1	0.2
XI Epithelial	259	1.5	0.8	1.4	3.8	1.9	0.6
Adrenocortical carcinoma	27	0.6	0.5	0.1	0.1	0.3	0.4
Thyroid carcinoma	48	–	0.1	0.3	0.8	0.3	0.4
Nasopharyngeal carcinoma	38	–	0.1	0.2	0.7	0.3	1.4
Other carcinoma	146	1.0	0.2	0.8	2.2	1.1	0.6
XII Other	29	0.4	0.2	0.2	0.3	0.2	1.1

* Including Burkitt's and unspecified lymphoma.
† Including malignant fibrous histiocytoma and neurofibrosarcoma.
– No registrations in this age group.

Registry and western Germany suggest that the annual incidence is around 2.5–4 per million; incidence is highest in the first year of life, and boys are affected one and a half times as often as girls. The second group not included in Table 1.1 is malignant melanoma. The age-standardized annual registration rate in Great Britain during 1971–1980 was 0.8 per million but it now seems likely that many of the 102 children registered had non-malignant tumours. In Manchester the incidence was 0.3 per million; the incidence increased with age and there were twice as many girls registered as boys.

Different diagnostic groups have distinctive age distributions. The incidence of ALL is highest among children aged 2–4. Early age peaks in incidence are found also for the embryonal tumours; indeed, for neuroblastoma, retinoblastoma and hepatoblastoma the highest incidence is found in the first year of life. By contrast, Hodgkin's disease, osteosarcoma, Ewing's sarcoma and malignant melanoma show a marked increase in incidence with age that continues into early adulthood. A third pattern of incidence related to age is seen in fibrosarcoma, where a peak in infancy is followed by very low incidence, which then increases in the 10–14 age group. The apparently similar pattern for gonadal germ cell tumours is in fact a combination of different age distributions for the two sexes. In boys the incidence is highest in early childhood and then falls sharply; the start of the postpubertal rise through adolescence is barely discernible before the age of 15. In girls, incidence is lower in early childhood, but the increase in the years following puberty takes place at an earlier age than in boys.

Overall, childhood cancer is about one-third more common among boys than among girls. The male predominance is greatest in the lymphomas, and less marked in leukaemia, brain tumours, neuroblastoma, and sarcomas of bone and soft tissue. The two sexes have similar incidence of retinoblastoma and Wilms' tumour. Only for germ cell tumours and some carcinomas, notably those of the adrenal cortex and thyroid, is there an excess of girls. The markedly different age distributions of gonadal germ cell tumours in the two sexes have been mentioned previously. For the other main diagnostic groups the sex ratio varies relatively little with age.

The patterns of incidence described above are typical of those found in mainly White populations throughout Europe, North America and Oceania. The principal systematic exceptions occur with the lymphomas.

Childhood Hodgkin's disease is more common in the warmer countries close to the tropics; NHL, and especially abdominal Burkitt's lymphoma, have a higher incidence in a large area around the Mediterranean including North Africa and the Middle East, and apparently extending into Europe as far as Spain and Greece (Stiller and Parkin, 1990). Published data on variations in incidence with ethnic group in Western countries almost entirely concern comparisons between Blacks and Whites in the USA. Overall, the incidence of childhood cancer in Blacks is lower than in Whites. This is largely accounted for by the fact that the incidence of ALL in Blacks is only half that in Whites (Parkin *et al.*, 1988b). Several other diagnostic groups have a slightly lower incidence in American Blacks, and Ewing's sarcoma is hardly ever seen. Wilms' tumour, retinoblastoma and osteosarcoma, however, each have an incidence in Blacks around 1.2 to 1.5 times greater than that in Whites.

Greater variations in incidence are found between other regions of the world. The most striking and probably the most well-known example is the extremely high incidence of Burkitt's lymphoma in some parts of tropical Africa and in Papua New Guinea where it is by far the commonest cancer among children.

Data on socioeconomic status and childhood cancer were reviewed by Greenberg and Shuster (1985). Several studies have shown a higher risk of leukaemia with high socioeconomic status, though others, including Birch *et al.* (1981), have found no effect. The lower incidence of childhood ALL in American and African Blacks may be at least partly due to a social class effect. There is a higher incidence of Hodgkin's disease in young children in many developing countries and this seems to be linked to poor socioeconomic conditions. In a small American study, younger children with Hodgkin's disease also tended to come from lower social class backgrounds (Gutensohn and Shapiro, 1982). It is possible that rhabdomyosarcoma (Grufferman *et al.*, 1982) and neuroblastoma (Carlsen, 1986; Davis *et al.*, 1987) are also slightly more common in children of lower socioeconomic status.

There is no evidence of any major change in the incidence of childhood cancer during recent years. There was, however, a small increase in the rates for ALL during the 1970s, which was more marked among children aged under five (Stiller and Draper, 1982). A rise in the incidence of germ cell tumours has also been reported from Manchester (Birch *et al.*, 1980).

Although there is little international variation in incidence among the industrialized Western countries, there have been many reports of small areas with an unexpectedly large number of leukaemias and other cancers in children. There is currently intense interest in the frequency and possible causes of such aggregations and this topic is discussed in the final section of this chapter.

1.2 ENVIRONMENTAL AETIOLOGY

Very little is known about the aetiology of most childhood cancer. For many diagnostic groups, the occurrence of the highest incidence at an early age and the cell type of origin strongly suggest that the causative factors operate before birth and possibly even before conception. As a result, many aetiological studies of childhood tumours have been concerned largely with exposures occurring during the mother's pregnancy, though postnatal factors have also been investigated.

The only environmental factor well established as the cause of more than a handful of cases is radiation. The relationship between antenatal obstetric irradiation and subsequent cancer in the child was first established over 30 years ago through the pioneering work of Alice Stewart and her colleagues (Stewart *et al.*, 1958). At that time, exposure to diagnostic

x-rays in pregnancy may have caused as many as 5% of all childhood malignant neoplasms, but reductions both in the frequency of x-raying and in the dose of radiation used at each examination will have reduced the proportion substantially. Ultrasound has now largely superseded obstetric x-ray examination in pregnancy. Two studies have concluded that there is no increased risk of cancer or leukaemia associated with obstetric ultrasound (Kinnier Wilson and Waterhouse, 1984; Cartwright *et al.*, 1984).

The use in the past of x-rays to treat various benign childhood conditions, including 'enlarged thymus', tinea capitis and haemangioma, has also caused subsequent malignant neoplasms. The groups of persons thus irradiated represented a small proportion of the total population of the countries concerned, and the great majority of the resulting cancers occurred during adulthood. In consequence, the proportion of childhood cancers induced by postnatal medical irradiation must be minute.

Radiotherapy for cancer can in turn give rise to second primary neoplasms. Although the cumulative risk can be high, childhood cancer is itself rare and many of the second primaries occur in later life, and so the number of childhood tumours caused by radiotherapy for a previous cancer is very small.

Excessive exposure to the ultraviolet component of sunlight is known to increase the risk of skin cancer (predominantly in adults), but there is no conclusive evidence that other non-ionizing radiations can cause cancer.

There has, however, been increasing public concern about the possible health effects of the low-frequency alternating electromagnetic fields (EMF) emitted by electrical sources such as power transmission lines and domestic wiring. The epidemiological literature has recently been reviewed by Coleman and Beral (1988) and Cartwright (1989). Some studies concentrated on occupational exposure to electrical equipment, often in contexts

5

where there was also exposure to possibly carcinogenic chemicals. Others have been concerned with ambient EMF in and near the home. Some, but not all, of the latter group of studies have shown an increased risk of childhood leukaemia or cancer associated with higher EMF dose. It is very hard to decide from these studies whether EMF is a risk factor for childhood cancer, but any excess risk is unlikely to be very large. A point which does emerge clearly is that, if these questions are to be investigated any further, then it is essential that more accurate ways of measuring EMF doses are used.

There have been reports of the possible carcinogenic effects of many different drugs taken by mothers during pregnancy. The only one of these agents firmly established as a transplacental carcinogen is diethylstilboestrol (DES), a hormone which was given to pregnant women with threatened abortion. Exposure to this drug *in utero* caused clear cell adenocarcinoma of the vagina or cervix predominantly in young women, though a few cases have been observed in girls aged under 15. The data on DES and cancer have been reviewed by Vessey (1989). DES was more widely prescribed in the USA than in much of Europe, though it appears to have been used on a larger scale in the Netherlands. The cumulative risk of clear cell adenocarcinoma of the vagina or cervix during the first 35 years of life among DES-exposed females is about 1 in 1000, with over 90% of cases occurring between the ages 15–27. During 1971–1980 in the UK there were three girls aged under 15 with clear cell adenocarcinoma, representing 0.02% of all childhood cancers over that decade. Exposure to exogenous oestrogens *in utero* has also been linked to gonadal germ cell tumours in adults of both sexes, but no such association has so far been reported for these tumours in children, possibly because of their much lower incidence.

Over the past decade, there have been six case reports of neuroblastoma in the offspring of mothers who took the antiepileptic drug phenytoin during pregnancy. This association has not been confirmed in any large series, possibly because of the low overall frequency of use of phenytoin. None of 188 children with neuroblastoma diagnosed previously at the same hospital as the most recent case had been exposed to phenytoin *in utero* (Koren *et al.*, 1989). In a matched case-control study, none of 104 children with neuroblastoma nor of the controls had been exposed to phenytoin (Kramer *et al.*, 1987).

Various other drugs taken during pregnancy have been associated with a raised risk of particular childhood cancers in individual case-control studies. These associations include barbiturates, diuretics and antihistamines with brain tumours (Gold *et al.*, 1979; Preston-Martin *et al.*, 1982), narcotic analgesics with ALL (McKinney *et al.*, 1987), diuretics and 'neurally active drugs' in general with neuroblastoma (Kramer *et al.*, 1987), analgesics, antipyretics and antibiotics with all diagnostic groups combined (Gilman *et al.*, 1989) and marijuana with acute non-lymphoblastic leukaemia (ANLL) (Robison *et al.*, 1989). None of these findings has been replicated. The highest relative risk was for the association of marijuana with ANLL, which moreover predominantly involved the myelomonocytic and monocytic subtypes. It was suggested, however, that if the association was real this may be the result of pesticide contamination rather than the drug itself.

Drugs given to children themselves have occasionally been reported as conferring an increased risk of malignant disease. In a recent study in Shanghai (Shu *et al.*, 1988), an association was found between use of the antibiotic chloramphenicol by children and subsequent risk of acute leukaemia of both lymphoblastic and non-lymphoblastic types. Chloramphenicol is less widely used in Western countries and this finding has not so far been repeated.

In a series of 40 children with juvenile rheumatoid arthritis who were given the alkylating agent chlorambucil, three (7.5%) developed acute non-lymphoblastic leukaemia (Buriot *et al.*, 1979). Alkylating agents used in the chemotherapy of cancer are also themselves carcinogenic but, as with radiotherapy, the number of childhood cancers caused by these drugs must be very low.

The offspring of mothers who smoke during pregnancy have an increased risk of adverse effects, including low birth weight and perinatal mortality, but the evidence on parental smoking and cancer in children has been inconclusive. Increased risks of rhabdomyosarcoma and brain tumours have been found with fathers' (but not mothers') cigarette smoking (Grufferman *et al.*, 1982; Preston-Martin *et al.*, 1982). In a more recent study from Sweden there was an increased risk of childhood cancer with maternal smoking during pregnancy (Stjernfeldt *et al.*, 1986), but in subsequent published correspondence other studies were reported in which no association was found (Buckley *et al.*, 1986; and McKinney and Stiller, 1986), and doubts were raised over the design of the original study.

Various other domestic environmental exposures have been linked with childhood cancers. Associations with pesticides (Infante *et al.*, 1978; Lowengart *et al.*, 1987; Buckley *et al.*, 1989), incense (Preston-Martin *et al.*, 1982; Lowengart *et al.*, 1987), hair dyes (Kramer *et al.*, 1987; Bunin *et al.*, 1987) have each been reported in at least two studies. Several other factors have been reported in one study each and there is little overall consistency in the findings. The principal exception is that several of the substances for which there was an increased risk of brain tumours following maternal exposure in pregnancy contain nitrosamines (Preston-Martin, 1989). The association of brain tumours with *in utero* exposure to N-nitroso compounds is supported by experimental evidence and the relationship is

being examined further in a large international case-control study of childhood brain tumours. Maternal use of incense, one of the nitrosamine-containing substances with an elevated risk of brain tumours, has also been associated with an increased risk of leukaemia (Lowengart *et al.*, 1987), but this latter association, if real, might be attributable to other constituents of incense such as aldehydes or polycyclic aromatic hydrocarbons.

The results of 14 studies on parental occupations and cancer were reviewed by Arundel and Kinnier Wilson (1986). Several reports showed significant associations with occupations involving exposure to lead, hydrocarbons (variously defined) and other chemicals, while others showed no such association. Since then, reports have appeared of at least 18 further studies in which occupational factors were examined. Numerous statistically significant associations were found in these analyses, but a clear picture of the role of occupational exposure is no more apparent than before.

The possible role of environmental exposure of children to radiation and of occupational exposure of their parents in the causation of childhood cancer, especially leukaemia, is highly controversial. This topic is reviewed in the final section of the present chapter.

Exposure to infections certainly plays a part in the aetiology of some childhood cancers. The classic example is that of Burkitt's lymphoma in the tropics, where the incidence of this tumour is very high. Children with Burkitt's lymphoma in these regions generally have raised antibody titres for Epstein-Barr virus (EBV), whereas in temperate regions, where Burkitt's lymphoma has a much lower incidence, few patients have raised EBV titres. In the high-incidence regions malaria is endemic and it is believed that this causes a continuous, intense antigenic stimulus which alters response to EBV infection so that the latter gives rise to Burkitt's lymphoma. In Tarime District, Tanzania, a malaria suppression programme apparently contributed to, but was not wholly responsible for, a temporary reduction in Burkitt's lymphoma incidence (Geser *et al.*, 1989). Epstein-Barr virus infection has also been related to the high incidence of nasopharyngeal carcinoma in North African children.

Hepatocellular carcinoma is most frequently found among children in regions where the same tumour has a high incidence in adults. The association of hepatocellular carcinoma with hepatitis B infection is well known, and in areas where hepatitis B is common a large proportion of children with hepatocellular carcinoma are chronic HBsAg carriers. In European countries, where hepatocellular carcinoma is very rare in children, a large proportion of patients also appear to be HBsAg positive (de Potter *et al.*, 1987; Leuschner *et al.*, 1988).

Greaves (1988) has proposed a hypothesis linking the 'common' immunophenotype of ALL, the commonest childhood cancer, with exposure to infection during infancy. Under this hypothesis, common ALL is the result of a sequence of two spontaneous mutations. The first would be associated with proliferation of B-cell precursors *in utero* and their associated self-mutagenic activity. If immune stimulation of mature lymphoid tissue generates a positive feedback proliferation signal to the B-cell precursors, and turnover of B-cell precursor cells in bone marrow is highest in early infancy, then the greater immunological challenge resulting from delayed exposure to infection may produce a less regulated proliferative stress. This in turn would bring about the second mutation in a cell belonging to a clone which had already expanded as a result of the first mutation, and it is that second mutation that would precipitate clinically overt leukaemia. If this model for the causation of common ALL is correct, then children with ALL might be expected to have relatively few infections in the first months of life and correspondingly more shortly before the onset of leukaemia; the risk of ALL could also vary with the number of immunizations in infancy and the duration of breastfeeding.

Epidemiological evidence on specific infections in early childhood has so far been equivocal. In one study (van Steensel-Moll *et al.*, 1986), children with leukaemia had fewer infections requiring hospitalization during the first year of life than did their controls, while in another (McKinney *et al.*, 1987) there was an excess of virus infections under the age of six months among children with leukaemia or lymphoma. Two studies (Kneale *et al.*, 1986; Hartley *et al.*, 1988) have found immunizations to have a protective effect, but in both of them this effect obtained for all diagnostic groups and not just for leukaemia. One case-control study showed a significantly reduced risk of cancer for children who were breastfed for more than six months (Davis *et al.*, 1988); the effect was highly significant among lymphomas, though there was a non-significant halving of the relative risk for ALL with prolonged breastfeeding. In three other studies containing larger numbers of children with leukaemia and NHL, there was no evidence for a protective effect of breastfeeding (McKinney *et al.*, 1987; van Duijn *et al.*, 1988; Magnani *et al.*, 1988).

It has been suggested that leukaemia might be a rare response to some unidentified, possibly subclinical, viral infection and that variations in incidence are related to variations in the level of herd immunity to the infection. This theory is discussed further in the final section of this chapter.

Possible relationships between maternal infections during pregnancy and childhood cancer have been investigated in a large number of epidemiological studies, and the literature was recently reviewed by Preston-Martin (1989). One of the most common viral infections, and the one most frequently studied in this context, is influenza; as with several of the other putative risk factors considered above, there has been a variety of positive and negative findings and no clearly unequivocal associations have emerged. Some of the mothers of HBsAg-positive children with hepatocellular carcinoma are themselves infected with hepatitis B (Leuschner *et al.*, 1988) but the infection need not have been transmitted to the children antenatally.

Infection with human immunodeficiency virus (HIV) carries an enormously increased risk of Kaposi's sarcoma and certain types of lymphoma. Children who become infected, whether by direct maternal transmission or through external sources such as contaminated blood products, might also be expected to be at high risk of cancers associated with acquired immune deficiency syndrome (AIDS) in adults. In a New Jersey hospital series of 100 HIV-infected children, 3% had already developed primary lymphoma of the central nervous system (CNS) within 18 months of follow-up (Epstein *et al.*, 1988). Kaposi's sarcoma has also been reported (Buck *et al.*, 1983). With current and anticipated levels of HIV infection these tumours are expected to remain rare in children, though it is possible that small aggregations of cases will occur in localities where there is a relatively high prevalence of HIV among women of childbearing age.

The role of various environmental exposures in the aetiology of childhood cancer is far from clear. Obstetric x-ray examination is certainly carcinogenic, but accounts for well under 5% of all current cases of childhood cancer. The only well-established environmental causes in Western populations, other than ionizing radiation, are intrauterine DES exposure and infection with hepatitis B and HIV, which together can account for only a tiny fraction of all cases. Large numbers of other risk factors for childhood cancer have been reported, each one yielding a positive finding in at most a handful of studies, with negative findings for the same factor in other studies. It is impossible to tell from published reports how much of this inconsistency is due to causal factors being missed because of the small numbers of cases in many of these studies, how much to other variations in study design and how much to chance in the absence of causation. It seems very likely, however, that for most of the factors studied either the associated excess risk is small or exposure is rare, and consequently studies of very large numbers of cases would be required to establish them conclusively as agents in the causation of childhood cancer.

A great many case-control studies have been carried out or are in progress, involving tens of thousands of cases. It is highly desirable that a detailed overview be performed of all studies carried out to date in the hope that this might resolve some of the many contradictions between individual studies and in the virtual certainty that it would at least generate well-defined hypotheses for further investigation.

1.3 GENETIC EPIDEMIOLOGY

Epidemiologically, genetic factors in the aetiology of childhood cancer may be detected in two ways: namely, through familial aggregations of childhood cancers and other diseases and through the presence of some constitutional genetic abnormality which may be manifested in distinctive associations of cancer with other conditions such as congenital abnormalities in the affected child. Many of the data quoted in this section are derived from a recent study of genetic conditions in a 13-year series of over 16 000 children in the National Registry of Childhood Tumours.

The clearest example of a childhood cancer due to an inherited genetic condition is retinoblastoma. Many families have been identified with retinoblastoma in several members, and often in more than one generation. In a large proportion of these familial cases both eyes are affected. An unusually early age of onset can often distinguish heritable from non-heritable forms of a cancer, and the median age at diagnosis for bilateral retinoblastoma is seven months, compared with 25 months for unilateral tumours. The usual definition of heritable retinoblastoma is any case in which there are bilateral tumours or a positive family history. By these criteria around 40% of cases in Western populations are heritable, though two-thirds of children with this form have no previous family history (Sanders *et al.*, 1988). These findings of frequent bilateral involvement and early age of onset accord well with the 'two-hit' mutational model of Knudson (1971), whereby retinoblastoma can be explained as the result of two mutations. In sporadic cases the first mutation is postzygotic, whereas in heritable cases it is prezygotic, being either inherited itself or as a rare germ cell mutation which can then be inherited by future generations. A few patients with retinoblastoma but without a family history of the tumour suffer from mental retardation, and in these patients a deletion was found in the long arm of chromosome 13. Subsequently, the 'retinoblastoma gene' locus was assigned to 13q14. This gene is strictly speaking an 'antioncogene', since the presence of the gene prevents the development of retinoblastoma, which only appears when both copies of the gene are lost. The characteristic deletion of 13q may be present constitutionally in around 5% of patients with otherwise apparently sporadic retinoblastoma (Bunin *et al.*, 1989). Adding these cases to those already classed as heritable by virtue of bilaterality or family history yields a proportion of retinoblastoma that is genetic in origin of about 45%. The pattern of inheritance is essentially Mendelian autosomal dominant with almost complete (about 90%) penetrance. Thus the offspring of survivors of heritable retinoblastoma themselves have a risk of nearly one-half that they will develop retinoblastoma, as was confirmed by a follow-up study in which 23 out of 52 (44%) offspring of survivors did so (Hawkins *et al.*,

1989). Survivors also have an extremely high risk of developing a second primary tumour, which in many cases cannot be ascribed to the treatment given for the original retinoblastoma. The relative risk is highest of all for osteosarcoma, for which the incidence among heritable retinoblastoma patients is hundreds of times that in the general population (Draper *et al.*, 1986). Many other types of second primary have also been observed, and the elevated risk of a second malignant neoplasm persists well into adulthood (Sanders *et al.*, 1989).

In comparison with retinoblastoma, familial aggregations of other childhood embryonal tumours are rare, and a correspondingly much smaller proportion of cases can be regarded as genetic on the basis of family history. In the National Wilms' Tumour Study in the USA, a family history of Wilms' tumour was found in only 37 out of 3442 cases (1.1%) (Breslow *et al.*, 1988). As survival rates are substantially higher than they were a generation ago, the proportion of Wilms' tumour cases with family history will presumably rise, but will nevertheless fall well short of the proportion of retinoblastoma patients with other family members affected (Li *et al.*, 1988).

Familial aggregations of neuroblastoma and hepatoblastoma are even more rare, and there is little published information other than case reports. There is, however, a well-documented association between hepatoblastoma and familial adenomatous polyposis coli (Kingston *et al.*, 1983).

A remarkable syndrome in which unusually large numbers of several types of cancer occur among members of the same family was first described by Li and Fraumeni (1969). The original report mentioned soft tissue sarcoma, adrenocortical carcinoma, premenopausal breast carcinoma and brain tumours, but the syndrome has also been found to include osteosarcoma and carcinomas of the larynx and lung. It is estimated that

0.7% of all childhood cancers are part of the Li-Fraumeni syndrome.

Several other familial neoplastic syndromes can give risk to cancer in childhood. The most numerous group of cases consists of those associated with von Recklinghausen's neurofibromatosis (NF-1). Among children with NF-1 the most frequent cancers are tumours of the CNS. Overall, the risk of brain and spinal tumours is over 40 times that in the general population; the risk of optic nerve glioma is increased about 1000-fold. Neurofibrosarcoma can develop at the site of a neurofibroma, and the majority of childhood neurofibrosarcomas are associated with neurofibromatosis. There is also an increased risk of rhabdomyosarcoma, and the relative risk for all types of soft tissue sarcoma combined is over 50. Various other cancers can occur in children with NF-1, and of these the commonest are the leukaemias: the risk overall for leukaemia is four times that in the rest of the population but chronic myeloid leukaemia has a relative risk of about 70. In total, NF-1 appears to account for 0.5% of all childhood cancers, slightly less than the Li-Fraumeni syndrome. It is inherited as an autosomal dominant, but many cases may be the result of new mutations.

Other familial syndromes characterized by the occurrence of tumours in affected members of a kindred account for considerably fewer cases of cancer before the age of 15. They include: multiple endocrine neoplasia type 2, associated with medullary carcinoma of the thyroid; dysplastic naevus syndrome (malignant melanoma); basal cell naevus syndrome or Gorlin's syndrome (medulloblastoma and basal cell carcinoma); Turcot's syndrome (brain tumours and carcinoma of the colon).

If a child has cancer without known family history, then the risk of childhood cancer also developing in a sibling of that child is approximately doubled (Draper *et al.*, 1977). A considerable proportion of pairs of childhood cancers within a sibship are associated with known genetic conditions including the cancer family syndromes described above, but familial aggregations can also occur in the absence of any defined genetic syndrome. The causes of the increased cancer risk among siblings are presumably mainly genetic, though common environmental exposures should not be ruled out. Twins are a particularly interesting, though very small, subgroup of childhood cancer sib pairs. The concordance rate among twins is especially high for leukaemia occurring in the first four years of life, and again it is very plausible that such cases should be genetically determined. Sometimes the same cytogenetic abnormalities are found in both of identical twins who develop leukaemia in early childhood, particularly strongly indicating that the origin of their disease is antenatal, though it need not be prezygotic as the twins have shared circulation *in utero* (Chaganti *et al.*, 1979). Twins, of course, share all antenatal and many postnatal environmental exposures, but it seems unlikely that the former practice of x-ray examination of suspected twin pregnancies can have accounted for many twin pairs of childhood cancers.

Among genetic conditions which are not themselves neoplastic, the one most frequently associated with childhood cancer is Down's syndrome. The risk of leukaemia is increased about 20-fold in Down's syndrome children, and 2–2.5% of children with leukaemia have Down's syndrome. Of this total, 55–60% are ALL and 35–40% are ANLL. Thus, although a majority of children with Down's syndrome and leukaemia have ALL, the relative risk of ANLL is higher. Within the broad category of ANLL, the relative risk for a rare subtype, megakaryoblastic leukaemia, is very much greater: of a total of 26 cases of megakaryoblastic leukaemia in the National Registry, half have occurred in children with Down's syndrome. The incidence of most other cancers among children with

11

Down's syndrome is unremarkable, but there is evidence that boys have an increased risk of malignant testicular germ cell tumours. Overall, 0.8% of children with cancer also have Down's syndrome.

Tuberous sclerosis affects an estimated 1 in 15 000 children. These children have a relative risk of 75 for brain tumours and 50 for rhabdomyosarcoma, resulting in an 18-fold risk for all cancers combined. About 0.1% of childhood cancers are associated with tuberous sclerosis.

Certain genetically determined immune deficiency syndromes carry an increased risk of cancer, though as these syndromes are themselves very rare they account for less than 0.1% of all cases of childhood cancer. Most of these cancers are lymphomas occurring in children with ataxia telangiectasia, and more than one-tenth of all children with this condition develop cancer before the age of 15. Leukaemia, lymphoma and other childhood cancers have also occasionally been seen in association with Wiskott-Aldrich syndrome, Chediak-Higashi syndrome, hypogammaglobulinaemia, IgA deficiency and severe combined immunodeficiency.

A number of associations have been reported between various childhood cancers and congenital abnormalities. One of these, retinoblastoma with mental retardation and a deletion on chromosome 13q, has already been mentioned.

There are several congenital abnormalities that occur in association with Wilms' tumour (Breslow and Beckwith, 1982). Slightly more than 1% of cases of Wilms' tumour are diagnosed in children with aniridia. One third of such children in the British Registry had bilateral Wilms' tumour, compared with 5% among children with Wilms' tumour who did not have aniridia. Some children with aniridia and Wilms' tumour also have genitourinary abnormalities, hemihypertrophy or mental retardation. The Wilms' tumour-aniridia syndrome is now known to be associated with a chromosomal deletion at 11p13. Wilms' tumour is also associated with hemihypertrophy, either alone or as part of the Beckwith-Wiedemann syndrome, and with isolated genitourinary abnormalities. An 11-fold excess of cardiac septal defects with Wilms' tumour was reported in an earlier study from the National Registry (Stiller *et al.*, 1987) but this association has yet to be confirmed in other large series.

Hemihypertrophy and Beckwith-Wiedemann syndrome are also associated with hepatoblastoma and adrenocortical carcinoma. Neural tube defects are more common among children with germ cell tumours.

At present, under 5% of childhood cancers can be directly attributed to genetic conditions. Variations in incidence between ethnic groups, however, as discussed in the first section of this chapter, suggest that a much larger proportion of childhood cancers may result from hereditary factors.

1.4 OTHER BIRTH CHARACTERISTICS

Several possible risk factors for childhood cancer are considered here which cannot with confidence be classified exclusively as either environmental or genetic in origin.

In one case-control study, several possible indicators of maternal fertility problems were associated with ALL (van Steensel-Moll *et al.*, 1985). A history of repeated miscarriage and hospital consultation for subfertility were both reported more frequently by case mothers, and they also had a longer interval between discontinuation of oral contraceptives and the index pregnancy.

Parental ages have been investigated in several studies but no consistent results have emerged.

In a case-control study of fatal cases of neuroblastoma, a significant protective effect was found for gestation of under 37 weeks but there was a significant excess risk for low birth weight among children born after 37 weeks or more (Cole Johnson and Spitz, 1985); these findings were not repeated in another study of incident cases (Neglia *et al.*, 1988). A case-control study of osteosarcoma among persons aged under 25 showed excess risks associated with preterm delivery and with length at birth below the 25th percentile (Operskalski *et al.*, 1987). In a series covering all diagnostic groups, children with germ cell tumours had a slightly longer period of gestation than their controls but no association was found for any other type of cancer (Hartley *et al.*, 1988).

Daling *et al.* (1984) reviewed the literature on birth weight and childhood cancer while reporting the results of their own study of 681 cases. In their study and in the majority of published series there was an increased risk in heavier babies which applied in various studies to several diagnostic groups, but was possibly limited to the first two years of life. Many of the series reviewed were small, however, and in one of the largest studies (Salonen and Saxen, 1975) there was no association. Subsequently, in addition to the studies of neuroblastoma and osteosarcoma mentioned above, an increased risk of Ewing's sarcoma for children with low birth weight (Hartley *et al.*, 1988) was the only association found in another series drawn from all diagnostic groups. For most types of childhood cancer the results from studies of birth weight are inconclusive, but a significantly raised relative risk for birth weight exceeding 4 Kg in children with ALL (Robison *et al.*, 1987) was in agreement with a number of earlier reports. If any of these associations are real, then it seems likely that birth weight is a marker for some other risk factor rather than affecting the risk of childhood cancer in its own right.

1.5 SURVIVAL RATES

In 1960, the age-standardized annual mortality rate for neoplasms among children aged 1–14 in England and Wales was 86 per million.

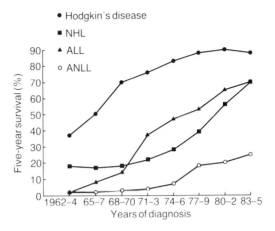

Fig. 1.1 Trends in five-year survival rates for children with ALL, ANLL, Hodgkin's disease and NHL diagnosed 1962–1985 (National Registry of Childhood Tumours data).

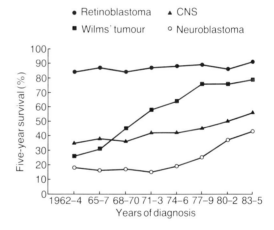

Fig. 1.2 Trends in five-year survival rates for children with CNS tumours, neuroblastoma, retinoblastoma and Wilms' tumour diagnosed 1962–1985 (National Registry of Childhood Tumours data).

Neoplasms accounted for 16% of all deaths in this age group and were the second most important cause after accidents. By 1987, the mortality had halved to 41 per million, though, as mortality from all causes had also halved, neoplasms still accounted for 16% of deaths

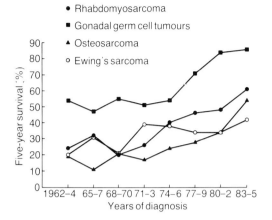

Fig. 1.3 Trends in five-year survival rates for children with osteosarcoma, Ewing's sarcoma, rhabdomyosarcoma and malignant gonadal germ-cell tumours diagnosed 1962–1985 (National Registry of Childhood Tumours data).

and ranked second after accidents. This dramatic reduction in mortality reflects an equally dramatic improvement in survival rates for children with cancer.

In the 1960s, survival rates were generally low. Retinoblastoma, Hodgkin's disease, astrocytoma, craniopharyngioma and fibrosarcoma were the only major diagnostic groups with a five-year survival rate of over 50%. Towards the end of the 1960s the five-year survival rate for childhood leukaemia was still only around 10%. Since then, there have been great advances in the treatment of most childhood cancers, and these have resulted in markedly higher survival rates. A detailed analysis of survival rates has recently been completed for a population-based series of over 15 000 children diagnosed during 1971–1985 and included in the National Registry (Stiller and Bunch, 1990). Figures 1.1–1.3 show the five-year survival rates for the principal diagnostic groups in that study together with the rates for 1962–1970, also derived from Registry data. Between the early 1960s and mid-1980s there have been substantial improvements in sur-

vival for almost every diagnostic group. During the 1960s, the main beneficiaries were children with Hodgkin's disease and Wilms' tumour. Since 1970, there have been further improvements for both these diagnostic groups but increases in survival rates also occurred over a much wider range of childhood cancers. The most spectacular improvements were in ALL and NHL, for both of which more than two-thirds of patients can expect to survive over five years. Large rises in the survival rate also took place for rhabdomyosarcoma, gonadal germ cell tumours, ANLL and neuroblastoma, though for these last two groups the survival rate is still below 50%. In the most recent period there was a substantial improvement in survival for osteosarcoma.

Undoubtedly these improvements in the survival rates are directly related to advances in treatment, as described in detail in other chapters. During this period of great technical developments in childhood cancer treatment there were also major changes in patterns of referral. At one time the majority of children with cancer were treated at local hospitals, there were few clinicians specializing in paediatric oncology and opportunities for participation in collaborative studies of treatment were limited. Treatment has gradually become more centralized and larger numbers of children have been entered in national and international clinical trials and studies. During the past two decades an increasing proportion of children with leukaemia has been entered in successive Medical Research Council (MRC) trials. In 1977 the United Kingdom Children's Cancer Study Group (UKCCSG) was formed and most regions now have a paediatric oncology centre whose consultant staff are UKCCSG members. The proportion of children treated at these centres, either exclusively or with their care shared between the centre and local paediatricians, has risen to about 70% overall, and nearly all children in some diagnostic groups, including neuroblastoma,

Wilms' tumour and rhabdomyosarcoma, are now treated at paediatric oncology centres.

In addition to the time trends in survival rates that are attributable to the development of more effective treatment, analyses of the Registry data have shown that for several diagnostic groups survival was related to patterns of referral and entry to clinical trials. For ALL diagnosed during 1971–1984, the survival rate was substantially higher for children who were included in the MRC UKALL trials (Stiller and Draper, 1989). The survival rate was also higher at hospitals seeing a larger number of cases of childhood ALL, though this effect was restricted to non-trial patients: for children in the trials, the survival rates were similar at small centres with few patients and at major centres with larger numbers.

Survival rates for patients with several types of childhood cancer diagnosed during 1977–1984 were compared between paediatric oncology centres and other hospitals (Stiller, 1988). For NHL, Ewing's sarcoma and rhabdomyosarcoma throughout this period there were higher survival rates at paediatric oncology centres than elsewhere. For ANLL the survival rates were similar at the paediatric centres and other teaching hospitals, but lower at non-teaching hospitals. The sizeable improvement in survival rates for osteosarcoma since 1980 was limited to patients at paediatric oncology centres. No significant variation was found between types of hospital for Hodgkin's disease, Wilms' tumour or neuroblastoma, though it is likely that the paediatric centres had proportionately more patients with advanced stage neuroblastoma.

1.6 STUDIES OF LONG-TERM SURVIVORS

As a consequence of the improved survival rates described above, the number of adult survivors of childhood cancer has greatly increased. Figure 1.4 shows the numbers of persons in the UK who were aged 18 and over

at the end of successive calendar years and were known to have had cancer in childhood. By 1971 there were already over 1000 such survivors. Since then, the numbers have increased steadily and there are now nearly 8000 adult survivors, equivalent to the adult population of a small town. Even with no further improvement in survival rates, this total would be expected to increase to over 14 000 by the year 2000.

As the number of long-term survivors has risen, there has been a correspondingly increased interest in their subsequent health, and several studies of large series of survivors of childhood cancer are in progress. These studies focus on several questions: whether the patients are really cured, their quality of life, their risk of developing a second malignant neoplasm, the likelihood of their having children of their own, and the health of those children.

Late effects and long-term follow-up are discussed in detail in other chapters. The following brief review of the epidemiological data is based largely on studies of survivors in Britain carried out at the Childhood Cancer Research Group (CCRG).

Although there is a small risk of very late relapse, the great majority of five-year survivors do appear to be cured in the sense that their mortality is only slightly higher than that of the general population (Hawkins, 1989). In general the quality of life of the survivors appears to be good. Some survivors have disabilities as a result of their disease or its treatment, including blindness and other visual impairment following retinoblastoma, a variety of handicaps following brain tumours and physical disability following bone tumours. It is expected that such disabilities will be less prevalent among future survivors, particularly as a result of more conservative treatment for retinoblastoma and the less frequent use of amputation for bone tumours. Current indications are that the risk of developing a second primary neoplasm within 25

15

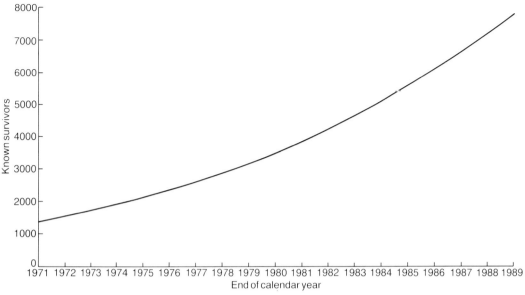

Fig. 1.4 Number of known adult survivors of childhood cancer in the UK at the end of successive calendar years, 1971–1989 (National Registry of Childhood Tumours data).

years following treatment for childhood cancer is about 4% (Hawkins *et al.*, 1987). The risk depends partly upon the treatment given for the original tumour; some second tumours are almost certainly radiation-induced, and there is an increased risk of leukaemia among survivors who were treated with alkylating agents (Tucker *et al.*, 1987). There is also a genetic element in the aetiology of some second tumours, exemplified by the enormously increased risk of osteosarcoma and high risk of various other cancers among survivors of the heritable form of retinoblastoma, as mentioned in an earlier section. The incidence of second tumours among survivors of childhood cancer may alter in the future. This may result partly from the changing distribution of original tumour types among survivors as improvements in survival rates have not been uniform across all diagnostic groups, and partly from alterations in methods of treatment for most childhood cancers. Vir-

tually nothing is known about the risk of second malignant neoplasms among very long-term survivors as they reach ages of 40 and above, the period of life during which the incidence of many of the common cancers rises markedly in the general population. These questions will be investigated through continuing follow-up studies of large series of childhood cancer survivors in the UK, the USA and elsewhere.

Some survivors are rendered infertile by their treatment but many others will have children. Among about 900 female survivors treated mainly before 1970 there were 57% of the expected number of live births (Hawkins *et al.*, 1988). Until recently the number of survivors of reproductive age was small, but around 4000 children born to survivors are now included in systematic studies. Many of these children are as yet very young and few have been followed up for a long period, and at present only tentative conclusions can be

16

drawn regarding their health. Women given abdominal radiotherapy have an increased risk of low birth weight babies, apparently because of a direct effect of radiation on the uterus rather than a genetic effect (Smith and Hawkins, 1989). The risk of malignant neoplasms among the offspring of survivors may in general be slightly increased to around the level experienced by siblings of children with cancer (Hawkins *et al.*, 1989). The only group known to have a markedly higher risk consists of the children born to survivors of the genetic form of retinoblastoma, as described above. The incidence of congenital malformations in the offspring of childhood cancer survivors appears to be little different from that observed in the population (Hawkins *et al.*, 1988). The longer-term health of the offspring of survivors and the health of children born to survivors who received more modern treatment for their cancers are currently under investigation.

1.7 TOPICAL ISSUES

There is a long history of reports of unexpectedly large numbers of children with leukaemia and other cancers in small geographical areas. The present heightened interest in this subject began with the observation of a possible high incidence of leukaemia in young persons in the vicinity of the Sellafield nuclear reprocessing plant and especially in the village of Seascale 3 km away. An independent advisory committee investigated this claim and confirmed that the incidence of leukaemia among children aged under ten in Seascale was ten times the national rate, though this was based on only five cases (Black, 1984). On the basis of current radiobiological knowledge, the measured levels of environmental radiation around the plant could not account for such a large increase. Nevertheless, attention was bound to centre on the reprocessing plant as a possible source of risk, though the precise nature of any risk

factor and the mechanism by which it might operate were unknown.

Suspicion that the presence of a nuclear plant could somehow be associated with a high risk of cancer was further intensified by reports of increased incidence in areas close to other establishments. Those which have been most thoroughly investigated are Dounreay in northern Scotland, the only other nuclear reprocessing plant in the UK, and two military sites in Berkshire, the Atomic Weapons Research Establishment at Aldermaston and the Royal Ordnance Factory at Burghfield. In both areas the presence of an excess of childhood leukaemia cases was verified (Committee on Medical Aspects of Radiation in the Environment, 1988, 1989) but, as with Sellafield, the levels of radioactive discharges into the environment could not account for the raised incidence on the basis of current risk estimates for radiation leukaemogenesis. In the two health districts closest to Aldermaston and Burghfield there was also found to be a raised incidence of childhood cancers other than leukaemia.

In each of these areas, the number of cases occurring over the whole of the time period studied was substantially higher than expected, though at Dounreay this was the result of a very much greater excess in more recent years. A high incidence of leukaemia has also been reported in other areas near to nuclear installations. In western Scotland, a region with two nuclear power stations and whose coastal waters are brought north past Sellafield by Irish Sea currents, an excess of myeloid leukaemia was detected in some areas during 1968–1974, and an overall excess of leukaemia in a different area during 1975–1981 (Heasman *et al.*, 1984); a subsequent analysis showed no significant excess near to nuclear installations and no evidence of consistently higher incidence in coastal areas (Hole and Gillis, 1986). A study in the vicinity of Hinkley Point power station, Somerset (Ewings *et al.*, 1989), produced results that were hard to interpret, with a high incidence of leukaemia in the decade following commissioning of the station, but low rates thereafter; in the five years before the power station was commissioned rates throughout Somerset, including the Hinkley Point area, were higher than those recorded nationally. A national study of mortality during 1969–1978 in relation to proximity to 15 nuclear installations in England and Wales was reported by Cook-Mozaffari *et al.* (1989a). They found that in districts near to an installation there was significant excess mortality from leukaemia (especially lymphoid) and Hodgkin's disease among persons aged 0–24. A subsequent study (Cook-Mozaffari *et al.*, 1989b) examined mortality over the same period in areas where the construction of nuclear installations had been considered but had occurred not at all or only after 1978. Excess mortality due to leukaemia and Hodgkin's disease among young people who lived near these 'potential' sites was very similar to that previously found among those who lived near the existing sites though, because the populations at risk were smaller, some of these results were not statistically significant.

From time to time, unusually high rates of childhood cancer (usually leukaemia) have been reported in other areas, some of them not linked to nuclear installations (Alexander *et al.*, 1990) or indeed to any obvious focus of risk (Gerrard *et al.*, 1986).

For any rare disease, such as childhood cancer, aggregations of unexpectedly large numbers of cases will occur in particular geographical areas or calendar periods even if the underlying risk is constant and cases arise independently. It is as yet unknown whether such aggregations in general occur more frequently than could be expected by chance. Published investigations based on incidence rates have concerned relatively small regions (Craft *et al.*, 1985; Alexander *et al.*, 1990) or very short time periods (McKinney *et al.*, 1989). A great variety of statistical methods has also been used on different data sets. Work is now in progress for the first time on studies of the patterns of incidence of childhood leukaemia and NHL during an 18-year period over the whole of Great Britain in which several methods of analysis will be applied to the same body of data. The results of these studies are expected to be published during 1991. It is hoped that they will provide by far the most detailed assessment to date of departures from randomness in the distribution of cases of this group of diseases. A comparative evaluation of the various methods of analysis is also in progress.

Even if it transpires that there is a large degree of non-randomness in the geographical distribution of childhood leukaemia cases, variations occurring on a national scale might still not account entirely for the markedly higher incidence around several nuclear installations. Fortunately these aggregations of cases have mostly occurred in sparsely populated areas and hence, although the incidence rate is considerably increased, the actual numbers of children affected tend to be small. Nevertheless, there is much legitimate public concern over the apparently high risks associated with nuclear plants and detailed studies have been undertaken in these areas in order to elucidate the nature of the association.

Two follow-up studies investigated the risk among children born to mothers resident in Seascale ('birth cohort' – Gardner *et al.*, 1987a) and among children who were born elsewhere but attended schools in Seascale ('schools cohort' – Gardner *et al.*, 1987b). The 'birth cohort' children had a leukaemia mortality 9.4 times that expected from national rates and an incidence of other cancers around three times that expected, but these results were based on 12 cases, eight of which were known to Black (1984). By contrast, in the 'schools cohort' there was no evidence of any excess of leukaemia or other cancers. These results pointed towards the possibility of a causative factor operating at the latest in infancy, and possibly antenatally or even before conception, rather than environmental exposure occurring in later childhood.

The next study was a very detailed case-control investigation of young people born in the West Cumbria district (which includes Sellafield) and diagnosed with leukaemia or lymphoma while living there (Gardner *et al.*, 1990). The main finding, which was given a great deal of sensational publicity, was that there was a significantly high relative risk for children whose fathers were employed at Sellafield at the time of their conception. Most strikingly, for five of the six patients with leukaemia or NHL whose fathers worked at Sellafield and for whom dose information was obtained, the fathers in each case had higher radiation doses before their child's conception than all of the matched control fathers. This result suggested that exposure of men to ionizing radiation may be leukaemogenic in their offspring. Whether there is in fact such an effect, however, is highly controversial. A wide range of putative risk factors was covered and some statistically significant results would be expected to arise by chance. No excess cancer risk had previously been found in the offspring of men who had received radiotherapy or who had been exposed to radiation from atomic bombs, though the timing of exposure relative to the conception of offspring may have differed. But no previous study of occupational exposure had access to dose records or had detected a dose–response relationship. In Shanghai a significant trend was found in risk of leukaemia with number of paternal preconception diagnostic x-ray exposures (Shu *et al.*, 1988). The need now is for a larger study of the offspring of persons with occupational radiation exposure at known dose levels.

Other explanations of the raised incidence around nuclear installations have been put forward that do not involve radiation and thus are also potentially applicable to unusual aggregations of cases occurring in other areas. Kinlen (1988) has suggested that leukaemia may be a rare response to a postulated widespread virus infection and that the incidence of leukaemia is inversely correlated with the level of herd immunity. This hypothesis differs from that of Greaves (1988) in that the significance of the infection lies in its leukaemogenic potential rather than its antigenicity. The communities around Sellafield and Dounreay are isolated and, in connection with the nuclear plants, have experienced large movements of population, factors which could lead to an unusually high exposure to infection among children with low immunity. The New Town of Glenrothes was selected as the only other area in Scotland which had experienced comparable isolation and population growth, and a significant excess of leukaemia below age 25 was found, with a greater excess below the age of five (Kinlen, 1988). Even after development as a New Town, Glenrothes had a fairly small population and the study included only 15 cases of leukaemia or lymphoma within that district. A significant excess mortality from leukaemia below the age of five has since been found in a group of four New Towns in England and Wales which, like Glenrothes, did not acquire their populations from a nearby conurbation, making them comparable in respect of population mixing (Kinlen *et al.*, 1990). In a study of childhood leukaemia in the Wessex region, incidence tended to be highest in outer suburbs of towns (Barclay, 1987). This result may be a reflection of variations in risk with social class but it could also be related to population mixing. Kinlen's hypothesis is now being further investigated by larger studies of areas which have experienced different levels of population movement.

Discharges from nuclear installations are the source of environmental radiation which has most frequently been considered in relation to the aetiology of childhood cancer. However, even in areas near to such installations, the contribution of these discharges to total environmental exposure is small in comparison to. natural background radiation. Background radiation varies geographically: for example, levels of terrestrial gamma radiation tend to be higher in areas where the local rock contains a large proportion of granite. One large study relating geographical patterns in mortality to terrestrial gamma radiation levels suggested that background radiation may be an important cause of childhood cancer (Knox *et al.*, 1988), but the report of this study mentioned some unsolved methodological questions; an analysis based on more modern incidence data might also shed more light on this issue. Henshaw *et al.* (1990) found significant correlation between national mean radon exposure and childhood cancer incidence rates across 13 countries. These associations cannot be regarded as proven, however, as the cancer data were for relatively small areas in several of the countries and the radon exposure for these areas was not quoted. Furthermore, similar correlations were found for all childhood cancer combined and for several individual diagnostic groups, raising the possibility that radon exposure might be correlated with rates of ascertainment by cancer registries as much as with true incidence rates.

The radioactive discharges into the atmosphere resulting from the accident in 1986 at the Chernobyl nuclear power station affected background radiation levels over much of Europe. According to current radiobiological theory the predicted increase in childhood cancer incidence attributable to the contamination would be too small to detect by comparison with normal variability. Nevertheless, some uncertainty remains concerning the validity of the risk predictions, and the Chernobyl accident offers a unique opportunity to investigate the role of background radiation in the causation of childhood leukaemia since background levels effectively doubled in parts of Central and Eastern Europe. Already there has been concern that the occurrence of an unusually large number of cases of leukaemia among infants in Scotland may be linked to Chernobyl (Gibson *et al.*, 1988). In order to investigate these questions, the International Agency for Research on Cancer is coordinating a study of childhood leukaemia incidence in Europe following the Chernobyl accident, and preliminary results are expected by 1991.

ACKNOWLEDGEMENTS

I am very grateful to Mrs E.M. Roberts for secretarial assistance and to Mrs P.A. Brownbill for producing the graphs. The Childhood Cancer Research Group is supported by the Department of Health and the Scottish Home and Health Department.

REFERENCES

Alexander, F., Cartwright, R., McKinney, P.A. and Ricketts, T.J. (1990) Investigation of special clustering of rare diseases: childhood malignancies in North Humberside. *J. Epidemiol. Community Health*, **44**, 39–46.

Arundel, S.E. and Kinnier Wilson, L.M. (1986) Parental occupations and cancer: a review of the literature. *J. Epidemiol. Community Health*, **40**, 30–6.

Barclay, R. (1987) Childhood leukaemia in Wessex. *Community Medicine*, **9**, 279–85.

Birch, J.M. and Marsden, H.B. (1987) A classification scheme for childhood cancer. *Int. J. Cancer*, **40**, 620–4.

Birch, J.M., Marsden, H.B. and Swindell, R. (1980) Incidence of malignant disease in childhood: a 24-year review of the Manchester Children's Tumour Registry data. *Br. J. Cancer*, **42**, 215–23.

Birch, J.M., Swindell, R., Marsden, H.B. and Morris Jones, P.H. (1981) Childhood leukaemia in north-west England 1954–77: epidemiology, incidence and survival. *Br. J. Cancer*, **43**, 324–9.

Black, E. (1984) *Investigation of the Possible Increased Incidence of Cancer in West Cumbria*, HMSO, London.

Breslow, N.E. and Beckwith, J.B. (1982) Epidemiological features of Wilms' tumor: results of the National Wilms' Tumor Study. *J.N.C.I.*, **68**, 429–36.

Breslow, N., Beckwith, J.B., Ciol, M. and Sharples, K. (1988) Age distribution of Wilms' tumor: report from the National Wilms' Tumor Study. *Cancer Res.*, **48**, 1653–7.

Buck, B.E., Scott, G.B., Valdes-Dapena, M and Parks, W.P. (1983) Kaposi sarcoma in two infants with acquired immune deficiency syndrome. *J. Pediatrics*, **103**, 911–3.

Buckley, J.D., Hobbie, W.L., Ruccione, K., Sather, H.N., Woods, W.G. and Hammond, G.D. (1986) Maternal smoking during pregnancy and the risk of childhood cancer. *Lancet*, **ii**, 519–20.

Buckley, J.D., Robison, L.L., Swotinsky, R. *et al.* (1989) Occupational exposures of children with acute nonlymphocytic leukaemia: a report from the Children's Cancer Study Group. *Cancer Res.*, **49**, 4030–7.

Bunin, G.R., Kramer, S., Marrero, O. and Meadows, A.T. (1987) Gestational risk factors for Wilms' tumor: results of a case-control study. *Cancer Res.*, **47**, 2972–7.

Bunin, G.R., Emanuel, B.S., Meadows, A.T., Buckley, J.D., Woods, W.G. and Hammond, G.D. (1989) Frequency of 13q abnormalities among 203 patients with retinoblastoma. *J.N.C.I.*, **81**, 370–4.

Buriot, D., Prieur, A-M., Lebranchu, Y., Messerschmitt, J. and Griscelli, C. (1979) Leucémie aigue chez trois enfants atteints d'arthrite chronique juvenile traités par le Chlorambucil. *Arc. Franc. Pédiat.*, **36**, 592–8.

Carlsen, N.L.T. (1986) Epidemiological investigations on neuroblastomas in Denmark 1943–1980. *Br. J. Cancer*, **54**, 977–88.

Cartwright, R.A. (1989) Low frequency alternating magnetic fields and leukaemia: the saga so far. *Br. J. Cancer*, **60**, 649–51.

Cartwright, R.A., McKinney, P.A., Hopton, P.A. *et al.* (1984) Ultrasound examinations in pregnancy and childhood cancer. *Lancet*, **ii**, 999–1000.

Chaganti, R.S.K., Miller, D.R., Mayers, P.A. and German, J. (1979) Cytogenetic evidence of the intrauterine origin of acute leukaemia in monozygotic twins. *N. Engl. J. Med.*, **300**, 1032–4.

Cole Johnson, C. and Spitz, M.R. (1985) Neuro-blastoma: case-control analysis of birth characteristics. *J.N.C.I.*, **74**, 789–92.

Coleman, M. and Beral, V. (1988) A review of epidemiological studies of the health effects of living near or working with electricity generation and transmission equipment. *Int. J. Epidemiol.*, **17**, 1–13.

Committee on Medical Aspects of Radiation in the Environment (1988) *Second Report: Investigation of the Possible Increased Incidence of Leukaemia in Young People near Dounreay Nuclear Establishment, Caithness, Scotland*, HMSO, London.

Committee on Medical Aspects of Radiation in the Environment (1989) *Third Report: Report on the Incidence of Childhood Cancer in the West Berkshire and North Hampshire Area, in which are Situated the Atomic Weapons Research Establishment, Aldermaston and the Royal Ordnance Factory, Burghfield*, HMSO, London.

Cook-Mozaffari, P.J., Darby, S.C., Doll, R. *et al.* (1989a) Geographical variation in mortality from leukaemia and other cancers in England and Wales in relation to proximity to nuclear installations, 1969–78. *Br. J. Cancer*, **59**, 476–85.

Cook-Mozaffari, P., Darby, S. and Doll, R. (1989b) Cancer near potential sites of nuclear installations. *Lancet*, **ii**, 1145–7.

Craft, A.W., Openshaw, S. and Birch, J.M. (1985) Childhood cancer in the Northern Region, 1968–82: incidence in small geographical areas. *J. Epidemiol. Community Health*, **39**, 53–7.

Daling, J.R., Starzyk, P., Olshan, A.F. and Weiss, N.S. (1984) Birth weight and the incidence of childhood cancer. *J.N.C.I.*, **72**, 1039–41.

Davis, M.K., Savitz, D.A. and Graubard, B.I. (1988) Infant feeding and childhood cancer. *Lancet*, **ii**, 365–8.

Davis, S., Rogers, M.A.M. and Pendergrass, T.W. (1987) The incidence and epidemiologic characteristics of neuroblastoma in the United States. *Am. J. Epidemiol.*, **126**, 1063–74.

Draper, G.J., Heaf, M.M. and Kinnier Wilson, L.M. (1977) Occurrence of childhood cancers among sibs and estimation of familial risks. *J. Med. Genet.*, **14**, 81–90.

Draper, G.J., Sanders, B.M. and Kingston, J.E. (1986) Second primary neoplasms in patients with retinoblastoma. *Br. J. Cancer*, **53**, 661–71.

van Duijn, C.M., van Steensel-Moll, H.A., van der

Does-van den Berg, A. *et al.* (1988) Infant feeding and childhood cancer. *Lancet*, **ii**, 796–7.

Epstein, L.G., Di Carlo, F.J., Joshi, V.V. *et al.* (1988) Primary lymphoma of the central nervous system in children with acquired immunodeficiency syndrome. *Pediatrics*, **82**, 355–63.

Ewings, P.D., Bowie, C., Phillips, M.J. and Johnson, S.A.N. (1989) Incidence of leukaemia in young people in the vicinity of Hinkley Point nuclear power station, 1959–86. *Br. Med. J.*, **299**, 289–93.

Gardner, M.J., Hall, A.J., Downes, S. and Terrell, J.D. (1987a) Follow up study of children born to mothers resident in Seascale, West Cumbria (birth cohort). *Br. Med. J.*, **295**, 822–7.

Gardner, M.J., Hall, A.J., Downes, S. and Terrell, J.D. (1987b) Follow-up study of children born elsewhere but attending schools in Seascale, West Cumbria (schools cohort). *Br. Med. J.*, **295**, 819–22.

Gardner, M.J., Snee, M.P., Hall, A.J., Powell, C.A., Downes, S. and Terrell, J.D. (1990) Results of case-control study of leukaemia and lymphoma among young people near Sellafield nuclear plant in West Cumbria. *Br. Med. J.*, **300**, 423–9.

Gerrard, M., Eden, O.B. and Stiller, C.A. (1986) Variations in incidence of childhood leukaemia in South East Scotland (1970–1984). *Leuk. Res.*, **10**, 561–4.

Geser, A., Brubaker, G. and Draper, C.C. (1989) Effect of a malaria suppression program on the incidence of African Burkitt's lymphoma. *Am. J. Epidemiol.*, **129**, 740–52.

Gibson, B.E.S., Eden, O.B., Barrett, A., Stiller, C.A. and Draper, G.J. (1988) Leukaemia in young children in Scotland. *Lancet*, **ii**, 630.

Gilman, E.A., Kinnier Wilson, L.M., Kneale, G.W. and Waterhouse, J.A.H. (1989) Childhood cancers and their association with pregnancy drugs and illnesses. *Paediatric Perinatal Epidemiol.*, **3**, 66–94.

Gold, E., Gordis, L., Tonascia, J. and Szklo, M. (1979) Risk factors for brain tumors in children. *Am. J. Epidemiol.*, **109**, 309–19.

Greaves, M.F. (1988) Speculations on the cause of childhood acute lymphoblastic leukemia. *Leukemia*, **2**, 120–5.

Greenberg, R.S. and Shuster, J.L. (1985) Epidemiology of cancer in children. *Epidemiologic Reviews*, **7**, 22–48.

Grufferman, S., Wang, H.H., DeLong, E.R., Kimm, S.Y.S., Delzell, E.S. and Falletta, J.M. (1982) Environmental factors in the etiology of rhabdomyosarcoma in childhood. *J.N.C.I.*, **68**, 107–13.

Gutensohn, N.M. and Shapiro, D.S. (1982) Social class risk factors among children with Hodgkin's disease. *Int. J. Cancer*, **30**, 433–5.

Hartley, A.L., Birch, J.M., McKinney, P.A. *et al.* (1988) The Inter-Regional Epidemiological Study of Childhood Cancer (IRESCC): past medical history in children with cancer. *J. Epidemiol. Community Health*, **42**, 235–42.

Hawkins, M.M. (1989) Long term survival and cure after childhood cancer. *Arch. Dis. Child.*, **64**, 798–807.

Hawkins, M.M., Draper, G.J. and Kingston, J.E. (1987) Incidence of second primary tumours among childhood cancer survivors. *Br. J. Cancer*, **56**, 339–47.

Hawkins, M.M., Smith, R.A. and Curtice, L.J. (1988) Childhood cancer survivors and their offspring studied through a postal survey of general practitioners: preliminary results. *J. R. Coll. Gen. Pract.*, **38**, 102–5.

Hawkins, M.M., Draper, G.J. and Smith, R.A. (1989) Cancer among 1348 offspring of survivors of childhood cancer. *Int. J. Cancer*, **43**, 975–8.

Heasman, M.A., Kemp, I.W., MacLaren, A.M., Trotter, P., Gillis, C.R. and Hole, D.J. (1984) Incidence of leukaemia in young persons in west of Scotland. *Lancet*, **i**, 1188–9.

Henshaw, D.L., Eatough, J.P. and Richardson, R.B. (1990) Radon as a causative factor in induction of myeloid leukaemia and other cancers. *Lancet*, **335**, 1008–12.

Hole, D.J. and Gillis, C.R. (1986) Childhood leukaemia in the west of Scotland. *Lancet*, **ii**, 524–5.

Infante, P.F., Epstein, S.S. and Newton, W.A. (1978) Blood dyscrasias and childhood tumours and exposure to chlordane and heptachlor. *Scand. J. Work. Environ. Health*, **4**, 137–50.

Kingston, J.E., Herbert, A., Draper G.J. and Mann, J.R. (1983) Association between hepatoblastoma and polyposis coli. *Arch. Dis. Child.*, **58**, 959–62.

Kinlen, L. (1988) Evidence for an infective cause of childhood leukaemia: comparison of a Scottish

New Town with nuclear reprocessing sites in Britain. *Lancet*, **ii**, 1323–7.

Kinlen, L.J., Clarke, K. and Hudson, C. (1990) Evidence from population mixing in British New Towns 1946–85 of an infective basis for childhood leukaemia. *Lancet*, **336**, 577–82.

Kinnier Wilson, L.M. and Waterhouse, J.A.H. (1984) Obstetric ultrasound and childhood malignancies. *Lancet*, **ii**, 997–9.

Kneale, G.W., Stewart, A.M. and Kinnier Wilson, L.M. (1986) Immunizations against infectious diseases and childhood cancers. *Cancer Immunol. Immunother.*, **21**, 129–32.

Knox, E.G., Stewart, A.M., Gilman, E.A. and Kneale, G.W. (1988) Background radiation and childhood cancers. *J. Radiol. Prot.*, **8**, 9–18.

Knudson, A.G. (1971) Mutation and cancer: statistical study of retinoblastoma. *Proc. Nat. Acad. Sci. USA*, **68**, 820–3.

Koren, G., Demitrakoudis, D., Weksberg, R., Rieder, M. *et al.* (1989) Neuroblastoma after prenatal exposure to phenytoin: cause and effect? *Teratology*, **40**, 157–62.

Kramer, S., Ward, E., Meadows, A.T. and Malone, K.E. (1987) Medical and drug risk factors associated with neuroblastoma: a case-control study. *J.N.C.I.*, **78**, 797–804.

Leuschner, I., Harms, D. and Schmidt, D. (1988) The association of hepatocellular carcinoma in childhood with hepatitis B virus infection. *Cancer*, **62**, 2363–9.

Li, F.P. and Fraumeni, J.F. (1969) Rhabdomyosarcoma in children: epidemiologic study and identification of a familial cancer syndrome. *J.N.C.I.*, **43**, 1365–73.

Li, F.P., Williams, W.R., Gimbrere, K., Flamant, F., Green, D.M. and Meadows, A.T. (1988) Heritable fraction of unilateral Wilms' tumor. *Pediatrics*, **81**, 147–9.

Lowengart, R.A., Peters, J.M., Cicioni, C. *et al.* (1987) Childhood leukemia and parents' occupational and home exposures. *J.N.C.I.*, **79**, 39–46.

McKinney, P.A. and Stiller, C.A. (1986) Maternal smoking during pregnancy and the risk of childhood cancer. *Lancet*, **ii**, 519.

McKinney, P.A., Cartwright, R.A., Saiu, J.M.T. *et al.* (1987) The inter-regional epidemiological study of childhood cancer (IRESCC): a case control study of aetiological factors in leukaemia and lymphoma. *Arch. Dis. Child.*, **62**, 279–87.

McKinney, P.A., Alexander, F.E., Cartwright, R.A. and Ricketts, T.J. (1989) The Leukaemia Research Fund Data Collection Study: descriptive epidemiology of acute lymphoblastic leukemia. *Leukemia*, **3**, 880–5.

Magnani, C., Pastore, G. and Terracini, B. (1988) Infant feeding and childhood cancer. *Lancet*, **ii**, 1136.

Neglia, J.P., Smithson, W.A., Gunderson, P., King, F.L., Singher, L.J. and Robison, L.L. (1988) Prenatal and perinatal risk factors for neuroblastoma: a case-control study. *Cancer*, **61**, 2202–6.

Operskalski, E.A., Preston-Martin, S., Henderson, B.E. and Visscher, B.R. (1987) A case-control study of osteosarcoma in young persons. *Am. J. Epidemiol.*, **126**, 118–26.

Parkin, D.M., Stiller, C.A., Bieber, A., Draper, G.J., Terracini, B. and Young, J.L. (eds) (1988a) *International Incidence of Childhood Cancer*, IARC Scientific Publications No. 87, Lyon.

Parkin, D.M., Stiller, C.A., Draper, G.J. and Bieber, C.A. (1988b) The international incidence of childhood cancer. *Int. J. Cancer*, **42**, 511–20.

de Potter, C.R., Robberecht, E., Laureys, G. and Cuvelier, C.A. (1987) Hepatitis B related childhood hepatocellular carcinoma. *Cancer*, **60**, 414–8.

Preston-Martin, S. (1989) Epidemiological studies of prenatal carcinogenesis, in *Perinatal and Multi-generation Carcinogenesis*, (eds N.P. Napalkov, J.M. Rice, L Tomatis and H Yamasaki), IARC Scientific Publications No. 96, Lyon, 289–314.

Preston-Martin, S., Yu, M.C., Benton, B. and Henderson, B.E. (1982) N-nitroso compounds and childhood brain tumours: a case-control study. *Cancer Res.*, **42**, 5240–5.

Robison, L.L., Codd, M., Gunderson, P., Neglia, J.P., Smithson, W.A. and King, F.L. (1987) Birth weight as a risk factor for childhood acute lymphoblastic leukemia. *Pediatr. Hematol. Oncol.*, **4**, 63–72.

Robison, L.L., Buckley, J.D., Daigle, A.E. *et al.* (1989) Maternal drug use and risk of childhood nonlymphoblastic leukemia among offspring: an epidemiologic investigation implicating marijuana (A report from the Children's Cancer Study Group). *Cancer*, **63**, 1904–11.

Salonen, T. and Saxen, T. (1975) Risk indicators in childhood malignancies. *Int. J. Cancer*, **15**, 941–6.

Sanders, B.M., Draper, G.J. and Kingston, J.E.

(1988) Retinoblastoma in Great Britain 1969–80: incidence, treatment and survival. *Br. J. Ophthalmol.*, **72**, 576–83.

Sanders, B.M., Jay, M., Draper, G.J. and Roberts, E.M. (1989) Non-ocular cancer in relatives of retinoblastoma patients. *Br. J. Cancer*, **60**, 358–65.

Shu, X.O., Gao, Y.T., Brinton, L.A. *et al.* (1988) A population-based case-control study of childhood leukemia in Shanghai. *Cancer*, **62**, 635–44.

Smith, R.A. and Hawkins, M.M. (1989) Pregnancies after childhood cancer. *Br. J. Obstet. Gynaecol.*, **96**, 378–80.

van Steensel-Moll, H.A., Valkenburg, H.A., Vandenbroucke, J.P. and van Zanen, G.E. (1985) Are maternal fertility problems related to childhood leukemia? *Int. J. Epidemiol.*, **14**, 555–60.

van Steensel-Moll, H.A., Valkenburg, H.A. and van Zanen, G.E. (1986) Childhood leukemia and infectious diseases in the first year of life: a register-based case-control study. *Am. J. Epidemiol.*, **124**, 590–4.

Stewart, A., Webb, and Hewitt, D. (1958) A survey of childhood malignancies. *Br. Med. J.*, **1**, 1495–508.

Stiller, C.A. (1988) Centralisation of treatment and survival rates for cancer. *Arch. Dis. Child.*, **63**, 23–30.

Stiller, C.A. and Bunch, K.J. (1990) Trends in survival for childhood cancer in Britain diagnosed 1971–85. *Br. J. Cancer*, **62**, 806–15.

Stiller, C.A. and Draper, G.J. (1982) Trends in childhood leukaemia in Britain 1968–1978. *Br. J. Cancer*, **45**, 543–51.

Stiller, C.A. and Draper, G.J. (1989) Treatment centre size, entry to trials and survival in acute lymphoblastic leukaemia. *Arch. Dis. Child.*, **64**, 657–61.

Stiller, C.A. and Parkin, D.M. (1990) International variations in the incidence of childhood lymphomas. *Paediatr. Perinatal Epidemiol.*, **4**, 302–23.

Stiller, C.A., Lennox, E.L. and Kinnier Wilson, L.M. (1987) Incidence of cardiac septal defects in children with Wilms' tumour and other malignant diseases. *Carcinogenesis*, **8**, 129–32.

Stjernfeldt, M., Berglund, K., Lindsten, J. and Ludvigsson, J. (1986) Maternal smoking during pregnancy and risk of childhood cancer. *Lancet*, **i**, 1350–2.

Tucker, M.A., Meadows, A.T., Boice, J.D. *et al.* (1987) Leukemia after therapy with alkylating agents for childhood cancer. *J.N.C.I.*, **78**, 459–64.

Vessey, M.P. (1989) Epidemiological studies of the effects of diethyl-stilboestrol, in *Perinatal and Multigeneration Carcinogenesis*, (eds N.P Napalkov, J.M. Rice, L. Tomatis and H. Yamasaki), IARC Scientific Publications No. 96, Lyon, 335–48.

Chapter 2

The genetic basis of children's cancers

J.K. COWELL and C.D. MITCHELL

2.1 INTRODUCTION

All cancers arise as a result of disturbance of the genetic material. Thus, genes may be expressed at inappropriate times or in inappropriate tissues. Alternatively, mutations may occur in genes normally regulating orderly cell growth and differentiation. Whatever the genetic lesion, it is passed on to all daughter cells and, therefore, at the cellular level, the cancer phenotype is genetically determined. A major challenge to biologists today is to identify and isolate the genes involved in these processes and, by understanding their normal function, address questions such as population screening and gene therapy. Cancer, however, is a multistep process and the cells in the tumours are constantly undergoing clonal evolution and expansion such that better-adapted cells emerge. Merely observing genetic changes in the end-stage tumour may mask information about critical events in tumour initiation and progression. Cancer can also be familial, where the inheritance is from parent to child. In these cases the mutation precedes the onset of the tumour and is therefore likely to be responsible for the initiation of tumorigenesis.

There is a class of cancer genes that apparently act in a dominant manner – the cellular oncogenes. These oncogenes, on their own, cannot transform primary cells but in combination they can (Land *et al.*, 1983). Since oncogenes are the mutated forms of normal cellular genes – proto-oncogenes – a simple model predicts that, because they control only a limited subset of the cellular regulation mechanism controlling growth, their successive mutation forms the basis of multistep carcinogenesis. The *ras* genes, for example, control cytoplasmic processes, whereas the *myc* oncogenes specify nuclear proteins. *Myc* induces premalignant phenotypes, which makes these cells responsive to transformation by *ras* oncogenes (Weinberg, 1989). Realization of the direct involvement of these genes in human cancer came from the observation that oncogenes were frequently located near to the breakpoint in chromosome translocations consistently found in some tumours, in particular the leukaemias.

2.2 LEUKAEMIA

Cytogenetic abnormalities in leukaemia may

be either numerical or structural. Numerical abnormalities are common in both acute myeloblastic leukaemia (AML) and acute lymphoblastic leukaemia (ALL). Thus, in AML 15–20% of patients have gain or loss of a single chromosome as the only detectable abnormality, particularly trisomy 8 or monosomy 7. In ALL, by contrast, there is no clear pattern discernible in the reported solitary numerical changes. However, if numerical changes seen in addition to structural alterations are considered, then +21, +6, +8, +18 and −7 and −20 are non-random changes. Two other recognizable groups of patients with ALL are the near-haploid (26–28 chromosomes) and hyperdiploid (>50 chromosomes) groups. About 20% of L1 morphology cases are hyperdiploid and this group has lower than average age, moderate tumour load and tends to have a good prognosis.

A variety of consistent structural chromosomal abnormalities has been described in leukaemias and lymphomas (Heim and Mitelman, 1987). Each chromosomal rearrangement is associated with a specific form of leukaemia and thus cytogenetic abnormalities are now used as an aid to classification. In addition, the rearrangements almost certainly represent one of the genetic events resulting in malignancy; identification of the genes involved in such rearrangements will provide further knowledge about leukaemogenesis and, possibly, novel forms of treatment. The best characterized chromosomal rearrangements seen in haematological malignancies are in chronic myeloid leukaemia (CML) and Burkitt's lymphoma (BL). So far, few of the rearrangements seen in acute leukaemias have been characterized at the molecular level.

2.2.1 CHRONIC MYELOID LEUKAEMIA

The first consistent cytogenetic abnormality to be described in a human malignancy was

the presence of a minute chromosome in CML, subsequently named the Philadelphia chromosome (Ph') (Nowell and Hungerford, 1960). With the newly discovered technique of G-banding, it was then realized that the Ph' chromosome was the derivative chromosome 22 of a balanced reciprocal 9;22 translocation (Rowley, 1973). This translocation is now one of the most intensively studied at both the cytogenetic and molecular levels.

During the chronic phase of the disease a single Philadelphia chromosome can be identified. In the subsequent accelerated phase, and during blast crisis, additional cytogenetic abnormalities may be identified, such as an additional chromosome 8, an isochromosome 17 or a further Philadelphia chromosome.

At the molecular level the important initial finding was that the c-*abl* oncogene was located on the long arm of chromosome 9 (Heisterkamp *et al.*, 1982). This gene is the cellular homologue of the Abelson leukaemia virus, responsible for some cases of leukaemia in cats. Analysis of a series of somatic cell hybrids containing either the 9q+ or the 22q− (Ph') chromosome, demonstrated that all or a major part of the c-*abl* gene had been translocated from chromosome 9 to chromosome 22 (de Klein *et al.*, 1982). It was then shown that the breakpoint on chromosome 9 lay within 14 kilobases (kb) of the 5′ end of the c-*abl* gene (Heisterkamp *et al.*, 1983). As the breakpoint on chromosome 9 lies in the most telomeric band of the chromosome, 9q34, this means that the c-*abl* gene must be translocated on a very small fragment of chromosome 22. Studies in further CML patients showed that there was quite a wide variation in the position of the chromosome 9 breakpoint within the c-*abl* gene. In contrast, the breakpoints on chromosome 22 were very tightly clustered within a region of only 5.8 kb (Groffen *et al.*, 1984), now called '*bcr*' (for breakpoint cluster region). Subsequent work has demonstrated that CML cells and cell lines contain a novel c-*abl* RNA transcript of 8.2 kb, larger than the normal 7.4 and 6.8 kb transcripts (Collins *et al.*, 1984). This abnormal transcript encodes a protein of 210 kilodaltons (kD), far larger than the normal 145 kD product. In addition, the CML protein product has tyrosine kinase activity, a property not possessed by the normal c-*abl* protein, but often a property of transforming retroviral proteins (Konopka *et al.*, 1985).

How does the 9;22 translocation result in a c-*abl* transcript of abnormal size and with an abnormal biochemical activity? Schtivelman *et al.* (1985) were able to show that the abnormal protein was a fusion protein, consisting of c-*abl* sequences at the 3' end but with novel sequences at the 5' end. The implication of this finding is that the *bcr* must lie within a gene on chromosome 22. Thus the molecular consequence of c-*abl* sequences being placed in juxtaposition to sequences from the *bcr* gene is the production of a chimeric *bcr-abl* protein with enhanced tyrosine kinase activity. Figure 2.1 indicates the structures of the *abl* and *bcr* genes, and the chimeric gene resulting from the Ph' chromosome rearrangement.

Subsequent work on the molecular genetics of the Ph' chromosome suggests that there is a correlation between the exact position of the breakpoint within *bcr* and the length of the chronic phase of the disease (Mills *et al.*, 1988). Patients with breakpoints in the 5' region of the *bcr* gene had a four times longer chronic phase than those with 3' breakpoints. The reasons for this apparent correlation will require further investigation.

About 10% of CML patients lack cytogenetic evidence of the Philadelphia chromosome (Ph⁻). Some of these patients behave in an identical fashion typical to Ph patients, but, in others, clinical or haematological features suggest that Ph⁻ disease is different. There have now been several reports of Ph⁻ CML in which molecular techniques have succeeded in demonstrating rearrangements around the

bcr sequence (Morris *et al.*, 1988; Bartram and Carbonelli, 1986; Zaccaria *et al.*, 1990). In a

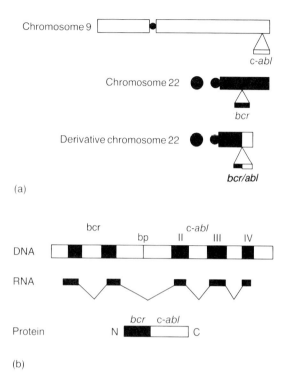

Fig. 2.1 (a) The c-*abl* gene is located near the telomere on the long arm of chromosome 9, and the *bcr* gene on the long arm of chromosome 22. The Philadelphia chromosome (which is the derivative chromosome 22) consists of the short arm, centromere and proximal part of the long arm of chromosome 22, and a small fragment of chromosome 9. The derivative chromosome is smaller than the normal chromosome 22. (b) At the DNA level the *bcr* and c-*abl* genes are in direct apposition. Exons are represented by filled boxes and introns by open boxes. The breakpoint on chromosome 9 is within the first intron of c-*abl*, so that exons II, III and IV are translocated intact, leaving exon I behind on chromosome 9. The primary RNA transcript includes both *bcr* and c-*abl* sequences; the intron sequences are subsequently spliced out to produce a mature mRNA. Translation of the mRNA results in a fusion protein encoded by *bcr* at its N-terminal and c-*abl* at its C-terminal end.

27

further Ph⁻ case, rearrangements of both *bcr* and *c-abl* have been detected; in yet another case, *bcr* rearrangement was detected but without a detectable *c-abl* abnormality or expression of a novel *c-abl* transcript (Bartram, 1985). Expression of the *bcr-abl* fusion protein has been detected in two cases of Ph⁻CML (Wiedemann *et al.*, 1988).

The main problem with these studies of Ph⁻ CML is the clinical heterogeneity of the condition and the lack of unequivocal diagnostic criteria. Thus, the results outlined above might well reflect the different molecular pathology of disparate diseases.

2.2.2 BURKITT'S LYMPHOMA

The best-understood chromosomal rearrangement in a lymphoma is the reciprocal translocation t(8;14) seen in the majority of cases of Burkitt's lymphoma. There are also variant translocations, t(2;8) and t(8;22), seen in about 15% of Burkitt's lymphoma patients. Identical rearrangements are also seen in B-cell ALL. The c-*myc* cellular oncogene lies at the breakpoint on chromosome 8 and the immunoglobulin heavy chain locus, and kappa and lambda light chain loci lie at the breakpoints on chromosomes 14, 2 and 22 respectively. The t(8;14) translocation results in the coding portion of the c-*myc* gene being interposed within immunoglobulin gene sequences. The consequences of the variant translocations are less clear (review in Heim and Mitelman, 1987).

The c-*myc* oncogene was originally identified by its homology with its viral counterpart, v-*myc*, which is the transforming oncogene of the avian myelocytomatosis virus MC29 (review in Varmus, 1984). There is strong conservation of the c-*myc* DNA sequence across many species. The human c-*myc* gene consists of three exons, the second and third of which are homologous to v-*myc*, and which encode the *myc* protein (Bernard *et al.*, 1983). The first exon provides a long untrans-

lated sequence. There is marked conservation of the coding regions, especially for exon 3, where there is 94% amino acid homology between human and murine proteins, and 76% between avian and mammalian proteins (Bernard *et al.*, 1983; Watson *et al.*, 1983). Homology between human and murine sequences in exon 1 is also high, and this homology extends at least 2 kb 5' to the exon (Fahrlander *et al.*, 1985).

Both c-*myc* and v-*myc* products are nuclear phosphoproteins that are able to bind double-stranded DNA *in vitro* (Donner *et al.*, 1982). The protein contains a region of leucine repeat motifs which is required for tetramerization and transformation of primary cells. The C-terminal region of the protein, encoded by exon 3, is very basic, which accounts for the DNA binding properties of the protein. These features are compatible with the c-*myc* protein being a transcriptional regulator (review in Mitchell and Tjian, 1989).

If serum-starved quiescent fibroblasts are treated with platelet-derived growth factor, or lymphocytes are treated with a mitogen, there is a 10–40-fold increase in c-*myc* mRNA within 3 h (Kelly *et al.*, 1983). Subsequently, though, both c-*myc* mRNA and protein are expressed at a constant rate throughout the cell cycle. It seems then, that c-*myc* expression is necessary for arrested cells to enter the cell cycle, but expression is then maintained irrespective of the cell cycle stage, provided that appropriate growth factors are present (Hann *et al.*, 1985). Down-regulation of c-*myc* appears to accompany differentiation in several cell types. For example, the induction of mouse erythroleukaemia cells to differentiate rapidly leads to a decline in c-*myc* mRNA, followed by a wave of increased expression and then a further decline. Furthermore, rather than being expressed throughout the cell cycle, as is the case in terminally differentiated cells, c-*myc* expression occurs primarily during the G_1 phase of the cell cycle. Thus, the level of c-*myc* expression at specific stages of the cell cycle may control the balance between self-renewal and differentiation within a cell population.

Understanding the illegitimate recombination between c-*myc* and immunoglobulin loci seen in Burkitt's lymphoma is helped by knowledge of the normal process of recombination needed to produce a functional immunoglobulin gene. Each immunoglobulin locus, in its germ line (unrearranged) configuration, consists of clusters of C (constant), J (junction), D (diversity) and V (variable) regions. Assembly of a complete gene capable of heavy chain production requires recombination between V, D and J elements, with deletion of intervening DNA. Production of other heavy chain classes requires further recombination using switch regions, iterated DNA sequences lying within the intron just 5' to the relevant constant region loci (Fig. 2.2). All immunoglobulin gene rearrangements involve only one allele, the other allele remaining silent or 'excluded'.

In BL cells the chromosome translocations are illegitimate recombination events resulting from aberrant immunoglobulin gene re-

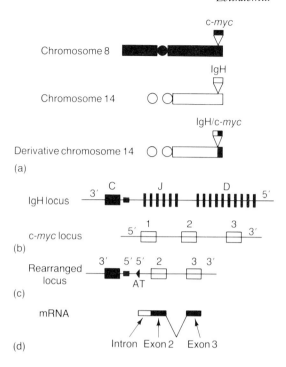

(a)

(b)

(c)

(d)

Fig. 2.3 (a) The c-*myc* genes lies near the telomere on the long arm of chromosome 8, and the immunoglobulin heavy chain gene (IgH) near the telomere on the long arm of chromosome 14. As a result of the balanced t(8;14) translocation the c-*myc* gene is translocated to chromosome 14, adjacent to the immunoglobulin heavy chain gene. (b) The germ line immunoglobulin heavy chain gene is shown with the 3' end to the left and the 5' end to the right, with C, J and D regions as filled boxes. The switch region is the small box. The c-*myc* gene is shown in the opposite orientation with exons 1, 2 and 3 indicated. (c) The translocation breakpoint on chromosome 8 lies between the first and second exons of c-*myc*. The second and third exons, together with part of the first intron, are translocated to chromosome 14, usually just 5' to the switch region. There is an alternative transcription start site for the truncated c-*myc* gene in the first intron, indicated by AT. (d) The mature mRNA includes sequences from the first intron because of the loss of the normal splice sites at the first exon/intron boundary.

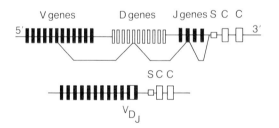

Fig. 2.2 (a) A germ line immunoglobulin gene is depicted with its 5' end to the left and 3' end to the right. The V (variable), D (diversity), J (joining) and C (constant) regions are indicated as vertical bars. S is the mu heavy chain switching region. In order for the gene to be functional the germ line configuration must be rearranged so that V, D and J sequences are adjacent. The intervening sequences, including redundant V, D and J sequences, are excised. The rearranged gene can then be transcribed.

arrangements, and usually involve the silent or excluded allele (Erickson *et al.*, 1982; Erickson *et al.*, 1983). The precise rearrangement varies among patients and can be classified according to the location of the breakpoint around the c-*myc* locus. To date no breakpoints have been described within the c-*myc* coding region. Instead, intragenic breakpoints cluster within the first exon or intron, relocating the normal c-*myc* promoters onto the other derivative chromosome. Breakpoints lying 5' to the gene usually lie within the 2.0 kb DNase hypersensitive region. These translocations leave the entire c-*myc* transcriptional unit intact, but have probably disrupted other 5' regulatory sequences, in particular disturbing the normal negative feedback mechanism. In the absence of the normal promoter and first exon sequences, transcription is initiated from a cryptic promoter in the first intron, which results in an abnormally sized c-*myc* mRNA (Fig. 2.3). Distant breakpoints generally remain uncharacterized.

Translocation breakpoints occur at a number of sites in the immunoglobulin heavy chain locus. Frequent targets are the switch regions. Most Burkitt's lymphomas are composed of relatively immature cells that express surface immunoglobulin; the heavy chain switch region is a frequent breakpoint site in these tumours. In some lymphomas the breakpoint is not at a switch region; for example, in the Burkitt's cell line 'Daudi', the breakpoint lies among the V genes (Erickson *et al.*, 1982) and in the 'Manca' and 'BL31' cell lines it lies near the J region (Wiman *et al.*, 1984; Siebenlist *et al.*, 1984; Cory *et al.*, 1983). However, in the latter two cases the breakpoints do not lie at the normal sites of recombination but several hundred base pairs away.

The variant translocations t(2;8) and t(8;22) have been less well characterized than the major t(8;14) group. *In situ* hybridization studies confirmed that the translocation breakpoints lay within bands 2p12 and 2q11, the

sites of kappa and lambda genes respectively. By analogy with the t(8;14) group, it seemed reasonable to expect that the variant translocations were the result of aberrant recombination between c-*myc* and an immunoglobulin light chain locus. It transpires, however, that in the variant translocations the chromosome 8 breakpoint lies 3' to c-*myc*, rather than 5'. Thus, the light chain constant region locus is translocated from its normal position on chromosome 2 (kappa) or 22 (lambda), to the 8q+ chromosome, while the c-*myc* gene remains in its normal position (Erickson *et al.*, 1983).

How could the knowledge of the molecular anatomy of the c-*myc* translocation be used in treatment for patients with Burkitt's lymphoma? A 'molecular' therapy could entail switching off protein production of the translocated c-*myc* gene. As already noted, initiation of transcription from a cryptic promoter within the first intron leads to an abnormally large mRNA because of intron sequences that are not removed during processing. This extra sequence is not translated into a protein product since it lies 5' to the AUG initiation codon. Thus, the mRNA transcript from the translocated c-*myc* gene is specifically 'tagged' in a readily identifiable way. Production of a protein can be inhibited if the ribosomes necessary for translation are unable to associate with the mRNA. An 'antisense' mRNA oligonucleotide, which has a sequence homologous to the 5' 'tag' on the abnormal c-*myc* mRNA transcript, will bind to the transcript by complementary base-pairing and so prevent the association of the ribosomes. Protein synthesis from the abnormal mRNA transcript will specifically be inhibited. That such a manoeuvre could be successful has now been demonstrated *in vitro* by McManaway *et al.* (1990). By using an appropriate antisense RNA oligonucleotide sequence they have been able to demonstrate a reduction in cell proliferation and in c-*myc* protein synthesis in Burkitt's lymphoma cell lines in culture. The specificity of their approach was emphasized by the failure of the oligonucleotide to influence the behaviour of a BL cell line in which the translocation breakpoint lay 5' to the first exon. In this situation, the mRNA transcript is not tagged by the intron sequences necessary for binding of the antisense RNA. Thus, ribosomes were still able to bind to the mRNA molecule and initiate translation.

2.2.3 ACUTE LYMPHOBLASTIC LEUKAEMIA

Although a number of structural abnormalities are consistently reported in ALL, few of them have been characterized at the molecular level. An ALL-associated rearrangement that has recently been characterized is a reciprocal translocation between chromosomes 1 and 19 [t(1;19) (q23;p13)]. This rearrangement is seen in up to 6% of paediatric acute leukaemias and in approximately 30% of leukaemias with a pre-B-cell phenotype. Both the insulin receptor gene which lies at 19p13.2–p13.3 and the cellular oncogene c-*ski* lying at 1q22–24 were candidate genes by virtue of their chromosomal localization, but neither gene lies in the region of the translocation. This finding exemplifies the point that the cytogenetic abnormality provides only a crude indication of the chromosomal location of an abnormality, and that molecular analysis is considerably more refined. However, another gene, E2A, which encodes proteins with the properties of immunoglobulin enhancer binding factors and which is located in the chromosome region 19p13.2–p13.3, was found to be rearranged in the majority of leukaemias and cell lines carrying the t(1;19) (q23;p13) abnormality (Mellentin *et al.*, 1989). The rearrangements of the E2A gene resulted in the synthesis of a transcript which was larger than that of the normal E2A gene. It remains unclear how such an abnormality is related to the genesis of leukaemia.

The single most common group of chromosomal abnormalities in T-cell ALL involve inversions or balanced translocations with breakpoints in the chromosome region 14q11–13. This region contains the subunit of the T-cell antigen receptor, and the involvement of this gene in the rearrangement has been confirmed. A functional T-cell receptor is a sulphide-linked heterodimer of alpha and beta chains. Like the immunoglobulin genes, the T-cell receptor genes must undergo rearrangement of V, J and C regions before the gene is capable of producing a peptide. In rearrangements associated with T-cell malignancy, the breakpoint on chromosome 14 lies within the alpha-subunit gene, between the V and C regions, a situation analogous to the breakpoint in the immunoglobulin heavy chain locus seen in Burkitt's lymphoma.

2.2.4 ACUTE MYELOID LEUKAEMIA

A reciprocal translocation t(15;17) (q22;q11.2–12) is characteristic of acute promyelocytic leukaemia (APL) (FAB type M3). This translocation is not associated with any other malignancy. The region on chromosome 17 has now been cloned and studied by Borrow *et al.* (1990). The breakpoints in ten cases of APL clustered within a 12 kb region of chromosome 17. This region is the first intron of the retinoic acid receptor. Since this gene is interrupted in an intron it is likely that the product of the translocation is a fusion protein, a situation analogous to that found in CML.

It will be clear from the preceding discussion of genetic changes in leukaemias that activation/aberrant expression of a particular gene may be important in tumorigenesis. There is, however, another class of cancer genes, termed 'tumour suppressor genes', whose function is to promote normal tissue development and loss of whose function gives rise to the malignant phenotype.

2.3 SOLID TUMOURS

Histopathological analysis of the majority of children's solid tumours reveals an embryonic-like organization. This suggests an arrest in development whereby the normal differentiation signals are overridden, resulting in continued, uncontrollable division of embryonic cells. Tumour cells usually express specific genes which may identify the stage of development at which this arrest occurred and, although usually committed to a particular pathway of differentiation, are still relatively undifferentiated. Since most tissues are fully differentiated at, or soon after, birth the mutations responsible for the initiation of tumorigenesis probably occur during embryogenesis. Once the cells are fully differentiated they can no longer be part of the pool of potential tumour precursor cells. What is not clear is the stage during embryogenesis, the 'window of differentiation', in which cancer-causing mutations are effective. After initiation tumours go through repeated rounds of clonal evolution where better adapted cells, as a result of genetic reorganization, gain growth advantages and eventually dominate the tumour. Progression therefore continues at different rates, is characterized by secondary genetic changes and accounts for variation in the time of presentation. Several embryonal tumours show familial aggregation implying a genetic predisposition. Although rare, it has generally been the analysis of these patients which has led to the pinpointing of the predisposing mutation. In particular, the study of retinoblastoma established many of the precedents for the analysis of other children's cancers.

2.4 RETINOBLASTOMA

2.4.1 GENETICS

Retinoblastoma (Rb) has proved to be the prototype for the analysis of the inherited cancer predisposition syndromes. With improved survival of patients, it soon became clear that there were both genetic and sporadic forms of Rb (Vogel, 1979). Approximately 25–30% of cases have a family history. In the familial form the Rb phenotype segregates in an autosomal dominant fashion. That is, it appears as though inheritance of a single mutant gene is sufficient for tumorigenesis. Thus, the offspring of individuals carrying the mutant Rb gene have a 50:50 chance of inheriting it. In rare cases individuals will inherit the defective gene but not develop the tumour. These are examples of 'incomplete penetrance', which occurs in an estimated 10% of cases (Vogel, 1979). From these observations it is clear that it is only the predisposition to tumour development that is inherited and that, at the cellular level, the mutation behaves in a recessive manner. This suggestion is further supported by the observation that, in gene carriers, not all retinal cells develop into cancers.

Clearly, if the Rb mutation is a recessive trait, a second mutation is required in the homologous normal gene. In a mathematical treatise of Rb, Knudson (1971) formulated a hypothesis that contended that only two genetic events were required for tumour initiation. Since in hereditary cases the first 'hit' is inherited, only a single additional random event is required. Hereditary tumours are usually multifocal and tend also to have an early age (mean = 10 months) of onset compared with sporadic ones, since as soon as the second hit occurs the tumour is initiated. In non-familial cases both hits occur as sporadic, random events in a retinal precursor cell. Since the chance of the same gene in the same cell experiencing a mutational event is low, sporadic tumours are usually unilateral, unifocal and have a later age of onset (mean = 18 months). Most tumours, whether hereditary or sporadic, occur before the age of five years and rarely, if ever, occur after the age of 11 years.

It is clear from the preceding discussion that, if the tumours are detected early, they can be treated successfully and the patient will survive. But carriers of the Rb predisposition gene run other risks; in particular, they are at a significantly higher risk than the general population of developing second, non-ocular tumours with a peak between the ages of 15–25. Second malignant tumours in Rb patients usually occur in mesenchymal tissues (Abramson *et al.*, 1976; Meadows *et al.*, 1985; Draper *et al.*, 1986) of which 66% are osteosarcomas and soft tissue sarcomas. In a study of 693 cases of bilateral Rb (Abramson *et al.*, 1984), 15% were shown to develop second primary tumours, most commonly osteosarcoma. More than one-third of these tumours develop in an unirradiated site. Osteosarcomas and soft tissue sarcomas are also the tumours most frequently seen within the irradiated field in treated individuals. It is clear, therefore, that the gene essential to normal retinal development also plays a role in bone and muscle development during puberty.

Early detection of Rb tumours in familial cases is relatively straightforward since the 'at risk' individuals can be clearly identified. Because the presence of multiple tumours in both eyes is not a chance occurrence, as described by Knudson (1971), the children of bilaterally affected individuals, together with those with a proven family history, are screened regularly during the first five years of life. Although Knudson's prediction is that unilaterally affected individuals represent sporadic cases it soon became clear that, occasionally, these individuals could also have affected children. Since there is currently no means of discriminating between which of these individuals have truly sporadic disease and those who can transmit the predisposition gene, the children of all Rb patients must be screened. That 10% of gene carriers may not develop the tumour means that relatives of gene carriers must also be screened. In addition to the observation that gene carriers may not develop the disease it has also been reported that Rb tumours can spontaneously regress. In these cases a small scar is left on the retina characteristic of that seen after successful treatment of the tumours. Others have suggested that these scars may represent a more benign form of the disease called retinomas (Gallie and Phillips, 1982). Parents of affected individuals, therefore, should undergo thorough retinal examination; if scars are detected the predisposition gene is present and offspring have a 50% risk of tumour development. In some families, individuals who were apparently examples of incomplete penetrance have retinal scars. The genetic basis of this manifestation of the disease is not known but may imply different types of mutation in the Rb gene compared with individuals who develop multifocal disease.

In some families there are several affected sibs born to unaffected parents. Again, genetic predisposition is probable. In some cases this family pattern could be due to the inheritance of an unbalanced chromosome abnormality (Strong *et al.*, 1981; Dudin *et al.*, 1984) or that one of the parents is a tissue mosaic, transmitting the gene through the germ line while the mutation is not present in retinal cells. The identification of these families again raises the question of whether to screen all sibs of affected individuals. Clearly the ability to determine exactly who is a carrier of the predisposition gene and who is not would have major advantages to all concerned. An important step towards this goal was taken with the identification of the exact location of the Rb predisposition gene.

2.4.2 13q- SYNDROME

It was noted in the early 1960s (Stallard, 1962; Lele *et al.*, 1963) that some Rb patients also had other congenital abnormalities, notably mental retardation and particular dysmorphic features (Motegi *et al.*, 1983). Analysis of chromosomes in lymphocytes from these patients showed that they carried chromosome abnormalities, most usually a deletion from the long arm of chromosome 13. The larger the deletion the more severe the associated congenital abnormalities. In the smaller deletions usually the only phenotypic consequence was Rb. As the number of cases reported increased it became clear that chromosome region 13q14 was always involved.

Although chromosome deletions were by far the most common constitutional chromosome abnormality in Rb patients, translocations have also been reported (Ejima *et al.*, 1988; Turleau *et al.*, 1985; Blanquet *et al.*, 1987). In some cases these rearrangements involved breakpoints in region 13q14, presumably constituting the first hit (see later). In translocations also involving the X chromosome, however, the breakpoints on chromosome 13 were not always in 13q14 (Hida *et al.*, 1980; Nichols *et al.*, 1980; Ejima *et al.*, 1982). In these cases, which were always in females, it is assumed that the spreading of X-chromosome inactivation during development extended to the relocated chromosome 13 and included the Rb predisposition gene. Thus, functional inactivation constituted the first 'hit' rather than physical mutation within the predisposition gene.

Analysis of chromosome 13 deletions in Rb patients was refined by the demonstration that the gene for esterase-D (ESD) was also located on this chromosome (Van Heyningen *et al.*, 1975). Sparkes *et al.* (1980) demonstrated that even the smallest 13q-deletion involved the ESD gene and that cells from these patients showed only 50% of the enzyme activity seen in normal cells. We were able to extend these observations to establish a screening programme using a modified ESD quantitation method (Cowell *et al.*, 1986; Cowell *et al.*, 1989) from which we identified 18 deletions (3.5%). In eight of these patients the deletions were small and

had only been identified by ESD quantitation. At least half of these deletion patients developed only unilateral tumours, which apparently contradicts Knudson's hypothesis and it appears that some deletions are associated with a lower penetrance (Matsunaga, 1980), possibly due to the lethal consequences of other gene mutations within the deletion (Dryja *et al.*, 1984). The identification of deletions such as these, pinpointing the site of the Rb gene, was to prove vital in its characterization.

The close proximity of the ESD and Rb genes allowed a linkage analysis in Rb families using the previously well-characterized ESD protein polymorphism (Hopkinson *et al.*, 1973; Cowell *et al.*, 1987). The frequency of the rarer 2-allele meant that the Rb phenotype could only be followed in 10% of the families but, despite this limitation, Sparkes *et al.* (1983) were able to demonstrate that the hereditary, non-deletion form of Rb was located in region 13q14. Several other groups have been able to confirm these observations (Halloran *et al.*, 1985; Mukai *et al.*, 1984; Cowell *et al.*, 1987). There have been no reported cases, to date, of recombination between these two genes.

2.4.3 HOMOZYGOSITY

Knudson's hypothesis (Knudson, 1971) predicts that the Rb gene is recessive at the cellular level. Both copies, therefore, have to be inactivated for tumour initiation. These mutations include deletions, translocation or point mutation, provided they result in loss of function of the Rb gene. Since the normal function of the Rb gene prevents tumour formation, this recessive cancer gene has been termed a 'tumour suppressor gene' (Knudson, 1985). Gallie and colleagues (Godbout *et al.*, 1983) identified Rb patients who were constitutionally heterozygous for the ESD protein polymorphism and demonstrated loss of alleles in the tumours from a proportion of these individuals; i.e. they became homozygous for one or other allele. The same phenomenon was recorded by several groups (Cavenee *et al.*, 1983; Dryja *et al.*, 1984; Benedict *et al.*, 1987) using chromosome-13-specific DNA probes which recognized restriction fragment length polymorphisms (RFLPs). Analysis of DNA/gene markers from other chromosomes in these tumour/normal pairs demonstrated the specificity of loss of heterozygosity for markers on chromosome 13. Karyotype analysis in these cases showed that chromosome 13 was grossly intact. Where karyotypic analysis was not possible the presence of two copies of chromosome 13 was determined using quantitation of the hybridization signal on Southern blots. By analysing flanking markers, Cavenee *et al.*, (1983) presented formal proof for mitotic recombination and non-disjunction as mechanisms for the generation of homozygosity in tumour cells. In all cases it was assumed that the chromosome region containing the normal Rb gene was lost with duplication of the mutant allele. Later this was confirmed by showing that, in familial Rb, it was the chromosome which was transmitted from an affected parent that was retained in the tumour in the affected offspring (Cavenee *et al.*, 1985). Small homozygous deletions were later shown to be another means by which loss of function of the Rb gene was achieved (Dryja *et al.*, 1986).

Traditionally, the molecular analysis of a particular hereditary disorder was possible if the biochemical basis for the disease was understood and a gene product was available. A typical example was the understanding achieved about the mutations in thalassaemia patients following the identification and cloning of the globin genes (review in Orkin and Kazazian, 1984). More recently the combined technologies of cell and molecular biology has given rise to the field of 'reverse genetics' (Orkin, 1986) where the gene responsible for

a particular well-defined phenotype is isolated in the absence of any protein product. This strategy, however, requires that the location of the responsible genetic locus be known, either through chromosome deletion/translocation analysis or genetic linkage studies. In practice, candidate genes are isolated from the relevant chromosome region and, in the first instance, authentication of the identity of the gene then depends on demonstrating specific mutations within these genes in the relevant tissues.

2.4.4 ISOLATION OF THE Rb GENE

The overwhelming evidence for a single Rb gene encouraged several groups to try to isolate it. The approaches used followed the standard protocols of reverse genetics whereby chromosome-13-specific DNA sequences were isolated at random from either chromosome 13 flow-sorted chromosomes (Lalande *et al.*, 1984) or somatic cell hybrids containing only 13 or a limited group of chromosomes (Cavenee *et al.*, 1984; Dryja *et al.*, 1984; Scheffer *et al.*, 1986). These randomly isolated DNA sequences were then mapped along the length of the chromosome using deletions derived from Rb patients. From a limited series of chromosome 13 DNA sequences Lalande *et al.* (1984) identified one, H3-8, which mapped to the critical region of 13q14. Using this probe Dryja *et al.* (1986) isolated an adjacent sequence which showed both homozygous and heterozygous deletions in different Rb tumours and which showed sequence conservancy between species, suggesting that it was located within the coding region of a gene.

Friend *et al.*, (1986) subsequently isolated a cDNA, 4.7R, from a transformed fetal retina cell line. mRNA transcripts of this sequence were absent in tumour cells. More extensive analysis by Lee *et al.* (1987a) and Fung *et al.* (1987), who had independently isolated the same gene, suggested that few, if any, Rb tumours had normal transcripts from the 4.7R gene, now called RB1. In their analysis transcripts were either absent or, if present, had a smaller transcript size, indicating deletions from the mRNA (Lee *et al.*, 1987a; Fung *et al.*, 1987). By contrast, Goddard *et al.*, (1988) reported that the majority of tumour cell lines had normal length transcripts.

The authenticity of 4.7R as the Rb predisposition gene was still based on evidence derived from analysis of tumour cells and somewhat surprising in this respect was the apparent ubiquitous expression of this gene (Friend *et al.*, 1986) in normal cells. Analysis of the genomic structure of RB1 showed that it spanned approximately 200 kb (Friend *et al.*, 1987; Bookstein *et al.*, 1988). Complete sequencing of the gene has identified 27 exons, of which 26 are only 50–150 base pairs (bp) long, the last exon measuring approximately 1.9 kb. The exons tend to cluster in two major groups separated by large introns.

Abnormal gene expression in tumours provided strong evidence for the authenticity of the RB1 gene, but did predisposing mutations also involve this gene? One Rb patient carried a constitutional reciprocal translocation between chromosomes 1 and 13. Somatic cell hybrids, which retained the derivative t(13;1) chromosome (Mitchell and Cowell, 1989) were analysed using DNA probes from the 5' and 3' end of the genomic sequence. The 13q14 breakpoint of the translocation was shown to lie in the middle of the RB1 gene. Cavenee and colleagues (Higgins *et al.*, 1989) reported several other translocations from Rb patients with breakpoints interrupting the RB1 gene. Others were able to demonstrate more subtle abnormalities in predisposed individuals by analysis of the mRNA products in tumour cells (Dunn *et al.*, 1988) and direct sequencing (Yandell *et al.*, 1989). Although the numbers analysed by these methods are small, the emerging picture is that no specific exon is consistently involved.

2.4.5 THE Rb PROTEIN

The availability of the RB1 cDNA sequence (Lee *et al.*, 1987a; Friend *et al.*, 1987) allowed the prediction of the amino acid sequence of the Rb protein (pRB). No motifs common to classes of genes which had membrane localization or ATP-binding domains, for example, were detected; neither was there any structural homology with known oncogenes or developmental genes.

Using specific antibodies against the Rb gene product (see below) studies have shown that, even though transcription occurs in some tumours, translation did not; no detectable gene product was found in tumour cells (Whyte *et al.*, 1988).

The precise function of the Rb gene is, however, still uncertain except that, by inference, it appears to be important in the control of the normal development of the retina. Lee *et al.* (1987b) presented evidence which suggested that the Rb gene product was a nuclear protein that binds DNA. In cell cycle studies Mihara *et al.* (1989) showed that pRB is produced throughout the cell cycle but its activity is regulated by phosphorylation. In quiescent cells only the unphosphorylated form is present. At the G_1/S boundary, and throughout S phase, the phosphorylated form appears; during G_2/M the unphosphorylated form again predominates. This suggests that the hypophosphorylated form inhibits cell proliferation, although quite how this effect is mediated is not known. Presumably, the hypophosphorylated form is inactivated by phosphorylation and this is a prerequisite for the cell's entry into S phase. Such a model is supported by the observation that cells induced to terminally differentiate, and that hence lose their proliferation potential, lose their ability to phosphorylate pRB. Recently Whyte *et al.*, (1988) demonstrated that pRB bound to the early protein, E1A, of adenovirus. DNA tumour viruses encode a set of proteins capable of overriding normal regulations of cellular growth. E1A can

36

immortalize cells on its own or can interact with the *ras* oncogene to transform cells in culture. E1A also regulates gene expression. It can activate transcription of other early viral genes and cellular genes and can also repress transcription of genes linked to certain viral or cellular enhancers (review in Berk, 1986). E1A has also been shown to associate with host cell proteins, possibly mediating some physiological effects induced by E1A.

Specific E1A mutations affecting binding of E1A to the RB1 protein (pRB) ablate the transforming powers of E1A (Whyte *et al.*, 1988, Horowitz *et al.*, 1989; Whyte *et al.*, 1989). The demonstration that the products of oncogenes and tumour suppressor genes can form protein complexes prompted investigation of the products of other oncogenes. Thus it was shown that pRB also binds to large-T antigen (LT) in SV40 transformed cells (Moran, 1988). In the J82 bladder carcinoma cell line the exon deletion in the Rb-cDNA precludes binding to either E1A or SV40 LT (Horowitz *et al.*, 1989) but can still bind to DNA. Neither SV40 nor Ad12, however, have been directly linked with human cancer. The E7 transforming protein from human papilloma virus-16 has many features in common with E1A; it is sufficient and necessary to transform rodent cells and is present in more than half of human cervical cancers (Dyson *et al.*, 1989). E7 also binds to the pRB, further suggesting that its binding of oncogene transforming proteins may be a common feature. LT only binds the underphosphorylated form of pRB, and it is presumed that it thereby interferes with the growth-suppressive effect of the Rb protein. pRB becomes phosphorylated just before entry into S phase; indeed this phosphorylation is thought to be permissive for S phase entry. It may thus be that viral transforming proteins that bind pRB prevent or curtail this phosphorylation-mediated relief of Rb's antiproliferative action. Whyte *et al.*, (1988) proposed that pRB is part of a signalling pathway allowing cells to respond to environmental signals. By binding proteins such as E1A the normal function of pRB is lost and hence an essential link in signal transduction which promotes cell proliferation. By antagonizing pRB the constraints of normal growth are removed. Hu *et al.* (1990) showed that there are two distinct regions of the protein, between amino acids 393–572 and 646–772, which are essential for binding of E1A and LT. The same regions of the Rb protein are also common sites for spontaneously occurring mutations of Rb found in tumours not associated with DNA tumour virus infection. These observations lend further support for the theory that the various viral proteins are targeting domains which are essential for the normal growth-suppressive function of the Rb protein.

2.4.6 PRENATAL SCREENING

The cloning of the Rb gene raised the possibility of using natural variations in DNA structure at this locus for prenatal screening. The relatively rare polymorphism associated with the ESD enzyme had previously been the only option available (Sparkes *et al.*, 1983; Cowell *et al.*, 1987). The 4.7R cDNA, however, failed to identify RFLPs that could be used for this purpose. Unique sequences, isolated from the introns of RB1 (Wiggs *et al.*, 1988), recognized RFLPs with fairly high frequencies and, in an analysis of 20 Rb families, no recombination was observed between the Rb phenotype and any of these probes. We (Onadim *et al.*, 1990) and others (Scheffer *et al.*, 1989) have extended this analysis. In a further 46 families from the UK we have failed to detect any recombinants. The single most useful probe, RS2.O, recognizes a variable number tandem repeat (VNTR) within the large (80 kb) intron in the 4.7R genomic sequence. The RFLP is based on a 53 base pair repeat and is identified using the RSAI enzyme, which recognizes an 8-allele system. In our analysis over 70% of families were informative using this probe alone. Of the remaining families only 8% were uninformative for any of the other probes. Thus, it will be possible to offer prenatal screening to 92% of Rb families in the UK. Practical application of this system has already been demonstrated (Mitchell *et al.*, 1988; Onadim *et al.*, 1990). There is, however, clearly still a requirement to generate other probes from either within the 4.7R genomic sequence or from flanking regions so that the same service can be offered to all families. A comprehensive panel of DNA probes would (a) eliminate fetuses/infants not at risk for Rb and (b) allow clinical attention to be focused on those 'at risk' children who need them.

In the absence of a family history it is still difficult to distinguish whether newly diagnosed cases are gene carriers or not. DNA sequence data now available for RB1 (McGee *et al.*, 1989) means that, using the polymerase chain reaction (PCR) and sequencing of the amplified products, specific mutations might be revealed in hereditary cases. There are still problems, however, since, if lymphocytes are used as the source of DNA, the mutation will only be heterozygous in gene carriers, making the identification of single base pair changes difficult. Furthermore, not all of the genomic structure of the Rb gene can be analysed in this way and some mutations will not be detected. If tumour material is available from the patient, identification of mutations becomes easier because the majority of tumours will be homozygous for the causative mutation. This analysis can now be extended to formalin-fixed and paraffin-embedded tissue. If the mutation found in the tumours is present in the patient's lymphocytes they can be confirmed as gene carriers.

2.4.7 MUTATIONS IN OTHER TUMOURS

Approximately 70% of Rb tumours demonstrably develop homozygosity at chromosome 13 loci (Zhu *et al.*, 1989), although probably all Rb tumours carry loss-of-function mutations in both copies of RB1. Using the technique of RNase protection, which is sensitive enough to recognize point mutations, Dunn *et al.* (1989) found aberrations in 13/22 tumours and, although their location appeared to be random, exons 1 and 19 were most frequently involved. In hereditary cases small deletions and insertions were most often seen whereas, point mutations, usually affecting the splice acceptor/donor site producing whole exon deletions, were more common in sporadic cases. In one patient the predisposing mutation found in constitutional cells was a 9 base pair deletion in exon 19. It was possible to isolate tumour cells from three individual foci in the eye and, in each case, the second mutation was different.

Epidemiological studies have shown that individuals carrying germ line mutations are also predisposed to other tumours (Abramson *et al.*, 1976), 66% of which are osteosarcomas and soft tissue sarcomas. Deletions of Rb gene function have been found in these classes of tumours even in patients without Rb (Friend, 1987). In the ten osteosarcoma cell lines studied by Horowitz *et al.* (1990), five had lost expression of pRB or produced abnormal forms. The majority of those are normal length but under- or unphosphorylated, suggesting that they carry mutations that result in a failure to be recognized by modifying proteins. This may be an important feature in the development of osteosarcoma. It is still not clear, however, why inactivation of such a widely expressed gene results in only a narrow spectrum of tumour types.

Abnormalities of RB1 have also been examined in a variety of tumours not normally associated with Rb predisposition. Small cell lung carcinoma (SCLC) often shows abnormalities involving chromosome 13 (Wurster-Hill *et al.*, 1984). Approximately 60% of SCLC lack RB1 message or have defective messages (Harbour *et al.*, 1988). In 8/9 tumours with normal RB1 message gene mutations were presumed since pRB was absent in five cases and in the other three aberrant proteins were seen, which is similar to the observations of

Yokato *et al.* (1987). The array of other tumours showing aberrations of RB1 is somewhat confusing. Approximately 30% of bladder cell lines do not produce pRB. In one bladder carcinoma cell line, Horowitz *et al.* (1989) found a homozygous mutation in a splice-acceptor site resulting in the deletion of exon 21 from the mRNA. The translated protein fails to bind E1A. Breast carcinomas show a low frequency of abnormalities in RB1 (Lee *et al.*, 1988; T'Ang *et al.*, 1989; Horowitz *et al.*, 1989) and no abnormalities were seen in 11 colon cancers or 10 melanomas. The rare inactivation of RB1 in breast and bladder tumours may simply be important for the proliferation of these individual malignancies rather than being a common event in this class of tumours. Since the Rb gene is relatively large, and therefore may be particularly susceptible to mutation, which in some cell types confers a selective growth advantage, it is perhaps not surprising that individual tumours within any one histological subgroup show mutation of this gene.

The fact that constitutional mutations of the Rb gene consistently lead only to the development of retinoblastoma suggests that the specific function provided by this gene is essential for the normal development of these cells, whereas the infrequent, inconsistent association with other tumours may imply a role in tumour progression.

The use of chromosome deletions to map randomly isolated chromosome-specific DNA sequences led to the isolation of the Rb predisposition gene. This same approach is now being applied to a variety of other cancers, considered below. However, where the genetics present a more complex pattern than that seen for Rb, such as in Wilms' tumour, for example, it is unlikely that this approach will be so straightforward.

affecting 1 in 10 000 children each year and accounts for around 6% of all children's tumours. Although often considered a hereditary tumour, conforming to a two-hit hypothesis (Knudson and Strong, 1972), the genetic component is not as obvious as in Rb, for example, with less than 1% having a family history. In a few cases (Miller *et al.*, 1964) WT is associated with the sporadic form of aniridia – congenital absence of irises – as well as mental retardation and/or abnormal genitalia (Riccardi *et al.*, 1978) – the AGR syndrome. These patients invariably have a constitutional chromosome deletion involving region 11p13 which confers a 50% risk to tumour development (Narahara *et al.*, 1984). The fact that only half of the deletion patients develop a tumour suggests that the second hit may be a rarer event than in Rb. In patients with the smallest sub-band deletions aniridia (AN) and WT may be the only associated phenotypes placing these genes in the proximal part of the 11p13 band. Cytogenetic analysis of the patient described by Turleau *et al.* (1984b), who had WT and retardation but not aniridia, placed WT proximal to AN.

The 11p13 deletion can also be transmitted by carriers of balanced translocations (Yunis and Ramsay, 1980; Hittner *et al.*, 1979). The inheritance of the unbalanced form of this rearrangement leads to the WAGR phenotype. Wilms' tumour is not the only malignancy associated with deletion of region 11p13. Andersen *et al.* (1978) reported one AGR patient, a girl, who developed bilateral gonadoblastoma at age 21 months. Both kidneys and gonads are of mesodermal origin and derive from embryologically adjacent sites involving the mesonephros, implying that the same gene in 11p13 may act in a pleiotropic fashion and affect the development of a number of different tissues.

2.5 WILMS' TUMOUR

Wilms' tumour (WT) is a kidney tumour

2.5.1 LOSS OF HETEROZYGOSITY

The loss of chromosome 11 alleles in Wilms'

tumours was demonstrated by several groups (Orkin *et al.*, 1984; Fearon *et al.*, 1984; Koufos *et al.*, 1984), supporting the two-hit hypothesis and the candidacy of WT as a tumour suppressor gene. Homozygosity can result from mitotic recombination, non-disjunction or chromosome deletion. The frequency in WT, however, is much lower than that seen for retinoblastoma, at around 30%, although 11p13 is not always involved. Allele loss restricted to 11p15 and 11p13 has been reported (Mannens *et al.*, 1988; Reeve *et al.*, 1989; Wadey *et al.*, 1990). This demonstration possibly implies that there are two genes on the short arm of chromosome 11 that are important in Wilms' tumorigenesis. Alternatively, a gene in 11p15, promoting tumour progression, may account for the development of homozygosity in this region as well as in a small percentage of other tumours (review in Wadey *et al.*, 1990). Recently, several WT families have been reported (Grundy *et al.*, 1988; Huff *et al.*, 1988) in whom it was possible to carry out linkage analysis using probes from the short arm of chromosome 11. The unanimous finding was that the WT phenotype in these families was not linked to 11p DNA markers. Although the familial incidence of WT (<1%) is even lower than that of 11p deletions it is clear that there may be other genes associated with WT predisposition.

Loss of heterozygosity on the short arm of chromosome 11 has since been reported in several laboratories (Schroeder *et al.*, 1987; Dao *et al.*, 1987; Williams *et al.*, 1989; Mannens *et al.*, 1988; Wadey *et al.*, 1990) and Schroeder *et al.* (1987) have shown that the paternally derived allele is retained in 5/5 tumours. Others have confirmed this observation (Reeve *et al.*, 1984; Mannens *et al.*, 1989; Williams *et al.*, 1989; Pal *et al.*, 1990).

Wilkins (1988) proposed a theory of genomic imprinting to try to explain these observations. According to Comings (1973), inactivation of a diploid pair of regulatory genes which normally suppress function of a trans-forming gene would be required to release cells from normal growth controls. It also appears, in many cases, that the maternal genome largely determines embryonic development (review in Solter, 1988) and expression of some genes differs depending on their maternal or paternal origin. Wilkins suggested that the transforming gene for WT is on chromosome 11 but only active on the paternal chromosomes, the maternal allele having been inactivated by genomic imprinting. Thus, only the paternal transforming gene would respond to the absence of the suppressing gene product and expression of the transforming gene would only occur if the paternal chromosome is retained. The exact mechanism of genomic imprinting is still unclear but one possibility is that gene inactivation could result from selective methylation of genes. Williams *et al.*, (1989) claimed a reduction in the degree of methylation of the HRAS locus in WT compared with normal tissues from the same patients. Our own studies show that in WT the degree of methylation appears to be reduced, but not eliminated, for most loci along the length of chromosome 11p.

2.5.2 BECKWITH-WIEDEMANN SYNDROME

The presence of a second tumour predisposition gene in 11p15 was supported by the observation in Beckwith-Wiedemann syndrome (BWS), a somatic overgrowth condition (Beckwith, 1963; Wiedemann, 1964) with a complex phenotype. One feature of this syndrome is that there is often an associated predisposition to the development of rare paediatric tumours, most usually WT but also hepatoblastoma, rhabdomyosarcoma, adrenal carcinomas, pancreatoblastomas and non-Hodgkin's lymphoma (Wiedemann, 1983). In rare cases patients with BWS have constitutional chromosome abnormalities involving the distal tip of the short arm of chromosome

11 (Waziri *et al.*, 1983; Turleau *et al.*, 1984a; Henry *et al.*, 1989). Linkage in the familial form of BWS (Ping *et al.*, 1989; Koufos *et al.*, 1989) also implicates region 11p15 in the aetiology of BWS. In some patients, combinations of these tumours have been reported, suggesting a common aetiological event arising as a result of a mutation at the same locus. Koufos *et al.*, (1986) analysed three hepatoblastomas and showed that in two there was a loss of heterozygosity for chromosome 11 markers, while in a third tumour heterozygosity was retained. There were similar findings in two rhabdomyosarcomas. Scrable *et al.* (1987) have shown that loss of heterozygosity in embryonal rhabdomyosarcomas was restricted to the distal half of the short arm of chromosome 11 and mitotic recombination mapping suggests that the predisposition locus is in the 11p15.5-pter region. Markers from other chromosomes were the same in tumour and normal tissues.

2.5.3 MOLECULAR ANALYSIS OF 11p13

Molecular cloning strategies, similar to that described for Rb, have been designed to try to identify the WT predisposition gene. They mostly involve random mapping strategies of chromosome-11-specific DNA sequences, isolated from a variety of chromosome-specific DNA libraries (Porteous *et al.*, 1987; Lewis *et al.*, 1988; Davis *et al.*, 1988; Gessler *et al.*, 1989; Rose *et al.*, 1990). Recently a candidate gene (WT33) has been isolated from the 11p13 region (Call *et al.*, 1990; Gessler *et al.*, 1990). This candidate gene was shown to have a 'zinc-finger' motif, a feature which is associated with DNA binding function, and raises the possibility that it may regulate the expression of other genes. WT33 is also only expressed in fetal kidney, the gonads and the spleen. The specific localization to the kidney and the gonads might have been expected because of their common embryological origin. Why expression is also found in the spleen is

not clear. A detailed analysis of the temporal expression pattern of WT33 showed that it was most highly expressed in cells making the transition between mesenchymal and epithelial cells (Pritchard-Jones *et al.*, 1990), further supporting the idea that WT33 controls aspects of normal development. The next step is to determine whether structural abnormalities of this gene, implicating it in tumorigenesis, can be detected in tumour cells. The only way of truly demonstrating the involvement of a particular gene in tumour predisposition would be to show that introduction of a normal copy of that gene restores the non-malignant phenotype in the cells. Stanbridge and colleagues were able to suppress malignancy of a WT cell line by the introduction of a whole copy of chromosome 11p (Weissman *et al.*, 1987). These experiments have been extended to show that when the WT33 gene is deleted from this chromosome, by X-irradiation prior to its introduction in the WT cell line, malignancy is not suppressed (Stanbridge, pers. comm). While this strongly supports a role for a tumour suppressor gene in 11p13 it cannot be proved that other genes on chromosome 11 are not contributing to the suppression. Strong circumstantial evidence for the involvement of the gene in tumorigenesis can be provided by the demonstration of mutations which are restricted to the candidate gene in tumour cells. Southern blotting experiments, however, will only identify relatively large rearrangements. Homozygous deletions of WT33 have been reported in a small percentage of tumours (Gessler *et al.*, 1990) involving the whole gene and flanking regions. In these cases it was possible that adjacent genes might also be candidates. We have recently detected a partial homozygous deletion of this gene involving only the 3' end and not adjacent genes, which is reminiscent of observations with the Rb gene (Friend *et al.*, 1986). Heterozygous rearrangements were noted in four other tumours involving the 5' end of the gene. Histopathological analysis of these tumours showed that they were all advanced-stage tumours. It is possible, therefore, that mutations in this gene lead to the development/progression of aggressive tumours. The low percentage of rearrangements of WT33 in tumour cells may reflect the fact that this gene is only involved in tumorigenesis in a proportion of cases. Detailed sequencing of the WT33 gene in tumour cells will allow its involvement to be assessed more critically.

At the time of writing these two genes, RB1 and WT33, are the only cancer predisposition genes which have been molecularly cloned but inevitably others will soon follow.

2.5.4 CHROMOSOME ANALYSIS OF TUMOUR CELLS

Chromosome analysis of tumour cells can often be overinterpreted since these cells are highly evolved. They arise from successive clonal evolution, during which time advantageous rearrangements leading to tumour progression have occurred. Chromosome analysis of tumour cells alone would not have identified the relevant regions in Rb and WT, for example. Given this caveat the presence of consistent chromosome abnormalities may reflect important events in tumorigenesis. Thus, although early reports on Rb tumour cells suggested frequent involvement of 13q in cytogenetic abnormalities, subsequent detailed analysis of many more tumours failed to confirm this (Squire *et al.*, 1985). In the course of these studies it became clear that chromosomes 1 and 6 were also frequently involved in structural abnormalities (Squire *et al.*, 1985). Chromosome analysis of WT shown the same overall pattern as seen in Rb. Thus, although abnormalities involving the short arm of chromosome 11 may be the most frequently observed single abnormality (Douglass *et al.*, 1985; Slater 1986; Solis *et al.*, 1988), this does not always involve

11p13 and the majority of tumours have two normal copies of chromosome 11 (Kaneko *et al.*, 1983; Kondo *et al.*, 1984). Again chromosomes 1 and 16 were frequently abnormal. We now know that the development of homozygosity in WT is an important event in tumorigenesis which does not alter the gross appearance of the chromosome.

2.6 OTHER TUMOURS

The location of hereditary cancer predisposition genes can only be assigned unequivocally through linkage analysis. Although constitutional chromosome abnormalities usually imply that the breakpoints interrupt the critical gene this may not always be the case since substantial deletions may also be associated with these rearrangements. The development of somatic homozygosity for particular regions of chromosomes directs attention to potential sites. These observations, however, cannot be used reliably to pinpoint cancer genes since many chromosomes may show loss of alleles in the same tumour or be seen only in advanced tumours. Thus, these genetic changes are more likely associated with tumour progression rather than with tumorigenesis. Tumour chromosome analysis may also be misleading as to the site of predisposition genes since, although consistent abnormalities may be noted, they may have no relevance to tumorigenicity. Given this caveat there is fragmentary information about a variety of other paediatric tumours which are reviewed below. For many of these tumours there are rare cases of familial aggregations but insufficient for linkage studies. Relatively poor survival of patients with these cancers has been a contributing factor.

Medulloblastoma is the most common malignant primary brain tumour of children and arises from primitive cells in the neuroepithelium. There have been a few cytogenetic studies but, although chromosome 1q is implicated, no clear pattern emerges (Bigner *et al.*, 1988; Griffin *et al.*, 1989). In Ewing's sarcoma, a primary sarcoma of osseous and non-osseous origin, chromosome analysis has shown a consistent translocation between chromosomes 11 and 22, t(11;22) (q23;q12), in tumour cells (see Griffin *et al.*, 1986). It is hard to interpret the importance of these rearrangements since it appears that the exact position of the breakpoints is variable. There has also been a consistent rearrangement recorded in rhabdomyosarcomas, t(2;13) (q35;q14), where the consistent breakpoint is on chromosome 2 (Douglass *et al.*, 1987; Hayashi *et al.*, 1988; Moriyama *et al.*, 1986) despite the suggestion of a critical locus on the short arm of chromosome 11 from loss of heterozygosity studies (Scrable *et al.*, 1987).

2.6.1 NEUROBLASTOMA

Neuroblastoma (Nb) arises from primitive neural crest cells and is the most common neoplasm diagnosed in infancy. There have been a few reported cases of familial Nb although, as for WT, they are rare. To date the only indication as to the location of the Nb predisposition gene comes from chromosome analysis of tumour cells. In the majority of cases abnormalities involving the short arm of chromosome 1 have been reported, specifically region 1p31–36. Family pedigrees have not, so far, been suitable for linkage analysis. Homozygosity studies have implicated 1p in advanced-stage tumours (Fong *et al.*, 1989), although chromosome 14q also frequently shows allele loss. Cytological evidence for gene amplification in the form of double minutes (DM) and homogeneously staining regions (HSR) have been frequently reported in Nb (Cowell, 1982) and represent amplification of the N-*myc* oncogene, which is often associated with translocation from the normal position on chromosome 2 to the p31–36 region of chromosome 1.

It has been suggested that N-*myc* amplifi-

cation is an indication of advanced-stage disease in Nb (Brodeur *et al.*, 1984; Seeger *et al.*, 1985; Kaneko *et al.*, 1987), although amplification appears to be more related to the capacity for progression rather than to a particular stage. In tumours where cells have only a single copy of N-*myc* at diagnosis, 94% had progression free survival and generally did better after therapy regardless of stage. In contrast, 50% of tumours with elevated N-*myc* levels, regardless of stage, go on to metastasize and kill the patient. Seeger *et al.*, (1985) also noted that, while Stage IV and Stage IVS disease are both widely disseminated at diagnosis, the better prognosis IVS tumours did not show amplification of N-*myc*, whereas stage IV disease did. Thus, N-*myc* amplification is a reasonable indicator of poor prognosis, identifying 50% of cases. A better prognostic indicator, however, was reported to be the presence of abnormalities involving the short arm (p) of chromosome 1 (Christiansen and Lampert, 1988). In their study, 83% of poor prognosis patients had 1p abnormalities, whereas only 33% of those tested had N-*myc* amplification. This observation was in contrast to that of Kaneko *et al.* (1987), where 60–70% of poor prognosis tumours had both 1p abnormalities and elevated N-*myc* levels. The significance of these observations remains to be determined but it is clear that molecular pathology of this kind is providing better indications for prognosis.

2.7 CONCLUSION

The analysis of childhood tumours offers a unique opportunity to study not only the cancer phenotype but also, possibly, genes which are important in normal embryonic development. To date only the Rb predisposition gene, and a candidate for the WT gene, have been isolated, although it seems likely that others will soon follow. The availability of these genes will mean that mutations in individual patients can be characterized in the tumours. The demonstration of a mutation in constitutional cells defines the patient as a gene carrier. As patterns emerge it may be that particular mutations will be associated with a particular course of the disease, thereby allowing predictions to be made about invasiveness, prognosis and susceptibility to other tumours, for example. This analysis is already available for the leukaemias where, although their significance in tumour initiation is uncertain, specific genetic rearrangements can classify the disease and indicate prognosis. If these objectives are realized generally then molecular pathology will become increasingly important in clinical practice but will depend on the careful collection and processing of tumour and normal tissue from each patient.

REFERENCES

Abramson, D.H., Ellesworth, R.M. and Zimmerman, L.E. (1976) Nonocular cancer in retinoblastoma survivors. *Trans. Am. Acad. Ophthalmol. Otolaryngol.*, **81**, 454–7.

Abramson, D.H., Ellsworth, R.M., Kitchin, F.D. and Tung, G. (1984) Second nonocular tumours in retinoblastoma survivors. Are they radiation-induced? *Ophthalmology*, **91**, 1351–5.

Andersen, S., Geertingen, P., Larsen, H.W. *et al.* (1978) Aniridia, cataract and gonadoblastoma in a mentally retarded girl with deletion of chromosome 11. *Ophthalmologica*, **176**, 171–7.

Bartram, C.R. (1985) bcr rearrangement without juxtaposition of c-abl in chronic myeloid leukaemia. *J. Exp. Med.*, **162**, 2175–9.

Bartram, C.R. and Carbonelli, F. (1986) bcr rearrangement in Philadelphia-negative CML. *Cancer Genet. Cytogenet.*, **21** 183–4.

Beckwith, J.P. (1963) Extreme cytomegaly of the adrenal fetal cortex, omphalocele hyperplasia of kidneys and pancreas, and Leydig-cell hyperplasia: another syndrome? *Western Soc. Pediatr. Res.* Los Angeles, Nov 11th:

Benedict, W.F., Srivatsan, E.S., Mark, C. *et al.* (1987) Complete or partial homozygosity of chromosome 13 in primary retinoblastoma. *Cancer Res.*, **47**, 4189–91.

Berk, A.J. (1986) Adenovirus promoters and E1A transactivation. *Ann. Rev. Genet.*, **20**, 45–79.

Bernard, O., Cory, S., Gemdakis, S. *et al.* (1983) Sequence of murine and human cellular myc oncogenes and two modes of myc transcription resulting from chromosome translocation in 3-lymphoid tumours.*EMBO J.*, **2**, 2375–83.

Bigner, S.H., Mark, J., Friedman, H.S. *et al.* (1988) Structural chromosomal abnormalities in human medulloblastoma. *Cancer Genet. Cytogenet.*, **30**, 91–101.

Blanquet V., Turleau C., Creau-Goldberg, N. *et al.* (1987) De novo t(2;13) (p24.3;q14.2) and retinoblastoma. Mapping of two 13q14 probes by in situ hybridisation. *Hum. Genet.*, **76**, 102–5.

Bookstein, R., Lee, E.Y.-H.P., To, H. *et al.* (1988) Human retinoblastoma susceptibility gene: Genomic organization and analysis of heterozygous intragenic deletion mutants. *Proc. Nat. Acad. Sci. USA*, **85**, 2210–4.

Borrow, J., Goddard, A., Sheer, D. and Solomon, E. (1990) Molecular analysis of acute promyelocytic leukaemia breakpoint cluster region on chromosome 17. *Science*, **249**, 1577–80.

Brodeur, G.M., Seeger, R.C., Schwab, M. *et al.* (1984) Amplification of N-myc in untreated human neuroblastomas correlates with advanced disease stage. *Science*, **224**, 1121–4.

Call, K.M., Glaser, T., Ito, C.Y. *et al.* (1990) Isolation and characterisation of a zinc finger polypeptide gene at the human chromosome 11 Wilms' tumour locus. *Cell*, **60**, 509–20.

Cavenee, W.K., Dryja, T.P., Phillips, R.A. *et al.* (1983) Expression of recessive alleles by chromosomal mechanisms in retinoblastoma. *Nature*, **305**, 779–84.

Cavenee, W., Leach, R., Mohandas, T. *et al.* (1984) Isolation and regional localisation of DNA segments revealing polymorphic loci for human chromosome 13. *Am. J. Hum. Genet.*, **36**, 10–24.

Cavenee, W.K., Hansen, M.F., Nordenskjold, M. *et al.* (1985) Genetic origin of mutations predisposing to retinoblastoma. *Science*, **228**, 501–3.

Christiansen, H. and Lampert, F. (1988) Tumour karyotype discriminates between good and bad prognostic outcome in neuroblastoma. *Br. J. Cancer*, **57**, 121–6.

Collins, S.J., Kubonishi, I., Myoski, I. and Groudine, M.T. (1984) Altered transcription of the c-abl oncogene in K562 and other chronic myelogenous leukaemia cells. *Science*, **225** 72–4.

Comings, D.E. (1973) A general theory of carcinogenesis. *Proc. Nat. Acad. Sci. USA*, **70**, 3324–8.

Cory, S., Gerondakis, S. and Adams, J.M. (1983) Interchromosomal recombination of the cellular oncogene c–myc with the immunoglobulin heavy chain locus in murine plasmacytomas is a reciprocal exchange. *EMBO J.*, **2**, 697–703.

Cowell, J.K. (1982) Double minutes and homogeneously staining regions: Gene amplification in mammalian cells. *Ann. Rev. Genet.*, **16** 21–59.

Cowell, J.K., Rutland, P., Jay, M. and Hungerford, J. (1986) Deletions of the esterase-D locus from a survey of 200 retinoblastoma patients. *Hum. Genet.*, **72**, 164–7.

Cowell, J.K., Jay, M., Rutland, P. and Hungerford, J. (1987) An assessment of the usefulness of electrophoretic variants of esterase D in the antenatal diagnosis of retinoblastoma in the United Kingdom. *Br. J. Cancer*, **55**, 661–4.

Cowell, J.K., Hungerford, J., Rutland, P. and Jay, M. (1989) Genetic and cytogenetic analysis of patients showing reduced esterase-D levels and mental retardation from a survey of 500 individuals with retinoblastoma. *Ophthal. Ped. Genet.*, **110**, 117–27.

Dao, D.D., Schroeder, W.T., Chao, L.Y. *et al.* (1987) Genetic mechanisms of tumour-specific loss of 11p DNA sequences in Wilms' tumour. *Am. J. Hum. Genet.*, **41**, 202–17.

Davis, L.M., Stallard, R., Thomas, G.H. *et al.* (1988) Two anonymous DNA segments distinguish the Wilms' tumour and aniridia loci. *Science*, **241** 840–2.

De Klein, D., Van Kessel, A.G., Grosveld, G. *et al.* (1982) A cellular oncogene is translocated to the Philadelphia chromosome in chronic myelocytic leukaemia. *Nature*, **300**, 765–7.

Donner, P., Greiser-Wilke, I. and Moeling, K. (1982) Nuclear localisation and DNA binding of the transforming gene product of avian myelocytomatosis virus. *Nature*, **296**, 262–6.

Douglass, E.C., Wilimas, J.A., Green, A.A. and Look, A.T. (1985) Abnormalities of chromosome 1 and 11 in Wilms' tumour. *Cancer Genet. Cytogenet.*, **14**, 331–8.

Douglass, E.C., Valentine, M., Etcubanas, E. *et al.* (1987) A specific chromosomal abnormality in

rhabdomyosarcoma. *Cytogenet. Cell Genet.*, **45**, 148–55.

Draper G.J., Sanders, B.M. and Kingston, J.E. (1986) Second primary neoplasms in patients with retinoblastoma. *Br. J. Cancer*, **53**, 661–71.

Dryja, T.P., Cavenee, W.K., White, R. *et al.* (1984) Homozygosity of chromosome 13 in retinoblastoma. *N. Engl. J. Med.*, **310**, 550–3.

Dryja, T.P., Rapaport, J.M., Joyce, J.M. and Petersen, R.A. (1986) Molecular detection of deletions involving band q14 of chromosome 13 retinoblastomas. *Proc. Nat. Acad. Sci. USA*, **83**, 7391–4.

Dudin, G., Nasr, A., Traboulsi, E. *et al.* (1984) Hereditary retinoblastoma and 13q- mosaicism. *Cytogenet. Cell Genet.*, **38**, 335–7.

Dunn, J.M., Phillips, R.A., Becker, A. and Gallie, B.L. (1988) Identification of germline and somatic mutations affecting the retinoblastoma gene. *Science*, **241**, 1797–1800.

Dunn, J.M., Zhu, X., Gallie, B.L. and Phillips, R.A. (1989) Characterization of mutations in the RB1 gene, in *Recessive Oncogenes and Tumor Suppression*, (eds W. Cavenee, N. Hastie and E. Stanbridge), Cold Spring Harbor Laboratory Press, Cold Spring Harbor, pp. 93–100.

Dyson, N., Howley, P.M., Munger, K. and Harlow, E. (1989) The human papilloma virus-16 E7 oncoprotein is able to bind to the retinoblastoma gene product. *Science*, **243**, 934–6.

Ejima, Y., Sasaki, M.S., Kaneko, A. *et al.* (1982) Possible inactivation of part of chromosome 13 due to 13qXp translocation associated with retinoblastoma. *Clin. Genet.*, **21**, 357–61.

Ejima, Y., Sasaki, M.S., Kaneko, A. and Tanooka, H. (1988) Types, rates, origin and expression of chromosome mutations involving 13q14 in retinoblastoma patients. *Hum. Genet.*, **79**, 118–23.

Erickson, J., Finan, J., Nowell, P.C. and Croce, C.M. (1982) Translocation of immunoglobulin VH genes in Burkitt lymphoma. *Proc. Nat. Acad. Sci. USA*, **79**, 5611–5.

Erickson, J., Ar-Rushdi, A., Drwinga, H. *et al.* (1983) Transcriptional activation of the translocated c-myc oncogene in Burkitt lymphoma. *Proc. Nat. Acad. Sci. USA*, **80**, 820–4.

Fahrlander, P.D., Piechaczyk, M. and Marcu, K.B. (1985) Chromatin structure of the murine c-myc locus: implications for the regulation of normal and chromosomally translocated genes. *EMBO J.*, **4**, 3195–202.

Fearon, E.R., Vogelstein, B. and Feinberg, A.P. (1984) Somatic deletion and duplication of genes on chromosome 11 in Wilms' tumours. *Nature*, **309**, 176–8.

Fong, Chin-To, Dracopoli, N.C., White, P.S. *et al.* (1989) Loss of heterozygosity for the short arm of chromosome 1 in human neuroblastomas: Correlation with N-myc amplification. *Proc. Nat. Acad. Sci.*, **86**, 3753–7.

Friend, S.H., Bernards, R, Rogelj, S. *et al.* (1986) A human DNA segment with properties of the gene that predisposes to retinoblastoma and osteosarcoma. *Nature.* **323** 643–6.

Friend, S.H., Horowitz, J.M., Gerber, M.R. *et al.* (1987) Deletions of a DNA sequence in retinoblastomas and mesenchymal tumors: Organization of the sequence and its encoded protein. *Proc. Nat. Acad. Sci. USA*, **84**, 9059–63.

Fung, Y.T., Murphree, A.L., T'Ang, A. *et al.* (1987) Structural evidence for the authenticity of the human retinoblastoma gene. *Science*, **236**, 1657–61.

Gallie, B.L. and Phillips, R.A. (1982) Multiple manifestations of the retinoblastoma gene. *Birth Defects: Original Article Series*, **18**, 689–701.

Gessler, M. and Bruns, G.A.P. (1989) A physical map around the WAGR complex on the short arm of chromosome 11. *Genomics*, **5**, 43–55.

Gessler, M., Poustka, A., Cavenee, W. *et al.* (1990) Homozygous deletion in Wilms' tumours of a zinc-finger gene identified by chromosome jumping. *Nature*, **343**, 774–8.

Godbout, R., Dryja, T.P., Squire, J. *et al.* (1983) Somatic inactivation of genes on chromosome 13 is a common event in retinoblastoma. *Nature*, **304**, 451–3.

Goddard, A.D., Balakier, H., Canton, M. *et al.* (1988) Infrequent genomic rearrangement and normal expression of the putative Rb1 gene in retinoblastoma tumors. *Mol. Cell. Biol.*, **8**, 2082–8.

Griffin, C.A., McKeon, C., Israel, M.A. *et al.* (1986) Comparison of constitutional and tumor-associated 11;22 translocations: Nonidentical breakpoints on chromosomes 11 and 22. *Proc. Nat. Acad. Sci. USA*, **83**, 6122–6.

Griffin, C.A., Hawkins, A.L., Packer, R.J. *et al.* (1989) Chromosome abnormalities in pediatric brain tumours. *Cancer Res.*, **40**, 175–9.

Groffen J., Stephenson, J.R., Heisterkamp, N. *et al.* (1984) Philadelphia chromosomal breakpoints are clustered within a limited region, bcr, on chromosome 22. *Cell*, **36**, 93–9.

Grundy, P., Koufos, A., Morgan, K. *et al.* (1988) Familial predisposition to Wilms' tumour does not map to the short arm of chromosome 11. *Nature*, **336**, 375–6.

Halloran, S.L., Boughman, J.A., Dryja, T.P. *et al.* (1985) Accuracy of the detection of the retinoblastoma gene by esterase-D linkage. *Arch. Ophthalmol.*, **103**, 1329–31.

Hann, S.R., Thompson, C.B. and Eisenman, R.N. (1985) C-myc oncogene protein synthesis is independent of the cell cycle in human and avian cells. *Nature*, **314**, 366–9.

Harbour, J.W., Lai, S.-L., Whang-Peng, J. *et al.* (1988) Abnormalities in structure and expression of the human retinoblastoma gene in SCLC. *Science*, **241**, 353–7.

Hayashi, Y., Inaba, T., Hanada, R. and Yamamoto, K. (1988) Translocation 2;8 in a congenital rhabdomyosarcoma. *Cancer Genet. Cytogenet.* **30**, 343–5.

Heim, S and Mitelmann, F. (1987) *Cancer Cytogenetics*, Alan R. Liss Inc., New York, p.309.

Heisterkamp, N., Groffen, J., Stephenson, J.R. *et al.* (1982) Chromosomal localisation of human cellular homologues of two viral oncogenes. *Nature*, **299**, 747–9.

Heisterkamp, N., Stephenson, J.R., Groffen, J. *et al.* (1983) Localisation of the c-abl oncogene adjacent to a translocation breakpoint in chronic myelocytic leukaemia. *Nature*, **306**, 239–42.

Henry, I., Jeanpierre, M., Couillin, P. *et al.* (1989) Molecular definition of the 11p15.5 region involved in Beckwith-Wiedemann syndrome and probability in predisposition to adrenocortical carcinoma. *Hum. Genet.*, **81**, 273–7.

Hida, T., Kinoshita, Y., Matsumoto, R., Suzuki, N. and Tanaka, H. (1980) Bilateral retinoblastoma with 13qXp translocation. *J. Paediatr. Ophthalmol. Strab.*, **17** 144–6.

Higgins, M.J., Hansen, M.F., Cavenee, W.K. and Lalande, M. (1989) Molecular detection of chromosomal translocations that disrupt the putative retinoblastoma susceptibility locus. *Mol. Cell Biol.*, **9**, 1–5.

Hittner, H.M., Riccardi, V.M. and Francke, U. (1979) Aniridia caused by a heritable chromosome 11-deletion. *Opthalmologica*, **86**, 1173–83.

Hopkinson D.A., Mestriner, M.A., Cortner, J. and Harris, H. (1973) Esterase-D: a new human polymorphism. *Ann. Hum. Genet*, **37**, 119–37.

Horowitz, J.M., Yandell, D.W., Park, S. *et al.* (1989) Point mutational inactivation of the retinoblastoma antioncogene. *Science*, **243**, 937–40.

Horowitz, J.M., Park, S.-H., Yandell, D.W. and Weinberg, R.A. (1990) Frequent inactivation of the retinoblastoma anti-oncogene is restricted to a subset of human tumour cells. *Proc. Nat. Acad. Sci. USA*, **87**, 101–7.

Hu, Q., Dyson, N. and Harlow E. (1990) The regions of the retinoblastoma protcin needed for binding to adenovirus E1A or SV40 large T antigen are common sites for mutations. *EMBO J.*, 1147–55.

Huff, V., Compton, D.A., Chao, L.-Y. *et al.* (1988) Lack of linkage of familial Wilms' tumour to chromosomal band 11p13. *Nature*, **336** 377–8.

Kaneko, M., Saito, S., Tsuchida, Y. *et al.* (1983) Wilms' tumour, nephron disorder and ambiguous genitali *Z. Kinderchir.*, **38**, 345–9.

Kaneko, Y., Kanda, N., Maseki, N. *et al.* (1987) Different karyotypic patterns in early and advanced stage neuroblastomas. *Cancer Res.*, **47**, 311–8.

Kelly, K., Cochran, B.H., Stiles, C.D. and Leder, P. (1983) Cell-specific regulation of the c-myc gene by lymphocyte mitogens and platelet derived growth factor. *Cell*, **35**, 603–10.

Knudson, A.G. (1971) Mutation and cancer: statistical study of retinoblastoma. *Proc. Nat. Acad. Sci. USA*, **68**, 820–3.

Knudson, A.G. (1985) Hereditary cancer, oncogenes, and antioncogenes. *Cancer Res.*, **45**, 1437–43.

Knudson, A.G. and Strong, L.C. (1972) Mutation and cancer: a model for Wilms' tumour of the kidney. *J.N.C.I.*, **40**, 313–24.

Kondo, K., Chilcote, R.R., Maurer, H.S. and Rowley, J. (1984) Chromosome abnormalities in tumour cells from patients with sporadic Wilms' tumour. *Cancer Res.*, **44**, 5376–81.

Konopka, J.B., Watanabe, S.M., Singer, J.W. *et al.* (1985) Cell lines and clinical isolates derived from Ph'-positive chronic myelogenous leukaemia patients express c-abl proteins with a structural alteration. *Proc. Nat. Acad. Sci. USA*, **82**, 1810–14.

Koufos, A., Hansen, M.F., Lampkin, B.C. *et al.* (1984) Loss of alleles at loci on human chromosome 11 during genesis of Wilms' tumour. *Nature*, **309**, 170–2.

Koufos, A., Hansen, M.F., Copeland, N.G. *et al.* (1986) Loss of heterozygosity in 3 embryonal tumours suggests a common pathogenetic mechanism. *Nature*, **316**, 330–4.

Koufos, A., Grundy, P., Morgan, K. *et al.* (1989) Familial Wiedemann-Beckwith syndrome and a second Wilms' tumour locus both map to 11p15.5. *Am. J. Hum. Genet.*, **44**, 711–9.

Lalande, M., Dryja, T.P., Schreck, R.R. *et al.* (1984) Isolation of human chromosome 13-specific DNA sequences cloned from flow sorted chromosomes and potentially linked to the retinoblastoma locus. *Cancer Genet. Cytogenet.*, **13** 283–95.

Land, H., Parada, L.F. and Weinberg, R.A. (1983) Tumorigenic conversion of primary embryo fibroblasts requires at least two cooperating oncogenes. *Nature* **300**, 596–602.

Lee, E.Y.-H.P., To, H., Shew, J.-H. *et al.* (1988) Inactivation of the retinoblastoma susceptibility gene in human breast cancers. Science, **241**, 218–21.

Lee, W.H., Bookstein, R., Hong, F. *et al.* (1987a) Human retinoblastoma susceptibility gene: cloning identification and sequence. *Science*, **235**, 1394–9.

Lee, W.H., Shew, J.Y., Hong, F.D. *et al.* (1987b) The retinoblastoma susceptibility gene encodes a nuclear phosphoprotein associated with DNA binding activity. *Nature*, **329**, 642–5.

Lele, K.P., Penrose, L.S. and Stallard, H.B. (1963) Chromosome deletion in a case of retinoblastoma. *Ann. Hum. Genet. Lond.*, **27**, 171–4.

Lewis, W.H., Yeger, H., Bonetta, L. *et al.* (1988) Homozygous deletion of a DNA marker from chromosome 11 in sporadic Wilms' tumour. *Genomics* **3**, 25–31.

Mannens, M., Slater, R.M., Heytig, C. *et al.* (1988) Molecular nature of genetic changes resulting in loss of heterozygosity of chromosome 11 in Wilms' tumours. *Hum. Genet.*, **81**, 41–8.

Matsunaga, E. (1980) On estimating penetrance of the retinoblastoma gene. *Hum. Genet.* **56**, 127–8.

McGee, T.L., Yandell, D.W. and Dryja, T.P. (1989) Structure and partial genomic sequence of the human retinoblastoma susceptibility gene. *Gene*, **80**, 119–28.

McManaway M.E., Neckers L.M., Loke, S.L. *et al.*

(1990) Tumour-specific inhibition of lymphoma growth by an antisense oligodeoxynucleotide. *Lancet*, **i**, 808–11.

Meadows, A.T., Baum, E., Fossati-Bellani, F. *et al.* (1985) Second malignant neoplasms in children: An update from the late effects study group. *J. Clin. Oncol.* **3**, 532–8.

Mellentin, J.D., Murre, C., Donlon, T.A. *et al.* (1989) The gene for enhancer binding proteins E12/E47 lies at the t(1;19) breakpoint in acute leukemias. *Science*, **246**, 379–82.

Mihara, K., Cao, X.-R., Yen, A. *et al.* (1989) Cell cycle-dependent regulation of phoshorylation of the human retinoblastoma gene product. *Science*, **246**, 1300–3.

Miller, R.W., Fraumeni, J.R. and Manning, M.D. (1964) Association of Wilms' tumour with aniridia, hemihypertrophy, and other congenital malformations. *N. Engl. J. Med.*, **27**, 922–7.

Mills, K.I., MacKenzie, E.D. and Birnie, G.D. (1988) The site of the breakpoint within the bcr is a prognostic factor in Philadelphia-positive CML patients. *Blood*, **72**, 1237–41.

Mitchell, C.D., Nicolaides, K., Kingston, J. *et al.* (1988) Prenatal exclusion of hereditary retinoblastoma. *Lancet*, **i**, 826.

Mitchell, C.D. and Cowell, J.K. (1989) Predisposition to retinoblastoma due to a translocation within the 4.7R locus. *Oncogene*, **4**, 253–7.

Mitchell, P. and Tjian, R. (1989) Transcriptional regulation in mammalian cells by sequence-specific DBA binding proteins. *Science*, **245**, 371–8.

Moran, E. (1988) A region of SV40 large T antigen can substitute for a transforming domain of the adenovirus E1A products. *Nature*, **334**, 168–70.

Moriyama, M., Shuin, T., Kubota, Y. *et al.* (1986) A case of rhabdomyosarcoma of the bladder with a 2;5 translocation in peripheral lymphocytes. *Cancer Genet. Cytogenet.*, **22**, 177–81.

Morris, C.M., Rosman, I., Archer, S.A. *et al.* (1988) A cytogenetic and molecular analysis of five variant Philadelphia translocations in chronic myeloid leukaemia. *Cancer Genet. Cytogenet.*, **35**, 179–97.

Motegi, T., Kaga, M., Yanagawa, Y. *et al.* (1983) A recognizable pattern of the midface of retinoblastoma patients with interstitial deletion of 13q. *Hum. Genet.*, **64**, 160–2.

Mukai, S., Rapaport, J.M., Shields, J.A. *et al.* (1984) Linkage of genes for human esterase-D and

hereditary retinoblastoma. *Am. J. Ophthalmol.*, **97**, 681–5.

Narahara, K., Kikkawa, K., Kimira, S. *et al.* (1984) Regional mapping of catalase and Wilms' tumour-aniridia, genitourinary abnormalities, and mental retardation triad loci to the chromosome segment 11p1305–p1306. *Hum. Genet.*, **66**, 181–5.

Nichols, W.W., Miller, R.C., Sobel, M. and Hoffman, E. (1980) Further observations of a 13qXp translocation associated with retinoblastoma. *Am. J. Ophthalmol.*, **89**, 621–7.

Nowell, P.C. and Hungerford, D.A. (1960) A minute human chromosome in human granulocytic leukemia. *Science*, **132**, 1497.

Onadim, Z., Mitchell, C.D., Rutland, P.C. *et al.* (1990) Application of intragenic DNA probes in prenatal screening for retinoblastoma gene carriers in the United Kingdom. *Arch. Dis. Child.*, **65**, 651–6.

Orkin, S.H. (1986) Reverse genetics and human disease. *Cell*, **47**, 845–50.

Orkin, S.H. and Kazazian, H.H. (1984) Mutation and polymorphism of the human b-globin gene and its surrounding DNA. *Ann. Rev. Genet.*, **18**, 131–71.

Orkin, S.H., Goldman, D.S. and Sallan, S.E. (1984) Development of homozygosity for chromosome 11p markers in Wilms' tumour. *Nature*, **309**, 172–4.

Pal, N., Wadey, R.B., Buckle B. *et al.* (1990) Preferential loss of maternal alleles in sporadic Wilms' tumour. *Oncogene*, **5**, 1665–8.

Ping, A.J., Reeve, A.E., Law, D.J. *et al.* (1989) Genetic linkage of Beckwith-Wiedemann syndrome to 11p15. *Am. J. Hum. Genet.*, **44**, 720–3.

Porteous, D.J., Bickmore, W., Christie, S. *et al.* (1987) HRAS-1 selected chromosome transfer generates markers that colocalise aniridia- and genitourinary dysplasia- associated translocation breakpoints and the Wilms' tumour gene within band 11p13. *Proc. Nat. Acad. Sci. USA* **84**, 5355–9.

Pritchard-Jones, K., Fleming, S., Davidson, D. *et al.* (1990) The candidate Wilms' tumour gene is involved in genitourinary development. *Nature*, **346**, 194–7.

Reeve, A.E., Housiaux, P.J., Gardner, R.J.M. *et al.* (1984) Loss of a harvey ras allele in sporadic Wilms' tumour. *Nature*, **309**, 174–6.

Reeve, A.E., Sih, S.A., Raizis, A.M. and Feinberg, A.P. (1989) Loss of alleleic heterozygosity at a second locus on chromosome 11 in 'sporadic Wilms' tumour cells. *Mol. Cell Biol.*, **9**, 1799–1803.

Riccardi, V.M., Sujansky, E., Smith, A.C. and Francke, U. (1978) Chromosome imbalance in the aniridia-Wilms' tumour association: 11p interstitial deletion. *Pediatrics*, **61**, 604–10.

Rose, E.A., Glaser, T., Jones, C. *et al.* (1990) Complete physical map of the WAGR region of 11p13 localizes a candidate Wilms' tumour gene. *Cell*, **60**, 495–508.

Rowe, D., Gerrard, M., Gibbons, B. and Malpas, J.S. (1987) Two further cases of t(2;13) in alveolar rhabdomyosarcoma indicating a review of the published chromosome breakpoints. *Br. J. Cancer*, **56**, 379–80.

Rowley, J.D. (1973) A new consistent chromosomal abnormality in chronic myelogenous leukaemia identified by quinacrine fluorescence and Giemsa staining. *Nature*, **243**, 290–3.

Scheffer, H., Van Der Lelie, D., Aanstoot, G.H. *et al.* (1986) A straightforward approach to isolate DNA sequences with potential linkage to the retinoblastoma locus. *Hum. Genet.*, **74**, 249–55.

Scheffer, H., Te Meerman, G.J., Kruize, Y.C.M. *et al.* (1989) Linkage analysis of families with hereditary retinoblastoma: nonpenetrance of mutation, revealed by combined use of markers within and flanking the RB1 gene. *Am. J. Hum. Genet.*, **45**, 252–60.

Schroeder, W.T., Chao, L.-Y., Dao, D.T. *et al.* (1987) Nonrandom loss of maternal chromosome 11 alleles in Wilms' tumours. *Am. J. Hum. Genet.*, **40**, 413–20.

Schtivelman, E., Lifshitz, B., Gale, R.P. and Canaani, E. (1985) Fused transcript of abl and bcr genes in chronic myelogenous leukaemia. *Nature*, **315**, 550–9.

Scrable, H.J., Witte, D.P., Lampkin, B.C. and Cavenee, W.K. (1987) Chromosomal localisation of the human rhabdomyosarcoma locus by mitotic recombination mapping. *Nature*, **329**, 645–7.

Seeger, R.C., Brodeur, G.M., Sather, H.N. *et al.* (1985) Association of multiple copies of the N-myc oncogene with rapid progression of neuroblastomas. *N. Engl. J. Med.*, **311**, 1111–6.

Siebenlist, U., Hennighausen, L., Battey, V. and Leder, P. (1984) Chromatin structure and protein binding in the putative regulatory region of the c-myc gene in Burkitt lymphoma. *Cell*, **37**, 381–91.

Slater, R.M. (1986) The cytogenetics of Wilms' tumour. *Cancer Genet. Cytogenet.*, **19**, 37–41.

Solis, V., Pritchard, J. and Cowell, J.K. (1988) Cytogenetics of Wilms' tumours. *Cancer Genet. Cytogenet.*, **34**, 223–34.

Solter, D. (1988) Differential imprinting and expression of maternal and paternal genomes. *Ann. Rev. Genet.*, **22**, 127–46.

Sparkes, R.S., Sparkes, M.C., Wilson, M.G. *et al.* (1980) Regional assignment of genes for human esterase D and retinoblastoma to chromosome band 13q14. *Science*, **208**, 1042–4.

Sparkes, R.S., Murphree, A.L., Lingua, R.W. *et al.* (1983) Gene for hereditary retinoblastoma assigned to human chromosome 13 by linkage to esterase-D. *Science*, **217**, 971–3.

Squire, J., Gallie, B.L. and Phillips, R.A. (1985) A detailed analysis of chromosomal changes in heritable and non-heritable retinoblastoma. *Hum. Genet.*, **70**, 291–301.

Stallard, H.B. (1962) The conservative treatment of retinoblastoma. Doyne Memorial Lecture, 1962. *Trans. Ophthalmol. Soc.*, **83**, 473–535.

Strong, L.C., Riccardi, V.M., Ferrel, R.E. and Sparkes, R.S. (1981) Familial retinoblastoma and chromosome 13 deletion transmitted via an insertional translocation. *Science*, **213**, 1501–3.

T'Ang, A., Wu, K.-J., Hashimoto, T. *et al.* (1989) Genomic organization of the human retinoblastoma gene. *Oncogene*, **4** 401–7.

Turleau, C., De Grouchy, J., Chavin-Colin, F. *et al.* (1984a) Trisomy 11p15 and Beckwith-Wiedemann syndrome. A report of two cases. *Hum. Genet.*, **67**, 219–21.

Turleau, C., De Grouchy, J., Tournade, M.F. *et al.* (1984b) Del 11p/aniridia complex. Report of three patients and review of 37 observations from the literature. *Clin. Genet.*, **26**, 356–62.

Turleau, C., De Grouchy, J., Chavin-Colin, F. *et al.* (1985) Cytogenetic forms of retionoblastoma: Their incidence in a survey of 66 patients. *Cancer Genet. Cytogenet.*, **16**, 321–34.

Van Heyningen, V., Bobrow, M., Bodmer, W.F. *et al.* (1975) Chromosome assignment of some human enzyme loci. Mitochondrial malate dehydrogenase to 7, mannosphosphate isomerase and pyruvate kinase to 15, and probably, esterase-d to 13. *Ann. Hum. Genet.*, **38**, 295–305.

Varmus, H.E. (1984) The molecular genetics of cellular oncogenes. *Ann. Rev. Genet.*, **18**, 553–612.

Vogel, W. (1979) The genetics of retinoblastoma. *Hum. Genet.*, **52**, 1–54.

Wadey, R.B., Pal, N.P., Buckle, B. *et al.* (1990) Loss of heterozygosity in Wilms' tumour involves two distinct regions of chromosome 11. *Oncogene*, **5**, 901–7.

Watson, D.K., Psallidoupoulos, M.C., Samuel, K.P. *et al.* (1983) Nucleotide sequence analysis of human c-myc locus, chicken homologue and myelocytomatosis virus MC29 transforming gene reveals a highly conserved gene product. *Proc. Nat. Acad. Sci. USA*, **80**, 3642–5.

Waziri, M., Patil, S.R., Hanson, J.W. and Bartley, J.A. (1983) Abnormality of chromosome 11 in patients with features of Beckwith-Wiedemann syndrome. *J. Pediatr.*, **102**, 873–6.

Weinberg, R.A. (1989) Oncogenes, antioncogenes, and the molecular bases of multistep carcinogenesis. *Cancer Res.*, **49**, 3713–21.

Weissman, B.E., Saxon, P.J., Pasquale, S.R. *et al.* (1987) Introduction of a normal human chromosome 11 into a Wilms' tumour cell line controls its tumorigenic expression. *Science*, **236**, 175–80.

Whyte, P., Buchkovich, K., Horowitz, J.M. *et al.* (1988) Association between an oncogene and an anti-oncogene: the adenovirus E1A proteins bind to the retinoblastoma gene product. *Nature*, (1988) **334**, 124–9.

Whyte, P., Williamson, N.M. and Harlow, E. (1989) Cellular targets for transformation by the adenovirus E1A proteins. *Cell*, **56**, 67–75.

Wiedemann, H.R. (1964) Complexe malformatif familial avec hernie ombilicle et macroglossie; un syndrome nouveau? *J. Genet. Hum.*, **13**, 223–32.

Wiedemann, H.R. (1983) Tumours and hemihypertrophy associated with Wiedemann-Beckwith syndrome. *Eur. J. Pediatr.*, **141**, 129.

Wiedemann, L.M., Karhi, K.K., Shivji, M.K.K. *et al.* (1988) The correlation breakpoint cluster region rearrangement and p210 phl/abl expression with morphological analysis of Ph-negative chronic myeloid leukemia and other myeloproliferative diseases. *Blood*, **71**, 349–55.

Wiggs, J., Nordenskjeld, M., Yandell, D. *et al.* (1988) Prediction of the risk of hereditary retinoblastoma using DNA polymorphisms within the retinoblastoma gene. *N. Engl. J. Med.*, **318**, 151–7.

Wilkins, R.J. (1988) Genomic imprinting and carcinogenesis. *Lancet*, **1**, 329–30.

Williams, J.C., Brown, K.W., Mott, M.G. and Maitland, N.J. (1989) Maternal allele loss in Wilms' tumour. *Lancet*, **1**, 283–4.

Wiman, K.G., Clarkson, B., Hayday, A.C. *et al.* (1984) Activation of a translocated c-myc gene: role of structural alterations in the upstream region. *Proc. Nat. Acad. Sci. USA*, **81**, 6798–6802.

Wurster-Hill, D.H., Cannizzaro, L.A., Pettengill, O.S. *et al.* (1984) Cytogenetics of small cell carcinoma of the lung. *Cancer Genet. Cytogenet.*, **13**, 303–30.

Yandell, D.W., Campbell, T.A., Dayton S.H. *et al.* (1989) Oncogenic point mutations in the human retinoblastoma gene: their application to genetic counseling. *N. Engl. J. Med.*, **321**, 1689–95.

Yokato, J., Wada, M., Shimostao, Y. *et al.* (1987) Loss of heterozygosity on chromosomes 3, 13 and 17 in small cell carcinoma and on chromosome 3 in adenocarcinoma of the lung. *Proc. Nat. Acad. Sci. USA*, **84**, 9252–6.

Yunis, J.J. and Ramsay, K.C. (1980) Familial occurrence of the aniridia-Wilms' tumour syndrome with deletion 11p13–14.1. *J. Pediatr.*, **96**, 1027–30.

Zaccaria, A., Testoni, N., Tassinari, A. *et al.* (1990) Molecular and cytogenetic studies of a patient with Philadelphia-negative, bcr-positive chronic myeloid leukemia and t(12;12) (q13;p12). *Genes. Chroms. Cancer*, **1**, 284–8.

Zhu, X., Dunn, J.M., Phillips, R.A. *et al.* (1989) Preferential germline mutation of the paternal allele in retinoblastoma. *Nature*, **340**, 312–3.

Chapter 3

Tumour pathology

T.J. TRICHE

3.1. INTRODUCTION

Childhood cancer treatment represents one of the great success stories of oncology. Thirty years ago, due to the advent of chemotherapy, the first cures of leukaemia in children, previously unheard of, were being recorded (Hammond, 1986). Since that time, protocols that allow the majority of children with cancer to survive have been developed. The success of multimodality therapy, especially chemotherapy combined with surgery and radiotherapy, has become the paradigm for all oncology.

Despite these gratifying successes, there remains a major problem that is almost unique to paediatric cancer: accuracy of diagnosis. Difficulty in pinpointing the histogenetic phenotype remains a rather too frequent problem – witness the problem of small, round cell tumours of childhood. Even reliable distinction between malignant and benign is often confounded – as, for example, in fibromatosis versus fibrosarcoma.

3.2 DEFINING CHILDHOOD CANCERS

3.2.1 INCIDENCE

The total incidence of childhood cancer (that is, in patients less than 15 years of age) is

about 1% of that in adults. The incidence in children is about 100 new cases per year per million population in the United States, about 6000 new cases per year (Young *et al.*, 1986). This is a paltry figure compared to the nearly one million new cases of cancer that will be diagnosed in adults in the same time frame. Despite this vast difference in incidence, the combination of superior survival coupled with an anticipated normal life expectancy results in a steadily growing population of childhood cancer survivors that is disproportionate to their relative numbers at the outset. These children are surviving into adulthood with normal or near-normal life expectancy and productive lives. It is thus appropriate that those involved in their diagnosis and therapy make every effort to maximize survival and minimize morbidity and long-term complications. This goal can only be realized when there is an exhaustive understanding of the unique features of childhood as opposed to adult cancer.

3.2.2 COMPARISON OF CHILDHOOD/ ADULT CANCER

Cancer in adults, in an overwhelming number of cases, is carcinoma; over 80% of serious cancer falls into this category, and an even larger percentage if the relatively trivial malignancies such as basal cell carcinoma are included in the total. In contrast, cancer in children is rarely carcinoma (less than 6%), even when of epithelial origin. Thus, for example, liver cancer in adults is virtually always hepatocellular carcinoma, while in children it is generally hepatoblastoma, at least in younger patients. Even in older patients, unique childhood forms of carcinoma, such as fibrolamellar carcinoma, with intermediate prognosis, are the rule. Hepatocellular carcinoma is the exception.

The majority of childhood cancer is accounted for by three groups of malignancy: leukaemia, lymphoma, and brain tumours; together these are responsible for about two-thirds of all childhood cancer. The remaining third, however, in aggregate, represents some of the most biologically unique and interesting of human tumours. At the same time, these tumours certainly represent unique diagnostic and therapeutic problems.

Perhaps more so than in any form of adult cancer, malignancy in children – after exclusion of the obvious leukaemias and brain tumours – is typically of unclear histogenesis, grade of malignancy, or treatment responsiveness. Because of the overall excellent prognosis, more so than in most forms of adult cancer, it is imperative to distinguish subsets or subtypes of childhood cancer with varying prognosis, as for example the following:

(a) Embryonal rhabdomyosarcoma

This has a greater than 80% survival rate with adequate therapy; it is virtually a different disease from the alveolar type, which, treated identically, has a survival rate as low as 30%.

(b) Fibrosarcoma

In the first quinquenium, this is essentially curable by simple surgical excision; fibrosarcoma in an adolescent can be a highly malig-

nant soft tissue sarcoma akin to those in adults.

(c) Neuroblastoma

In the first year of life this often spontaneously regresses, or at least responds completely to therapy in the vast majority of cases; the apparently same disease after one year of age, especially if Stage IV, is virtually incurable short of highly aggressive not to say experimental therapy.

These few examples typify a recurring theme that is almost unique to childhood cancer: simple diagnosis alone is an inadequate therapeutic guideline. Factors such as histologic subtype, age, site, stage, and tumour-specific parameters (such as amplification of the N-*myc* oncogene in neuroblastoma) profoundly affect an individual patient's treatment responsiveness and prognosis.

It is thus incumbent on the pathologist involved in the diagnosis of children with cancer to evaluate not just the histological appearance but the ancillary parameters as well. Increasingly, this will include information from specialized diagnostics such as ploidy determination, cytogenetics, molecular cytogenetics, gene expression, growth factor receptor expression, oncogene amplification, and inherited or acquired mutations in key regulatory genes. The remainder of this chapter will be devoted to a consideration of each of these issues in turn.

3.3 SOME NOVEL FEATURES OF CHILDHOOD CANCER

3.3.1 CHILDHOOD CANCER TYPES

Based on data from the US National Cancer Institute SEER Programme, haematopoietic malignancy accounts for nearly half of all childhood cancer, and together with brain tumours, two-thirds of malignancy in

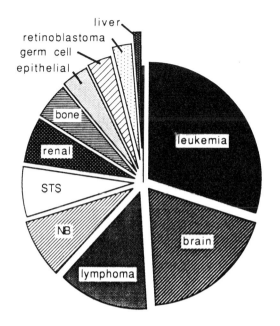

Fig. 3.1 Incidence of childhood cancer by type: depicted in US white males in descending order of frequency in a clockwise fashion from the top. Leukaemia is by far the single largest category, followed closely by CNS tumours, lymphoma, neuroblastoma (NB), soft tissue sarcomas (STS), and Wilms' tumours (renal). The remaining tumours (osteosarcoma and Ewing's sarcoma in bone, various epithelial malignancies [generally carcinoma or melanoma], germ cell tumours, retinoblastoma, liver tumours [primarily hepatoblastoma, as well as hepatocellular carcinoma and sarcomas of liver]), and a very small number of miscellaneous tumours, account for less than a quarter of the total. (*Note* rates vary by age, race, and geography. Data from SEER Study, 1973–82).

patients less than 16 years of age is accounted for (Young *et al.*, 1986; Parkin *et al.*, 1988). With neuroblastoma, this makes up nearly three quarters of the total. The remaining tumours consist of six readily recognized tumour groups, specifically (in order of decreasing incidence) soft tissue sarcoma,

renal tumours, bone tumours, various epithelial tumours, germ cell tumours, retinoblastoma, liver, and miscellaneous tumours (Fig. 3.1).

One immediate point that emerges from these data is the obvious paucity of epithelial malignancies in children. Although epithelial malignancies are more common than germ cell tumours, retinoblastoma, or hepatic tumours, even these epithelial tumours are not akin to the usual carcinomas of adults; tumours such as melanoma or related pigmented lesions are disproportionately frequent, while common adult carcinomas such as lung, renal cell, breast, colon, bladder, pancreatic, and skin are extremely uncommon. Thus, true carcinoma in children is vanishingly rare.

3.3.2 GESTATIONAL/INHERITED MALIGNANCY

The age incidence of childhood tumours is also highly characteristic and is unlike that of adults. Although the incidence of cancer in adults increases with age, it decreases rather sharply after the first quinquenium in children; overall incidence is greatest in the first year of life. This clearly implicates aetiologic factors that are quite different from those in adults, and strongly suggests that many cases of childhood cancer represent gestational-related defects in tissue growth and differentiation.

In general, other than in leukaemia, most of the common forms of childhood cancer mimic developing or embryonal tissue development. The lymphomas of childhood are dominated by blastic tumours such as B and T cell lymphoblastic lymphoma. In the brain, children have a disproportionately large percentage of PNETs, or primitive neuroectodermal tumours, that resemble fetal brain. Neuroblastoma has no analogue in adults, and is indistinguishable from the fetal adrenal medulla; neuroblastoma *in situ* and spontaneously regressing 'neuroblastoma' are likely to be two faces of the same process of delayed developmental maturation (Beckwith and Perrin, 1963; Haas *et al.*, 1988). The majority of childhood soft tissue tumours are rhabdomyosarcoma, which closely parallels the normal development of myogenic mesenchyme, but which is unheard of in adult soft tissue sarcomas where the majority are malignant fibrous histiocytoma, a tumour with no known parallel to a normal tissue (Harms *et al.*, 1985). Wilms' tumour, the only common renal tumour in children, so closely resembles developing kidney that in some cases the two cannot be distinguished (Beckwith *et al.*, 1990). Finally, bone tumours are dominated by osteosarcoma, a clear analogue of normal bone differentiation. (Miller and Dalager, 1974).

Clearly, the development of cancer in children closely parallels normal tissue development. This is not true of adult cancer, where malignancy is routinely superimposed on pre-existing tissues, the vast majority of which are epithelial, thereby giving rise to carcinoma.

These unique features of cancer in children suggest that rather precise genetic factors might underlie at least some, if not all, cases, particularly in the newborn age group. Recent work by Malkin *et al.* (1990) not only lends credence to this theory, but implicates mutations in the p53 suppressor gene in the development of certain adult cancers as well, an unexpected consequence of inherited mutations that cause childhood cancer.

In the case of Wilms' tumour, recent work has documented not just one inherited genetic defect, but several all grouped on the short arm of chromosome 11, from 11p13 to p *ter* (Francke, 1990). These observations are particularly interesting in that the distinction between clusters of genes important in normal tissue development (in this case the renal and gonadal mesenchyme) and tumour genes effectively ceases to exist (van Heyningen *et al.*, 1990; Huang *et al.*, 1990; Pritchard-Jones

et al., 1990). Deregulation of a gene or genes necessary for normal kidney development appears to lead directly to Wilms' (and related) tumours, but seemingly by more than one route.

One imagines that the rapidly accumulating body of data on the inherited basis of childhood malignancy will inexorably lead to a fundamental reappraisal of the relationship between ontogenesis and oncogenesis; it now seems the two are, at least in some cases, mediated by the same genes, albeit under the influence of normal versus defective control mechanisms. If we dissect the details of developmental regulation we are likely to have discerned the genetic basis of at least some malignancies, particularly in children.

3.3.3 BORDERLINE MALIGNANCY AND BENIGN TUMOURS

In view of the above, it should come as no surprise that it is all too frequently impossible to distinguish benign from malignant tumours. This is especially true of tumours in the very young, particularly in the first year of life. The majority of the latter are in fact benign in their clinical behavior, but morphologic criteria are frequently insufficient to distinguish the two (Coffin and Dehner, 1990). Furthermore, there is no clear distinction between the two in many tumour systems, where tumours may display intermediate behaviour, from locally aggressive and recurrent, to invasive and metastatic, despite a similar histological appearance. This principle is perhaps best exemplified by fibromatosis and fibrosarcoma. The two are generally interpreted, respectively, as the benign and malignant counterparts of the same tumour. In practice, the two cannot be reliably separated, as noted by Stout (1962), who originally defined the two. In this seminal paper, even Stout notes a similar incidence of pulmonary metastases with both tumours – hardly an encouraging sign that anyone else is likely to do better.

Fortunately for the pathologist, but unfortunately for the patient, the ambiguity progressively diminishes with age. After one year, there are no more 'neuroblastomas *in situ*'; a tumour in the adrenal gland with neuroblastoma histology is malignant, with no equivocation. Likewise, fibrous tumours are likely to be aggressive, if not outright malignant, particularly after the age of five. Nephroblastomatosis effectively disappears; the cytologically and histologically identical tumour in older patients is now considered as nephroblastoma, or Wilms' tumour. Even in germ cell tumours the shift is from benign, sacrococcygeal teratomas to obviously malignant germ cell tumours of ovary or testis.

Even though it will become progressively more apparent with age that a given tumour is malignant, the problem of predicting prognosis among obviously malignant tumours persists. Generally, adolescents are prone to more aggressive tumours. Age, for example, is an independent prognostic variable, along with stage and site, in rhabdomyosarcoma. Older patients appear to do poorly compared to younger patients with similar or identical tumours.

It should be clear that histological criteria alone are not sufficient for accurate diagnosis among these patients, particularly in the absence of an accurate and up-to-date clinical history. Clinically useful diagnosis in this patient population requires not only a knowledge of the histological and cytological appearance of a given tumour, but, having arrived at a diagnosis, correlative data and knowledge of unique features of individual tumours are also necessary before making a treatment recommendation. This is well exemplified by neuroblastoma, where the diagnosis is generally straightforward, but where histological parameters alone are not prognostic, even with highly refined histological classification schemes such as that described by

Shimada *et al.* (1984) in which both age and histology/cytology are required for determining prognosis.

3.3.4 HISTOGENESIS

Carcinoma of the lung in an adult is generally a straightforward diagnosis; histogenesis is rarely an issue, unless hybrid forms between the three common forms of lung carcinoma (adeno-, squamous cell, and small cell) are present. In any event, the origin from bronchial epithelium, and the classification, therefore, as carcinoma, is universally accepted.

Would that this were the case with cancer in children. Here, the histogenesis is all too often unclear. With no clear tissue of origin, or at least a normal tissue counterpart, a diagnosis is virtually impossible. As discussed above, the preponderant gestational nature of paediatric cancer virtually ensures that a large proportion of tumours will be composed predominantly of undifferentiated cells. This in turn dictates that a diagnosis will often turn on the finding of scattered foci or, in worst case scenarios, a single cell with tissue-specific phenotypic traits. This is not an easy task, and makes it likely to miss those cells committed to a tissue lineage by virtue of patterns of gene expression, but which have not yet manifested the consequent characteristic morphological sequelae.

Rhabdomyosarcoma is a perfect example of this conundrum. It is generally acknowledged that few cells in a typical rhabdomyosarcoma show sufficient evidence of myogenesis to be identified morphologically, yet how can a diagnosis of rhabdomyosarcoma reasonably be applied to a purely mesenchymal tumour? Numerous innovative solutions have been proposed and implemented, from PTAH stains common a decade ago to immunocytochemistry so common today. These methods succeed where the eye fails because they either render single cells with the requisite rhabdomyogenic phenotype more apparent

(PTAH) or they detect a larger percentage of cells within the tumour that express a requisite gene product (protein), such as skeletal muscle myosin (immunocytochemistry).

For the purist, this approach is hardly commensurate with the principles of developmental biology. The developing limb is, after all, certainly composed of myogenic mesenchyme – as well as of osteogenic, angiogenic, and neurogenic cells, to name only the obvious possibilities. Why, then, is a mesenchymal tumour a rhabdomyosarcoma because fewer than 1% of the cells express a muscle-specific protein? We assume for the purposes of the discussion to follow that historical precedent prevails, but the reader is alerted to the fact that the widespread adoption of diagnostic methods discussed below would almost certainly compel major revision of our existing histogenetic concepts and nosological terms.

3.4 TRADITIONAL DIAGNOSTIC METHODS

Given the special problems attendant upon diagnosis of cancer in the paediatric age group, it is no wonder that an inordinate number of methods exist (and are being developed) to optimize diagnostic accuracy. In many cases, they may offer insight into aetiology and refine prognosis in the process.

The problem becomes acute when the tumour in question lacks any discernable morphological differentiation. These so-called 'small round blue cell tumours' are often not particularly small, round, or blue (or all three), but they are definitely morphologically undifferentiated, at least by routine light microscopy (Triche, 1988).

The major routine diagnostic methods are light microscopy of paraffin embedded, hematoxylin and eosin stained cells. This is the one universal method that must be applied to every case, with or without special stains. The second and third methods are

immunocytochemistry which is often confused with special stains (but is *not* a special stain), and electron microscopy – which does not simply make one's ignorance bigger, as pundits have suggested.

3.4.1 LIGHT MICROSCOPY

It is unfortunate that such a powerful diagnostic tool has been so poorly implemented. The means exist to vastly improve the quality of routine light microscopy, but are rarely used. For example:

(a) fixation with formaldehyde is probably the least effective fixation commonly in use yet generally it remains the method of choice;

(b) paraffin is an inferior matrix to various synthetic ('plastic') polymers, but virtually all tissue is embedded in paraffin or paraffin/plastic mixtures:

(c) nuclei are generally about 7 to 10 microns in diameter, yet superimposition of nuclear images is commonplace in putative 4 micron sections, a physical impossibility best explained by 'efficiency' of volume as opposed to attention to detail in the histology laboratory;

(d) haematoxylin and eosin essentially stain only nuclei distinctly; cytoplasm, acellular extracellular matrix, and most other structures stain more or less homogeneously pink. Cytoplasmic structure, the usual basis for histogenetic determination is poorly visualized if at all;

(e) coverslips and mounting media that in aggregate exceed the limits of refraction of most X40 objective lenses are the rule rather than the exception, thereby rendering fine detail unresolved and uninterpretable.

It is remarkable that diagnosis proceeds as well as it does, given the routine handicaps encountered in everyday practice.

This author views the rather favourable result that eventuates despite these impediments as certain evidence that the human mind is far more resourceful than we commonly credit it with. One need only observe the average pathologist adjusting the condenser and manipulating the field diaphragm on his or her microscope to realize the extent of sub-optimal preparation of histology slides. Imagine our success if all were optimal.

3.4.2 SPECIAL STAINS

In part to compensate for the shortcomings described above, and in part to reveal truly new information, most paediatric pathologists utilize a small group of special stains that add some objectivity to tissue interpretation. A few particularly useful ones will be considered here.

1. PAS

Detection of glycogen, glycoproteins, and glycolipids (any that manage to resist extraction by routine embedding solvents such as alcohol and xylene) is possible with this stain (which is really not a stain *per se*, but rather an acid hydrolysis followed by Schiff's base reduction with resultant chromogenesis). Digestion with diastase removes glycogen, leaving only glycolipids and glycoproteins. This is useful information when considering certain tumours known to differentially lack or possess glycogen, such as lymphoma and neuroblastoma versus Ewing's sarcoma and soft tissue sarcomas, respectively. Unfortunately, glycogen is evanescent in routinely processed tissue, and tumours that are supposed to contain glycogen sometimes don't (Triche *et al.*, 1986). Worse, some that shouldn't, do (Triche and Ross, 1978). Though useful, then, the stain's value is scarcely unequivocal.

2. PTAH

Because detection of myogenesis is not an uncommon problem, particularly in the evaluation of sarcomas and small round cell tumours, methods were developed before the advent of immunocytochemistry or EM to provide evidence of rhabdomyogenesis. Phosphotungstic acid pretreatment of tissue sections renders Z discs (and even the smooth muscle equivalents, fusiform densities) stainable by routine hematoxylin. Cross striations are thus accentuated, or so it is thought. In reality, if cross striations are already evident, the tumour shouldn't be a particular diagnostic problem.

3. Trichrome

Synthesis of a collagenous extracellular matrix (ECM) is almost uniquely a function of sarcomas. Detection of an ECM is sometimes difficult in routine H and E sections. The trichrome stain is widely used for this purpose.

It should be noted that collagens are to varying degrees glycoproteins. They are thus readily detected by the PAS stain, even (or more so) after diastase digestion. A PAS with and without diastase is frequently all that is necessary to rule out a lymphoma, for example.

3.4.3 IMMUNOCYTOCHEMISTRY

Antibody mediated detection of proteins (and therefore gene products) has within the past decade virtually revolutionized tumour and tissue diagnosis, but not without considerable error and misguided enthusiasm. The initial enthusiasm coupled with unwarranted faith in seemingly reliable results has been supplanted by the sobering realization that the technique is in fact fraught with false positive and negative results, irreproducible results, uncontrollable or uncontrolled variables that determine the results, and a basic misconception regarding the specificity of antibodies in the first place (Erlandson, 1984). Despite this, immunocytochemistry remains the single most useful and sensitive means of assaying gene expression. The foibles inherent in the technique only require that the results be interpreted with a degree of scepticism and most importantly, interpreted within the context of clinical information and the results of histopathological examination.

1. Fixation

Formalin, though at best a mediocre fixative for morphology, in practice is a nearly ideal fixative for immunocytochemistry. Precisely the features that render it so marginal for preservation of structures (poor and reversible fixation) are ideal for retention of antigenicity. The lack of denaturation and alteration in tertiary configuration allow near optimal binding of antibody to target antigen. The only superior method may be alcohol. The best means of antigenic preservation, though, is no fixation at all, but in practice this is not feasible. Air drying of frozen sections may be the closest thing; in this case, the only fixation is denaturation by dessication. With rehydration, the antigens are very nearly returned to their native state.

2. Antibodies

Two major antibody preparations are used, polyclonal and monoclonal. Esoteric preparations such as Fab fragments, bifunctional antibodies, and bacterially expressed antibodies, though useful for specific purposes, are not particularly useful for diagnostic work.

Although monoclonal antibodies theoretically offer the advantage of superior apparent specificity, this is often not borne out in practice. Although every antibody molecule is theoretically identical, and therefore of precisely the same specificity, two practical problems and at least one theoretical problem obviate the superficially apparent superiority of monoclonal antibodies:

(a) Antibody specificity relates to an epitope, or antibody binding site, that may appear on proteins, glycolipids, or glycoconjugates of diverse origin. This has been a very real problem with antibodies such as Leu7 (HNK-1), originally raised against human natural killer cells, then found to bind myelin associated glycoprotein, and more recently realized to bind a number of neural cell adhesion molecule (NCAM) isomers. Specific, yes, but bound to only one gene product, no.

(b) Most antigens that induce an antibody response do so on the basis of multiple epitopes scattered over the surface of the antigen moiety. In general these number in dozens, and the antibodies that bind them are derived from dozens if not hundreds of clones, each with potentially different affinities for the antigens in question. A monoclonal antibody possesses but one, and it may not be particularly high. More importantly, binding that is mediated by a single epitope can't begin to compare with multi-site binding. Thus, the number of monoclonal antibody molecules bound to an antigen are usually limited.

(c) Theoretically, today's and tomorrow's clone in a hybridoma culture should be the same. In reality, changes do occur over time, and they are generally not an improvement. The same monoclonal today may lack affinity or even be lost over time. Change over time has been seen with hybridomas, though usually reversion to earlier passages of the cell line will obviate the problem. It remains at least a theoretical consideration, however.

Polyclonal antibodies, although theoretically inferior to monoclonal on several counts (absolute lack of identity over time to name one), are in practice the preferred antibody for most antigens. They offer multipoint, multiepitope binding with antibody molecules derived from innumerable clones, each with slightly different affinity, and derived from multiple immunoglobulin classes. The benefit is usually rather dense labelling of the antigen with antibody, and therefore enhanced detection. The detriment is the propensity of the antibody preparation, even when purified to a single subclass (such as $IgG_{1, 2}$, etc.) to react with other constituents of the cell or tissue. This generally cannot be predicted in advance, and is often highly dependent on antibody dilution. For this reason, polyclonals must be 'fine tuned' at the outset with each new preparation to optimize conditions and hence reliability.

3. Chromogens

Preservation of antigens and binding of antibody are two critical factors in immunocytochemistry. Detection of the complex is critical to the end result, as there is otherwise no visible result of antigen-antibody interaction.

Several methods of detecting antigen-antibody complex formation have been developed over time. Radioactive antibodies have been detected by autoradiography, but this is impractical for diagnostic purposes. Immunofluorescence using fluorescein-labelled antibodies were first used on tissue sections, and are still in use for renal biopsy interpretation and flow cytometry, but have been supplanted by peroxidase or related methods for routine diagnosis.

Sternberger's peroxidase-antiperoxidase (PAP) method with diaminobenzidine (DAB) chromogen was the first widely adopted peroxidase method (Sternberger, 1979). More recently, more sensitive techniques such as avidin-biotin detection, with peroxidase coupled to avidin and biotinylated antibodies, has become the *de facto* standard (Hsu *et al.*, 1981). Alkaline phosphatase-anti-alkaline phosphatase (APAAP) with non-DAB chromogens (generally water soluble) offers superior sensitivity but has not been widely adopted (Davey *et al.*, 1987).

4. Controls

Superior sensitivity achieved with improved methods of detection are not a substitute for controls which, though obligatory, are all too often omitted. Lack of well chosen and appropriate controls is probably the single most common cause of trivial and unreliable results. This does not mean normal tissue controls; the only appropriate control is a tumour known to be reactive for the antibody in question. Batch controls are often employed as an economy measure, but individual cases often deviate from the parameters established for the controls and thereby may test spuriously positive or negative. A ubiquitously positive antibody such as vimentin (which reacts with normal blood vessels, even within a tumour) is a useful safeguard to rule out negativity due to poor preservation or tumour viability. If vimentin is positive, negative results on the same tumour block is more believable.

Ultimately, observer judgement is imperative in the interpretation of results. Lack of uniformity throughout the section, 'edge effects' (where local hyperconcentration of antibody, secondary to evaporation at the edge of the section, may yield false positive results), and completely spurious positivity in single cells (presumably due to artefactual precipitation of antibody or chromogen) are only a few of the pitfalls that the wary pathologist must guard against. These caveats notwithstanding, the method remains the single most useful adjunct to straightforward tissue diagnosis currently in use.

59

Table 3.1 Ultrastructural features of selected childhood tumours

Feature	Neuroblastoma		Ewing's/PNET	Rhabdomyosarcoma		Lymphoma
	Primitive	*Differentiated*		*Primitive*	*Differentiated*	
Glycogen	Common	Less common	Abundant	Routinely present	Less common	Very rarely
Dense-core granules	Sparse	Numerous	Not typical ones	Never	Never	Never
Thin (actin) filaments	None visible	None visible	Rare	Common	Always	Almost never
Neurofilaments	Occasional	Common	Rare	Never	Never	Never
Intermediate filaments	Uncommon	Uncommon	Scattered	Routine	Always present	Very rare
Thick (myosin) filaments	Never	Never	Never	Never	Necessary for diagnosis	Never
Z-bands	Never	Never	Never	Rare or absent	Virtually always	Never
Cell–cell attachments	Common	Common and elaborate	Universal	Common	Routinely present	Almost never
Microtubules	Not uncommon	Numerous	Not uncommon	Not uncommon	Rare	Sometimes
Basal lamina	Absent	Common	Never	Rarely	Routinely present	Never
Collagen stroma	Not between cells	Septae	Virtually absent	Routinely present	Generally conspicuous	Never (tumour origin)
Dense lysosomes	Often	Often	Occasional	Some	Rare	Sometimes prominent

3.4.4 ELECTRON MICROSCOPY

Electron microscopy was, in the minds of some, the first major advance in pathological diagnosis since the time of Virchow or before. For the first time, tumour cells could be examined at extraordinary magnification. Structures previously beyond detection by light microscopy were seen, and became useful indices of histogenesis or even specific disease diagnosis: disorganized Z bands in primitive rhabdomyosarcoma were easily found and cemented the diagnosis; cell junctions excluded a diagnosis of haematopoietic malignancy (since haematopoietic cells lack cell junctions – recent reports notwithstanding); neurites and dense core granules, however scant, were irrevocable evidence of neuroblastoma.

It is difficult for this author to fully comprehend the apparent backlash against EM that has developed with widespread adoption of immunocytochemistry. This rather abrupt abandonment of EM as a diagnostic tool was perhaps precipitous and ill conceived. More recently, the increasing awareness of pitfalls in immunocytochemical diagnosis seems to have ushered in renewed appreciation of the synergy that can occur between the two in difficult-to-diagnose cases. Each depends on separate, generally exclusive parameters (the presence of antigen in immunocytochemistry; the presence of specific structures in EM) and are mutually supportive in these cases. Renal pathology has recognized this for years; it seems tumour pathology has, of late, also rediscovered the obvious.

This chapter is not the place to consider EM findings of use in the diagnosis of childhood tumours in any detail, but Table 3.1 provides an overview of some of the more useful findings among the common childhood tumours.

3.5 NEWLY DEVELOPING DIAGNOSTIC METHODS

The widely recognized revolution in biomedical research has predictably provided a host of possible new diagnostic techniques of use in tumour diagnosis. Perhaps of greater potential value will be their application to individual tumours to predict proliferative capacity, responsiveness to growth factors, propensity for metastasis, treatment resistance (and to which modalities), aetiology, and predisposition. These parameters are obviously beyond the reach of current diagnostic methods, but they are often intrinsic to several of the newer methods now appearing.

The following sections will consider six of the more promising (at least in the author's opinion) techniques that are particularly applicable to tumour diagnosis. It should be emphasized that these are only a limited number of techniques; many others are in development, and a seemingly infinite number of variations on each of the main methods have already been described. This section seeks only to introduce the basic concepts.

3.5.1 CYTOGENETICS

Numerical or structural chromosomal aberrations have long been recognized to be a fundamental defect in cancer cells. Within the past decade, however, a series of tumour-specific abnormalities have been identified, with the number seeming to increase daily (Sandberg *et al.*, 1988). At this point, then, there seems to be no doubt that cytogenetic analysis of a tumour is a diagnostic procedure.

The frequent hurdle faced in many cases is lack of suitable fresh tumour tissue. This has not been a problem in leukaemia, where cytogenetic analysis has been a diagnostic mainstay for years. Solid tumours have only recently become viable candidates, particularly

Table 3.2 Genetic abnormalities in childhood cancer

Tumour	Cytogenetics	Relevant locus	Gene(s)	Class	Other tumours
Chronic myelogenous leukemia	t(9;22) (Philadelphia chromosome)	q34;q11	*bcr/abl* fusion gene	Oncogene	ANLL, ALL, some lymphomas
Burkitt's lymphoma	t(8;2 or 14 or 22)	8q24	c-*myc* + lg enhancer	Oncogene	Non-Burkitt's
Neuroblastoma	1) HSR; DMs* 2) del lp	1p36.1? ?	N-*myc*;	Oncogene; suppressor?	Wilms', Alveolar RMS
Retinoblastoma	del(13q)	13q14	RB-1	Suppressor	Osteosarcoma, some soft tissue sarcomas
Osteosarcoma, rhabdomyosarcoma	None at this level	17p12–13.3	p53	Suppressor	Scope unknown, but likely many others
Wilms'	del(11p)	11p13–11p15.5	WT-1, LK15	Suppressor	?Embryonal RMS (speculative)
Alveolar RMS	t(2;13)(q37;q14)	q14 (proximal to RB)	Unknown	Unknown	
Ewing's sarcoma, PN, PNET, EOE	t(11;22), t(17;22)	22q12	Unknown	Unknown	Rhabdoid tumours, ? RMS
Synoviosarcoma	X;18	?	?	Unknown	None to date

* HSR homogeneously staining region; DMs double minutes, extrachromosomal material.

with improvements in short-term culture that have allowed reproducible metaphase spreads for analysis. Without metaphases, conventional cytogenetics is impossible.

The large number of reported cytogenetic abnormalities in paediatric cancers, some of which are present in greater than 85% of cases, has led to greater utilization of the method. Neuroblastoma, rhabdomyosarcoma, Wilms' tumour, retinoblastoma, leukaemias, (Biedler *et al.*, 1983; Douglass *et al.*, 1987; Koufos *et al.*, 1984; Balaban *et al.*, 1982; Sandberg, 1990, respectively), lymphoma and certain bone and soft tissue tumours have all been noted to frequently display diagnostically useful abnormalities. These are summarized in Table 3.2.

Despite its usefulness, cytogenetic analysis is only useful when successful, which is considerably less than 100% of cases. This, coupled with the less than 100% occurrence of diagnostic abnormalities within a given tumour category, has limited the use of the method. Nevertheless, a positive result is diagnostic in most cases.

3.5.2 MOLECULAR CYTOGENETICS

While only some cytogenetic analyses result in the creation of useful metaphase preparations, all such preparations harbour interphase nuclei. Since individual chromosomes remain somewhat discrete even within interphase nuclei, it is possible to separately label particular DNA sequences. This has recently been used, for example, to identify the Philadelphia translocation, using two different complementary probes labelled with two different fluorescent markers, one for the *bcr* locus on chromosome 22, the other for the *abl* oncogene on chromosome 9 (Tkachuk *et al.*, 1990). In cells lacking the translocation, two discrete spots of fluorescence are identified in most interphase nuclei. Cells with the translocation fuse the two loci (*bcr/abl*), and a single locus of intermediate colour results.

Although still in the earliest stages of development, this technique will clearly emerge in the near future as a viable alternative, or at least an enhancement to, conventional cytogenetics. It also represents a useful bridge between the gross level analysis characteristic of conventional cytogenetics and the small scale analysis true of conventional DNA (Southern) blots.

Perhaps the most exciting prospect inherent in the technique is the opportunity to unequivocally document any of the tumour-specific translocations, once they are identified and cloned. Armed with such knowledge, one cannot only detect these tumour-specific translocations, one can do so on individual cells. Such information cannot be derived from conventional Southern analysis, nor even from *in situ* hybridization of tissue sections. Recent work with aneuploidy determinations on bladder cancer using archival paraffin-embedded tissue sections suggest that many analyses will be feasible on routinely processed tissue as well. This is important as it is the first example of DNA-based diagnostics that can be applied to routinely processed tissue without recourse to intermediate steps such as polymerase chain reaction (PCR) amplification (see below).

Despite its newness, this technique is the single technique most likely to enjoy widespread adoption by pathologists as soon as it is technologically proven.

3.5.3 DNA DIAGNOSTICS

1. Southern analysis

Routine use of high molecular weight DNA from cells (theoretically only 46 molecules per cell) is not feasible. Instead, orderly and reproducible reduction of chromosomal DNA awaited the introduction of restriction enzymes, or DNA endonucleases (REs), that allow reduction of total cellular DNA to reasonable-sized fragments that could be manipulated. Electrophoresis through agarose provided a means of size separating the fragments, and Southern's introduction of a solid membrane support to which the DNA could be transferred following electrophoresis provided a means of analysing DNA sequences, using complementary DNA probes for sequences of interest (Southern, 1975).

The immediate advantages of the technique for evaluation of tumour DNA are many: absolute specificity of hybridization, sensitive to even single base mismatches (under appropriate hybridization conditions); detection of underlying genetic abnormalities in tumour versus normal tissue, including deletion, mutation, and amplification (extra gene copies); and reproducibility of results sufficient for diagnostic use.

One of the immediate diagnostic applications to emerge from the refinement of this technique is analysis of immunoglobulin gene rearrangements that occur in all lymphoid cells, uniquely in each cell. Given that a lymphoma or lymphocytic leukaemia is by

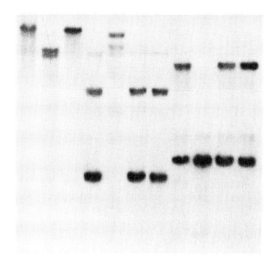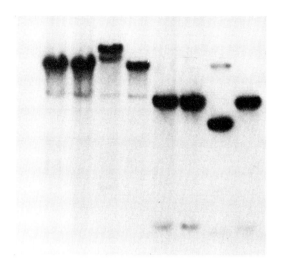

Fig. 3.2 Southern analysis of immunoglobulin gene rearrangement: high molecular weight DNA extracted from a patient with lymphadenopathy and suspected lymphoma. Patient (lanes 4 and 8 in panels A and B) and controls (negative: lanes 6, 7, 10, and 11, panel A; 1, 2, 5 and 6, panel B; positive: lanes 5 and 9, panel A; 3 and 7, panel B). DNA digested with *Bam*H1 (group 1, panels A and B) and *Hind*III (group 2, panels A and B). DNA was electrophoresed in agarose, blotted, and hybridized with probes for T-cell antigen receptor, beta subunit (panel A) and the immunoglobulin joining region for kappa heavy chain (panel B). Note that the patient material is identical to germ line bands (negative control) and distinct from the positive control. This is reliable evidence for a lack of monoclonality, and therefore no lymphoma. (Kindly provided by Dr Paul Pattengale and Jean Sanders, Children's Hospital, Los Angeles.)

definition a monoclonal proliferation, each cell in the tumour should harbour the identical immunoglobulin gene (B cells) or T cell receptor gene rearrangement, depending on T or B lineage of the neoplasm. This is manifest as unique bands on a Southern blot that are distinct from the germ line (or unrearranged) band pattern that is routinely detected in all lymphoid cells. Existence of such a pattern, detected with either an immunoglobulin gene (J_H) or a T cell receptor (T_γ) specific probe, provides unequivocal evidence that a monoclonal population of cells exists within the specimen analysed. This is tantamount to a diagnosis of malignancy with better than 97% reliability – certainly at least on a par with, if not superior to, pathologists' routine diagnostic accuracy (Cossman *et al.*, 1991).

An illustrative example will be found in Figure 3.2, where the germ line configuration is seen for T cell receptor, and a rearranged band is seen for immunoglobulin heavy chain joining region.

2. RFLP analysis

A standard method of DNA analysis in research laboratories, restriction fragment length polymorphism (RFLP) studies, have not yet penetrated to general use by pathologists, other than in specific situations.

Geneticists have adopted the technique, for numerous reasons, especially the enormous value of the technique to detect carrier states, and to determine heterozygosity versus homozygosity.

The underlying principle of RFLP analysis is that each person inherits one copy, or allele, of a gene from each parent. Although each copy of the gene may be identical, intervening or flanking sequences are generally not. As a result, restriction endonucleases (REs) with sequence specificity will cleave the DNA at different points. When a labelled complementary probe is hybridized with these fragments (after Southern blotting), many genes will display two or more different sized fragments, derived from different parents.

These length polymorphisms secondary to differential cutting by REs (thus RFLPs) are also an index of genetic constitution. In the context of tumour analysis, hybridization with probes for genes (or even anonymous DNA sequences) that flank a tumour gene (or putative gene) of interest often reveals not the polymorphism expected, as compared to normal tissue from the same patient, but instead a loss of heterozygosity (LOH), indicative of loss of genetic material. By using a series of probes of known location relative to the gene of interest, the extent of loss can be estimated, and by using probes proximal and distal to the gene of interest, it can be confirmed that at least one copy of the gene in question has been lost.

This method of analysis particularly identifies genes, the loss of which, as opposed to amplification, are key to development of a tumour. These have been categorized as tumour suppressor genes, although they are certainly not solely so; rather, they represent genes important in regulation of development or control of cell cycle. This principle is exemplified by studies of Wilms' tumour, where cytogenetic abnormalities on chromosome 11p were first noted among these

patients (Kaneko *et al.*, 1981; Glaser *et al.*, 1989). Later work using RFLP analysis to detect LOH on 11p confirmed loss of sequence in the region of 11p13 to 11p15 (Koufos *et al.*, 1984; Reeve *et al.*, 1989; Wadey *et al.*, 1990; Mannens *et al.*, 1990). Most recently, at least one (WT1) of what are probably several regulatory genes has been cloned and shown to be important in the aetiology of both Wilms' tumour and the developing kidney (Call *et al.*, 1990; Bonetta *et al.*, 1990). This is emerging as a general principle in several tumour systems.

3.5.4 RNA DIAGNOSTICS

As useful as analysis of DNA may be, it provides no information about patterns of gene expression in a cell or tissue. Since immunocytochemistry is ultimately an index of gene expression, it might seem that an intermediate method is unnecessary. On the contrary, the problems that plague antibody mediated detection of gene products dictate that confirmatory methods be considered. Analysis of messenger RNA (mRNA), the next most proximal step in the pathway of gene expression, is the method of choice. It has the added advantage that information which cannot be gleaned from immunocytochemistry is readily obtained, including detection of abnormal message that translates to abnormal protein – usually not discriminated from normal by antibodies.

1. Northern blot

Analysis of mRNA has developed somewhat in parallel with routine methods of DNA analysis. Just as DNA blotting has made genomic DNA analysis routine, blotting of RNA (Northern blot, by analogy) has become standard for detection of gene expression (Alwine *et al.*, 1977). Alternatives such as slot blots are used, but fail to distinguish trunc-

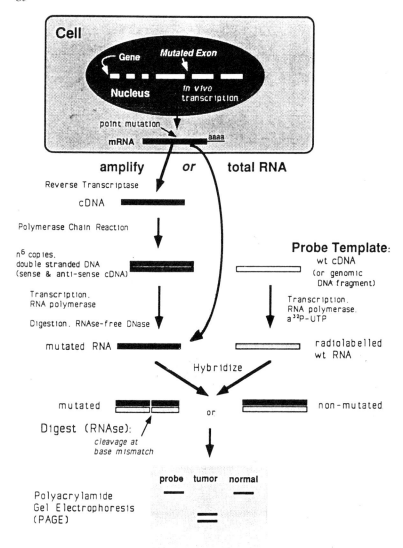

Fig. 3.3 Diagram of RNAse protection assay: with complete identity between the probe RNA and the target RNA, the RNA-degrading enzyme RNAse is incapable of attacking perfectly hybridized double-stranded RNA (right, and lane 3 of gel). However, under carefully controlled conditions, even a single base mismatch is susceptible to enzymatic degradation, resulting in the formation of two or more lower molecular weight fragments (left, and lane 2 of gel). Lane 1 depicts mobility of unlabelled wt probe. Ideally, even a single base mutation, deletion, or other sequence abnormality can be detected.

ated, fused, or other such abnormalities in mRNA. The size separation by electrophoresis that precedes blotting in Northern analysis renders these abnormalities apparent.

2. RNAse protection assay

The relative sensitivity of Northern blotting is sufficient for many purposes, but the procedure does present two major deficiences: it requires a significant tissue sample (a large fragment of a lymph node, for example) and it does not detect point mutations or small deletions within the mRNA.

The RNAse protection assay offers greatly enhanced sensitivity as well as the possibility of detecting point mutations and other minute abnormalities in a tumour's mRNA (Zinn *et al.*, 1983; Cox *et al.*, 1984). In this method, a radiolabelled RNA probe is hybridized in solution with target mRNA under conditions that promote RNA:RNA hybrid formation. The complexes are then digested with RNAse A to remove irrelevant RNA and the remaining RNA:RNA hybrids are electrophoresed in polyacrylamide under denaturing conditions. Persistent RNA by definition is protected by duplex formation with complementary RNA, thereby providing absolute proof of the presence of even minute amounts of message.

A derivative technique, now under development, will offer additional information, based on the exquisite susceptibility of single stranded RNA to RNAse. Even a single base outloop may be sufficient to allow enzymatic degradation at that site. In this case, the resultant RNA from each strand will be cleaved by the RNAse, resulting in two or more smaller fragments, compared to full length mRNA (Fig. 3.3). These two bands will be readily detectable on the gel, much as are rearranged bands in Southern blots of malignant lymphoid cells (see above).

3. Relevance to routine diagnostics

The major disadvantage of RNA analysis is its inordinate susceptibility to ubiquitous RNA-degrading enzymes (RNase). Because preventive measures must be taken immediately after harvesting of tissue, only fresh or fresh frozen tissue is useful for analysis. This is a major handicap, but increasing availability of fresh tumour tissue, mandatory in many current cooperative group protocols, prom-

ises to offset the problem in a proportion of cases. The inevitable lack of fresh tissue in other cases will however limit the utility of RNA analysis.

Conversely, the extraordinary information content of RNA analysis is likely to compel adoption of the methodology for certain clinical situations. Northern analysis will be imperative for confirmation of predicted abnormalities of gene expression, such as overexpression or lack of expression of important oncogenes (as has been proposed for *myc* family oncogenes, to name only one). RNAse protection assay, on the other hand, is likely to be useful as an alternative to direct sequencing for detection of point mutations and deletions. It has already been proposed as a means of detecting minimal residual disease in leukaemia (Veelken *et al.*, in press).

3.5.5 AMPLIFICATION METHODOLOGY

An adequate source of starting material is an ever-present problem in DNA and RNA diagnostics. Generous amounts of ideally handled, rapidly excised and processed fresh tumour tissue are an endangered species, particularly with the increasing popularity of limited incisional biopsies, fine needle aspiration cytology, and non-surgical therapy. The unfortunate consequence of these developments is a dearth of adequate specimens. To offset this problem, methods that amplify target DNA or RNA have come to enjoy extraordinary popularity within the past few years. The polymerase chain reaction (PCR) has become the method of choice for this purpose.

1. PCR

Since its introduction in 1985, over 600 publications utilizing the method had appeared by 1990. The number has increased almost exponentially since then. Clearly, this is an extremely useful technique. It offers great potential for diagnostic applications, certain shortcomings notwithstanding. The major concerns from a diagnostic viewpoint are the known reproducible misincorporation of nucleotides during repeated amplification cycles and the propensy of spurious DNA (either exogenously introduced or adventitiously amplified in a crude specimen) to be amplified. Various methods to confirm PCR results have correspondingly been adopted, and are mandatory for clinical diagnosis by this method.

The principle of PCR is straightforward. By annealing (binding) two oligonucleotide primers that flank a genomic DNA sequence of interest to both strands of denatured, double stranded DNA, complementary copies of each strand can be synthesized in the presence of a heat stable DNA polymerase derived from the thermophilic bacterium *Thermus aquaticus*. The process is repeated, after heat denaturation, reannealing of additional primers, and primer extension, up to 40 or 50 cycles, routinely resulting in million-fold amplifications of the target sequence between the two primers (Saiki, 1990).

The product of PCR will thereby ideally consist of millions of copies of the same size DNA fragments, determined by the number of nucleotides lying between the primer pair chosen at the outset. From these data, the size can be predicted (generally in the few hundred nucleotide range) and checked on a sizing agarose gel. The presence of a single band after ethidium bromide staining is reliable evidence of a successful result. It does not, however, guarantee that the aforementioned artefacts have not occurred.

The amplified DNA from PCR can be used for a host of purposes, from direct sequencing and hybridization reactions to use as a probe itself. The possibilities are virtually endless and will not be discussed in detail here. Suffice it to say that information of importance to tumour diagnosis, from point mutations in suppressor genes to gross dele-

tions of important genes, can be readily detected with the method.

2. Detection of mRNA by PCR

PCR is not limited to amplification of genomic DNA. By first creating a complementary cDNA copy of mRNA with reverse transcriptase, it is possible to create subsequent DNA copies by conventional PCR, using the mRNA:cDNA duplex as the starting material. The end product will be a faithful DNA copy of the portion of the mRNA between appropriately chosen primer pairs (Kawasaki, 1990).

Further refinements have also been introduced. Particularly useful is asymmetric PCR (APCR) whereby single stranded copies can be produced by using gross excess (50 or more fold) of one of the primers in the original primer pair. This results in a gross excess of the sense or anti sense strand of the original starting material (depending on which primer is added in excess). This is adapted for studies of gene expression resulting in highly enriched product for either mRNA or its complementary sequence. The two can be analysed (from separate reactions) to verify one another, as when directly sequencing the PCR products for point mutations or deletions.

3.5.6 PROTEIN DETECTION

Given the fact that, although analysis of RNA may offer superior specificity of information, protein analysis offers its own unique advantages, it is worth reconsidering methods of protein detection. The major advantage of proteins is their abundance and stability compared to DNA. The disadvantage is the lack of usable detection methodology with similar specificity. Ideally, protein sequence information derived from microsequencing could provide comparable data, but such methodology is arduous and impractical for diagnostic

68

purposes. Other biochemical methods rely on non-specific parameters such as apparent molecular mass (SDS-PAGE), charge (ion exchange chromatography and isoelectric focusing), or binding to ligands (affinity chromatography), but none of these is unique to a single protein.

Realistically, the only method that approaches the specificity of sequence-specific hybridization of nucleic acids is protein-antibody complex formation. A method somewhat analogous to Southern and Northern blotting was consequently developed, and (not surprisingly) christened Western blotting (Towbin *et al.*, 1979).

1. Western blotting

As the name implies, this method immobilizes size-separated protein on a support membrane, like DNA and RNA blotting.

Unlike the latter methods, individual proteins are detected with antibodies as opposed to complementary, sequence-specific DNA or RNA probes. Although the interaction is protein-protein, the fundamental basis for recognition is totally different, as discussed previously under immunocytochemistry. As a consequence, the reliability of information is less, particularly in view of the profound detergent-driven denaturation of proteins that occurs during the preceding gel electrophoresis. Many antibodies simply fail to bind to such denatured protein, as the interaction is based primarily on three-dimensional (tertiary) configuration, not amino acid sequences.

2. Correlation with immunocytochemistry

Despite these shortcomings, Western blot-

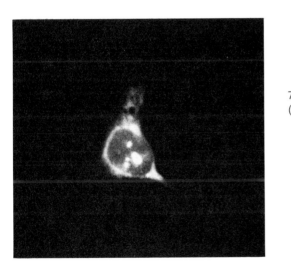
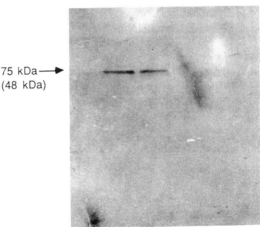

Fig. 3.4 Immunodetection of gene products: Panel A depicts a single cell reactive with antibody for chromogranin amongst a field of many non-reactive cells. The significance of this result is suspect without confirmation. Panel B is a Western immunoblot of a protein extract from the same tumour tissue, reacted with anti-chromogranin. Here the positive reactivity with patient sample (lane 2) and positive control (lane 3), as a single band of appropriate molecular mass, and coupled with a lack of reactivity with negative controls (lanes 1, 4, and 5), supports the result in A.

ting has proved to be an important adjunct to immunocytochemistry as well as a stand-alone application. By itself, the method has not enjoyed wide acceptance as a tumour diagnostic tool. As a means of confirming the results of immunocytochemistry, it is uniquely valuable. Figure 3.4A illustrates a single tumour cell in a field of many that has reacted with an antibody to chromogranin. The reliability of this immunocytochemical result is suspect at best, at least without independent corroboration. Figure 3.4B is a Western blot of extracted proteins from the same tumour in which the identical antibody was used to detect the target protein. The reaction with a single band of appropriate molecular weight provides rather compelling evidence that the reaction seen in panel A can only be explained by the presence of chromogranin in that cell.

It was precisely this methodology that was first used to document the presence of chromogranin in tumours previously thought to lack chromogranin expression. The same approach has now documented innumerable examples of 'inappropriate' (at least to our preconceived notions) gene expression of diverse type by numerous tumours. Often, the paucity of expression or limited numbers of cells within the tumour expressing the gene has precluded reliable detection by RNA blotting. In that the stoichiometry of gene expression dictates that there will be an exponentially greater amount of protein than mRNA, and the biological half-life of protein is likewise many fold greater than for RNA, not to mention the relative resistance of proteins to proteolytic degradation compared to the ephemeral resistance of RNA to ubiquitous RNA degrading enzymes, it should be abundantly clear that protein detection is easier than detection of RNA.

3.6 SUMMARY AND CONCLUSIONS

It should be apparent from the preceding discussion that a host of new techniques, coupled with existing ones, promise to forever alter the manner in which we diagnose tumours. Perhaps more importantly, it is also likely to change our fundamental concepts of tumour relationships and origins. Most relevant from the perspective of clinical oncology, however, is the potential for tailoring protocols to specific, homogeneous tumour entities likely to respond homogeneously to specific agents or treatment protocols.

The ultimate goal of the approach to tumour characterization and diagnosis outlined here is the ability to diagnose and to predict treatment responsiveness, and ultimate prognosis in individual tumours. It is likely that the more parameters that are known in connection with a given tumour, the better the chances of predicting precise factors in that patient's outcome. As a sufficient body of information regarding the genetic composition and defects of individual tumours is assembled, knowledge of the biological behaviour and clinical aggressiveness, not to mention treatment responsiveness, should inevitably follow.

REFERENCES

Alwine, J.C., Kemp, D.J. and Stark, G.R. (1977) Method for detection of specific RNAs in agarose gels by transfer to diazobenzyloxymethyl-paper and hybridization with DNA probes. *Proc. Natl. Acad. Sci. U.S.A.*, **74**, 5350.

Balaban, G., Gilbert, F., Nichols, W. *et al.* (1982) Abnormalities of chromosome No. 13 in retinoblastomas from individuals with normal constitutional karyotypes. *Cancer Genet. Cytogenet.*, **6**, 213.

Beckwith, J.B., Kiviat, N.B. and Bonadio, J.F. (1990) Nephrogenic rests, nephroblastomatosis, and the pathogenesis of Wilms' tumour, in *Forefront of Pediatric Pathology: A Festschrift for Benjamin H. Landing*, (Eds R. Jaffe, B.B. Dahms, H.F. Krous, E. Lieberman and T.J. Triche) Hemisphere Publishing, Philadelphia. p. 1.

Beckwith, J.B. and Perrin, E.V. (1963) *In situ* neuroblastomas: A contribution to the natural history of neural crest tumors. *Am. J. Pathol.*, **43**, 1089.

Biedler J.L., Meyers M.B. and Spengler, B.A. (1983) Homogeneously Staining Regions and Double Minute Chromosomes, Prevalent Cytogenetic Abnormalities of Human Neuroblastoma Cells, in *Advances in Cellular Neurobiology*, Academic Press, New York, p. 267.

Bonetta, L., Kuehn, S.E., Huang, A. *et al.* (1990) Wilms' tumor locus on 11p13 defined by multiple CpG island-associated transcripts. *Science*, **250**, 994.

Call, K.M., Glaser, T., Ito, C.Y. *et al.* (1990) Isolation and characterization of a zinc finger polypeptide gene at the human chromosome 11 Wilms' tumor locus. *Cell*, **60**, 509.

Coffin, C.M. and Dehner, L.P. (1990) Soft tissue tumors in first year of life: a report of 190 cases. *Pediat. Pathol.*, **10**, 509.

Cossman, J. Zehnbauer, B., Garrett, C.T. *et al.* (1991) Gene rearrangements in the diagnosis of lymphoma leukemia. *Am. J. Clin. Pathol.*, **95**, 347.

Cox, K.H., DeLeon, D.V., Angerer, L.M. and Angerer, R.C. (1984) Detection of mRNAs in sea urchin embryos by in situ hybridization using asymmetric RNA probes. *Dev. Biol.*, **101**, 485.

Davey, F.R., Erber, W.N., Gatter, K.C. and Mason, D.Y. (1987) Immunophenotyping of acute myeloid leukemia by immuno-alkaline phosphatase (APAAP) labeling with a panel of antibodies. *Am. J. Hematol.*, **26**, 157.

Douglass, E.C., Valentine, M., Etcubanas, E. *et al.* (1987) A specific chromosomal abnormality in rhabdomyosarcoma [published erratum appears in *Cytogenet. Cell Genet.*, 1988; **47** (4): following 232]. *Cytogenet. Cell Genet.*, **45**, 148.

Erlandson, R.A. (1984) Diagnostic immunohistochemistry of human tumors. *Am. J. Surg. Pathol.*, **8**, 615.

Francke, U. (1990) A gene for Wilms' tumour? *Nature*, **343**, 692.

Glaser, T., Jones, C., Douglass, E.C. and Housman, D. (1989) Constitutional and somatic mutations of chromosome 11p in Wilms' tumor. *Cancer Cells*, **7**, 253.

Haas, D., Ablin, A.R., Miller, C. *et al.* (1988) Complete pathologic maturation and regression of stage IVS neuroblastoma without treatment. *Cancer*, **62**, 818.

Hammond, G.D. (1986) Keynote address: The cure of childhood cancers. *Cancer*, **58** (suppl) 407.

Harms, D., Schmidt, D. and Treuner, J. (1985) Soft tissue sarcomas in childhood. A study of 262 cases including 169 cases of rhabdomyosarcoma. *Z. Kinderchir*, **40**, 140.

Hsu, S.M., Raine, L. and Fanger, H. (1981) Use of the Avidin-Biotin-complex (ABC) in immunoperoxidase technique: a comparison between ABC and unlabelled antibody (PAP) procedure. *J. Histochem. Cytochem.*, **29**, 577.

Huang, A., Campbell, C.E., Bonetta, L. *et al.* (1990) Tissue, developmental, and tumor-specific expression of divergent transcripts in Wilms' tumor. *Science*, **250**, 991.

Kaneko, Y., Egues, M.C. and Rowley, J.D. (1981) Interstitial deletion of short arm of chromosome 11 limited to Wilms' tumor cells in a patient without aniridia. *Cancer Res.*, **41**, 4577.

Kawasaki, E.S. (1990) Amplification of RNA, in *PCR Protocols. A Guide to Methods and Applications*, (eds M.A. Innis, D.H. Gelfand, J.J. Sninsky and T.J. White), Academic Press, San Diego, p. 21.

Koufos, A., Hansen, M.F., Lampkin, B.C. *et al.* (1984) Loss of alleles at loci on human chromosome 11 during genesis of Wilms' tumour. *Nature*, **309**, 170.

Malkin, D., Li, F.P., Strong, L.C. *et al.* (1990) Germ line p53 mutations in a familial syndrome of breast cancer, sarcomas, and other neoplasms. *Science*, **250**, 1233.

Mannens, M., Devilee, P., Bliek, J. *et al.* (1990) Loss of heterozygosity in Wilms' tumors, studied for six putative tumor suppressor regions, is limited to chromosome 11. *Cancer Res.*, **50**, 3279.

Miller, R.W. and Dalager, B.S. (1974) U.S. childhood cancer deaths by cell types, 1960–68. *J. Pediatr.*, **85**, 664.

Parkin, D.M., Stiller, C.A., Draper, G.J. *et al.* (1988) International incidence of childhood cancer, Lyon, Oxford University Press, **87**, pp. 101–7.

Pritchard-Jones, K., Fleming, S., Davidson, D. *et al.* (1990) The candidate Wilms' tumour gene is involved in genitourinary development. *Nature*, **346**, 194.

Reeve, A.E., Sih, S.A., Raizis, A.M. and Feinberg, A.P. (1989) Loss of allelic heterozygosity at a second locus on chromosome 11 in sporadic Wilms' tumor cells. *Mol. Cell. Biol.*, **9**, 1799.

Saiki, R.K. (1990), Amplification of genomic DNA,

in *PCR Protocols. A Guide to Methods and Applications*, (eds M.A. Innis, D.H. Gelfand, J.J. Sninsky and T.J. White), Academic Press, San Diego, p. 13.

Sandberg, A.A., Turc, C.C. and Gemmill, R.M. (1988) Chromosomes in solid tumors and beyond. *Cancer Res.*, **48**, 1049.

Sandberg, A.A. (1990) *The chromosomes in human cancer and leukemia*. 2 edn. Elsevier North Holland, New York, 1315.

Shimada, H, Chatten, J., Newton, W.A.J. *et al.* (1984) Histopathologic prognostic factors in neuroblastic tumors: definition of subtypes of ganglioneuroblastoma and an age-linked classification of neuroblastomas. *J. Natl. Cancer Inst.*, **73**, 405.

Southern, E.M. (1975) Detection of specific sequences among DNA fragments separated by gel electrophoresis. *J. Mol. Biol.*, **98**, 503.

Sternberger, L.A. (1979) Immunocytochemistry. 2nd edn. Vol. 1. John Wiley & Sons, Chichester, UK, p. 354.

Stout, A.P. (1962) Fibrosarcoma in Infants and Children. *Cancer*, **15**, 1028.

Tkachuk, D.C., Westbrook, C.A., Andreeff, M. *et al.* (1990) Detection of *bcr-abl* fusion in chronic myelogeneous leukemia by *in situ* hybridization. *Science*, **250**, 559.

Towbin, H., Staehelin, T. and Gordon, J. (1979) Electrophoretic transfer of proteins from polyacrylamide gels to nitrocellulose sheets: procedure and some applications. *Proc. Natl. Acad. Sci. U.S.A.*, **76**, 4350.

Triche, T.J. (1988) Diagnosis of small round cell tumors of childhood. *Bull. Cancer*, (Paris), **75**, 297.

Triche, T.J. and Ross, W.E. (1978) Glycogen-containing neuroblastoma with clinical and histopathologic features of Ewing's sarcoma. *Cancer*, **41**, 1425.

Triche, T.J., Askin, F.B. and Kissane, J.M. (1986) Neuroblastoma, Ewing's sarcoma, and the differential diagnosis of small-, round-, blue-cell tumors in *Pathology of Neoplasia in Children and Adolescents*, (ed. M. Finegold) W.B. Saunders, Philadelphia, p. 145.

Veelken, H., Tycko, B. and Sklar, J. (in press) Sensitive detection of clonal antigen receptor gene rearrangements for the diagnosis and monitoring of lymphoid neoplasia by a polymerase chain reaction-mediated ribonuclease protection assay. *Blood*.

van Heyningen, V., Bickmore, W.A., Seawright, A. *et al.* (1990) Role for the Wilms' tumour gene in genital development? *Proc. Natl. Acad. Sci. U.S.A.*, **87**, 5383.

Wadey, R.B., Pal, N., Buckle, B. *et al.* (1990) Loss of heterozygosity in Wilms' tumour involves two distinct regions of chromosome 11. *Oncogene*, **5**, 901.

Young, J.J., Ries, L.G., Silverberg, E. *et al.* (1986) Cancer incidence, survival, and mortality for children younger than age 15 years. *Cancer*, **58**, 598.

Zinn, K. DiMaio, D. and Maniatis, T. (1983) Identification of two distinct regulatory regions adjacent to the human beta-interferon gene. *Cell*, **34**, 865.

Chapter 4

The radiation biology of paediatric tumours

G.G. STEEL and T.E. WHELDON

4.1 BASIC CONCEPTS OF RADIATION BIOLOGY

4.1.1 CONCEPT OF CLONOGENIC CELLS

All tumours contain both neoplastic and non-neoplastic cells, and not all of the neoplastic cells are capable of perpetuating the tumour. It is clear, especially in well-differentiated tumours, that under undisturbed conditions neoplastic cells undergo differentiation. In the tissue of origin, cells originate in a stem-cell compartment, then become committed to maturation, finally passing through an end-cell state before being lost from the tissue (Potten, 1983). That such a process also often occurs in tumours is clear from their histological structure, from the high rates of cell death that are known to occur especially in carcinomas (Steel, 1977), and from the relatively small proportion of tumour cells that show evidence of being stem cells. Only a minority of the cells in a tumour have a proliferative capacity that threatens the life of the patient. If these can be killed, the tumour cannot continue to grow.

The term 'clonogenic' is used to describe cells extracted from tumours that have the ability to produce a large family of descendents under the artificial conditions of a laboratory assay. The belief is that they may be representative of the stem cells within the tumour. A variety of assays have been developed for clonogenic cells from tumours in rodents; for human tumours it is common to use tissue culture methods.

A typical *in vitro* clonogenic assay involves disaggregating the tumour to form a single-cell suspension, dividing it into samples, irradiating these to various radiation doses (but also keeping an untreated control sample), and finally plating the cells out under growth conditions that allow the formation of individual colonies to be detected. Some cells attach to plastic and will form monolayer colonies in sparse cultures; others require a semisolid culture medium to prevent the dispersal of the colonies. For any particular radiation dose the colony formation per 100 cells plated divided by the colony formation of the control sample gives a measure of the 'surviving fraction' of clonogenic cells. It is important to recognize that this describes the effect of radiation in abolishing colony-forming ability. Cells that fail to form colonies may not be killed immediately and they may in fact go on to divide a few times. But the assay regards them as unimportant with regard to tumour cure or the time of recurrence.

4.1.2 CELL SURVIVAL CURVES

A plot of the surviving fraction of clonogenic cells against radiation dose gives direct information on radiosensitivity. Some examples are shown in Fig. 4.1. Human tumour cells differ considerably in radiosensitivity and it has been found that the surviving fraction at 2 Gy (i.e. SF_2) discriminates best between sensitive and resistant cell lines (Deacon *et al.*, 1984). Since 2 Gy is also a commonly used dose per fraction in clinical radiotherapy, SF_2 is a practically useful parameter.

As can be seen from Fig. 4.1, cell survival

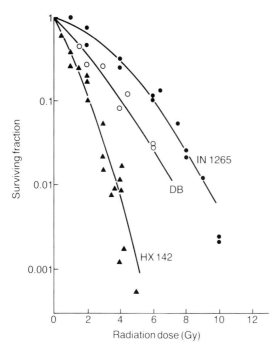

Fig. 4.1 Cell survival curves following high-dose-rate irradiation of three human tumour cell lines: HX142, a neuroblastoma (Peacock *et al.*, 1988); DB, a Wilms' tumour (Parkins and Edwards, unpublished); IN1265, a glioblastoma (Yang *et al.*, 1990).

curves following high dose rate irradiation are commonly curved, convex upwards on the semilogarithmic plot. The significance of this has been the subject of considerable radio-biological research. In some cell lines the data are consistent with a shoulder followed by an exponential decline with dose. Broadly speaking, the curvature could arise from:

1. the need to inactivate multiple targets within a cell before its proliferative capacity is abolished, the likelihood of this increasing as a non-linear function of dose:
2. the production by radiation of non-lethal lesions which by interaction can become lethal, the probability of this increasing with dose;
3. saturation of, or radiation damage to, repair systems, leading to less repair at high radiation doses.

It is not yet possible definitively to choose between these hypotheses. The shape of cell survival curves does not by itself allow such a choice to be made. Most investigators now specify the radiosensitivity of cells by reference to a survival equation of the form:

$$\text{surviving fraction} = \exp(-\alpha D - \beta D^2)$$

This is known as the linear-quadratic equation since on a semilogarithmic plot the first term describes a linear component (the 'α-component') and the second a quadratic component ('β'). The linear component defines the initial slope of the survival curve at low radiation doses. The ratio α/β determines the curvature of the survival curve; it has units of dose and is in fact the dose at which the α and β terms in the equation are equal. This ratio is also an important determinant of the steepness with which curves of total dose for an isoeffect in normal tissues increase with increasing dose per fraction.

As radiation dose rate is reduced, cell survival increases as shown in Fig. 4.2. This increase reflects the occurrence of repair dur-

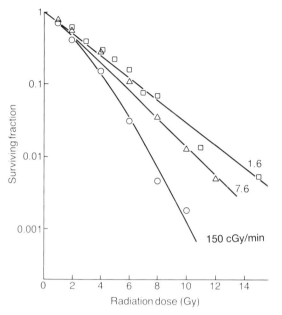

Fig. 4.2 Cell survival curves for a human melanoma cell line (HX118) irradiated at dose rates of 150, 7.6 or 1.6 cGy/min.

ing irradiation at reduced dose rate. Since at very low dose rate the slope of the survival curve approximates the initial slope of the high dose rate curve, it has been argued that the linear (α) component reflects the induction by radiation of non-repairable damage while the quadratic component (whose size is determined by β) describes the induction of repairable damage (Steel *et al.*, 1987). Radiosensitive cells tend to have high α values (section 4.2.3).

Fractionated irradiation with small dose per fraction produces similar radiobiological effects to low dose rate irradiation. In fact, the lowest dose rate in Fig. 4.2 (1.6 cGy/min) is roughly equivalent to treatment with 2 Gy fractions (Fowler, 1989a), provided the overall treatment times are similar, or sufficiently short to avoid differences in the extent of cellular repopulation. The effect of such fractionated irradiation is also dominated by the linear component of cell killing, which in radiosensitive tumours is steep.

4.1.3 RELATION OF CELL SURVIVAL TO GROSS TUMOUR RESPONSE

The reason why much radiobiological attention focuses on the abolition of colony-forming ability in clonogenic cells is because it is believed that this effect of radiation may relate most closely to the growth delay and cure of tumours. Local tumour control is envisaged as the result of eradicating the last clonogenic cell. This may not be true precisely for, in spite of the general failure of immunotherapy of cancer, there may be factors in the local environment of tumours that help to get rid of the last few undamaged clonogenic cells.

Each cubic centimetre of tumour tissue contains around 10^9 cells and if only 1% of these are clonogenic there are 10^7 to be killed. A 100 g tumour will therefore contain around 10^9 clonogenic cells. Killing 99% of these could lead to the tumour regressing to below 1 g, a size that may be clinically undetectable. If radiation cell killing is roughly exponential with dose it will require another 7 logs of cell kill (and therefore $7/2 = 3.5$ times more radiation dose) to eradicate this residual disease. This line of argument therefore leads to the view that complete remission may be far from tumour cure. Unless many more logs of cell kill can be induced the tumour will be likely to recur. The duration of the 'disease-free period' will increase with the extent of clonogenic cell depopulation. Precisely the same argument applies to the chemotherapy of cancer.

4.1.4 RADIATION DAMAGE TO NORMAL TISSUES

A basic fact of radiotherapy and chemotherapy is that normal-tissue damage increases with dose of radiation or drugs. Radiation induces a variety of types of damage. Damage to epithelia, especially of the intestine and mucous membranes, leads to early breakdown of these surface tissues (within days to a few weeks). The reason is that the rate of cell turnover is high: an interruption in cell production quickly leads to a serious cellular deficit. There are other tissues, for instance, connective tissue, liver, and the CNS system, in which the manifestation of radiation damage occurs much later (months to a year or more). Prominent among these 'late' radiation effects are those that result from damage to blood vessels. The radiobiological properties of early-reacting and late-reacting normal tissues differ in important respects. Some organs can manifest both early and late responses. The healing of the early reaction in irradiated skin may be followed by late effects that arise from damage to the dermis. A similar situation arises in the bone marrow, where proliferation-specific cytotoxic drugs tend to induce haemopoietic failure within a few weeks through damage to the rapidly proliferating elements but other agents may damage stem cells and thus compromise the long-term integrity of the marrow.

The distinction between 'early' and 'late' radiation damage to normal tissues may differ to some extent between adults and children. Particularly in very young children, connective tissue cells may proliferate significantly faster than in adults and this could lead to a less clear-cut difference between early and late reactions. This might, for instance, be manifested by a higher α/β ratio for late effects in children. Radiation effects on bone growth are an example of important age-related differences in late radiation effects.

Dose protraction (by multiple fractions or low dose rate) spares radiation damage to normal tissues. This is due to two main processes: repair of cellular damage, and repopulation. Repair is a fast process and it is almost complete within 4–6 h of a radiation dose. It occurs in almost all normal tissues,

although it is low in haemopoietic stem cells. The speed of repopulation depends on the kinetic properties of the target cells. Early-reacting tissues repopulate quickly, tissues like the lung much more slowly, and in the CNS this activity may be absent.

As a result of these processes the radiation dose that a normal tissue will tolerate increases as the dose is protracted. The steepness of this effect is a matter of considerable interest, both from the practical aspect of correctly adjusting dose for modifications in therapeutic schedule, and from the aspect of therapeutic gain. The reason why fractionation succeeds clinically is because it leads to an increase in the tolerance of normal tissues that exceeds the increase in local control dose for tumours.

As recently as 1982 it was recognized that the steepness of isoeffect curves for normal tissues differ between those that are early- and late-reacting. Based on the linear-quadratic model (section 4.1.2) it has been reasoned that the target cells for early reactions have a higher α/β ratio than for late reactions. This fits the experience that has been accumulated in experimental animals, and it leads to the prediction that if the radiation dose per fraction is reduced below the conventional level of 2 Gy there should be a relative increase in effects on tumours (and early-reacting normal tissues) as compared with the late normal-tissue reactions. This is the basis for current attempts to explore hyperfractionation (i.e. the use of multiple small fractions per day over a conventional overall treatment time).

Repopulation occurs not only in early-reacting normal tissues but also in tumours. If the tumour cells that survive radiation exposure can repopulate with a doubling time of 1 week, then over a 6 week course of radiotherapy each clonogenic cell could produce 2^6 (= 64) descendents. There is evidence that some human tumour cells, particularly in children, can proliferate rapidly and this is the foundation for interest in accelerated radiotherapy (i.e. the use of multiple fractions per day over a shortened treatment time, keeping the dose per fraction within the conventional range).

4.1.5 THE OXYGEN EFFECT

The most important physiological modifier of radiation sensitivity is oxygen. All mammalian cells are more sensitive in the presence than in the absence of oxygen. The ratio of the radiation dose for a given effect under hypoxia divided by the dose required under well-oxygenated conditions is termed the 'oxygen enhancement ratio' (OER). Values for the OER range up to about 2.5–3.0 for complete hypoxia. The oxygen effect arises from the role of oxygen in interacting with free radicals produced by radiation, increasing the fixation of damage.

Since tumours frequently contain ischaemic regions the average oxygen tension is often lower than in normal tissues; in addition, there is evidence for microscopic regions of tumours existing at very low oxygen tension. It has thus widely been supposed that failure of local tumour control by radiotherapy may be attributable to the presence of hypoxic tumour cells. This has led to a number of therapeutic strategies designed to overcome this problem:

1. Hyperbaric oxygen. It is possible to irradiate patients within a high-pressure oxygen tank, attempting to increase the oxygen tension in the blood and therefore in body tissues. This procedure is technically complicated and unattractive to the patient but clinical trials may have shown some benefit in head and neck cancers (Dische, 1979).
2. Chemical radiosensitizers. A number of electron-affinic compounds are known to resemble oxygen in conferring radiosensitivity on hypoxic cells. The best-known is misonidazole. This is very effective in sensitizing hypoxic cells, *in vitro* and in experimental tumours, to radiation. It has, however, been largely ineffective in clinical trials, the principal exception being the large DAHANCA trial on head and neck cancer (Overgaard, 1989). The search for more effective sensitisers continues (Stratford and Adams, 1989).
3. High linear-energy-transfer (LET) radiotherapy. Some radiations produced by particle accelerators are less influenced in their biological effects by the presence of oxygen than is the case with X-radiation, gamma-radiation or high-energy electrons. Heavy particles produce densely-ionized tracks within which the intensity of damage (or LET) is high. High LET radiations have a low OER and should therefore overcome the radioresistance conferred by hypoxia. Neutrons produced by a particle accelerator are most commonly used, the high LET tracks being those of the protons and other subatomic particles that they generate within the tissues. In a number of studies neutron therapy has led to serious late normal-tissue reactions and it may be that under truly isotoxic conditions the benefits in most tumour sites are small (Fowler, 1989b).

One possible reason for the lack of success achieved clinically with these manoeuvres designed to outwit the hypoxic tumour cells is the phenomenon of reoxygenation. An initial dose of radiation to a tumour will preferentially kill oxic cells and leave survivors that are predominantly hypoxic. A second dose given immediately afterwards will therefore be less effective. But after a period of hours or days, cells damaged by the first dose will die and the supply of oxygen to the survivors may improve. This can even lead to a hypoxic fraction below that of the untreated tumour. Reoxygenation has been demonstrated in experimental tumours and if it occurs in human tumours it will reduce the impact of hypoxic cells. The current view is that, although the importance of hypoxia as a cause of failure in radiotherapy may in the past have been overestimated, it still remains an important factor. There may be some tumour types in which reoxygenation is inadequate; furthermore, in accelerated radio-therapy protocols designed to overcome re-population (section 4.1.4) reoxygenation may be less adequate and the approaches listed above may give greater benefit.

4.1.6 RADIOSENSITIVITY OF TUMOUR CELLS

If hypoxia is less of a problem than has been thought, how do we explain the resistance of many common tumour types to radiotherapy? Repopulation has already been mentioned as a possible candidate. In some tumour types it has been postulated that the fraction of cells that can regrow the tumour after treatment may be small. This can be described as a low 'clonogenic fraction' (section 4.1.1) and would lead to tumour control at a lower radiation dose.

More important perhaps is the steepness of the cell survival curve. A simple calculation illustrates the importance of the cell kill per dose in determining the outcome of a multi-fraction schedule. The three cell survival curves shown in Fig. 4.1 have surviving fractions at 2 Gy of 0.19 (neuroblastoma), 0.33 (Wilms') and 0.64 (glioma). Imagine treating these with a course of 20 fractions of 2 Gy, allowing full recovery between them. The overall surviving fraction will be $(SF_2)^{20}$, which for the three tumour cell lines gives: 4×10^{-15}, 2×10^{-10} and 1.3×10^{-4}. The first of these corresponds to the eradication of over 1 kg of tumour cells, the last to less than 1 mg. This is of course a very crude calcula-tion that ignores hypoxia and many other factors that might influence response but it

does illustrate how critical the initial slope of the cell survival curve might be.

Deacon *et al.* (1984) reviewed the literature on the *in vitro* radiosensitivity of human tumours and demonstrated a correlation between SF_2 values and the level of clinical response of the various tumour types. The existence of such a correlation is evidence that the inherent radiosensitivity of oxic tu-mour cells may be an important reason for clinical failure: in spite of the crudeness of the above calculation it is difficult to see how the glioma cell line IN1265 could be responsive to conventional fractionated radiotherapy.

4.2 RADIOSENSITIVITY OF CELLS DERIVED FROM PAEDIATRIC TUMOURS

4.2.1 RADIOSENSITIVITY OF SOLID TUMOURS

How radiosensitive are the cells of childhood tumours? During the past ten years a number of investigators have attempted to examine this. Much of the available data are summar-ized in Tables 4.1 and 4.2. Table 4.1 includes data on four tumour types that occur predomi-nantly in childhood: neuroblastoma, med-ulloblastoma, Wilms' tumour, and Ewing's sarcoma. In addition, some data are also included in this table on osteosarcoma and glioma, tumours that do occur in children. It is not known whether the tissue samples that gave rise to these data came from children or adults. They have been included here in order to provide a comparison for those tumour types that are thought to be more radiosensitive.

A word of caution is appropriate in relation to these data. Since there is no reliable *in situ* method of measuring radiosensitivity, such studies begin by setting up cell cultures from tissue biopsies, passaging the cells that grow out from the explants, and establishing con-

78

Table 4.1 Radiation sensitivity of non-lymphoid paediatric tumours

Designation	Type	Alpha	Beta	SF_2	Source
NB-1	Neuroblastoma	1.07	0	0.15	Ohnuma *et al.* (1977)
LAN-1	"	0.45	0.020	0.37	Weichselbaum *et al.* (1980)
HX138	"	1.03	0.040	0.11	Deacon *et al.* (1984)
HX142	"	0.82	0.095	0.13	Deacon (1987)
HX143	"	0.89	0.17	0.085	Deacon (1987)
DB	Wilms'	0.55	0.023	0.33	Parkins and Edwards (unpublished)
TX-7	Medulloblastoma	0.55	0.019	0.31	Weichselbaum *et al.* (1976)
STSAR-10	Ewing's Sarcoma	0.39	0.064	0.36	Weichselbaum *et al.* (1989)
STSAR-11	"	0.46	0.055	0.32	"
STSAR-33	"	0.56	0.076	0.24	"
STSAR-34	"	0.31	0.059	0.58	"
5838	"	0.16	0.051		Kinsella *et al.* (1984)
4573	"	0.25	0.61		"
TX-14	"	0.53	0.024	0.32	
D283	"	0.68	0.080	0.19	Powell, S. (unpublished)
TE671	Rhabdomyosarcoma	0.25	0.029	0.54	"
STSAR-2	Osteosarcoma	0.33	0.070	0.39	Weichselbaum *et al.* (1989)
STSAR-6	"	0.69	0.011	0.24	"
STSAR-22	"	0.52	0.061	0.28	"
STSAR-23	"	0.51	0.093	0.25	"
STSAR-35	"	0.14	0.12	0.47	"
STSAR-43	"	0.50	0.016	0.34	"
TX-4	"	0.36	0.040	0.41	Weichselbaum *et al.* (1976)
SaOS	"	0.077	0.105	0.55	Weichselbaum *et al.* (1980)
A2	Glioma	0.41	0.035	0.38	Gerweck (1977)
A3	"	0.12	0.040	0.67	"
A7	"	0	0.069	0.86	"
TX13	"	0.58	0.010	0.30	Weichselbaum *et al.* (1976)
U118MG	"			0.76	Nilsson *et al.* (1980)
U118MG	"			0.71	Millar and Jinks (1985)
U251MG	"			0.71	"
IN859	"	0.31	0.033	0.57	Yang *et al.* (in press)
IN1265	"	0.042	0.053	0.73	"
SB	"	0.36	0.0077	0.47	"

tinuous cell lines whose radiosensitivity can then be examined by cell cloning techniques. Within this procedure there is inevitably a high degree of cellular selection. The cells that grow may be tumour (i.e. neoplastic) cells but stromal cells may also grow. Unfortunately, few investigators have carefully characterized their continuous cell cultures and it may well be that some of these did not in fact contain malignant cells. Whether those that do contain malignant cells are representative of the *in situ* tumour cell population is also open to question.

The data are shown graphically in Fig. 4.3. The osteosarcomas and gliomas have a surviving fraction at 2 Gy (SF_2) that ranges from 0.24 to 0.86. The data for medulloblastoma and Ewing's sarcoma, also the single values

Table 4.2 Radiation sensitivity of human leukaemic cells. AML, acute myeloblastic leukaemia. APL, acute promyelocytic leukaemia. ALL, acute lymphoblastic leukaemia. AMML, acute myelomonocytic leukaemia. CML, chronic myeloid leukaemia.

Designation	Type	Alpha	Beta	SF_2	Source
P3HR	Burkitt's	0.87	0.009	0.17	Fertil *et al.* (1980)
MOLT-4	Lymphobl.	2.04	0	0.015	Szekely and Lobreau (1985)
MOLT-3	Lymphobl.			0.07	Cohen *et al.* (1988)
JM	Lymphobl.			0.2	"
176	AML	0.013	0.22	0.40	Weichselbaum *et al.* (1981)
HL60	Promyelocytic	0.55	0.056	0.26	"
HL60		0.63	0	0.30	Lehnert *et al.* (1986)
2	APL	0.44	0.018	0.39	Ozawa *et al.* (1983)
KG+	Erythroleuk.	0.78	0.001	0.13	Lehnert *et al.* (1986)
K562	Erythroleuk.	0.27	0.061	0.46	Weichselbaum *et al.* (1981)
45	ALL	0.51	0.032	0.316	"
1	AMML	0.32	0.023	0.48	Ozawa *et al.* (1983)
3	AMML	0.38	0.019	0.43	"
4	AMML	0.63	0.029	0.26	"
8	AMML	1.25	0.036	0.070	"
9	AMML	1.33	0.020	0.064	"
10	AMML	1.82	0	0.26	"
5	AML	0.56	0.029	0.29	"
6	AML	0.64	0.031	0.25	"
7	AML	0.94	0.033	0.132	"
11	AML	2.0	0	0.018	"
12	AML	3.3	0	0.0013	"
Reh	ALL	0.81	0.001	0.12	Lehnert *et al.* (1986)
NALM-6	ALL	0.46	0.003	0.18	"
CEM	T-cell			0.073	Schimm *et al.* (1988)
Mean of 10	Acute non-lymph.	1.45	0.13	0.032*	Kimler *et al.* (1985)
Mean of 11	T-lineage			0.53*	Uckun and Song (1988)
Mean of 8	B-lineage			0.53*	"
K-562	CML	0.085	0.0007	0.70	Lehnert *et al.* (1986)

* Mean values

for rhabdomyosarcoma and Wilms' tumour, fall in the same range as the osteosarcomas. Only the neuroblastomas appear to be more radiosensitive.

4.2.2. RADIOSENSITIVITY OF LEUKAEMIAS

Table 4.2 summarizes data on leukaemias. The majority of these were acute non-lympho- cytic leukaemias. What is remarkable is the range of values that have been recorded. Kimler *et al.* (1985) studied ten acute non-lymphocytic leukaemias (ANLL) and found that they were quite radiosensitive, with D_0 values in the range 0.41–0.95 Gy and a mean extrapolation number of 1.0 (these parameter values correspond roughly to $SF_2 = 0.032$). The cases studied by Weichselbaum *et al.* (1981) were uniformly more resistant. The

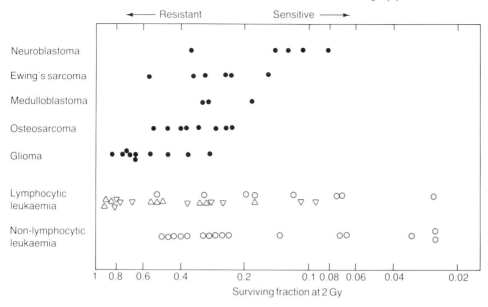

Fig. 4.3   The initial slope of cell survival curves for a variety of mainly paediatric tumours, as indicated by the surviving fraction at 2 Gy (SF₂). For the lymphocytic leukaemias, the triangles indicate the results of Uckun and Song (1988): △ B-cell, ▽ T-cell (SF₂ values have been derived from their parameter estimates).

extensive study by Ozawa *et al.* (1983) produced a wide range of values among myeloid leukaemias. Cohen *et al.* (1988) studied 19 lymphoblastic leukaemias. Once again there was a wide range of SF₂ values, ranging from 0.1 to 0.9, and the mean values for T-cell and B-cell tumours were the same (0.53 ± 0.3 SD). As can be seen from Fig. 4.3, the leukaemic SF₂ values altogether range from below 0.02 to above 0.5.

A study by Thomson *et al.* (1985) of the radiosensitivity of lymphocytes from patients with chronic myeloblastic leukaemia (CML) evaluated the time-dependent induction of pyknosis (not a cloning assay); these authors also found considerable differences in response from patient to patient.

What are we to conclude? It is clear that some cells that have been obtained from human leukaemias are highly radiosensitive,

but the majority are not. Studies of the radiosensitivity of normal haemopoietic precursor cells in man and in rodents have also shown considerable differences, which may reflect a variation in radiosensitivity among the various clonogenic subtypes in the marrow and peripheral blood (Hendry and Lord, 1983). It could be, therefore, that the wide range of results for leukaemic cells arises from differences from one patient (or one experimental design) to another in the cell type that grows out in tissue culture. But it is also possible that the culture conditions (especially for fresh tissue explants) were not satisfactory, and this may have led to overestimation of radiation resistance in some cases. At this stage it is difficult to make a confident statement about the radiosensitivity of leukaemic cells.

81

4.2.3 RECOVERY FROM RADIATION DAMAGE IN NEUROBLASTOMAS AND LEUKAEMIAS

The data reviewed above indicate that some tumours of childhood are very radiosensitive. These tumours have survival curves that are steep and almost shoulderless. It has often been supposed that such curves indicate 'repair deficiency', i.e. that cellular recovery after irradiation is small. Recent work in this department on neuroblastomas has questioned this conclusion.

The ability of cells to recover from radiation damage can be judged by:

1. The magnitude of the dose-rate effect. As radiation dose rate is reduced from the typical acute rates of around 1 Gy/min to 1 cGy/min (a factor of 100) the exposure times become long enough for recovery to proceed *during* irradiation. Cell survival increases and the bending dose–response curves seen at high dose rate tend to become straight and to extrapolate the initial slope of the high dose rate curve (Fig. 4.2). The change in steepness of the survival curves has been used as an indication of the extent of recovery (Steel *et al.*, 1987).
2. Dose-sparing due to fractionation. As fraction number is increased (in the absence of an increase in overall time) the total iso-effect dose increases.
3. Split-dose recovery experiments. If a dose of radiation is divided into two equal halves, separated by a few hours, recovery is allowed to occur in the interval and the overall level of cell survival is greater. The increase in survival at a given dose is indicated by a 'recovery ratio', the ratio of the surviving fractions.
4. Delayed-plating experiments. If cells are irradiated under conditions in which cell proliferation is inhibited and then passaged into fresh culture medium at intervals there-

after, the surviving fraction is often found to rise. This has widely been taken to indicate recovery from radiation damage.

Neuroblastomas show very little dose-rate effect and for radiation doses that give up to 2 logs of cell kill (survival = 0.01) little split-dose recovery is detectable (Deacon *et al.*, 1985; Wheldon *et al.*, 1986b; Holmes *et al.*, 1990). However, because of their high radiosensitivity these measurements are made after small radiation doses. As indicated in section 4.1.2, it may be valid to divide cell survival after irradiation into a linear 'α' component and a bending 'β' component. The β component is repairable, the α component not. Radiosensitive tumours tend to have high α values. Peacock *et al.* (1988) showed in 11 human tumour cell lines that split-dose recovery increased with the radiation dose at which it was measured and the rate of increase (surprisingly) was greater in neuroblastomas than in more radioresistant cell lines. This implied that on the basis of recovery at a given dose, or of the size of the β component, there was *more* recovery in the neuroblastomas.

This rather surprising conclusion leads to the view that neuroblastomas are not radio-sensitive because they fail to repair radiation damage, but because for a given radiation exposure they suffer a greater level of damage. There may be a higher incidence both of irreparable damage (leading to a large α component) and of reparable damage (leading to a large β component). Studies of the molecular aspects of radiation damage suggest that some cell lines may be more tolerant than others of a given degree of genetic damage (Powell and McMillan, 1990).

Few data are available on the dose-rate effect and recovery in leukaemias. Uckun and Song (1988) reported studies on three T-cell and one B-cell tumours. In each they found a substantial effect of lowering the dose rate down to 7 cGy/min, much larger than has been found for normal bone marrow cells. The cells that they used had SF_2 values ranging from 0.08 to 0.22, in the middle of the range shown in Fig. 4.3. Szekely and Lobreau (1985), using the highly radiosensitive MOLT-4 cell line were able to detect no split-dose recovery for survival down to 0.01. However, this required a split of only $1 + 1$ Gy and, as indicated above, this may be too low a dose to prove that the cells had no capacity to recover.

4.3 IMPLICATIONS FOR CLINICAL RADIOTHERAPY

The amount of firm data on the radiobiological properties of childhood tumours is small and, as illustrated in Fig. 4.3, the variations from one cell line to another are wide. Other factors that may influence clinical response are also poorly documented: hypoxia, rate of reoxygenation, proliferation rate (especially during regrowth after the start of treatment) and rate of repair of radiation damage. The collection of data cited in the figure does, however, support the view that the clonogenic cells of some childhood tumours are of high radiosensitivity and would be little affected by lowering the radiation dose rate or changing fraction size. From the available data, this is most clearly seen in the case of neuroblastoma. It has therefore been argued by Wheldon *et al.* (1986a, 1986b, 1987) that the treatment of neuroblastoma would be best done by hyperfractionation.

The reasoning behind this is that the normal tissues that limit radiotherapy are usually (though not always) late-responding tissues whose stem cells are turning over rather slowly. For example, with localized radiotherapy, radiation dosage is usually limited by risks of long-term damage to vascular endothelium and slowly proliferating parenchymal tissues. With total body irradiation, where bone-marrow rescue is used, it is the risk of damage to the lung which sets the

limit. These late-responding tissues show considerable dose recovery as a result of protraction. In terms of the linear-quadratic model this may be described as a low α/β ratio. The data on neuroblastomas, including the cell survival data as shown in Table 1, imply that for some tumour cells the α/β ratio is much higher. In this situation, lowering the dose per fraction should spare damage to late-responding normal tissues to a greater extent than damage to the tumour cells (Fowler, 1989c). Therefore, higher doses could be given using smaller doses per fraction and should be tolerated by late-responding tissues, while greater damage is done to the tumour. By the same argument, lowering the dose rate should also be beneficial. At a reduced dose rate the effect of fractionation is less and the same therapeutic gain should be obtained with fewer fractions (Steel *et al.*, 1987).

With any new fractionation schedule for childhood tumours, it will be important to keep the overall duration of treatment as short as possible. Repopulation is now perceived as a significant detriment to successful therapy in rapidly growing tumours (Fowler, 1989c) and the available evidence suggests that cell proliferation rates in paediatric tumours are high (Steel, 1977, and Table 4.2). For this reason, hyperfractionation should be given in the form of twice-daily treatments over a reduced overall time, a strategy known as 'accelerated hyperfractionation' (Thames *et al.*, 1983). Where this is done, it is important that the two fractions on any one day are sufficiently well separated that no significant interaction between them occurs. This probably requires a minimum separation of about 6 h, though a slightly greater separation (e.g. 8 h) would be desirable. Also, it should be appreciated that rapidly turning over tissues which give acute responses (skin, epithelia, bone marrow) will benefit less than late-responding tissues from the reduction of dose per fraction and are more likely to be affected

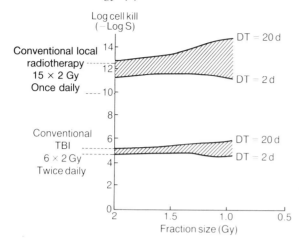

Fig. 4.4 Calculated values of log (surviving fraction) for the treatment of neuroblastoma by two radiotherapy schedules involving twice-daily treatments. Doubling time (DT) for repopulation assumed to range from 2 to 20 d (the shaded areas). Cellular sensitivity assumed typical of neuroblastoma. For each fraction size, the total dose was calculated as being radiobiologically equivalent to a standard regimen in terms of its effects on late-responding normal tissues (assumed $\alpha/\beta = 3$ Gy). The upper set of curves correspond to the case where the standard regimen is conventionally fractionated local radiotherapy (15 × 2 Gy); the lower curves are for a standard regimen of TBI (6 × 2 Gy) to be followed by bone-marrow rescue.

adversely by the shortened time-scale (Thames and Hendry, 1987). Acute-responding tissues should be closely monitored, where possible, to ensure that excessive reactions are not allowed to develop.

In the case of neuroblastoma, the possible benefits of accelerated hyperfraction may be demonstrated by some sample calculations. Firstly, consider a conventionally fractionated regimen which might be used for local radiotherapy: 15 treatments of 2 Gy, given daily (but excluding weekends). The linear-quadratic model may be used to calculate total doses, using different fraction sizes, which

should have the same effect on late-responding normal tissues (assuming $\alpha/\beta = 3$ Gy for those tissues). Overall time matters little in the case of late-responding tissues so the reduced time which will result if treatments are given twice daily should make little difference. However, neuroblastoma cells will be differently affected both by the reduced fraction size (and higher total dose) and by the reduced time. The effect of changing fraction size and total dose may be estimated for neuroblastoma from the data of Table 4.1. The average parameter values for the five neuroblastoma cell lines are $\alpha = 0.85$ Gy^{-1} and $\beta = 0.065$ Gy^{-2}. The effect of altered time depends on the assumed doubling time for repopulation in neuroblastomas; this is not reliably known but probably lies between 2 and 20 d.

The upper set of curves in Fig. 4.4 show the results of these calculations. Accelerated fractionation regimens (fraction size < 2 Gy, treatment time < 20 d) may be seen to have greater effects on tumour cells for equivalent effects on late-responding tissues. For a doubling time of 20 d, the superiority of the hyperfractionated regimen continues to increase as the fraction size decreases to less than 1 Gy. For the 2 d doubling time, the isoeffect curve is rather flat and fraction size may have little influence on outcome.

The lower set of curves in Fig. 4.4 shows the results of a similar set of calculations for the case of treatment using total body irradiation (TBI) and bone-marrow rescue. In this case, the standard regimen is taken to consist of 6 × 2 Gy, given twice daily over 3 d. The dose-limiting organ was taken to be lung, also with an α/β ratio of 3 Gy. The results again show that, for a doubling time of 20 d, the results might be better with a fraction size of 1 Gy rather than 2 Gy. For the 2 Gy doubling time, fraction size should again have little effect.

The results provide some support for the use of accelerated hyperfractionation, with a fraction size of 1.5 Gy or slightly less, in the treatment of neuroblastoma by local radio-therapy or TBI. It should be noted that the predicted advantage of the accelerated hyper-fractionation regimen is fairly modest, though it would probably be worthwhile clinically if it could be achieved in practice.

In the case of other solid paediatric tumours, the data are mostly insufficient to support similar calculations. For all the child-hood tumours, and especially for the leu-kaemias, there is evidence for considerable variation in radiosensitivity from one cell line to another. If similar variability occurs in the clinic, it points to the need for the develop-ment of methods of radiosensitivity testing leading to individualized radiotherapy as a way of optimizing radiotherapy fractionation.

REFERENCES

Cohen, J.D., Robins, H.I., Mulcahy, *R.T. et al.* (1988) Interactions between hyperthermia and irradiation in two human lymphoblastic leu-kemia cell lines in vitro. *Cancer Res.,* **48**, 3576–80.

Deacon, J. (1987). The radiobiology of human neuro-blastoma. Ph.D. thesis, University of London.

Deacon, J., Peckham, M.J. and Steel, G.G. (1984) The radioresponsiveness of human tumours and the initial slope of the cell survival curve. *Radiother. Oncol., 2*, 317–23.

Deacon, J.M., Wilson, P.A. and Peckham, M.J. (1985) The radiobiology of human neuroblastoma. *Radiother. Oncol., 3*, 201–9.

Dische, S. (1979) Hyperbaric oxygen: the Medical Research Council trials and their clinical signifi-cance. *Br. J. Radiol.,* **51**, 888–94.

Fertil, B., Deschavanne, P.J., Lachet, B. and Malaise, E.P. (1980) In vitro radiosensitivity of six human cell lines: A comparative study with different statistical models. *Radiat. Res.,* **82**, 297–309.

Fowler, J.F. (1989a) Dose-rate effects in normal tissues, in *Brachytherapy 2*, Proceedings of the 5th International SELECTRON Users' Meeting 1988 (ed R.F. Mould), Nucletron International BV, Leersum, The Netherlands, pp. 26–40.

Fowler, J.F. (1989b) Heavy particles in radiotherapy, in *The Biological Basis of Radiotherapy*, 2nd edn,

(eds G.G. Steel, G.E. Adams and A. Horwich), Elsevier Science Publishers BV, Amsterdam, pp. 249–66.

Fowler, J.F. (1989c) The linear-quadratic formula and progress in fractionated radiotherapy. *Br. J. Radiol.,* **62**, 679–94.

Gerweck, L.E., Kornblith, P.L., Burlett, P. *et al.* (1977) Radiation sensitivity of cultured human glioblastoma cells.*Radiology,* **125**, 231–4.

Hendry, J.H. and Lord, B.I. (1983) The analysis of the early and late response to cytotoxic insults in the haemopoietic cell hierarchy, in *Cytotoxic Insult to Tissue,* (eds C.S. Potten and J.H. Hendry), Churchill Livingstone, London.

Holmes, A., McMillan, T.J., Peacock, J.H. and Steel, G.G. (1990) The radiation dose-rate effect in two human neuroblastoma cell lines. *Br. J. Cancer,* **62**, 791–5.

Kimler, B.F., Park, C.H., Yakar, D. and Mies, R.M. (1985) Radiation response of human normal and leukemic hemopoietic cells assayed by in vitro colony formation. *Int. J. Radiat. Oncol. Biol. Phys.,* **11**, 809–16.

Kinsella, T.J., Mitchell, J.B., McPherson, S. *et al.* (1984) In vitro radiation studies on Ewing's sarcoma cell lines and human bone marrow: application to the clinical use of total body irradiation. *Int. J. Radiat. Oncol. Biol. Phys.,* **10**, 1005–11.

Lehnert, S., Rybka, W.B., Suissa, S. and Giam-battisto, D. (1986) Radiation response of haemato-poietic cell lines of human origin. *Int. J. Radiat. Biol.,* **49**, 423–31.

Millar, B.C. and Jinks, S. (1985) Studies on the relationship between the radiation resistance and glutathione content of human and rodent cells after treatment with dexamethasone in vitro. *Int. J. Radiat. Biol.,* **47**, 539–52.

Nilsson, S., Carlsson, J. and Larsson, B. (1980) Survival of irradiated glia and glioma cells studied with a new cloning technique. *Int. J. Radiat. Biol.,* **37**, 267–79.

Ohnuma, N., Kasuga., T., Nojiri, I. and Furuse, T. (1977) Radiosensitivity of human neuroblastoma cell line NB–1. *Gann,* **68**, 711–2.

Overgaard, J. (1989) Sensitisation of hypoxic tumour cells – clinical experience. *Int. J. Radiat. Biol.,* **56**, 801–11.

Ozawa, K., Miura, Y., Suda, T. *et al.* (1983) Radi-ation sensitivity of leukemic progenitor cells in acute nonlymphocytic leukemia. *Cancer Res.*, **43**, 2339–41.

Peacock, J.H., Cassoni, A.M. and McMillan, T.J. (1988) Radiosensitive human tumour cell lines may not be recovery deficient. *Int. J. Radiat. Biol.*, **54**, 945–53.

Potten, C.S. (1983) *Stem Cells*, Churchill Livingstone, London.

Powell, S. and McMillan, T.J. (1990) DNA damage and repair following treatment with ionizing radiation. (in press)

Schimm, D.S., Olson, S. and Hill, A.B. (1988) Radiation resistance in a multidrug resistant human T-cell leukemia line. *Int. J. Radiat. Oncol. Biol. Phys.*, **15**, 931–6.

Steel, G.G. (1977) *The Growth Kinetics of Tumours*, Oxford University Press.

Steel, G.G., Deacon, J.M., Duchesne, G.M. *et al.* (1987) The dose-rate effect in human tumour cells. *Radiother. Oncol.* **9**, 299–310.

Stratford, I.J. and Adams, G.E. (1989) Radiation sensitisers and bioreductive drugs, in *The Biological Basis of Radiotherapy*, 2nd edn, (eds G.G. Steel, G.E. Adams and A. Horwich), Elsevier Science Publishers BV, Amsterdam, pp. 145–62.

Szekely, J.G. and Lobreau, A.U. (1985) High radiosensitivity of the MOLT–4 leukaemic cell line. *Int. J. Radiat. Biol.*, **48**, 277–84.

Thames, H.D. and Hendry, J.H. (1987) *Fractionation in radiotherapy*, Taylor and Francis, London.

Thames, H.D., Peters, L.J., Withers, H.R. and Fletcher, G.H. (1983) Accelerated fractionation versus hyperfractionation: rationales for several treatments per day. *Int. Radiat. Oncol. Biol. Phys.*, **9**, 127–38.

Thomson, A.E.R., Vaughan-Smith, S., Peel, W.E. and Wetherley-Mein, G. (1985) The intrinsic radiosensitivity of lymphocytes in chronic lymphocytic leukaemia, quantitatively determined independently of cell death rate factors. *Int. J. Radiat. Biol.*, **48**, 943–61.

Uckun, F.M. and Song, C.W. (1988) Radiobiological features of fresh leukemic bone marrow progenitor cells in acute lymphoblastic leukemia. *Cancer Res.*, **48**, 5788–95.

Weichselbaum, R.R., Epstein, J., Little, J.B. and Kornblith, P.L. (1976) In vitro cellular radiosensitivity of human malignant tumors. *Eur. J. Cancer*, **12**, 47–51.

Weichselbaum, R.R., Nove, J. and Little, J. (1980) X-ray sensitivity of human tumor cells in vitro. *Int. J. Radiat. Oncol. Biol. Phys.*, **6**, 437–40.

Weichselbaum, R.R., Greenberger, J.S., Schmidt, A. *et al.* (1981) In vitro radiosensitivity of human leukemia cell lines. *Radiology*, 139, 485–7.

Weichselbaum, R.R., Rotmensch, J., Ahmed-Swan, S. and Beckett, M.A. (1989) Radiobiological characterization of 53 human tumor cell lines. *Int. J. Radiat. Biol.*, **56**, 553–60.

Wheldon, T.E., O'Donoghue, J., Gregor, A. *et al.* (1986a) Radiobiological considerations in the treatment of neuroblastoma by total body irradiation. *Radiother. Oncol.*, **6**, 317–26.

Wheldon, T.E., Wilson, L., Livingstone, A. *et al.* (1986b) Radiation studies on multicellular tumour spheroids derived from human neuroblastoma: Absence of sparing effect of dose fractionation. *Eur. J. Cancer Clin. Oncol.*, **22**, 563–6.

Wheldon, T.E., Berry, I., O'Donoghue, J.A. *et al.* (1987) The effect on human neuroblastoma spheriods of fractionated radiation regimes calculated to be equivalent for damage to late responding normal tissues. *Eur. J. Cancer Clin. Oncol.*, **23**, 855–60.

Yang, X., Darling, J.L., McMillan, T.J. *et al.* (1990) Radiosensitivity, recovery and dose-rate effect in three human glioma cell lines. *Radiother. Oncol.*, **19**, 49–56.

Chapter 5

Cancer chemotherapy and mechanisms of resistance

J.R. HARDY and C.R. PINKERTON

5.1 INTRODUCTION

Anticancer drugs can be classified into various groups according to their primary mode of action. Many drugs appear to have multiple mechanisms of cell kill and in any one tumour cell line or tissue, one or other mechanism may predominate. Within each group can be placed drugs which differ markedly with respect to their pharmacokinetic, toxic and metabolic profiles. The primary aim of this chapter is to discuss the primary mode of action of the agents in each group and how this relates to mechanisms of drug resistance. This is particularly relevant in that considerable emphasis has lately been placed on developing methods of overcoming the drug resistance that occurs when treating many common tumours rather than the often fruitless search for new anticancer agents. The most commonly used drugs are classified in Table 5.1. Table 5.2 lists the major side-effects of each of these and their pharmacokinetic characteristics are shown in Table 5.3.

5.2 GENERAL PRINCIPLES

Cytotoxic drugs are cell poisons which act indiscriminately on most cells, inhibiting cell division. Their clinical role relies on a differential killing effect between normal and malignant cells. The 'therapeutic index' of a particular drug, i.e. the tumour cell kill in relation to normal tissue damage, determines its clinical usefulness.

DNA synthesis is not a continuous process within the cell cycle but occurs in a relatively short space of time known as the S phase (Fig. 5.1). This is preceded and followed by apparent 'resting' phases G_1 and G_2, prior to mitosis (M phase) and cell division.

Phase-specific drugs affect only those cells in specific parts of the cell cycle. Those that exert their lethal effects only against proliferating cells are termed 'cycle-specific'. Most drugs act preferentially on rapidly dividing, or cycling, cells. Therefore, rapidly growing tumours are usually the most sensitive to chemotherapy and rapidly proliferating normal tissues, e.g. bone marrow and mucosa, suffer the most toxicity. Those cells within a tumour that are not actively dividing (G_0 cells) determine the tumour growth fraction, i.e. the ratio of the number of cycling cells compared to the total number of cells. Tumours with a large proportion of cells in G_0 tend to be relatively chemoresistant. An initial reduction in tumour cell population (e.g. by surgery or radiotherapy) may draw resting

Table 5.1 Classification of the commonly used cytotoxic agents

Agent type	*Substance name*	*Major clinical use*
1. Antimetabolites		
Antifolates	Methotrexate	Leukaemia, lymphoma, CNS, osteosarcoma
Fluoropyrimidines	5-Fluorouracil	Colorectal, liver
Purine analogues	6-Mercaptopurine (6-MP)	Leukaemia, lymphoma
	6-Thioguanine (6-TG)	Leukaemia, lymphoma
Pyrimide analogues	Cytarabine	Leukaemia, lymphoma, CNS
2. Alkylating agents	Nitrogen mustard	Hodgkin's disease
	Cyclophosphamide ⎱ Ifosfamide ⎰	Leukaemia, lymphoma, neuroblastoma, rhabdomyosarcoma, Ewing's sarcoma, germ cell
	Melphalan	Neuroblastoma, sarcomas, leukaemia, Hodgkin's disease
	Busulphan	Leukaemia
Nitrosoureas	BCNU (carmustine) ⎱ CCNU (lomustine) ⎰	Brain tumours, lymphomas
3. Platinum compounds	Cisplatin ⎱ Carboplatin ⎰	Germ cell tumours, neuroblastoma, sarcomas, CNS, liver
4. Vinca alkaloids	Vincristine	Leukaemia, lymphoma, Wilms' tumour, neuroblastoma, rhabdomyosarcoma, Ewing's sarcoma
	Vinblastine	Lymphoma
	Vindesine	Sarcomas
5. Epipodophyllotoxins	Etoposide (VP-16) ⎱ Teniposide (VM-26) ⎰	Leukaemia, lymphoma, neuroblastoma, germ cell tumours
6. Antitumour antibiotics	Doxorubicin	Leukaemia, lymphoma, neuroblastoma, rhabdomyosarcoma, Ewing's sarcoma, Wilms' tumour
	Daunorubicin	Leukaemia
	Epirubicin	Lymphoma, sarcoma
	Mitozantrone	Lymphoma, leukaemia
	Actinomycin D	Wilms' tumour, Ewing's sarcoma, rhabdomyosarcoma
	Bleomycin	Germ cell tumours, lymphoma
7. Miscellaneous	Dacarbazine	Sarcoma, Hodgkin's disease
	Procarbazine	Hodgkin's disease
	Amsacrine	Leukaemia
	L-asparaginase	Leukaemia
	Hydroxyurea	Chronic leukaemia
	Prednisolone	Leukaemia, lymphoma

Table 5.2 Toxicity of the commonly used cytotoxic agents.

Agent	Common/dose-limiting toxicities	Rare toxicities
1. Antimetabolites		
Methotrexate	BM, M, renal (HD)	Liver, lung, CNS
5-Fluorouracil	BM, M, diarrhoea	CNS, chest pain, conjunctivitis
6-MP	BM	liver
6-TG	BM	liver
Ara-C	BM, M, N & V, diarrhoea	liver, CNS, lung, conjunctivitis
2. Alkylating agents		
Nitrogen mustard	BM, N & V, V, A	cholinergic (HD), sterility
Cyclophosphamide	BM, N & V, A, haemorrhagic cystitis	SIADH, sterility, C, lung, heart (HD)
Ifosfamide	BM, cystitis, A, N & V	CNS, kidney, SIADH, C, sterility
Melphalan	BM, A (HD), V	C, sterility
Chlorambucil	BM	C, sterility
Busulphan	BM (cumulative), cutaneous	lung, Addisonian-like state, sterility
BCNU, CCNU	BM (delayed), N & V	lung, renal, C, sterility, liver
Platinum compounds		
Cisplatin	N & V, diarrhoea, renal, N	BM (HD), hypersensitivity
Carboplatin	BM, N & V (HD)	Renal (HD)
4. Vinca alkaloids		
Vincristine	N, constipation, V, jaw pain	SIADH
Vinblastine	BM, V, jaw pain	N, M
Vindesine	BM, V	N
5. Epidophyllotoxins		
Etoposide	BM, N & V (p.o.), A	N
Teniposide	BM, V, A	Lung
6. Antitumour antibiotics		
Doxorubicin	BM, N & V, A, M, V	C, radiation recall
Daunorubicin	BM, N & V, V, M, A	C, radiation recall
Epirubicin	BM, A, V	C
Mitoxantrone	BM	Cholestasis
Actinomycin D	BM, N & V, A, M, diarrhoea, V	Radiation recall
Bleomycin	Fever/chills, M, pigmentation	Lung, Raynaud's phenomena, hypertension, hypersensitivity
7. Miscellaneous		
Dacarbazine	N & V, BM, V	Flu-like syndrome, liver
Procarbazine	N & V, BM, alcohol intolerance	N, hypersensitivity, C
Amsacrine	BM, V,	C
L-asparaginase	Hypersensitivity, coagulopathy	Hypoalbuminaemia, hyperglycaemia, CNS, hyperamylasemia, liver

SIADH, syndrome of inappropriate antidiuretic hormone. BM, bone marrow. N & V, nausea and vomiting. M, mucositis. V, vesicant. A, alopecia. N, neurotoxicity. C, cardiac. (HD), high-dose regimen.

Table 5.3 Pharmacokinetics and specific information. i.v., intravenous. i.a., intra-arterial. i.m., intramuscular. s.c., subcutaneous. p.o., oral. i.t., intrathecal. M, metabolized. R, renal.

Agent	Routes of administration	Elimination	
Methotrexate (MTX)	i.v., i.m., i.t., p.o.	R	Reverse cytotoxic effect by giving reduced folates, e.g. folinic acid. Hyperhydration and urinary alkalinization is necessary with high-dose i.v. therapy. Erratic bio-availability at high oral doses. Distribution to and slow exit from 'third spaces', e.g. pleural fluid prolongs terminal phase of drug clearance and can increase toxicity. CSF concentrations 1/30 that of plasma following i.v. dose.
5-Fluorouracil (5-FU)	p.o., i.v., i.a.	M	Plasma levels vary considerably after p.o. administration. Good penetration into CSF and third spaces. Rapid metabolic breakdown in liver and extrahepatic tissues to dihydrofluorouracil (80%); 20% excreted unchanged in urine. Possibly greater efficacy when given with folinic acid (stabilizes drug/thymidylate synthetase complex).
6-Mercaptopurine (6-MP)	p.o.	M	Erratic oral absorption and first pass metabolism, less than 50% reaches systemic circulation, 50% excreted in urine. Individual methyltransferase levels influence concentration of active metabolites. Allopurinol may increase toxicity by reducing inactive metabolites.
6-Thioguanine (6-TG)	p.o.	M	Metabolized by methylation of the sulphur substituent. Excreted in urine and faeces.
Cytarabine	i.t., i.v., s.c., i.m.	M	Rapid distribution into total body water following i.v. dose and rapid deamination in liver, plasma and peripheral granulocytes. 70% excreted in urine as inactive metabolite (ara-U). Usually given as continuous infusion or repeated boluses because of rapid deactivation. CSF concentrations 50% that in plasma but can be given i.t. Minimal deamination in the CSF prolongs active half-life.
Nitrogen mustard	i.v., topical	M	Very unstable in aqueous solution, spontaneous decomposition to reactive intermediates.

Table 5.3 *continued*

Agent	Routes of administration	Elimination	
Cyclophosphamide	i.v., p.o.	M R	Metabolized by hepatic mixed-function oxidase system and converted to active metabolites in peripheral tissues. Haemorrhagic cystitis can be prevented by hyperhydration and the concurrent use of MESNA, which converts acrolein to an inert thioether. 90% bioavailability p.o.
Ifosfamide	i.v.	M R	Hepatic activation with excretion of metabolites in the urine. Usually given as 3–5 day i.v. infusion with an equivalent dose of MESNA. Renal tubular damage may lead to Fanconi syndrome. Encephalopathy reversible if detected early but can be fulminant if drug is not discontinued. Greater incidence in patients with renal impairment.
Melphalan	p.o., i.v.	M	15% excreted unchanged in the urine; dose reduction is necessary with impaired renal function. High-dose therapy possible because of dose–response relationship and relative lack of non-haematological toxicity.
Chlorambucil	p.o.	M	Eliminated following metabolic transformation.
Busulphan	p.o.	M	Cumulative bone-marrow toxicity may lead to bone-marrow 'burn-out'. Useful in high-dose combination due to lack of extramedullary toxicity, although seizures may occur if prophylactic anticonvulsant not given.
CCNU BCNU	p.o. i.v.	M M	Highly lipid soluble and therefore readily cross blood-brain barrier to give CNS concentrations of 30% that in plasma. Very short half-life with rapid hepatic metabolism. Delayed myelosuppression.
Cisplatin	i.v.	R	Rapid initial clearance from plasma followed by slow decline associated with extensive binding to serum proteins and tissues. Urinary excretion following glomerular filtration of unbound platinum coordinate complexes. Renal toxicity secondary to tubular damage can be reduced by hyperhydration with hypertonic saline and mannitol-induced diuresis.

Table 5.3 *continued*

Agent	Routes of administration	Elimination	
Carboplatin	i.v.	R	Less extensively protein-bound than cisplatin. 70% of administered dose excreted in the urine as intact drug. Renal clearance of drug is closely correlated with glomerular filtration rate. Dose calculations should be made according to renal function as the AUC (and hence the toxicity and therapeutic efficacy of the drug) is dictated primarily by the pretreatment GFR. Not nephrotoxic at standard dose, hyperhydration not required.
Vincristine	i.v.	M	70% excretion in faeces primarily as metabolites following hepatic metabolism and biliary excretion. Reduce dose in patients with hepatic dysfunction. Possibly increased toxicity in infants.
Vinblastine	i.v.	M	10% faecal excretion. Reduce dose in patients with hepatic dysfunction.
Vindesine	i.v.	M	
Etoposide	i.v., p.o.	M, R	Variable bioavailability (~50%), therefore need to give twice the i.v. dose p.o. Lipid-soluble, but poor penetration to the CNS. 30% excretion as unchanged drug. Clearance is lowered and terminal half-life prolonged in patients with renal insufficiency. Dose modification based on creatine clearance has been suggested.
Teniposide	i.v.	M, R	Metabolic elimination is primary route of elimination.
Doxorubicin Daunorubicin	i.v. i.v.	M M	} Hepatic metabolism to doxorubicinol and excretion in bile and urine. Dose reduction essential with hepatic dysfunction. Cardiotoxicity related to total cumulative dose. Can be reduced by administration of repeated small doses (weekly) or continuous infusions.
Epirubicin	i.v.	M	Reportedly less cardiotoxic than doxorubicin.
Actinomycin D	i.v.	M, R	Rapid plasma clearance secondary to tissue uptake and DNA binding. Excretion of

Table 5.3 *continued*

Agent	Routes of administration	Elimination	
			unchanged drug in bile and urine following slow release from tissue pools.
Bleomycin	i.v., i.m., s.c.	R	Biphasic plasma elimination curve. Drug excreted unchanged in urine. Pharmacokinetics altered markedly in patients with abnormal renal function, therefore reduce dose. May be injected into pleural, pericardial, or peritoneal space to control malignant effusions. 50% intracavitary dose enters systemic circulation. Pulmonary toxicity proportional to total dose, more common in patients with underlying lung disease, previous thoracic radiotherapy impaired renal function, e.g. cisplatin treated, and following exposure to high oxygen concentrations.
Dacarbazine	i.v.	M	Hepatic activation, 50% drug excreted unchanged in urine. Spontaneous decomposition in light.
Procarbazine	p.o.	M	Microsomal metabolic activation. Inhibitor of monoamine oxidase, therefore avoid food containing tyramine.
Amsacrine	i.v.	M	Metabolized in the liver, conjugated with GSH and excreted in bile. Decrease dose with liver dysfunction. Highly protein-bound.
L-asparaginase	i.m., s.c., i.v.		Reduced risk of anaphylaxis with i.m. administration. Often given on an alternate-day basis, over 2–3 weeks to maintain plasma levels.
Hydroxyurea	i.v., p.o.	R, M	

cells into cycle (recruitment), thus increasing the susceptibility of cells to subsequent chemotherapy.

Tumours tend to be become more heterogeneous after exposure to cytotoxic agents, containing clones of cells that develop or are inherently resistant to the action of the drug. This is the basis behind combination chemotherapy, whereby several different drugs with differing mechanisms of action are used concurrently to reduce the risk of developing a population of predominantly resistant cells.

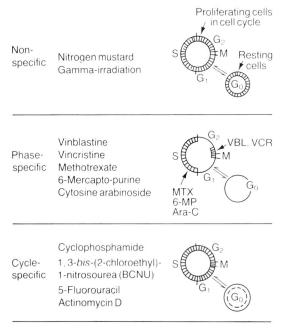

Non-specific	Nitrogen mustard Gamma-irradiation	
Phase-specific	Vinblastine Vincristine Methotrexate 6-Mercapto-purine Cytosine arabinoside	
Cycle-specific	Cyclophosphamide 1,3-*bis*-(2-chloroethyl)-1-nitrosourea (BCNU) 5-Fluorouracil Actinomycin D	

Fig. 5.1 Phases of cell cycle in dividing cell. The sites of action of phase- and cycle-specific agents are listed.

Tumour resistance usually arises following a 'genetic event' within the tumour cell, e.g. gene amplification, mutation, deletion or translocation. This in turn results in a number of different mechanisms of resistance, e.g. impaired drug transport, reduced intracellular drug activation, increased drug efflux.

The concept of drug scheduling is based on the need for recovery of critical normal tissues (e.g. bone marrow and intestinal or oral mucosa) between courses of chemotherapy. Tumour cells generally have less capacity for repair and repopulation following chemotherapy than normal cells, but if the interval between treatments is too short, normal stem cells will not have recovered sufficiently, resulting in cumulative toxicity. If the interval is too long, tumour cell recovery between cycles will allow the tumour to remain static or even increase in size.

5.3 MECHANISMS OF ACTION

5.3.1 ANTIMETABOLITES

Because of their resemblance to naturally occurring substances, these drugs act as fraudulent components in the synthesis of DNA and RNA.

(a) Antifolates

Although there has been much work into the development of new, 'improved' antifolates in recent years, methotrexate (MTX) remains the most commonly used agent in this class (Fig. 5.2). The synthesis of purine nucleotides, thymidylate and the amino acids serine and methionine is dependent on the presence of reduced folates, i.e. tetrahydrofolates (FH$_4$) (Fig. 5.3).

Dihydrofolate reductase (DHFR) is the enzyme responsible for maintaining the intracellular pool of FH$_4$. MTX is a potent inhibitor of DHFR and causes an accumulation of folate in the inactive oxidized form, thus inhibiting *de novo* purine synthesis with consequent cell death. The depletion of the reduced folate pool resulting from the inhibition of DHFR is only partial, however, and recently several other mechanisms of cytotoxic action

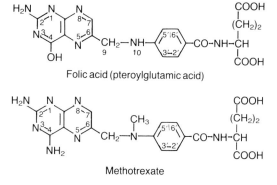

Fig. 5.2 Comparative structure of folic acid and the antagonist methotrexate showing the close homology.

94

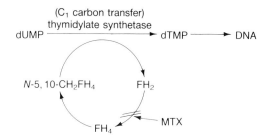

Fig. 5.3 Site of action of methotrexate within the pathway of folate metabolism. FH_2, dihydrofolate. FH_4, tetrahydrofolate. dUMP, deoxyuridine monophospate. dTMP, deoxythymidine monophosphate.

of MTX and its metabolites have become apparent.

The formation of polyglutamated metabolites of MTX and its derivatives within the cell results in the inhibition of a variety of folate-dependent enzymes in addition to DHFR. For example, thymidylate synthase and 5-aminoimidazole carboximide ribotide transformylase. Similarly, these enzymes appear to be inhibited by the folate by-products (e.g. dihydrofolate and 10-formyl dihydrofolate) that accumulate following DHFR inhibition.

There are a number of different mechanisms by which tumour cells can develop resistance to MTX:

1. Amplification of the DHFR gene results in increased levels of intracellular DHFR, thus overcoming the MTX inhibition of the enzyme.
2. The affinity of DHFR for MTX can be reduced by minor alterations in the structure of the enzyme.
3. Defective polyglutamation of MTX and its derivatives.
4. Impaired transport of MTX into the cell.
5. Salvage and re-use of preformed nucleosides that are transported into the cell and converted to nucleotides, thus bypassing the inhibition by MTX.

(b) Fluoropyrimidines

5-Fluorouracil (5-FU) remains the only uracil analogue in general clinical use. This drug requires intracellular conversion to its active components, which include fluorouridine triphosphate (FUTP) and 5-fluorodeoxy uridylate(5-FdUMP). The former is incorporated into nuclear RNA and inhibits RNA processing and function. The latter binds to the enzyme thymidylate synthase (TS), thus inhibiting the formation of deoxythimidine triphosphate (dTTP), an essential precursor of DNA. Resistance can develop following depletion of the enzymes required for 5-FU activation or following amplification of the TS gene, resulting in increased levels of the enzyme.

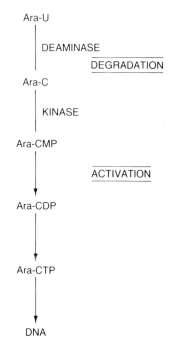

Fig. 5.4 Metabolism of cytarabine (ara-C). Both ara-C and its metabolite deoxycytosine monophosphate (ara-CMP) are inactivated by deaminase. A series of kinase enzymes metabolizes ara-C through the monophosphate (ara-CMP), and diphosphate (ara-CDP) compounds to the active triphosphate metabolite (ara-CTP).

(c) Cytarabine

Cytarabine (cytosine arabinoside, ara-C) is structurally very similar to the naturally occurring cytidine nucleoside, deoxycytidine. It is metabolized inside the cell by salvage pathway enzymes to its active form, ara-CTP, and competes with deoxycytidine triphosphate (dCTP), thus inhibiting DNA polymerase and interfering with DNA replication. It is also incorporated into DNA and interferes with DNA transcription. Ara-C is thus cell-cycle specific (killing cells selectively during the S phase of the cell cycle) and has its greatest effect during periods of rapid DNA synthesis (Fig. 5.4).

The exact mechanisms of resistance to cytarabine have not as yet been clearly defined. Possibilities include the depletion of activating enzymes, an increase in the intracellular pool of dCTP and increased ability of tumour cells to eliminate ara-CTP.

(d) Purine analogues

The purine analogues 6-mercaptopurine (6-MP) and 6-thioguanine (6-TG) differ from the purine nucleosides hypoxanthine and guanine only by the substitution of a thiol group in the place of a 6-hydroxyl group in the basic purine nucleus. Following intracellular activation by their conversion to 'fraudulent' nucleotides they are incorporated into DNA and result in faulty DNA replication and the development of strand breaks, the frequency of which is correlated with toxicity. They also appear to inhibit *de novo* purine biosynthesis by enzyme inhibition. 6-MP resistant cells lack the activating enzyme hypoxanthine guanine phosphoribosyl transferase (HGPRTase) (Fig. 5.5).

9-β-D-arabinofuranosyladenine (ara-A) is an analogue of adenosine which, as a triphosphate, ara-ATP, inhibits DNA polymerase. It is however rapidly deactivated *in vivo* by adenosine deaminase. 2'-deoxycoformycin is

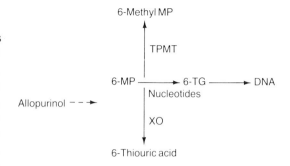

Fig. 5.5 Metabolism of 6-mercaptopurine (6-MP) to either the active 6-thioguanine nucleotides (6-TG) or the inactive 6-methyl mercaptopurine (6-methyl MP) and 6-thiouric acid. Allopurinol blocks xanthine oxidase (XO) and will increase toxicity. High levels of thiopurine methyltransferase (TPMT) reduce the number of 6-TG nucleotides and thus cytotoxicity.

a potent inhibitor of adenosine deaminase and greatly enhances the antitumour potency of ara-A.

5.3.2 ALKYLATING AGENTS

Nitrogen mustard was the first cytotoxic agent to come into clinical use but is now rarely used because of toxicity. Cyclophosphamide and its analogue ifosfamide are active against a wide range of solid and haematological malignancies. Both these agents are metabolized to their active forms (Figs 5.6 and 5.7). Other commonly used alkylating agents include chlorambucil, melphalan and busulphan.

The cytotoxicity of the alkylating agents is thought to relate to their ability to form covalent bonds with bases in DNA. Most have chemical structures which in aqueous solution form positively charged carbonium ions that bind to nucleophilic sites on nucleic acids. Ninety per cent of this alkylation occurs at the N7 position of guanine. It is not fully understood how the process of alkylation results in cytotoxicity but it is thought that

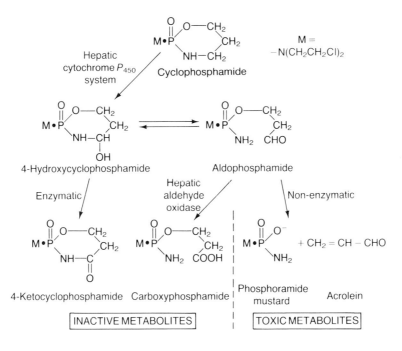

Fig. 5.6 Metabolism of cyclophosphamide to its inactive metabolites, the cytotoxic mustard derivative and the bladder-toxic acrolein.

the crosslinking and strand breaks in DNA that develop following exposure of cells to these agents interferes with the integrity of DNA, causing misreading of the DNA code and inhibition of DNA, RNA and protein synthesis.

The activity of alkylating agents within cells can be inhibited by conjugation to glutathione (GSH) or to other thiol-containing proteins. The glutathione system appears to be a major mechanism of resistance to alkylation mediated by glutathione-S-transferases (GST), multifunctional enzymes that catalyse the conjugation of GSH with electrophilic substances. It has been suggested that detection of high levels of GST or over-expression of the GST gene may correlate with drug resistance. Another mechanism of resistance involves

the rapid repair of DNA damage by DNA repair enzymes. Although the various alkylating agents have a common mechanism of action they are not uniformly crossresistant.

5.3.3 NITROSOUREAS

The nitrosoureas are generally classed as alkylating agents, but differ somewhat in their mode of action. In aqueous solution they are broken down into two reactive intermediates. The first forms a reactive chloroethyl carbonium ion that binds to a single strand of DNA, producing a second reactive site that results in DNA crosslinking. The second reactive species is an isocyanate that is thought to deplete GSH, inhibit DNA repair and interfere with RNA maturation by

97

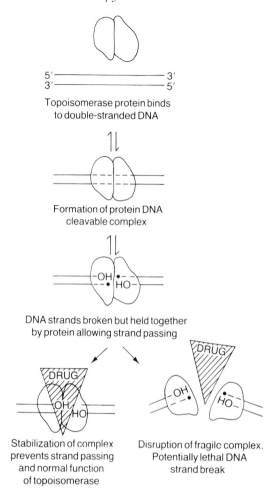

Topoisomerase protein binds
to double-stranded DNA

Formation of protein DNA
cleavable complex

DNA strands broken but held together
by protein allowing strand passing

Stabilization of complex
prevents strand passing
and normal function
of topoisomerase

Disruption of fragile complex.
Potentially lethal DNA
strand break

Fig. 5.7 Schematic representation of the action of topoisomerase II and the effect of drugs such as etoposide on its function.

a carbamoylation reaction. The alkylation reaction is probably the most important, however, in that some compounds in this class lack carbamoylation activity but still retain antimitotic activity.

These agents do not share crossresistance with the classical alkylators, although resistance can be similarly attributed to increased levels of GST and DNA repair enzymes.

5.3.4 PLATINUM COMPOUNDS

Cisplatin (cis (II) platinum diaminedichloride) is a tetravalent heavy metal compound with two chloride ions bound in transposition to two amine groups. Cisplatin can react with DNA or other nucleophilic sites (e.g. RNA or protein) only after at least one chloride ligand is replaced by water generating the positively charged reactive electrophilic monoaquo species. This occurs most readily in an environment of low chloride concentration, e.g. intracellularly or in urine. Following the replacement of both chloride groups a diaquo form is produced which forms both intra- and interstrand crosslinks, as seen with the alkylators. The cytotoxicity of cisplatin has been correlated with the formation of DNA interstrand crosslinks, changes in DNA conformation and inhibition of DNA synthesis. The interaction of cisplatin with two adjacent guanine nucleotides has been shown to block DNA polymerase.

Platinum compounds do not share crossresistance with the classic alkylating agents or nitrosoureas. Some platinum-resistant cell lines have been shown to form DNA crosslinks at a reduced rate, suggesting either slower drug uptake, impaired activation or rapid repair of DNA damage. Metallothioneine is a protein necessary for the detoxification of heavy metals in cells. Platinum resistance has been linked to high intracellular levels of this protein as well as to increased levels of glutathione and glutathione-S-transferase, which may also result in increased platinum detoxification.

Carboplatin (cis-diamino 1,1-cyclobutane-dicarboxiplatinum (II)) is an analogue of cisplatin that is structurally related but has a bidentate dicarboxylate chelate ligand replacing the two chlorine atoms. This drug has been shown to be as effective as cisplatin in several tumour types but is considerably less toxic. The two compounds appear to have the same mechanism of action and differ only in the kinetics of their interaction with DNA. Not surprisingly, tumours resistant to cisplatin are generally also resistant to carboplatin.

5.3.5 VINCA ALKALOIDS

The vinca alkaloids (vincristine, vinblastine and vindesine) are natural products derived from the plant *Vinca rosea*. Their mechanism of action relates to their ability to bind to tubulin, thus interfering with the function of the mitotic spindle during cell division and arresting cells in the metaphase of mitosis. The protein tubulin is found in the cytoplasm of all cells and is important for maintaining the cytoskeleton and for the formation of the mitotic spindle along which chromosomes migrate during mitosis. The vinca-tubulin complex appears to be more stable in tumour tissue compared to normal tissues which may contribute some selectivity towards malignant cells.

Mutations in tubular structure can result in altered drug binding and lead to drug resistance. The primary mechanism of resistance to the vinca alkaloids is probably due to decreased intracellular drug accumulation. This results from the increased efflux of drug secondary to the over-expression of a gene that codes for a P-glycoprotein efflux pump found in the cell membrane. An energy-dependent process, this can be blocked by inhibitors of ATP. The mechanism of multi-drug resistance (MDR), whereby tumour cells are resistant to several structurally unrelated drugs without necessarily having been exposed to them, is explained in this way.

The gene coding for the P-glycoprotein pump (MDR_1 gene) has been shown to be over expressed in certain multidrug-resistant cell lines. Various drugs can reverse MDR *in vitro*, including the calcium channel blockers verapamil, nifedipine and perhexilene and the calmodulin inhibitors (perfenazine and cyclosporin A). Several clinical trials are currently being undertaken to determine whether these agents might effectively overcome resistance *in vivo*.

5.3.6 EPIPODOPHYLLOTOXINS

The two commonly used epipodophyllotoxins, etoposide (VP-16) and teniposide (VM-26), are synthetic glycosidic derivatives of podophyllotoxin, an extract from the mandrake plant. Their precise mechanism of action is unknown. Whereas podophyllotoxin inhibits the assembly of microtubules and arrests cells in metaphase, as with the vinca alkaloids, etoposide prevents cells from entering mitosis and blocks cell-cycle progression in the late S and G_2 phases. The principal target of both etoposide and teniposide is cellular DNA and two mechanisms have been proposed to explain their cytotoxicity. The first involves the nuclear enzyme topoisomerase II, which functions to facilitate the relaxation, unwinding, controlled cleavage and rejoining of the DNA helix during replication and transcription. The enzyme forms a bridge across the double-stranded DNA break until continuity is restored. Topoisomerase inhibitors stabilize the DNA/protein 'cleavable complex' so that the normally rapid processes of strand division, strand passing and rejoining are arrested (Fig. 5.7).

Enzyme activity is greatest in metabolically active, rapidly dividing tissues. A definite relationship has been demonstrated between the production of strand breaks and the cytotoxicity of these agents, although DNA breaks can be detected at concentrations of drug well below those required to show inhibition of DNA synthesis. Moreover, strand breaks can be repaired rapidly after removal of the drug, suggesting that other mechanisms of cytotoxicity are involved. A second mechanism of action results from the metabolic activation of the drugs, either by cytochrome P_{450} or by peroxidases, to form highly reactive free radical intermediates that bind directly to DNA.

Resistance to the epipodophyllotoxins is therefore probably multifactorial. Possible mechanisms include:

1. decreased formation of topoisomerase II induced strand breaks secondary to changes in the amount of the enzyme present or its ability to function following mutational change;
2. increased repair of DNA strand breaks;
3. lack of drug activation to reactive species;
4. increased detoxification of reactive intermediates;
5. decreased drug accumulation secondary to increased drug efflux due to amplification of the MDR exit pump.

5.3.7 ANTITUMOUR ANTIBIOTICS.

These compounds were originally derived from bacteria and fungi and have both antimicrobial and antitumour activity. Subsequently, a number of analogues have been synthesized. The group therefore consists of a diverse range of drugs which differ in structure and mechanisms of action.

(a) Anthracyclines

Daunorubicin and doxorubicin are the anthracyclines most commonly used in clinical practice. Epirubicin (4'-epidoxorubicin) is structurally very similar and the best known of the many anthracycline analogues.

These compounds have a characteristic structure consisting of a planar anthracycline ring attached to an amino sugar. The planar ring allows the molecule to intercalate DNA, i.e. to insert itself within the DNA helix. The ring lies perpendicular to the long axis of the DNA helix and is stabilized by the binding of the amino group to the sugar phosphate backbone of DNA. This reaction is not, however, thought to be responsible for the cytotoxicity of these agents. There is consid-erable debate about the primary mechanism of action of these drugs. It is possible that there are multiple mechanisms of cell kill and that, in any one tumour cell line or tissue, one or other mechanism may predominate. There is good evidence that interference with topoisomerase II is responsible for the antitumour activity in some cell lines but the formation of free radicals is probably equally important. The anthracyclines can undergo both one- and two-electron reduction via a wide range of NADP reductases to yield the corresponding semi-quinone or dihydroquinone respectively. These in turn can reduce molecular oxygen to superoxide and/or hydrogen peroxide which may yield a hydroxyl radical that causes direct tissue injury. It has been shown in a number of cell systems that iron must be present for anthracycline free radical formation to result in significant damage. The iron drug complex is very reactive in catalyzing a variety of free radical reactions. This explains why superoxide dismutase, catalase, hydroxyl radical scavengers and iron chelators all lessen the toxicity of doxorubicin.

Tumour tissue with *in vitro* resistance to doxorubicin has been shown to express P-glycoprotein whereas only a small number of P-glycoprotein-negative tumours were resistant. Several experimental systems such as these have implicated the role of the MDR mechanism in clinical resistance to anthracyclines. Enhanced neutralization of anthracycline-induced free radicals by the glutathione redox system may also be involved.

Mitoxantrone is a synthetic compound classed as an anthracedione and is a hydroxy-quinone with a similar ring structure to the anthracyclines. It does not, however, cause free radical damage but does induce topoisomerase II mediated DNA damage.

(b) Bleomycin

Bleomycin is a mixture of low molecular

weight glycopeptides derived from a fungus. The constituent peptide bleomycin A_2 accounts for the majority of the drug used clinically. Its cytotoxicity results from the ability to bind to and degrade DNA. The molecule consists of a DNA-binding fragment (that binds preferentially to G–T or G–C sequences) and an iron-binding portion at the other end of the molecule. Bound ferrous iron (Fe^{2+}) undergoes spontaneous or enzymatic oxidation to the Fe^{3+} state, thus allowing the formation of active oxygen intermediates such as superoxide or hydroxyl radicals that attack and cleave the DNA strand.

Resistance can be related to enhanced DNA repair. Similarly, intracellular bleomycin-inactivating enzymes may be important determinants of tumour cell sensitivity. Reducing agents such as glutathione are necessary for the reactivation of Fe^{3+}-bleomycin to the active Fe^{2+} state and low glutathione levels may play a role in resistance of tumours to this agent.

(c) Mitomycin C

Mitomycin C alkylates and crosslinks double-stranded DNA following intracellular activation at three potential sites within the molecule. The drug also induces lipid peroxidation through the intermediate of oxygen radicals. Resistance to mitomycin C is poorly characterized, although the MDR system has been implicated in some cell lines.

(d) Actinomycin D

This drug consists of two identical cyclic polypeptides bound to a phenoxazone ring. Following intercalation of the ring structure into the DNA double helix, the polypeptide chains interact with deoxyguanosine and prevent the transcription of DNA blocking both DNA and RNA synthesis. Actinomycin D can

also form single-strand breaks following reduction of the molecule to radical intermediates or via topoisomerase II. The relevance of these strand breaks to the cytotoxicity of the drug is not, however, totally clear.

5.3.8 MISCELLANEOUS AGENTS

(a) Dacarbazine

Dacarbazine (DTIC) is a synthetic compound found by chance to have antimitotic activity. It functions as an alkylating agent following metabolic activation to an active species. In addition, one of the metabolites formed in the process inhibits the incorporation of purine nucleosides into DNA.

(b) Procarbazine

Procarbazine was discovered during a search for new monoamine oxidase inhibitors. Its exact mechanism of action is not completely understood although it is likely to involve alkylation following microsomal metabolic activation.

(c) Amsacrine

Amsacrine (mAMSA) was one of the first agents whose mechanism of action was shown to involve topoisomerase. It forms a tight complex with DNA and topoisomerase II and prevents the resealing of DNA breaks. The cytotoxicity of the drug correlates closely with the production of both single- and double-strand DNA breaks. Drug resistance appears related to altered topoisomerase II, which no longer cleaves DNA in the presence of amsacrine.

(d) L-asparaginase

This drug has a unique tumour-specific

mechanism of action. L-asparagine is an amino acid synthesized by the transamination of L-aspartic acid by L-asparagine synthetase. Certain malignant cells are unable to synthesize asparagine and rely on the body pool for the supply of this amino acid. L-asparaginase converts asparagine to aspartic acid and ammonia, thus depriving tumour cells of an essential nutrient. Its antitumour effect is therefore related to the depletion of circulating pools of L-asparagine, whereas resistance is related to an increase in L-asparagine synthetase activity following either mutation or enzyme induction.

(e) Hydroxyurea

Hydroxyurea is an analogue of urea. It acts by inhibiting the ribonucletide reductase enzyme system, thereby preventing DNA synthesis. It is one of the few specific S phase inhibitors.

(f) Corticosteroids

Steroid therapy is used for symptom relief, e.g. the management of raised intracranial pressure and bone pain. There is also a direct antitumour effect, however, particularly in haematological malignancies, via mechanisms that are not clearly understood but which may involve glucocorticoid receptors on the tumour cell.

5.4 CURRENT ISSUES

5.4.1 DEVELOPMENT AND USE OF ANALOGUES

In the last decade there have been few, if any, effective anticancer drugs with novel mechanisms of action. (Research directions in this field are reviewed in Chapter 25). This has led to the increased development and market-ing of analogues that differ little in terms of their anticancer spectrum but may have different toxicity profiles.

Three such drugs are ifosfamide, carboplatin and epirubicin. The minor structural variations compared to their predecessors are shown in Figs 5.8–5.10.

(a) Ifosfamide

Ifosfamide (Fig. 5.8), an oxazofospharine, was originally studied in adults more than 20 years ago but, because of the severe cystitis it produced, it did not enter clinical use following initial phase I and II studies. With the development of MESNA (sodium-2-mercapto-ethane sulphate) uroprotection the risk of cystitis was dramatically reduced. The advantage of ifosfamide compared with cyclophosphamide appears to be a superior therapeutic index with less myelosupression in relation to cytotoxicity. Initial phase II studies in children showed encouraging activity in a wide range of tumour types and there were responses in patients who had failed or progressed on conventional doses of cyclophosphamide (1–1.25 g/m^2) (Pinkerton, *et al.*, 1985; de Kraker and Voute, 1984). This led to the widespread introduction of ifosfamide for the management of soft tissue sarcomas, Ewing's sarcoma, brain tumours, leukaemia and lymphoma, and malignant germ cell tumours (Brade *et al.*, 1987). In recent years it has become clear that, although this drug may be less myelotoxic, thus allowing dose escalation, it has significant nephrotoxicity (Skinner *et al.*, 1990). This predominantly affects tubular function although glomerular function may also deteriorate on treatment. This toxicity appears to be related to age, dose and cumulative dose and in some patients a debilitating Fanconi syndrome has been reported. Only one single prospective randomized study in adults with sarcomas has been performed, which showed a marginal response advantage to ifosfamide,

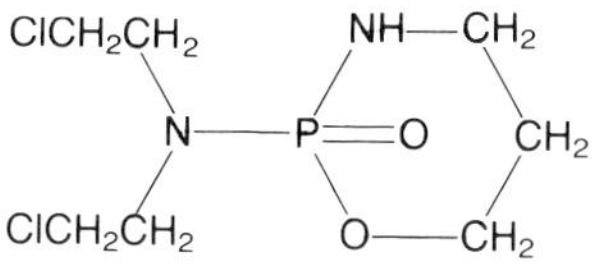

ClCH₂CH₂ ... (chemical structure)

Cyclophosphamide

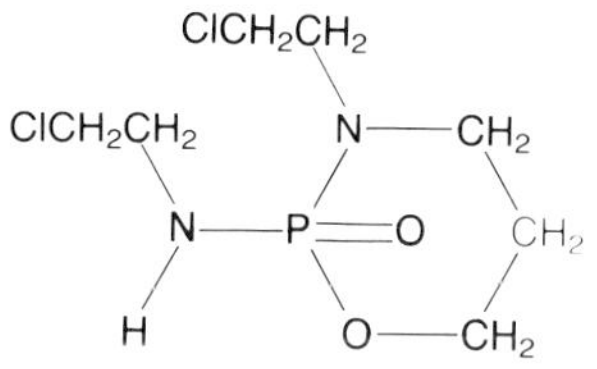

Ifosfamide

NH₃ Cl Pt NH₃ Cl (a)

NH₃ O—CO CH₂ ... (b)

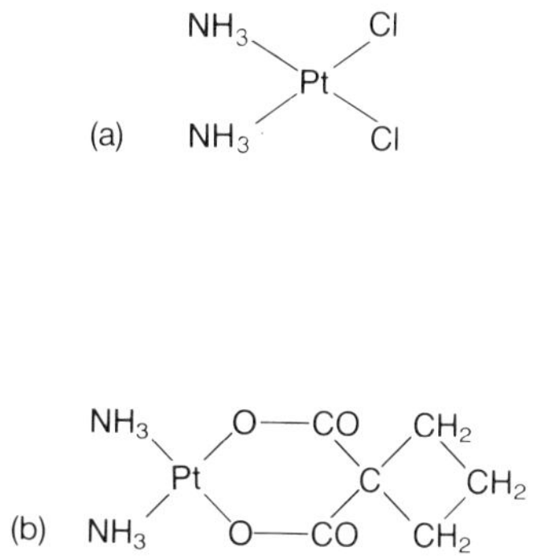

Fig. 5.9 Comparative structures of (a) cisplatin and (b) carboplatin.

Fig. 5.8 Structural similarities of cyclophosphamide and ifosfamide.

although the dose of cyclophosphamide given was comparatively small (Bramwell *et al.*, 1986). There has been no study comparing higher doses of cyclophosphamide, i.e. 2–3 g/m², which are tolerable with modern supportive care, particularly with the recent introduction of bone marrow growth factors.

Such studies are urgently required as the expense of ifosfamide, the inconvenience of giving a 3–5 d schedule that usually requires inpatient admission and concern about the long-term renal effects all weigh against its continued use unless there is clearly a superior antitumour effect (Shaw and Eden, 1990).

(b) Carboplatin

The nephrotoxicity and ototoxicity of cisplatin has been widely studied in both adults and children. This is related to dose, cumulative dose and method of drug administration. Despite all preventative measures a significant loss of high-tone hearing and a decline in glomerular filtration (^{51}CR EDTA clearance) is almost inevitable. Concern about this has led to the development and introduction of the analogue carboplatin (Fig. 5.9). This

drug is, at conventional doses, devoid of these toxicities, although both hearing and renal dysfunction have been reported at high doses (> 1 g/m²).

Unfortunately, the drug is significantly more myelosuppressive than cisplatin. Unlike the situation with ifosfamide, there are studies, for example in ovarian cancer and malignant germ cell tumours, which demonstrate equivalent therapeutic efficacy between the parent compound and its analogue, either alone or when combined with other myelosuppressive agents such as etoposide and cyclophosphamide (Gore *et al.*, 1989; Harstrick *et al.*, 1989). Compared to cisplatin, dose escalation is limited by myelosuppression and it is possible that the consequent antitumour effect is inferior. Moreover, because carboplatin kinetics are markedly affected by renal function, a simple dosage schedule based on surface area may lead to the undertreatment of small children with high EDTA clearance or conversely to excessive toxicity in patients with impaired renal function. (Calvert *et al.*, 1989). There have, however, never been randomized studies comparing carboplatin and cisplatin in any childhood tumour, although its introduction into first-line therapy for malignant germ cell tumours is logical on the basis of the adult data available. Because of patient numbers it is unlikely that such randomized studies will ever be possible but it is at least desirable that there is adequate phase II information regarding responses to carboplatin in other tumours where cisplatin is used, such as soft tissue sarcomas, brain tumours, neuroblastoma, osteosarcoma and hepatoblastoma. Although such studies have demonstrated encouraging activity in primitive neuroectodermal tumours and neuroblastoma, adequate information in other tumour types is awaited (Pinkerton *et al.*, 1989).

(c) Epirubicin

Epirubicin (Fig. 5.10) has replaced doxorubicin in some protocols for non-Hodgkin's lymphoma, Hodgkin's disease and soft tissue sarcomas (Ganzina, 1983). This drug was developed to provide an anthracycline of comparable antitumour efficacy with reduced cardiotoxicity. Prospective trials in adults incorporating detailed cardiac function studies and endomyocardial biopsy studies have shown that the drug is significantly less cardiotoxic (Jain *et al.*, 1985; Torti *et al.*, 1986). Unfortunately, to achieve comparable antitumour effect a higher dose is required than with the parent compound and consequently this advantage is reduced somewhat but still exists. This has led to the use of very high-dose epirubicin, i.e. up to 150 mg/m², in pulsed regimens for sarcomas. This has not been associated with unacceptable cardiotox-

icity and may have a therapeutic advantage. In chemosensitive tumours such as lymphomas and Hodgkin's disease, where the cure rates are high, the replacement of doxorubicin by epirubicin at conventional doses may be justified by a probable reduction in late cardiac toxicity.

5.4.2 IS THERE A ROLE FOR ROUTINE PHARMACOKINETIC STUDIES?

The routine measurement of serum MTX levels following administration of high-dose MTX is essential for the safe use of this strategy and of value in calculating the dose of folinic acid required. Details of serum or plasma levels after enteral and parenteral administration of most, if not all, of the agents currently in use in paediatric oncology are known. The number of compartments within which the drug is distributed, the primary organ involved in drug elimination, mechanisms of drug metabolism and elimination half-lives, have been determined. What is the clinical application of most of this information? Can these data be used to predict the likely efficacy of the drug or to predict the likelihood and the nature of organ toxicity or to provide a rational basis for the scheduling of drug administration?

In vitro studies with cell lines may provide a rough guide to the concentration required for cytotoxicity. Extrapolation to the *in vivo* situation where drug distribution and metab-

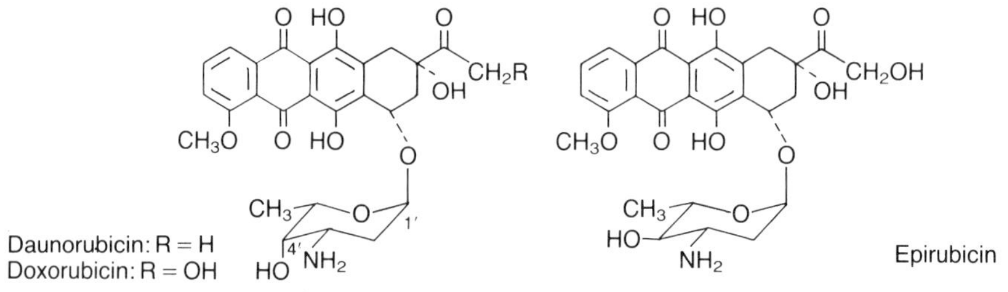

Fig. 5.10 Structures of the anthracyclines daunorubicin, doxorubicin and epirubicin.

olism occurs is difficult. Attempts to correlate *in vivo* with *in vitro* chemosensitivity using clonogenic assays, dye exclusion techniques and, more recently, the toluidine dye (MTT) assay have been of limited use (Von Hoff, *et al.*, 1990; Weisenthal and Lippman, 1985). There are, however, suggestions that both AUC and elimination half-life may correlate with response in the case of MTX and 6-MP in leukaemia treatment (Evans *et al.*, 1986; Koren *et al.*, 1990). This has not been demonstrated in any childhood solid tumour.

Although knowledge about tissue distribution and metabolic pathways of a drug are essential, prediction of toxicity is in general derived from clinical phase I and II studies rather than from pharmacokinetic characteristics. The relationship between drug scheduling or kinetic profile and either toxicity or efficacy needs to be clarified for many drugs. In the case of cytarabine prolonged infusion schedules have been shown to be more effective but also clearly more toxic. With high-dose MTX very large pulsed doses with folinic acid rescue can be given whereas prolonged low-dose oral therapy leads to mucosal toxicity (Pinkerton, 1987). It is important that future phase I and II studies build in questions regarding optimal scheduling.

The subject of pharmacogenetics is an expanding area of interest. 'Aldehyde dehydrogenase phenotype' appears to be linked with the metabolism of cyclophosphamide and probably ifosfamide and to lead to variations in the amount of active metabolite produced (Hadida Al-Hakam *et al.*, 1988). Similarly the thiopurine methyltransferase (TPMT) level will influence the conversion of 6-MP to an inactive metabolite (Fig 5.5). This appears to be sex-linked and high levels of TPMT correlate with treatment failure (Lennard and Lilleyman, 1989). The gene for bleomycin hydroxylase has recently been cloned and this may give a guide to the likelihood of drug toxicity (Sebti *et al.*, 1989). Work is underway looking at the relationship of cytochrome P_{450} and the active metabolism of a variety of anticancer drugs. In this way it may be possible to modify chemotherapy on the basis of predicted metabolism.

5.4.3 IS MULTIDRUG-RESISTANT PHENOTYPE RELEVANT IN CHILDHOOD TUMOURS?

The description of multidrug resistance (MDR) involving crossresistance between agents including vinblastine, vincristine, doxorubicin, daunorubicin, mitoxantrone, actinomycin D, etoposide and teniposide was followed by the cloning of the MDR gene responsible for this phenomenon (Goldstein *et al.*, 1989). Overexpression of this gene in certain tissues and tumour types has been demonstrated using Northern blotting and immunohistochemistry. The initial enthusiasm, with suggestions that MDR overexpression would correlate with chemosensitivity, have been somewhat dampened by recent observations that non-malignant tumour infiltrates such as monocytes may stain with MDR probes and normal stroma may also stain positively.

Attempts to reverse multidrug resistance using calcium channel blockers have also thus far been disappointing. Although there is a wealth of information showing the *in vitro* activity of drugs such as verapamil, nifedipine, cyclosporin and the phenothiazines, only verapamil has been shown to have an impact in a limited number of tumour types. Moreover, the dose of verapamil required to reverse MDR is close to or may exceed the threshold for cardiotoxicity (Durie and Dalton, 1988; Dalton *et al.*, 1989).

It may prove difficult to manipulate multidrug resistance in tumours but the demonstration of its existence could be of prognostic value. A striking difference in outcome has been reported in rhabdomyosarcoma with a highly significantly inferior outcome for those patients whose tumours were shown using immunocytochemistry to overexpress the MDR gene. Overexpression has also been described in advanced neuroblastoma (Chan, *et al.*, 1990; Goldstein *et al.*, 1990). It may be that, using this technique, patients should be allocated to treatment regimens containing non-MDR-linked drugs such as cisplatin or the alkylating agents. Alternatively, early dose escalation could be introduced specifically for patients likely to be at higher risk of multidrug resistance.

REFERENCES

Brade, W., Nagel, G.A. and Seeber, S. (eds) (1987) *Ifosfamide in Tumour Therapy*, Karger, Basle, Munich, Paris.

Bramwell, V.H.C., Mouridsen, H.T., Santoro, A. *et al.* (1986) Cyclophosphamide versus ifosfamide: preliminary report of a randomized phase II trial in adult soft tissue sarcomas. *Cancer Chemother. Pharmacol.*, **18**, (suppl 2), 13–6.

Calvert, A.H., Newell, D.R., Gumbrell, L.A. *et al.* (1989) Carboplatin dosage: prospective evaluation of a simple formula based on renal function. *J. Clin. Oncol.*, **7**, 1748–56.

Chan, H.S.L., Thorner, P.S., Haddad, G. and Ling, V. (1990) Immunohistochemical detection of P-glycoprotein: prognostic correlation in soft tissue sarcoma of childhood. *J. Clin. Oncol.*, **8**, 689–704.

Dalton, W.S., Grogan, T.M., Meltzer, P.S. *et al.* (1989) Drug-resistance in multiple myeloma and non-Hodgkin's lymphoma: detection of P-glycoprotein and potential circumvention by addition of verapamil to chemotherapy. *J. Clin. Oncol.*, **7**, 415–24.

de Kraker, J. and Voute, P.A. (1984) Ifosfamide and vincristine in paediatric tumours. A phase II study. *Eur. Paediatr. Haematol. Oncol.*, **1**, 47.

Durie, B.G.M. and Dalton, W.S. (1988) Reversal of drug-resistance in multiple myeloma with verapamil. *Br. J. Haematol.*, **68**, 203–6.

Evans, W.E., Crom, W.R., Abromowitch, M. *et al.* (1986) Clinical pharmacodynamics of high-dose methotrexate in acute lymphocytic leukemia. Identification of a relation between concentration and effect. *N. Engl. J. Med.*, **314**, 471–7.

Ganzina, F. (1983) 4-epi-doxorubicin, a new analogue of doxorubicin: a preliminary overview of preclinical and clinical data. *Cancer Treat. Rev.*, **10**, 1–22.

Goldstein, L.J., Galski, H., Fojo A. *et al.* (1989) Expression of a multidrug resistance gene in human cancers. *J.N.C.I.*, **81**, 116–24.

Goldstein, L.J., Fojo, A.T., Ueda, K. *et al.* (1990) Expression of the multidrug resistance, MDR1, gene in neuroblastomas. *J. Clin. Oncol.*, **8**, 128–36.

Gore, M.E., Fryatt, I., Wiltshaw, E. *et al.* (1989) Cisplatin/carboplatin cross-resistance in ovarian cancer. *Br. J. Cancer*, **60**, 767–9.

Hadidi Al-Hakam, F.A., Coulter, C.E.A. and Idle, J.R. (1988) Phenotypically deficient urinary elimination of carboxycyclophosphamide after cyclophosphamide administration in cancer patients. *Cancer Res.*, **48**, 5167–71.

Harstrick, A., Casper, J., Guba, R. *et al.* (1989) Comparison of the antitumor activity of cisplatin, carboplatin, and iproplatin against established human testicular cancer cell lines in vivo and in vitro. *Cancer*, **63**, 1079–83.

Jain, K.K., Casper E.S., Geller, N.L. *et al.* (1985) A prospective randomized comparison of epirubicin and doxorubicin in patients with advanced breast cancer. *J. Clin. Oncol.*, **3**, 818–26.

Koren G., Ferrazini, G., Sulh, H. *et al.* (1990) Systemic exposure to mercaptopurine as a prognostic factor in acute lymphocytic leukemia in children. *N. Engl. J. Med.*, **323**, 17–21.

Lennard, L. and Lilleyman, J.S. (1989) Variable mercaptopurine metabolism and treatment outcome in childhood lymphoblastic leukemia. *J. Clin. Oncol.*, **7**, 1816–23.

Pinkerton, C.R. (1987) Drug dose escalation in childhood cancer: the cost of cure? *Pediatr. Rev. Commun.*, **2**, 41–54.

Pinkerton, C.R., Rogers, H., James, C. *et al.* (1985) A phase II study of ifosfamide in children with recurrent solid tumours. *Cancer Chemother Rep.*, **15**, 258–62.

Pinkerton, C.R., Lewis I.J., Pearson, A.D.J. *et al.* (1989) Carboplatin or cisplatin? *Lancet*, **ii**, 161.

Sebti, S.M., Mignano, J.E., Jani, J.P. *et al.* (1989) Bleomycin hydrolase: molecular cloning, sequencing, and biochemical studies reveal membership in the cysteine proteinase family. *Biochemistry*, **28**, 6544–8.

Shaw, P.J. and Eden, T. (1990) Ifosfamide in paediatric oncology: tried but not tested? *Lancet*, **335**, 1022–3.

Skinner, R., Pearson, A.D.J., Price, L. *et al.* (1990) Nephrotoxicity after ifosfamide. *Arch. Dis. Child.*, **65**, 732–8.

Torti F.M., Bristow, M.M., Lum, B.L. *et al.* (1986) Cardiotoxicity of epirubicin and doxorubicin: Assessment by endomyocardial biopsy. *Cancer Res.*, **46**, 3722–7.

Von Hoff, D.D., Sandbach, J.F., Clarke G.M. *et al.* (1990) Selection of cancer chemotherapy for a patient by an in vitro assay versus a clinician. *J.N.C.I*, **82**, 110–6.

Weisenthal, L.M. and Lippman, M.E. (1985) Clonogenic and nonclonogenic in vitro chemosensitivity assays. *Cancer Treat. Rep.*, **69**, 615–32.

Chapter 6

Serum markers in tumour diagnosis and treatment

S.J. KELLIE

6.1 INTRODUCTION

The range and clinical applications of biological tumour-associated compounds found in the serum or urine of children with cancer have been refined and expanded during the past three decades. Tumour markers comprise molecules secreted into the circulation by tumour tissue, or they represent host-tissue-derived metabolic or immunologic products in response to neoplasia. This heterogeneous group of biological compounds consists of oncofetal proteins (alpha-fetoprotein, carcinoembryonic antigen), enzymes (neurone-specific enolase, alkaline phosphatase), hormones (human chorionic gonadotropin, catecholamines and their metabolites), carbohydrate antigens (CA125, CA19.9), and others, including neopterin and related compounds, neurotensin, and transcobalamin I.

Biological tumour markers have clinical utility in the differential diagnosis of paediatric tumours, and in detecting residual disease following apparent complete resection, thereby confirming clinical staging and as a means of evaluating response to therapy following surgery, chemotherapy or irradiation. Additionally, the detection of an elevated biological marker may indicate tumour recurrence before this is detected clinically or investigationally. However, tumour markers which are absolutely specific for a particular type of cancer or organ or tissue of origin, or markers which may identify tumour bearing individuals, do not exist. For this reason, the clinical applications of serum markers have been restricted largely to monitoring response to therapy or for detecting recurrence. The specificity and sensitivity of commonly used tumour markers in general paediatric use is suboptimal; the observation of 'false-positive' results in a number of non-malignant conditions and the variable rate of 'false-negative' results in children with cancer underline the importance of carefully evaluating marker results. The clinical applications of tumour markers in screening for cancer in adult or paediatric populations are controversial. Recently, the usefulness of screening whole populations of well infants for occult neuroblastoma using urinary catecholamine metabolites has generated a spirited debate on the economic, social and medical implications of mass screening.

This chapter reviews the range and clinical utility of biological tumour markers found in serum and urine, the role of physiological hormones and 'so-called' prognostic factors in paediatric tumour diagnosis and monitoring. The current status and opposing scientific viewpoints surrounding the controversial issue of screening infant populations for the presence of occult neuroblastoma are presented.

6.2 BIOLOGICAL TUMOUR MARKERS

6.2.1 ALPHA-FETOPROTEIN (AFP)

(a) Historical background

It was Hirszfeld *et al.* (1932) who first suggested the existence of an immunologic relationship between embryonic antigens and cancer tissue. AFP is the most thoroughly characterized oncodevelopmental antigen and serves as an important model of carcinofetal alteration in man. AFP was first described during the investigation of serum proteins in the human fetus by Bergstrand and Czar (1956). Abelev *et al.*'s description (1963) of an oncofetal antigen, immunologically identical to a normal fetal protein, arising in an experimental liver tumour represented the introduction of a potential 'cancer marker' in modern medicine and refocussed attention on the broad issue of carcinofetal reversion in malignancy. However, the biological reasons for observed changes in the structure or concentration of carcinofetal or oncodevelopmental gene products remains poorly understood, although gene activation, gene depression or other regulatory abnormality of protein synthesis have been suggested. Tatarinov (1964) reported high serum AFP concentrations in a patient with hepatocellular carcinoma. Human AFP was subsequently purified and characterized (Nishi, 1970; Alpert *et al.* 1972), and immunochemical studies, again by Nishi, and by Ruoslahti and Seppälä (1979) have shown that serum AFP isolated from human fetuses and from patients with liver tumours is immunologi-

cally identical. Since these early studies, the relationship between AFP production in humans and various physiological states and pathological alterations has been well documented.

Methodologies of AFP measurement have undergone considerable refinement since Abelev *et al.* (1963) first used the double diffusion method. The evolution of increasingly sensitive assays of serum AFP has paralleled this marker's expanding clinical role during the past three decades. Counter electrophoresis with a sensitivity of 0.25 to 0.5 µg/ml was described in 1971, followed by a latex agglutination inhibition technique with a sensitivity of 250 ng/ml in 1974, and immunoautoradiography with a sensitivity of 50 ng/ml in 1971. Radioimmunoelectrophoresis (1976), enzyme-linked immunosorbent assay (ELISA) (1976), and radioimmunoassay (1971), have improved sensitivity of AFP detection to 20 ng/ml, 3 ng/ml and 0.5 ng/ml respectively (Ruoslahti and Seppälä, 1979). These developments have been reflected in improved methods of measuring other tumour markers.

(b) Physiology

Physiological synthesis of AFP occurs in all three fetal tissues. Synthesis occurs in the human fetal yolk sac, hepatocytes and gastrointestinal mucosa during the early first trimester; however, AFP synthesis takes place predominantly in the hepatocytes after the eighth week (Gitlin *et al.*, 1972; Ruoslahti and Seppälä, 1979). AFP reaches a peak serum concentration of 3.0×10^6 ng/ml by the fifteenth week of gestation and declines thereafter, in part due to the rapid increase in fetal size. The AFP level ranges from 2.0×10^4 ng/ml to 5.0×10^4ng/ml at birth, falling to normal adult levels (<20 ng/ml) by approximately eight months of age (Brock *et al.*, 1975; Gitlin, 1975).

The rapid physiological fall in serum AFP

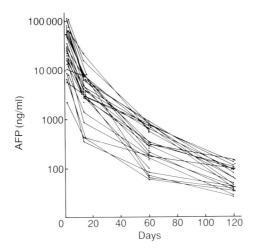

Fig. 6.1 Serum AFP levels of 32 normal babies measured consecutively at 2 or 3 days, 2 weeks, and 2 and 4 months after birth. (Reproduced with the permission of the editor of *Pediatric Research*).

concentration during the first eight months of postnatal life is a potential source of 'false-positive' error in interpretation in well infants in whom physiological elevations of AFP up to 200 times the normal adult range may be

observed. The clinician's dilemma is heightened by the high age-specific incidence of hepatoblastoma, testicular or sacrococcygeal teratomas observed during the first year of life. Fortunately, these neoplasms are most commonly associated with massive elevations of serum markers and this facilitates differentiation of these tumours from physiological elevations. Wu *et al.* (1981) monitored serum AFP levels consecutively from 2–3 days to 4 months after birth in 32 normal babies, and also measured serum AFP concentrations in 116 random specimens from infants with normal liver enzymes to establish age-related normal ranges. His study demonstrated that the half-life of AFP was approximately 5.5 days between birth and 2 weeks of age, 11 days between 2 weeks and 2 months of age, and 33 days between 2 and 4 months of age. Although the rate of decline was similar among paediatric patients of similar ages (Fig. 6.1) individual levels were highly variable and found to be independent of gestational age, weight or type of milk feeds

Table 6.1 Average normal serum AFP of infants at various ages

Age	No.	Mean ± S.D. (ng/ml)
Premature	11	134 734 ± 41 444
Newborn	55	48 406 ± 34 718
Newborn–2 weeks	16	33 113 ± 32 503
2 wk–1 month	43	9 452 ± 12 610
1 month	12	2 654 ± 3 080
2 months	40	323 ± 278
3 months	5	88 ± 87
4 months	31	74 ± 56
5 months	6	46.5 ± 19
6 months	9	12.5 ± 9.8
7 months	5	9.7 ± 7.1
8 months	3	8.5 ± 5.5

Reproduced with the permission of the editor of *Pediatric Research*.

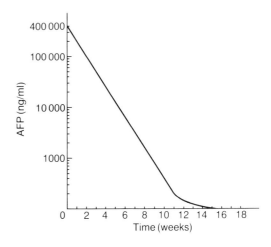

Fig. 6.2 Serum AFP levels following complete resection of an AFP-secreting tumour. The line depicts the expected rate of fall based on a half-life of 7 days.

(Table 6.1). The results indicate that the AFP level reaches adult levels after eight months of age. The change in the rate of AFP degradation during the first month of life implies that a considerable amount of AFP synthesis is maintained after birth. These results, which extend and confirm work by Masseyeff *et al.* (1975) are important in interpreting moderate elevations of serum AFP during the first year of life.

The biological half-life of AFP has been estimated to range from 3.5 to 7 days by serial measurements in children following complete resection of AFP-producing tumours (Gitlin *et al.*, 1966; Walhof *et al.* 1988). Figure 6.2 represents the expected rate of fall of serum AFP based on a half-life of 7 days, plotted on a logarithmic scale. Irrespective of the pretreatment concentration, the expected rate of fall following successful tumour treatment should be parallel to the line, and deviation away from the expected rate of fall should be regarded as evidence of persisting or recurrent AFP-secreting tumour.

AFP is neither specific for cancer of a particular site or histology, nor restricted to tumour-bearing individuals. Non-neoplastic conditions during infancy or later in life may result in elevated AFP concentrations. Elevated levels have been observed during the first six months of life in children with neonatal hepatitis, hepatic injury from biliary atresia, or congestive hepatomegaly (Alpert, 1972). Significant elevations of AFP beyond six months of age have been seen in children with viral hepatitis (Masopust *et al.*, 1970), ataxia-telangectasia (Waldmann *et al.*, 1972) or congential tyrosinosis (Belanger *et al.*, 1972). AFP values in children with benign hepatic disorders tend to be higher than those found in adults with similar pathology (Kew *et al.*, 1973; Bloomer *et al.*, 1975). AFP is not an acute-phase reactant, and, as might be expected, acutely elevated values following hepatic trauma or toxic injury have not been observed (Alpert *et al.*, 1971).

6.2.2. β-HUMAN CHORIONIC GONADOTROPHIC HORMONE (β-hCG)

Physiology

Human chorionic gonadotropin (β-hCG) is a glycoprotein hormone which comprises two dissimilar subunits designated alpha and beta. The alpha subunit of hCG shares structural homology with the alpha subunit of anterior pituitary hormones, including luteinizing hormone, follicle-stimulating hormone and thyroid-stimulating hormone. However, the recognition of antigenically distinct carboxyl terminals on the β chains of these hormones has enabled the development of a specific radioimmunoassay for the determination of the β subunit of hCG without interference from other hormones or the α subunit (Rosen *et al.*, 1975). The sensitivity of the widely available radioimmunoassay is approximately to 0.5–1 ng/ml. The normal serum half-life of β-hCG is approximately 24 hours (Vaitukaitis *et al.*, 1972; Zarate and MacGregor, 1982), indicating that blood

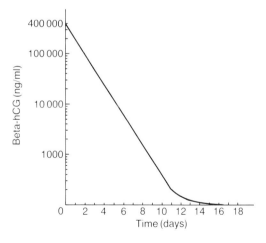

Fig. 6.3 Serum beta-hCG levels following complete resection of a beta-hCG secreting tumour. The line depicts the expected rate of fall based on a half-life of 24 hours.

levels should rapidly return to normal after complete resection of an hCG-producing tumour (Fig. 6.3).

6.3 CLINICAL APPLICATIONS OF AFP AND βhCG

The totipotential and pluripotential capabilities of germ cell tumours are phenotypically expressed by their diverse clinical, pathological and prognostic features. Pathologically, this group of tumours is comprised of germinomas, embryonal carcinomas, endodermal sinus tumours (yolk sac), choriocarcinomas, teratomas, polyembryomas and gonadablastomas. Most of the current classifications of germ cell tumours arising in both gonadal and extra-gonadal sites are essentially modifications of Teilum's concepts (1965). The schema illustrated in Fig. 6.4 restricts the term 'embryonal carcinoma' to tumours composed of undifferentiated, totipotential embryonal cells, with the potential to differentiate into extraembryonal neoplasms (endodermal

sinus tumours and choriocarcinomas) and tumours derived from all three germ layers (teratomas). Two-thirds of germ cell tumours in children are located in extragonadal sites; the majority of these are in the sacrococcygeal region in infants, the anterior mediastinum, and midline sites within the central nervous system, particularly the hypothalamic and pineal regions.

6.3.1 GERM CELL TUMOURS

(a) Germinomas

'Germinoma' is a general term used to designate a malignant germ cell tumour arising from the gonads or in an extragonadal site. Seminomas and dysgerminomas refer to germinomas arising in the testis and ovary respectively and are terms which have been replaced by the more generic term, germinoma. These tumours comprise approximately 15% of all paediatric germ cell tumours, and 11% of all ovarian tumours in

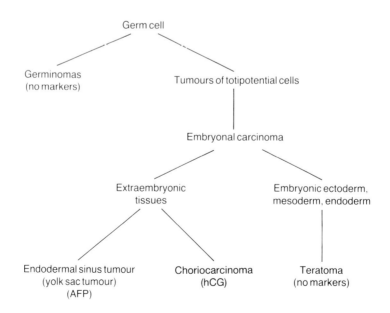

Fig. 6.4 Classification scheme of germ cell tumours, based on Teilum's classification.

children (Dehner, 1983). Germinomas in children are most commonly found in the ovary or in the pineal region in adolescent boys. Pure germinomas of the testis or anterior mediastinum are uncommon during the first two decades of life. Both immunohistochemical analysis of tumour tissue for AFP and serum AFP levels are negative in pure germinomas. Although β-hCG positivity has been noted, and elevated CSF levels of hCG have been demonstrated, these findings probably relate to the presence of multinucleated syncytiotrophoblasts in patients with mixed germ cell tumours rather than representing β-hCG secretion by 'pure germinoma'. Admixtures of other germ cell tumour types within germinomas is a more common observation than pure germinoma, underlining the importance of detailed histological examination of tumour material, and caution in interpreting raised biomarkers in patients with supposedly pure germinomas. Markers for AFP and β-hCG should be negative if there are no other malignant germ cell elements.

(b) Embryonal carcinomas

The clinical and histological relationship between embryonal carcinomas and endodermal sinus tumours (yolk sac carcinomas) is close but poorly defined. Embryonal carcinoma is a highly malignant neoplasm comprised of totipotential germ cells which may be regarded as the stem cells of teratomas, endodermal sinus tumours, and choriocarcinomas. Pure embryonal carcinoma is an uncommon finding in infants and children. This histological pattern is most frequently observed in association with other germ cell tumour elements including teratoma and endodermal sinus tumours. Endodermal carcinoma is found most frequently in the testes of young adults and commonly demonstrates positive immunostaining for AFP (Sharry *et al.*, 1985), and raised serum AFP levels have been documented in up to 70% of these

patients (Javadpour *et al.*, 1980). Raised serum and CSF β-hCG levels and immunopositivity for β-hCG have been demonstrated in patients with embryonal carcinoma (Packer *et al.*, 1984). However, it is possible that this represents a situation analogous to patients with so-called pure germinomas with raised hCG. It is probable that patients with embryonal carcinoma and immunopositivity for hCG or raised serum levels have tumours contains areas of syncytiotrophoblastic differentiation within embryonal carcinoma.

(c) Endodermal sinus tumours (yolk sac tumours)

Endodermal sinus tumours occur almost exclusively in children and they represent the most common malignant germ cell tumour in this age group. The ovary, testis and sacrococcygeal region are the commonest sites of involvement, with less common primary sites being, in paediatric patients, the anterior mediastinum, pineal region of the central nervous system, vagina, vulva, and liver (Green, 1983; Huntington *et al.*, 1970; Packer *et al.*, 1984). AFP synthesis in children with endodermal sinus tumours is analogous to the physiological AFP synthesis by the fetal yolk sac originally described by Gitlin *et al.* (1966). Endodermal sinus tumours represent the commonest testicular tumours in boys aged below three years. Serum AFP is elevated in approximately 75% of patients with endodermal sinus tumours. The serum levels of β-hCG is normal in patients with pure endodermal sinus tumour but may be elevated in patients with mixed germ cell tumours.

(d) Choriocarcinomas

These tumours are uncommon, highly malignant germ cell tumours characterized by syncytiotrophoblastic differentiation, the presence of multinucleated giant cells and immunopositivity for β-hCG. Choriocarcinomas occur in both gestational and non-gestational forms and the possibility of pregnancy mimicking an abdominal tumour in an adolescent female with a raised serum β-hCG must be considered before investigation with potentially hazardous ionizing radiation is pursued. Most choriocarcinomas in the paediatric age range are non-gestational and arise in the gonads, mediastinum, retroperitoneum or brain. Almost all extra-gonadal choriocarcinomas occur in males. Rarely, choriocarcinoma may present in infancy, with evidence of disseminated tumour features of gonadotropic stimulation and raised β-hCG, a complication of maternal-placental choriocarcinoma (Uctzelsen *et al.*, 1968). Patients with choriocarcinoma show strong tumour immunopositivity for β-hCG. Virtually all patients will show elevated levels of β-hCG, but not AFP (Javadpour, 1980).

(e) Germ cells arising within the CNS

Approximately 6% of germ cell tumours are found within the central nervous system and comprise 1 to 2% of all intracranial malignancies. The majority are located in midline sites with a preponderance in the pineal region. Tumours in this location often present with signs and symptoms of raised intracranial pressure, isosexual precocious puberty and Parinaud's syndrome (paralysis of upward gaze, absent or diminished pupillary reaction to light but not accommodation, and retraction nystagmus). These tumours may encompass a wide histological spectrum, making biopsy desirable. However, the risk of open or stereotaxic biopsy in patients with highly vascular, deeply located midline tumours may be unacceptable. In this situation, the assay of AFP and β-hCG in serum and CSF may identify the presence of immature germ cell elements. Although raised CSF biomarkers lack diagnostic specificity in the absence of tissue diagnosis, they provide the opportunity to monitor tumour response to irradiation or chemotherapy (Allen *et al.*, 1979; Edwards *et al.*, 1985).

(f) Monitoring markers

The detection and quantitation of AFP and β–hCG in tumour tissue and serum of patients with gonadal and extragonadal germ cell tumours are important for diagnosis and to monitor the response to therapy. Raised levels of AFP and/or β-hCG indicate the presence of endodermal sinus tumour elements or trophoblastic elements. Because of their relatively brief half-lives, the measurement of pre and post surgery levels have been useful in minimizing clinical staging errors. Although the majority of children with germ cell tumours have elevations of either AFP or β-hCG, there is a group in whom these markers are negative at the time of initial diagnosis and remain so throughout follow-up. A large group of patients with initially positive markers demonstrate falling serum levels of AFP and β-hCG in response to therapy. These biomarkers serve a particularly useful purpose for monitoring response to therapy, and for the early detection of recurrent disease often weeks or months before recurrence is apparent using modern diagnostic imaging techniques. The role of serum biomarkers in determining the duration of chemotherapy for children with germ cell tumours has not been resolved. Some groups, reporting excellent long-term outcome in patients with advanced germ cell tumours, continue treatment with cisplatin-based chemotherapy combinations for only two to three courses after complete remission, defined clinically, radiologically, and with serum markers (Pinkerton *et al.*, 1986). This approach, relying heavily on normalization of markers, contrasts with the traditional model of determining duration of therapy in advance, based on histology and stage, without reference to individual patient characteristics. Tumour recurrence unassociated with raised biomarkers in paediatric patients with raised serum AFP or β-hCG estimations at diagnosis has been documented (Pinkerton *et al.*, 1986).

6.3.2 HEPATIC MALIGNANCIES

Primary malignant liver tumours in children comprise up to 3% of paediatric malignancies (Alagille and Odievre, 1979). Over 90% of malignant liver tumours in children are hepatoblastomas or hepatocellular carcinomas (Wienberg and Feinegold, 1983). Diagnostic elevations of serum AFP or β-hCG are not seen in children with other types of primary malignant liver tumours including rhabdomyosarcoma, fibrosarcoma, angiosarcoma or secondary involvement by metastatic tumour or haemopoietic malignancy. Less than one-half of all liver tumours in children are benign (Mahour *et al.*, 1983), of these, mesenchymal haematoma and vascular tumours, particularly haemangiomas and haemangioendotheliomas, are observed most frequently.

(a) Hepatoblastoma

Hepatoblastomas are malignant tumours arising from the hepatic blastema and may contain both epithelial and/or mesenchymal elements. Of these tumours, 90% are diagnosed within the first three years of life at a median age of one year. The AFP level is raised, often to massive levels, in 90 to 95% of patients with hepatoblastoma and provides a reliable marker of complete resection when the fall in the serum AFP concentration is compared to the normal fall-off (Fig. 6.1, above). Approximately 3% of patients with hepatoblastoma secrete β-hCG (Murthy *et al.*, 1980; McArthur *et al.*, 1973; Nakagawara *et al.*, 1985), and may develop isosexual precocious puberty as a result of gonadotropic stimulation. These patients may demonstrate recurrence of their clinical endocrine abnormalities, in addition to raised tumour markers, at the time of recurrence.

(b) Hepatocellular carcinoma

The annual incidence of hepatocellular carcin-

oma in children is less than the incidence of hepatoblastoma. Histopathologically, hepatocellular carcinoma resembles its counterpart in adults. Hepatocellular carcinoma shows two age peaks during childhood and adolescence; the first before the age of four years and second between the ages of 12 to 15 years (Exelby *et al.*, 1974). This tumour is associated with cirrhosis significantly less frequently than in adults, but retains its strong aetiological association with hepatitis B infection (Lack *et al.*, 1983; Ohaki *et al.*, 1983). Serum AFP is elevated in up to 50% of children with hepatocellular carcinoma, and provides a valuable marker for monitoring the response to surgery or chemotherapy. Unfortunately, AFP is of limited value in patients with the fibrolamellar variant of hepatocellular carcinoma because levels of this biomarker are not usually informative (Maltz *et al.*, 1980; Paradinas *et al.*, 1982). The level of unsaturated vitamin-B_{12} binding protein (transcobalamin I) is elevated in most children with the fibrolamellar variant, and may be a useful marker of disease progression (Wheeler *et al.*, 1986).

6.3.3 OTHER NEOPLASMS WITH INFORMATIVE AFP OR β-hCG LEVELS

The value of AFP estimations in children with hepatic malignancies or germ cell tumours is well established. One of the major advantages of AFP is its high level of specificity (i.e. a low 'false-positive' rate). Elevated levels of AFP have been reported infrequently in association with malignant tumours of the gastrointestinal tract, most commonly in adult patients with tumours of the pancreas, biliary tract or stomach, and, less frequently, in patients with colorectal carcinoma, but not in association with oesophageal or small bowel carcinomas (McIntire *et al.*, 1975). These gastrointestinal neoplasms are commonly seen in the elderly, but rarely in adolescents. Elevated β-hCG levels have been reported in neoplasms involving the gastrointestinal tract

115

(stomach, liver, pancreas), the lung, breast, ovary, and rarely in lymphoproliferative disorders (Vaitukaitis *et al.*, 1976; Gailani *et al.*, 1976; Kahn *et al.*, 1977; Tormey *et al.*, 1977). These tumours are rare in adolescents and are usually associated with serum concentrations of less than 10 ng/ml. In contrast to North America, where paediatric oncologists care for patients aged up to 18 to 21 years, European and Australian oncologists rarely see newly diagnosed patients aged over 15 years and are even less likely to come across these typically 'adult' neoplasms.

6.4 CATECHOLAMINE METABOLITES IN NEURAL CREST TUMOURS

6.4.1 NORMAL CATECHOLAMINE METABOLISM

Adrenaline, noradrenaline and dopamine, the principle catecholamines found in the body, are synthesized by a sequence of hydroxyl-ation and decarboxylation steps from the amino acids phenylalanine and tyrosine. Tyrosine is converted to dopa and then to dopamine following transportation into the neuronal cytoplasm. Dopamine enters the granulated vesicles and is converted to nor-adrenaline by dopamine β-hydroxylase. Synthesis is regulated by feedback inhibition of tyrosine hydroxylase by noradrenaline and dopamine so that synthesis of dopa is coupled to catecholamine release. Noradrenaline is subsequently N-methylated by the phenyl-ethanolamine-N-methyltransferase to adrenaline. Both adrenaline and noradrenaline are metabolized by O-methylation to biologically inactive products with the enzyme catechol-O-methyltransferase (COMT) and by oxidative deamination with monoamine oxidase (MAO). The metanephrines and 3-methyoxy-4-hydroxymandelic acid (or vanillylmandelic acid, VMA) are the major metabolic end-products of noradrenaline and adrenaline metabolism. Homovanillic acid (HVA) is the major end-product of dopamine metablism (Fig. 6.5).

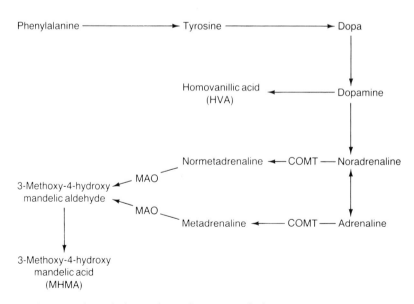

Fig. 6.5 Biosynthesis and catabolism of circulating catacholamines. COMT: Catechol-O-methyltransferase; MAO: Monoamine oxidase.

6.4.2 UNTIMED VERSUS 24-HOUR URINE COLLECTIONS

Twenty-four-hour urine collections have the advantage of taking into account diurnal variation in the rate of metabolite excretion and do not rely on a normal serum creatinine for interpretation. However, one of the issues not often discussed in the debate concerning the accuracy of a 24-hour urine collection versus an untimed collection, is the assumption that the former is complete. The difficulty in obtaining reliable 24-hour collections, particularly in young children, is well known, leading to delays and inaccuracies. Untimed collections are rapid, easy to collect, and provide a result that makes a correction for the rate of urine production, but not for diurnal variation of catecholamine metabolite or creatinine secretion (Mautalen, 1970). Although the adequacy of this approach has been questioned (Soldin and Hill, 1981) results obtained by Gitlow *et al.*. (1970) have been confirmed by others (Tuchman *et al.*, 1985; Kellie *et al.*, 1986). Analysis of the reliability of untimed urine specimens in the diagnosis of neural crest tumours point to results that are as good as, or better than, previously published data. This demonstrates the practical value of using catecholamine metabolite determinations expressed as 'creatinine equivalents' on untimed urine specimens in the diagnosis of these tumours (Tuchman *et al.*, 1985; Kellie *et al.*, 1986). Physiological, medication or dietary factors may influence the measurement of catecholamine metabolite excretion regardless of collection technique.

6.4.3 FACTORS AFFECTING URINARY CATECHOLAMINE METABOLITE EXCRETION

(a) Physiological factors

The 24-hour urinary excretion of catecholamines and their metabolites increases with age up to about 16 years, when the adult range is obtained. The ratio of urinary VMA and HVA excretion, expressed as μg/mg of creatinine, decreases steadily with age from infancy through to early adulthood. Increased physiological levels of adrenaline and noradrenaline secretion have been noted in ambulant subjects compared to hospitalized, recumbent patients. Moreover, increased noradrenaline secretion has been noted in response to raised autonomic sympathetic nervous activity related to physical stress, pain or cold, whereas mental stress may lead to increased secretion of adrenaline. Overall, the influence of physiological factors on the urinary excretion of catecholamines appears to be insignificant, and does not appear to result in false-positive elevations of catecholamine metabolite excretion in patients with suspected neural crest tumours.

(b) Pathophysiological factors

Essential hypertension has been associated with a slight to moderate elevation of noradrenaline secretion related to increased sympathetic tone. Patients with poorly controlled diabetes mellitus may excrete increased amounts of catecholamines probably related to severe ketoacidosis and hypoglycaemia. Occasionally, traumatic injury may result in pathophysiological secretion of catecholamines. Prescribed medications may increase or decrease catecholamine metabolite excretion. A number of anti-hypertensive drugs which affect catecholamine binding and release may produce a decrease in catecholamine secretion. Anti-hypertensive treatment with guanethidine, debrisoquine and the rauwolfia alkaloids may artificially diminish catecholamine metabolite excretion, whereas increased excretion may occur during treatment with catecholamine-containing drugs or sympathomimetics. Drugs in the former category include theophylline, L-dopa, chlorpromazine, prochlorperazine and caffeine. Treatment with sympathomimetics, including dextroamphetamine, ephedrine and methylphenidate, may elevate catecholamine excretion. A number of these agents are used commonly in children with asthma, severe vomiting, or behaviour disorders, and represent a potential source of 'false-positive' error depending on the analytic method used for assaying metabolite excretion.

(c) Dietary factors

The relevance of dietary restriction whilst assessing urinary biogenic amine excretion has been the source of some controversy. Dietary restrictions were once widely recommended and are still used by some centres today when a 24-hour urine collection for diagnostic purposes is in progress. This practice relates to concerns about possible 'false-positive' results due to the concentration of catecholamines in certain foods. Classically, children with neural crest tumours completing a 24-hour urine collection, have avoided a variety of foods for two days before and on the day of collection. The degree of dietary restriction varies greatly between centres. Common items of restricted foods include: avocados, bananas, plums, pineapples, walnuts, chocolate, vanilla-flavoured foods, vitamins and coffee. Feldman *et al.* (1987) investigated the dopamine, adrenaline, noradrenaline and serotonin content in 30 varieties of fruits and vegetables using a radioenzymatic assay technique. High concentrations of dopamine were identified in red and yellow bananas. Seven healthy volunteers consumed 1.6 kg of banana pulp in addition to their conventional diet; a mean increase in HVA excretion of 46% ± 9.8% over baseline values was observed. However, actual HVA excretion beyond the normal range was observed in only one of the seven volunteers. The impact of banana consumption on VMA excretion was not deter-

mined, due to the low adrenaline and noradrenaline concentrations in banana pulp. The absence of significant increases in VMA or HVA excretion, which may result in a 'false-positive' test result among children and young adults eating normal diets, has been confirmed by others (Rayfield *et al.*, 1972; Weetman *et al.*, 1976; Muscettola *et al.*, 1977). More recently, dietary interference in the determination of biogenic amines has been virtually eliminated by the development of specific and sensitive high performance liquid chromatographic methods of measurement (Potezny and Rosenblatt, 1986).

6.4.4 CLINICAL APPLICATIONS

(a) Neuroblastoma

Neuroblastoma is the commonest extracranial solid tumour in children and is derived from sympathetic neural crest tissue. Neuroblastoma is one of the 'small blue round' cell tumours of childhood and demonstrates a spectrum of maturation ranging from differentiated ganglioneuromas to highly undifferentiated neuroblastomas. Neuroblastoma cells lack the ability to store quantities of dopamine for further metabolism to noradrenaline. As a consequence, the major urinary metabolites are dopamine and its metabolite HVA, although some VMA is produced. A review of urinary excretion of these compounds using HPLC in 35 children with advanced neuroblastoma has confirmed HVA to be the diagnostic metabolite of choice. HVA was found to be elevated in 34 patients, with dopamine and VMA elevations in 29 patients (Rosano, 1984). The usefulness of urinary dopamine and/or HVA compared to VMA in the diagnosis of neuroblastoma have been documented by others (Kaser, 1965; Hinterberger and Bartholomew, 1969; Brewster *et al.*, 1977, Earl, 1986). Urinary VMA, HVA, dopamine or 3-methoxy-4-

hydroxy-phenylglycol (MHPG) are usually elevated beyond the normal range in almost 100% of patients with neuroblastoma (Gitlow *et al.*, 1970). HPLC measurement of HVA, the primary metabolite of dopamine, has shown this to be the most useful analyte for the detection of small primary tumours (Evans Stages I and II), in addition to being the most consistently elevated analyte in children with disseminated abdominal tumours (Rosano, 1984). LaBrosse and co-workers (1980) have examined the inter-relationships between the excretion of catecholamine metabolites, age at diagnosis, stage of disease, site of primary tumour and prognosis. They found elevated levels of VMA excretion in 71% of patients and HVA excretion in 75%. Additionally, they observed significantly higher levels of VMA excretion in patients with Stages IV and IV-S compared to patients with Stages I, II, or III disease. They found no significant relationship between VMA or HVA excretion and the primary site of the tumour, but noted that the VMA/HVA ratio was significantly related to survival in Stage IV patients although no correlation between levels of VMA or HVA excretion and prognosis was observed. Both LaBrosse *et al.*, (1980) and Laug *et al.* (1978) have demonstrated a statistically significant relationship between a high VMA/HVA ratio and a more favourable prognosis. However, this ratio does not reliably predict outcome in children with other stages of neuroblastoma.

False-positive elevations of catecholamine metabolite excretion suggesting the presence of a neural crest tumour in a patient without additional evidence of malignancy are rare. Gitlow *et al.* (1970) noted elevated HVA excretion, but diminished or normal excretion of other catecholamine metabolites in children with familial dysautonomia. Rosano (1984) reported elevated urinary catecholamine metabolites in two children with Duchenne-type muscular dystrophy without evidence of neural crest tumour. The elevated levels (expressed as mg/g of creatinine) in these patients may reflect the effect of muscular dystrophy on muscle mass and creatinine excretion. The high level of specificity (i.e. low 'false-positive' rate) of urinary catecholamine excretion for patients with neural crest tumours has reinforced the value of these assays for both diagnosis and follow-up. Refined assay techniques and broadening clinical applications, including mass screening of infants (see below), ensures that these markers will remain clinically useful as well as a potential source of controversy in the years to come.

The potential diagnostic roles of plasma catecholamines or their metabolites have received relatively little attention. Schuman *et al.* (1984) described the use of venous catecholamine sampling via selective venous caval catheterization in an infant with an occult ganglioneuroma secreting vasoactive intestinal peptide and catechoamines resulting in intractable diarrhoea. Elevated levels of plasma noradrenaline, adrenaline, and dopamine localized an otherwise unidentifiable tumour, permitting curative surgery. More recently, assays of plasma catecholamines in children with neuroblastoma have been reported (Boomsma *et al.*, 1989). Boomsma and co-workers investigated the relationships of noradrenaline, adrenaline, dopa, dopamine, and aromatic L-amino acid decarboxylase (ALAAD) to disease activity. The wide variation of plasma levels of noradrenaline, adrenaline and dopamine reported underscore the inconsistent relationship between these markers and disease activity. However, plasma dopa and ALAAD activity were clearly elevated in ten out of ten patients with active untreated neuroblastoma. ALAAD, and to a lesser extent dopa levels, fell with successful treatment and increased with relapse. The future role of these plasma markers in monitoring disease activity remains to be determined.

(b) Phaeochromocytoma

Phaeochromocytoma is a rare tumour in children, and fewer than 10% are malignant. The majority are associated with paroxysmal headache, sweating, palpitation and arterial hypertension. The metabolites of choice for the diagnosis of phaeochromocytoma are noradrenaline and adrenaline (Stenstrom *et al.*, 1983; Rosano, 1984). VMA alone should not be relied upon for diagnosis or monitoring, as levels of this metabolite are normal in approximately 10% of patients (Stenstrom *et al.*, 1983). HPLC and mass-spectroscopy, combined with gas chromatography, are both highly sensitive and specific methods although the latter is compromised by the high cost of instrumentation and the need for specialized support. Fluorescence techniques are subject to interference (and 'false-positive' results) from a variety of drugs and B-group vitamins. Urinary dopamine and HVA are usually normal in patients with these tumours.

(c) Carcinoid tumour

Carcinoid tumours arise from enterochromaffin cells which are thought to migrate from the neural crest to their final location in diverse organs. These tumours may be benign or malignant with the benign varieties most commonly found in the appendix. Extra-appendiceal carcinoids are rare in children (Anderson and Bergdahl, 1977). Carcinoid tumours and their metastases produce excessive amounts of 5-hydroxytryptamine (serotonin), histamine and other vasoactive peptides resulting in the 'carcinoid syndrome', characterized by tachycardia, hyperperistalsis, frequent watery stools, patchy cyanosis or vasodilatation of the skin, asthma, and valvular heart disease. Urinary excretion of a serotonin metabolite, 5-hydroxyindolacetic acid (5-HIAA) is elevated. At present there is a general consensus that the measurement of 5-HIAA in a 24-hour urine is the most appropriate initial test (Sampson, 1987). Although urinary serotonin excretion is not elevated in all carcinoid tumours, both this and urinary 5-HIAA may have a role in monitoring disease progress in some patients. The relative importance of various diagnostic markers for carcinoid tumours have been examined in some detail by Odelstad *et al.* (1982).

6.5 OTHER TUMOUR MARKERS

A large group of interesting tumour-derived molecules produced by cancer cells, and tumour associated metabolic or immunologic products from normal tissues, have been described. These products include oncofetal antigens such as carcinoembryonic antigen (CEA), carbohydrate antigens (CA125, CA19–9, and CA15–3). Also host response markers such as soluble interleukin 2, neopterin and related compounds, transcobalamin I, neurotensin and elements detected by proton nuclear magnetic resonance spectroscopy. In comparison to the tumour markers discussed earlier in this chapter, the remainder are of limited clinical application in paediatric oncology at the present time, although their roles are being examined in specialized centres.

6.5.1 NEURONE-SPECIFIC ENOLASE

The enolases are a group of glycolytic enzymes which exist as dimers composed of three immunologically distinct sub-units designated alpha, beta and gamma. The most acidic isoenzyme is composed of two gamma sub-units, and is termed neurone-specific enolase (NSE). NSE is distributed widely throughout the body in both neuronal and neuroendocrine cells, and has also been identified in non-neuronal tissue. The presence of NSE has been demonstrated, using immunostaining techniques, in all types of neurons, as well as in pinealocytes, pituitary glandular peptide-secreting cells, thyroid parafolli-cular cells, adrenal medullary chromaffin cells and in neuroendocrine cells found in lung and in other tissues which derive from the embryologic neural crest. The diversity of mature tissues expressing NSE has proven to be the major factor limiting its use to diagnose malignancies arising from specific tissues.

The major clinical application of serum NSE concentrations in paediatric oncology has been this marker's relationship between stage and treatment outcome in children with neuroblastoma (Odelstad *et al.*, 1982; Zeltzer *et al.*, 1986). Zeltzer *et al.* (1986) demonstrated a significant relationship between disease stage and NSE levels in 61 children with neuroblastoma. The median serum NSE values in patients with Stages I, II, III, IV and IV-S disease were 13, 23, 40, 214 and 40 ng/ml respectively. Although NSE is widely de-scribed as being a 'tumour marker', its greatest utility appears to be as a prognostic factor in patients with a confirmed diagnosis of neuroblastoma. Infants with Stage IV-S disease have significantly lower NSE levels than patients with Stage IV disease despite their extensive tumour burden. Zeltzer also reported a significantly inferior outcome for patients with pre-treatment NSE levels > 100 ng/ml (2-year disease-free survival of 10% versus 79% for those with values < 100 ng/ml).

Elevated NSE levels have been docu-mented in a variety of other paediatric tumours (Cooper *et al.* 1987), such as Wilms' tumour, acute leukaemia, non-Hodgkin's lymphoma, Ewing's sarcoma or soft tissue sarcomas (Table 6.2). Zeltzer *et al.* (1986) demonstrated significant NSE elevations in patients with leukaemia, hepatoblastoma and primitive neuroectodermal tumours. NSE has also been suggested as a marker for immature ovarian teratoma and dysgermin-oma (Kawata *et al.*, 1989); four out of eight patients with ovarian teratoma had values

between 10 and 50 g/ml, whereas four out of six patients with dysgerminoma had NSE values of > 50 g/ml. Raised serum NSE in patients with immature teratoma may reflect enzyme synthesized and released by neural components contained in these tumours. However, dysgerminomas are not generally considered to be of neural origin and the marked elevation of NSE in these patients is surprising. The value of serial NSE esti-mations in the subsequent management of these patients is not known (Kawata *et al.*, 1989). The presence of raised NSE in children with neuroblastoma or Wilms' tumour, and the recent demonstration of raised serum NSE in adults with renal cell carcinoma, con-firms this marker's lack of specificity in differ-

Table 6.2 Neurone-specific enolase levels at diag-nosis in children with cancer

| Tumour | No. | *Serum NSE ng/ml* | | | |
		<25	*25–50*	*51–100*	*100*
Controls a	27	27			
b	11	11			
Neuroblastoma					
Stages I & II	9	6	1	1	1
Stages III & IV	63	9	7	16	31
IV-s	3	2	1		
Ganglioneuroma	4	4			
Retinoblastoma	4	4			
Wilms' tumour					
Stages I & II	15	13	2		
Stages II & IV	14	5	3	4	2
Lymphoma	15	9	5	1	
Acute lymphoblastic leukaemia	23	20	2	–	1
Acute myeloblastic leukaemia	2	1	1		
Ewing's sarcoma	11	10	1		
Soft tissue sarcoma	23	19	3	1	

Controls (a): The Hospital for Sick Children, Great Ormond Street, London; Controls (b): Service d'Hemat-ologie Pediatrique, Cliniques Universitaires St. Luc, Brussels.
Reproduced with the permission of the editor of *Brit. J. Cancer.*

entiating between these tumours (Takashi *et al.*, 1989).

Raised serum levels of NSE in a variety of tumours have been reflected by immunohistochemical studies which have demonstrated its presence in neuroblastoma, ganglioneuroblastoma, neuroganglioma, phaeochromocytoma, retinoblastoma, and CNS tumours including medulloblastoma, primitive neuroectodermal tumours, paraganglioma, olfactory neuroblastoma, capillary haemangioblastomas, Merkel cell tumours and medullary thyroid carcinomas (Feldenzer and McKeever, 1987; Burger *et al.*, 1987; Touitou and Heshmati, 1988). The clinical relevance of increased NSE concentration in CSF has also been studied (Jacobi and Reiber, 1988). These workers detected NSE levels in the CSF of > 20 ng/ml in 33 of 172 patients with a variety of neurological disorders, including CNS tumours, cerebral infarctions, cerebral ischaemia, CNS inflammatory diseases and epilepsy. They confirmed that raised levels of NSE in CSF were not specific for a particular type of neurological disorder. Although the CSF NSE estimation may help identify patients with pathological organic CNS pathology, it lacks diagnostic usefulness (Jacobi and Reiber, 1988).

6.5.2 CARCINOEMBRYONIC ANTIGEN

Carcinoembryonic antigen is a glycoprotein moiety first described in fetal intestine, liver and pancreas during the first six months of gestation. CEA is elevated in approximately 70% of adult patients with adenocarcinoma of the colon. CEA concentration is more likely to be of assistance in determining tumour bulk at diagnosis, adequacy of initial therapy, particularly if surgical resection is thought to be complete, and to monitor response to subsequent therapy. The introduction of sensitive radioimmunoassays has shown that serum CEA may be elevated in diverse malignant and benign conditions.

Elevated serum CEA levels have been described in children with colon cancer (Pratt *et al.*, 1977; Rao *et al.*, 1985) and less frequently in children with Wilms' tumour, histiocytic lymphoma, hepatoblastoma, hepatocellular carcinoma, Stage IV neuroblastoma with hepatic involvement, germ cell tumour, pulmonary blastoma and retinoblastoma (Felberg *et al.*, 1976; Mann *et al.*, 1978; Melia *et al.*, 1981; Sculier *et al.*, 1987; Maeda *et al.*, 1988). Howell *et al.* (1988) demonstrated tissue CEA immunoreactivity in 68% of patients with ameloblastoma; serum CEA levels, however, were not reported. Although rare in paediatric neoplasms, CEA immunoreactivity may have potential value in diagnosis and follow-up. CEA has also been reported to be elevated in a variety of non-neoplastic conditions, including hepatic cirrhosis, hepatitis, inflammatory bowel disease and bronchitis (Mann *et al.*, 1978; Sculier *et al.*, 1987). This lack of specificity severely limits the utility of this marker in the diagnosis of paediatric malignancy and in differentiating malignant from non-malignant conditions.

6.5.3 SOLUBLE INTERLEUKIN-2

The interleukin-2 receptor is expressed on the cytoplasmic membrane of T-lymphocytes, on some B cells, and on monocytes following their activation. The same receptor has also been found on cell membranes in several lymphoproliferative disorders, including T-cell leukaemia, non-Hodgkin's lymphoma, hairy cell leukaemia, B-cell chronic lymphocytic leukaemia and Hodgkin's disease. Increased serum interleukin-2 receptor levels have been described in adults with various leukaemias, non-Hodgkin's lymphoma and Hodgkin's disease. Pui *et al.* (1987) and Wagner *et al.* (1987) have correlated raised serum interleukin-2 receptor levels with advanced disease, increased tumour burden, and an unfavourable prognosis in patients with non-Hodgkin's lymphoma. These findings have more recently been extended to children with non-T, non-B acute lymphoblastic leukaemia (Pui *et al.*, 1988), where higher interleukin-2 levels were also associated with a poor prognosis. Pui *et al.* (1989) have also demonstrated that higher levels of interleukin-2 receptor in children with Hodgkin's disease is associated with advanced disease, and, more importantly, this marker was found to be an independent predictor of treatment outcome after adjustment for other co-variables (Fig. 6.6). Raised levels of serum interleukin-2 have also been found in patients with immunological disorders such as acquired immunodeficiency syndrome (AIDS) and infectious mononucleosis (Kloster *et al.*, 1987). At the present time, the application of this marker in detecting residual tumour, or for monitoring the course of malignant disease, has not been studied prospectively.

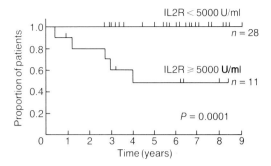

Fig. 6.6 Comparison of time-to-failure durations according to serum interleukin-2 receptor levels for patients with Stage III or IV Hodgkin's disease. Significantly worse treatment results were evident for patients with higher levels ($\geq$ 5000 u/ml). (Reproduced with the permission of the editor of *Leukemia*).

6.5.4 TRANSCOBALAMIN I AND NEUROTENSIN

The fibrolamellar variant of hepatocellular carcinoma is seen more commonly in adolescents and young adults than in younger children. In contrast to patients with classical hepatocellular carcinoma, the serum AFP is usually normal in patients with the fibrolamellar variant (McIntire *et al.*, 1975; Vaitukaitis *et al.*, 1976); however, the serum concentration of total unsaturated transcobalamin-binding capacity is often raised in such patients, and has been shown to rise in response to recurrent disease prior to clinical or radiological evidence of recurrence (Vaitukaitis *et al.*, 1976; Kahn *et al.*, 1977). Transcobalamin I alone appears to be a more sensitive and specific tumour marker than the total unsaturated vitamin B_{12} binding capacity. Carmel and Eisenberg (1977), in a retrospective survey of 139 patients, found that half of the patients with cancer had some abnormality of serum vitamin B_{12} or its binding

proteins, although the highest levels were most commonly observed in patients with primary or secondary liver involvement. These investigations are of limited value in diagnosis because of low selectivity and specificity. Elevated concentrations of neurotensin, a polypeptide hormone found in the gastrointestinal tract and CNS, has been found in four out of four patients with the fibrolamellar variant, but in only one out of sixteen patients with classic hepatocellular carcinoma (Collier *et al.*, 1984). Neurotensin may have a role as a tumour marker at diagnosis, or recurrence in patients with AFP negative fibrolamellar hepatocellular carcinoma.

6.5.5 NUCLEAR MAGNETIC RESONANCE SPECTROSCOPY (NMR)

Controversy surrounds the value of water-suppressed proton NMR spectroscopy for cancer detection (Fossel *et al.*, 1986; Wilding *et al.*, 1988; Berger *et al.*, 1989). Differences in the T_1 and T_2 values of the composite proton NMR signal between malignant and non-malignant tissues have prompted investigation into the application of this modality as a means of identifying patients with cancer using a sensitive and specific blood test. Fossel *et al.* (1986) analysed plasma from 337 people using water-suppressed proton nuclear magnetic resonance spectroscopy. Patients with malignant tumours were reliably distinguished from normal controls. Patients with benign tumours had statistically significant wider line widths compared to those with malignant tumours. Although the preliminary results demonstrated the potential value of this approach, other factors, including fasting, alcohol consumption, lactic acidosis and diabetic ketoacidosis may interfere with lipoprotein peaks, possibly invalidating the results. Wilding *et al.* (1988) investigated proton NMR spectra in healthy patients, patients with overt malignancy, and those with hypertriglyceridaemia. Contrary to the findings of Fossel *et al.*, they were unable to distinguish normal individuals from those with malignant tumours. Further work involving larger groups of patients with malignancies and non-malignant disorders, using NMR spectral information obtained from body fluids including urine, CSF and amniotic fluid, is necessary.

6.5.6 NEOPTERINS AND RELATED COMPOUNDS

Of the pterins, neopterin, first described in 1979 by Watcher *et al.* (1979) has been shown to be the most consistently raised in the presence of several malignancies, including the lymphoproliferative disorders. Neopterin is a metabolite derived from human macrophages following induction by gamma interferon and is produced in increased amounts by activated and rapidly proliferating cells. It appears to be a sensitive and specific activation marker of T-cell/macrophage interplay and can be detected in measurable quantities in plasma and urine. Abate *et al.* (1989) demonstrated

raised urinary neopterin excretion above the upper limit of normal in 85% in a series of adult patients with non-Hodgkin's lymphoma and found a relationship between the level of neopterin excretion with disease stage and the presence of constitutional symptoms. Regardless of stage, patients with lower neopterin excretion fared better than those with higher levels of excretion. Neopterin appeared to have prognostic significance, particularly in patients with limited disease. Raised neopterin levels in patients appeared to be a consequence of activation of the host immune system rather than a product of malignant cells. Unfortunately, raised levels have also been demonstrated in patients with viral infections and other malignant tumours, thereby diminishing its role as a specific tumour marker.

6.5.7 CARBOHYDRATE ANTIGENS (CA125, CA19.9, CA15.3)

CA125 is a glycoprotein associated with non-mucinous ovarian cancer. Elevated levels have also been found in adult patients with carcinoma of the endometrium, fallopian tube and breast. Elevated levels have been found during the first trimester of pregnancy, possibly reflecting CA125-associated glycoprotein production by the fetus, and also in patients with endometriosis, hepatitis, pelvic inflammatory disease, or during menstruation (Ruibal *et al.*, 1984; Pittaway and Foyez, 1987). Although the majority of ovarian tumours in children and adolescents are germ cell tumours, approximately one-third of malignant ovarian tumours occurring after the age of 15 years are of epithelial origin. Elevated CA125 is found in over 80% of patients with mucinous or non-mucinous ovarian carcinomas, and it is likely that this serum tumour marker will retain utility in diagnosis, assessing response to treatment and as a marker for early pre-clinical recurrence in a restricted number of adolescent patients.

CA19.9 is a carbohydrate cell surface antigen found in the sera of patients with colorectal, gastric or pancreatic cancer (Herlyn *et al.*, 1982). Unfortunately, elevated concentrations of this carbohydrate antigen have been found in a variety of non-malignant conditions, including inflammatory bowel disease, biliary disease, pancreatitis and hepatitis (Touitou and Bogdan, 1988). CA15.3 and CA50 are carbohydrate antigens found predominantly in adults with breast and other carcinomas. They appear to be of little relevance to paediatric oncologists at present and their usefulness is hampered, like the other carbohydrate antigens, by low specificity and sensitivity.

6.6 TUMOUR MARKERS AS 'PROGNOSTIC FACTORS'

Prognostic factors are indices derived from clinical and laboratory data which provide a prospective measure of the success of treatment. Traditionally, stage, site and extent of disease have provided the basis for prognostic classification. More recently, the value of tumour histology, immunologic techniques, cytogenetic and molecular analysis have been studied. The importance of individual prognostic factors may change with therapeutic refinement with some previously important risk factors losing their predictive value and new prognostic factors appearing. Circulating serum markers including LDH, ALP and ferritin lack both sensitivity and specificity for the presence of cancer in children, but retain clinical utility both as prognostic factors and as markers of tumour activity.

Lactic dehydrogenase, an enzyme that favours the reduction of pyruvate to lactate, is widely distributed throughout body tissue. Elevated serum levels have been reported in children with solid tumours including germ cell tumours, Ewing's sarcoma, neuroblastoma, non-Hodgkin's lymphoma and osteo-

sarcoma (Quin *et al.*, 1980; Bacci *et al.*, 1988; Link *et al.* 1988; Von Eyben *et al.*, 1988). Although LDH lacks tumour specificity, it has recently been found to be useful for following disease activity in patients with both neuroblastoma, Ewing's sarcoma and osteosarcoma (Quin *et al.*, 1980; Bacci *et al.*, 1988; Link *et al.*, 1988).

Serum alkaline phosphatase is a biological marker derived from the cell membrane of osteoblasts, and its value in diagnosis and monitoring response to therapy in adolescents with osteosarcoma remains unclear because of a lack of specificity. Elevated serum concentrations have been described in patients with liver disease, healing fractures, in association with normal growth, and may be elevated in patients receiving long-term parenteral nutrition therapy. Serum alkaline phosphatase levels may be elevated during treatment with antifungal agents, chlorothiazide, diazepam, gentamicin, phenytoin, phenobarbital, propranolol, sulphamethoxazole and aspirin. The prognostic significance of serum alkaline phosphatase levels was investigated in 116 children and adolescents with osteosarcoma treated at St. Jude Children's Research Hospital. Although WBC $>8 \times 10^9$/l, or LDH >300 U/l at diagnosis were correlated with shortened disease-free survival no prognostic significance was attached to pre-therapy alkaline phosphatase levels (Liddell *et al.*, 1988)

Ferritin is an iron storage protein present in most eukaryotic cells. Ferritin concentrations are particularly high in the liver, spleen and bone marrow. Raised serum ferritin levels may occur in association with a diversity of benign and malignant conditions including acute phase reactions to tissue injury, necrosis, inflammation or infection, liver disease, megaloblastic anaemia, haemolytic anaemia, sideroblastic anaemia, thalassaemia and iron overload (haemochromatosis, haemosiderosis). Raised levels have also been observed in children with Hodgkin's disease, hepatocellular carcinoma, neuroblastoma and germ cell tumours. Hann *et al.* (1980) investigated serum ferritin levels in 58 children with neuroblastoma and demonstrated that increased levels correlated with active disease, and confirmed these findings in a longitudinal study. The ferritin levels were found to return to normal in patients achieving remission. Their study suggested that increased serum ferritin in patients with neuroblastoma was tumour-derived and estimations of this marker could potentially provide a measure of disease activity. Almost 100% of children with hepatocellular carcinoma have elevated serum ferritin levels: the importance of this observation is nullified by the fact that more than three-quarters of patients with uncomplicated cirrhosis also have elevated levels. Although the serum ferritin level is of limited value diagnostically, it appears to fall with tumour response and rise with tumour recurrence or progression.

6.7 HORMONAL TUMOUR MARKERS

The endocrine manifestations of cancer in children and adolescents may result from the production of excessive amounts of hormone from a benign or malignant tumour arising in a gland normally associated with physiological synthesis. Ectopic hormone production may occur in tumours arising in endocrine glands which normally produce other hormones, or from hormones synthesized and secreted by tumours unrelated to endocrine tissue (Table 6.3). Biologically active hormones are found in age-related levels in the serum of normal persons. However, elevated levels provide a valuable biological marker in patients with functioning endocrine tumours due to the relative specificity for the organ of origin. Serial estimations offer a means of monitoring response to therapy and for detecting pre-clinical recurrence. Endocrine tumours in childhood are rare, comprising approximately 5% of neoplasms in this age

group. The majority are non-functioning. The presence of elevated hormone levels, or the degree of elevation, have generally been unhelpful in differentiating benign adenomas from their malignant counterparts.

6.8 CURRENT ISSUES – SCREENING FOR NEUROBLASTOMA IN INFANCY

Screening for disease offers the opportunity for early recognition, intervention, and initiation of treatment in patients with pre-clinical disease. Successful screening programmes for phenylketonuria, galactosaemia and neonatal hypothyroidism have encouraged paediatricians to critically examine a wide variety of childhood diseases for their suitability for early detection through screening programmes. In order to develop an effective screening programme, a number of principles and recommendations require consideration, as follows:

1. The human and economic cost of the condition to be investigated should be sufficiently serious to warrant justification of screening on a cost/benefit basis.
2. Diagnostic screening tests should be sufficiently sensitive (i.e. low 'false-negative' rate) in identifying affected individuals, and also have high specificity (i.e. low 'false-positive' rate) whereby non-affected individuals are not identified as having preclinical disease.
3. It should be expected that pre-clinical detection be associated with improved outcome. This principle is well illustrated by screening of newborns for metabolic disorders which, left untreated, could be associated with disastrous neuro-developmental consequences.
4. Effective treatment for the condition being screened for should be readily available.
5. The condition should be relatively prevalent in the selected population; an inverse relationship exists between the prevalence

Table 6.3 Hormones as tumour markers in paediatric oncology

Hormone-tumour marker	Syndrome	Tumour type	Ectopic-production
Cortisol, aldosterone androgen, oestrogen	Cushing's, Cohn's virilization feminization	Adrenal hyperplasia Adrenal adenoma Adrenal carcinoma	Adrenal rests (liver, testis, ovary)
Androgen	Isosexual precocity (male) Virilism (female)	Leydig cell tumour (testis) Sertoli-Leydig cell tumour (ovary)	
Oestrogen	Isosexual precocity (female) Feminization (male)	Granulosa cell tumour (ovary) Sertoli cell tumour (testis)	
Adrenaline, dopamine noradrenaline	Hypertension	Adrenal hyperplasia Adrenal adenoma Adrenal carcinoma	
Erythropoietin	Erythocytosis	Wilms' tumour Renal carcinoma Adrenal carcinoma	Cerebral haemangioblastomatosis Hepatoma Phaeochromocytoma
Renin	Hypertension	Wilms' tumour	
Thyrocalcitonin	Parathyroid hyperplasia diarrhoea MEN IIa & IIb	Medullary (C-cell) thyroid carcinoma	Carcinoid
T_3/T_4	Hyperthyroidism	Thyroid adenoma Thyroid carcinoma	Thyrotropin (pituitary)
PTH	MEN I, IIa	Parathyroid hyperplasia Parathyroid adenoma Parathyroid carcinoma	Hepatoma Renal carcinoma
Prolactin, ACTH Growth hormone, LH, FSH, TSH	Galactorrhea Cushing's syndrome Gigantism Precocious puberty Hyperthyroidism	Hormone secreting adenomas	Neuroblastoma Phaeochromocytoma Hepatoblastoma Choriocarcinoma
Insulin	Hypoglycaemia	Insulinoma	Carcinoid
Gastrin	Zollinger-Ellinson syndrome	Gastrinoma	
Glucagon	Hyperglycaemia	Glucagonoma	Carcinoid
VIP	Watery diarrhoea $\downarrow K^+$	VIPoma	Ganglioneuroblastoma
Somatastatin	Hyperglycaemia	Somatostatinoma	

of the condition and the cost of case finding.

6. Sufficient facilities should be available for the diagnosis, counselling and treatment of patients identified by the screening programme.

127

6.8.1 HISTORICAL BACKGROUND – THE JAPANESE EXPERIENCE

With the exception of screening for neuroblastoma, introduced by Japanese workers in 1973, the principal applications for tumour markers in paediatric oncology have been to assist in differential diagnosis, predict outcome, or monitor therapy. Controversy regarding screening infants for neuroblastoma has increased recently with the initiation of selective screening of infants for neuroblastoma in Europe, North America and Australia by a number of paediatric oncology groups. Interest in this approach has been stimulated by the results of the Japanese neuroblastoma mass screening programme.

In 1973, Sawada and colleagues (1984) first developed a 'mass' screening system involving six- to seven-month-old infants in Kyoto City, Japan. Assaying only VMA using a spot test methodology, a comparison was drawn between patients with neuroblastoma diagnosed before screening became available and those detected afterwards. Their results indicated a striking increase in the proportion of infants aged less than 12 months with neuroblastoma (12/22 patients; 54.6%) and a decrease in the proportion aged over two years at diagnosis (7/22 patients; 31.8%) during the eight years after initiation of mass screening in 1973 compared to the 12 years before 1973. These changes were reflected in improved survival after screening; before mass screening only 17.1% (6/35) survived, whereas 72.7% (16/22) of those diagnosed after 1973 were alive at the time of reporting in 1983. The authors claimed the improved prognosis was dependent on early diagnosis.

Nishi *et al.* (1987) evaluated the impact of screening six-month-old infants from Sapporo City, Hokkaido for neuroblastoma using HPLC determinations of VMA and HVA in filter paper urine. Improvement in three parameters after the initiation of mass screening were noted: (1) age at diagnosis; (2) clinical stage; and (3) survival. A significant increase in the proportion of cases diagnosed before 12 months of age (14.3%; 5/35) before screening compared to (66.7%; 12/18) after initiation of screening was reported. In addition, they observed a significant increase in the number of patients with Stages I, II, and IV-S disease since 1981. Their findings are reflected in a statistically significant improvement in survival when comparing patients diagnosed before screening became available with those diagnosed more recently. Parallel analysis of age, clinical stage at diagnosis, and survival rate in the remainder of the Hokkaido Prefecture, where neuroblastoma screening had not been available, showed no change in these parameters compared to the period before 1981. The programme in Hokkaido was expanded in October 1987 to include the entire island. Naito *et al.* (1990) reporting on the expanded experience in Hokkaido, noted that the proportion of patients with neuroblastoma aged less than 12 months had increased from 17% to 66%, and the proportion of Stage I and Stage II patients had increased from 9% to 26% and from 9% to 32% respectively. These findings were reflected by an improvement in the five-year survival rate from 23% to 66.7%.

6.8.2 MASS SCREENING – THE INTERNATIONAL CONTEXT

In Europe, North America and Australia, advocates of the development and implementation of mass screening programmes of infants for neuroblastoma point to the Japanese data to justify international expansion of the screening programme. Proponents of mass screening emphasize the statistically significant survival advantage which infants aged less than 12 months have compared with older children, and also to the increasing proportion of infants with limited stage disease, who have a more favourable prognosis compared to older children with disseminated disease at diagnosis. Do infants with 'good-prognosis' lower stage disease evolve into 'poor-prognosis' symptomatic children with disseminated neuroblastoma? Clearly, if such a hypothesis could be proven, the benefits of early detection and treatment would justify mass screening of infants for neuroblastoma, and could be expected to be associated with a reduction in late mortality from this disease. Neuroblastoma is, neither clinically nor biologically, a homogeneous disorder and evidence suggesting that infants detected by mass screening programmes may not necessarily be those who present at a later time with poor prognosis disease has promoted vigorous debate concerning the presuppositions and methodology of screening programmes.

Hayashi and co-workers (1988) recently studied solid tumour cytogenetics in 15 infants with neuroblastoma initially identified by urinary VMA mass screening. Interestingly, near triploidy or hyperdiploidy was found in each infant, a prognostic feature that Look and co-workers (1984) had previously demonstrated to be strongly predictive of a favourable outcome. Dr. Hayashi's results differ from the cytogenetic patterns commonly observed in neuroblastomas from children aged over one year. In this latter age group, diploidy or near diploidy, homogeneously staining regions, double minutes, and translocations of chromosome I were most commonly found. These cytogenetic features identify a subgroup of patients with a poor prognosis. One can speculate, therefore, that the cytogenetic abnormalities identified in infants diagnosed by mass screening further define a sub-group of patients who already have a favourable prognosis. Both Nishi (1987) and Hayashi (1988) have reported improved prognosis in children with neuroblastoma detected as a result of pre-clinical screening. Further population-based investigation will be required to determine whether screening is detecting 'good prognosis'

patients whose tumours may spontaneously regress. It may be that the tumour cell molecular biology, together with patterns of metastasis and drug resistance, are fundamentally different in these patients compared to children aged over one year at diagnosis. To date, there is no evidence supporting the hypothesis that infants with 'good-prognosis' disease develop 'poor prognosis' disease with the passage of time if they remain undetected during their first year of life. A preliminary report from the Quebec neuroblastoma screening project has examined the impact of screening infants for pre-clinical neuroblastoma on this tumour's population-based mortality (Tuchman *et al.*, 1990). A high rate of compliance during the first months (92%) and provision for a five-year study may permit answers to these important questions. Unfortunately, data from Japan thus far has focused on survival of the screened population, and population-based studies will be necessary to determine whether the increased number of infants detected by screening during the first year of life will be off-set by a corresponding reduction in the prevalence of 'poor-prognosis' neuroblastomas amongst children aged over two years, and that such a difference will be associated with a 'down-staging' of tumour stage.

The impact of spontaneous remission of neuroblastoma during the first year of life has been explored by Carlsen (1990). This study, undertaken with the dual aims of determining the frequency of spontaneous regression of neuroblastoma and the impact this has on the assessment of the benefits of screening, indicated that spontaneous regression occurred in less than 2% of cases. However Carlsen's epidemiological findings of increased incidence and survival rates in association with an unchanged mortality raised the possibility that the inclusion of borderline lesions among the pool of 'real' neuroblastomas has occurred during recent decades in Denmark, possibly as a result of low grade tumours diagnosed incidentally by abdominal palpation or routine chest radiograph.

Selection of metabolites and methods of analysis have been developed and refined since Sawada first assayed VMA using a qualitative spot test for screening in 1973 (Sawada *et al.*, 1984). Sequential studies have determined the relative importance of VMA, or HVA, or both, or the VMA/HVA ratio as the optimal metabolite, or combination, for evaluation. Overall, HVA is regarded as a better tumour marker than VMA for the presence of neuroblastoma. Pritchard *et al.* (1989) have demonstrated that approximately one-third of patients with low-stage disease have no evidence of raised urinary excretion of either VMA or HVA. Interestingly, these workers suggested that VMA may be the preferred urinary marker for neuroblastoma in infancy. This observation has more recently been supported by Tuchman *et al.* (1990). Refinements in assay techniques have reduced the rate of 'false-positive' detection of neuroblastoma from 3.8% of infants after initial evaluation using the VMA 'spot' test, to 0.016%, using a quantitative HPLC assay for VMA and HVA (Sawada *et al.*, 1984; Matsumoto *et al.* (1985). More recently, the development of HPLC, thin layer chromatography, gas chromatography/mass spectrometry, or enzyme-linked immunoassay have improved both the sensitivity and specificity of screening tests. The selection of screening methodology depends on the regional availability of the method in question as much as the philosophy regarding cost/effectiveness ratio. The Quebec neuroblastoma study, for example, is using a two-step approach employing initial qualitative screening with thin layer chromatography followed by gas chromatography/mass spectrometry in selected cases (Tuchman *et al.*, 1990).

A neuroblastoma screening programme hinges on the acceptance of screening by the infants' parents. Compliance rates ranging from 50% to 92% for population-based infant screening programmes have been reported. Information and education regarding the objectives of neuroblastoma screening are best introduced during the antenatal period, and reinforced shortly after delivery to maximize the overall level of compliance. Although compliance is likely to be higher in studies where urine is collected prior to initial discharge from hospital, later testing may be more appropriate if the hypothesis that screening at six months of age is likely to detect infants at risk of 'poor-prognosis' disease is true.

Whether or not the fundamental goals of screening infants at birth, six months or even later, will result in the pre-clinical detection of poor-prognosis neuroblastoma remains to be determined. Expanding clinical interest in neuroblastoma screening in Europe, North America and Australia, coupled with the continued refinement of neuroblastoma screening in Japan, will provide a novel insight into the overall significance of screening for malignancy in a paediatric population. In the meantime, controversy will continue until current projects yield mature data, and important epidemiological, clinical and biological questions can be answered in a scientific and statistically valid way.

REFERENCES

Abate G, Comella, P., Marfella, A. *et al.* (1989) Prognostic relevance of urinary neopterin in non-Hodgkin's lymphomas. *Cancer*, **63**, 484–9.

Abelev, G.I., Perova, S.D., Khramkova, N.I. *et al.*, (1963) Production of embryonal alpha-globulin by the transplantable mouse hepatomas. *Transplantation*, **1**, 174–80.

Alagille D, and Odievre, M. (1979) *Liver and Biliary Tract Disease in Children.* p. 311, John Wiley & Sons, New York.

Allen, J.C., Nissellbalum, J. and Epstein, F. (1979) Alpha-fetoprotein and human chorionic gonadotrophin determination in cerebrospinal fluid. *J. Neurosurg.*, **51**, 368–74.

Alpert, E. (1972) Alpha-1-fetoprotein: Serologic marker of human hepatoma and embryonal carcinoma. Conference on immunology of carcinogenesis. *Natl. Cancer Inst. Monogr.*, **35**, 415–20.

Alpert, E., Drysdale, J.W., Isselbacher, K.J. and Schur, P.H. (1972) Human AFP: Isolation, characterization and demonstration of microheterogeneity. *J. Biol. Chem.*, **247**, 3792–8.

Alpert, E., Starzl, T.E., Schur, P.H. and Isselbacher, J. (1971) Serum AFP in hepatoma patients after liver transplantation. *Gastroenterology*, **61**, 144–8.

Anderson, A. and Bergdahl, L. (1977) Carcinoid tumors of the appendix in children: a report of 25 cases. *Acta. Chir. Scand.* **143**, 173–5.

Bacci, G., Avella, M., McDonald, D. *et al.* (1988) Serum lactate dehydrogenase (LDH) as a tumor marker in Ewing's sarcoma. *Tumori*, **74**, 649–55.

Belanger C., Belanger, M. and Larochelle, J. (1972) Existence of d'alpha-foetoprotein circulate chez 8 patients souffrant de tyrosinemia hereditare. *Tame*, **101**, 877–8.

Berger, S., Pflüger, K.-H., Etzel, W.A. and Fischer J. (1989) Detection of tumours with nuclear magnetic resonance spectroscopy of plasma. *Eur. J. Cancer Clin. Oncol.*, **25**, 535–43.

Bergstrand, C.G. and Czar, B (1956) Demonstration of a new protein fraction in serum from the human fetus. Scandinav *J. Clin & Lab Investigation*, **8**, 174.

Bloomer, J.R., Waldmann, T.A., McIntire, K.R., and Klatskin, G. (1975) α-Fetoprotein in non-neoplastic hepatic disorders. *J.A.M.A.*, **233**, 38–41.

Boomsma, F., Ausema, L., Hakvoort-Cammel, F.G.A. *et al.* (1989) Combined measurements of plasma aromatic L-amino acid decarboxylase and DOPA as tumour markers in diagnosis and follow-up of neuroblastoma. *Eur. J. Cancer Clin. Oncol.*, **25**, 1045–52.

Brewster, M.A., Berry, D.H. and Moriarty, M. (1977) Urinary 3-methoxy-4-hydroxyphenylacetic (homovanillic) and 3-methoxy-4-hydroxymandelic acid (vanillylmandelic) acids: gas-liquid chromatographic methods and experience with 13 cases of neuroblastoma. *Clin. Chem.*, **23**, 2247–9.

Brock, D.J., Scrimgeour, J.B. and Nelson, M.M. (1975) Amniotic fluid alpha fetoprotein measurements in the early diagnosis of central nervous system disorders. *Clin. Genet.*, **7**, 163–9.

Burger, P.C., Grahmann, F.C., Bliestle, A. and Kleihves, P. (1987) Differentiation in the medulloblastoma. A histological and immunohistochemical study. *Acta. Neuropathologica*, **73**, 115.

Carlsen, N.L.T. (1990) How frequent is spontaneous remission of neuroblastomas? Implications for screening. *Brit. J. Cancer*, **61**, 441–6.

Carmel, R. and Eisenberg, L. (1977) Serum vitamin B_{12} and transcobalamin abnormalities in patients with cancer. *Cancer*, **40**, 1348–53.

Collier, N.A., Weinbren, K., Broom, S.G. *et al.* (1984) Neurotensin secretion by fibrolamellar carcinoma of the liver. *Lancet*: **1**, 538–40.

Cooper, E.H., Pritchard, J., Bailey C.C. and Ninane, J. (1987) Serum neuron-specific enolase in children's cancer. *Brit. J. Cancer* **56**, 65–7.

Dehner, L.P. (1983) Gondal and extragonadal germ cell neoplasia of childhood. *Human Pathol.*, **14**, 493–511.

Earl, J. (1986) Measurement of the acidic metabolites of biogenic amines, in *The Clinical Biochemist*, (ed D.C. Sampson) A.A.C.B. Monogr. pp. 57–62.

Edwards M.S.B., Davis R.L. and Laurent, J.P. (1985) Tumor markers and cytologic features of cerebrospinal fluid. *Cancer* **56** (Suppl), 1773–7.

Exelby, P.R., Filler, R.M. and Grosfeld, J.L. (1974) Liver tumors in children with particular reference to hepatoblastoma and hepatocellular carcinoma. American Academy of Pediatrics Surgical Section Survey 1974. *J. Pediatr. Surg.*, **10**, 329–37.

Felberg, N.T., Michelson, J.B. and Shields, J.A. (1976) CEA family syndrome. Abnormal carcinoembryonic antigen (CEA) levels in asymptomatic retinoblastoma family members. *Cancer* **37**, 1397–402.

Feldenzer, J.A. and McKeever, P.E. (1987) Selective localization of gamma-enolase in stromal cells of cerebellar hemangioblastomas. *Acta. Neuropathologica*, **72**, 281.

Feldman, J.M., Lee, E.M. and Castleberry, C.A. (1987) Catecholamine and serotonin content of foods: effect on urinary excretion of homovanillic acid and 5-hydroxyindoleacetic acid. *J. Am. Diet. Assoc.*, **87**, 1031–3.

Fossel, E.T., Carr, J.M. and McDonagh, J. (1986) Detection of malignant tumours. Water-suppressed proton nuclear magnetic resonance spectroscopy of plasma. *N. Engl. J. Med.*, **315**, 1369–76.

Gailani, S., Chu, T.M., Nussbaum, A. *et al.* (1976) Human chorionic gonadotrophins (hCG) in non-trophoblastic neoplasms. *Cancer,* **38**, 1684–6.

Gitlin, D., (1975) Normal biology of α-fetoprotein. *Ann. N.Y. Acad. Sci.,* **259**, 7–16.

Gitlin, D. and Boseman, M. (1966) Serum AFP, albumin and G-globulin in the human conceptus. *J. Clin. Invest.,* **45**, 1826–38.

Gitlin, D., Perricelli, A. and Gitlin, G.M. (1972) Synthesis of α-fetoprotein by liver, yolk sac and gastrointestinal tract of the human conceptus. *Cancer Res.,* **32**, 979–82.

Gitlow, S.E., Bertani, L.M., Rausen, A. *et al.* (1970) Diagnosis of neuroblastoma by qualitative and quantitative determination of catecholamine metabolites in urine. *Cancer,* **25**, 1377–83.

Gitlow, S.E., Bertani, L.M., Wilk, E. *et al.*, (1970) Excretion of catecholamine metabolites by children with familial dysautonomia. *Pediatrics,* **46**, 513–22.

Green, D.M. (1983) The diagnosis and treatment of yolk sac tumors in infants and children. *Cancer Treat. Rev.,* **10**, 265–88.

Hann, H.-W.L., Levy, H.M. and Evans, A.E. (1980) Serum ferritin as a guide to therapy in neuroblastoma. *Cancer Res.,* **40**, 1411–3.

Hayashi, Y., Inaba, T., Hanada, R. and Yamamoto, K. (1988) Chromosome findings and prognosis in 15 patients with neuroblastoma found by VMA mass screening. *J. Pediatr.* **112**, 567–71.

Herlyn, M., Sears, H.F., Steplewski, Z. *et al.* (1982) Monoclonal antibody detection of a circulating tumor associated antigen I. Presence of antigen in sera of patients with colorectal, gastric and pancreatic carcinoma. *J. Clin. Immunol.,* **2**, 135–41.

Hinterberger, H. and Bartholomew, R.J. (1969) Catecholamines and their acidic metabolites in urine and in tumour tissue in neuroblastoma, ganglioneuroma and phaechromocytoma. *Clin. Chem. Acta.,* **23**, 169–75.

Hirszfeld, L. and Halber, W. (1932) Untersuchungen über verwandtschaftsreaktionen zwischen embryonal – und krebsgewebe. I Mitteilung. Rattenembryonen und Menschentumoren. Z Immunitätsforsch **75**, 193–208.

Howell, R.E., Handlers, J.P., Aberle, AM. *et al.* (1988) CEA immunoreactivity in odontogenic

tumors and keratocysts. *Oral Surg. Oral Med. Oral Pathol.,* **66**, 576–80.

Huntington, R.W. and Bullock, W.K. (1970) Yolk sac tumors of extragonadal origin. *Cancer,* **25**, 1368–76.

Jacobi, C. and Reiber, H. (1988) Clinical relevance of increased neuron-specific enolase concentration in cerebrospinal fluid. *Clin. Chimica. Acta.,* **177**, 49–54.

Javadpour, N. (1980) The role of biologic tumor markers in testicular cancer. *Cancer,* **45**, 1755–61.

Kahn, C.R., Rosen, S.W., Weintraub, B.D. *et al.* (1977) Ectopic production of chorionic gonadotropin and its subunits by islet cell tumors. *N. Engl. J. Med.,* **297**, 565–9.

Kaser, H. (1965) Catecholamine-producing neural tumors other than pheochromocytoma. *Pharmacol. Rev.,* **18**, 659–64.

Kawata, M., Sekiya, S., Hatakeya, R. and Takamizawa, H. (1989) Neuron-specific enolase as a serum marker for immature teratoma and dysgerminoma. *Gynecol. Oncol.,* **32**, 191–7.

Kellie, S.J., Clague, A.E., McGeary, H.M. and Smith, P.J. (1986) The value of catecholamine metabolite determination on untimed urine collections in the diagnosis of neural crest tumours in children. *Aust. Paediatr. J.,* **22**, 313–5.

Kew, M.C., Purves, L.R. and Bersohn, I. (1973) Serum alpha-fetoprotein levels in acute viral hepatitis. *Gut,* **14**, 939–42.

Kloster, B.E., John, P.A., Miller, L.E. *et al.* (1987) Soluble interleukin-2 receptors are elevated in patients with AIDS or at risk of developing AIDS. *Clin. Immunol. Immunopathol.,* **45**, 440–6.

LaBrosse, E.H., Com-Nougué, C., Zucker J.-M. *et al.* (1980) Urinary excretion of 3-methoxy-4-hydroxymandelic acid and 3-methoxy-4-hydroxyphenylacetic acid by 288 patients with neuroblastoma and neural crest tumors. *Cancer Res.,* **40**, 1995–2001.

Lack, E.E., Neave, C and Vawter, G.F. (1983) Hepatocellular carcinoma: Review of 32 cases of childhood and adolescence. *Cancer,* **52**, 1510–5.

Laug, W.E., Siegel, S.E., Shaw, K.N.F. *et al.* (1978) Initial urinary catecholamine metabolite concentrations and prognosis in neuroblastoma. *Pediatrics,* **62**, 77–83.

Liddell, R.H.A., Meyer, W.H., Dodge, R.K. *et al.*, (1988) Prognostic indicators for patients with osteosarcoma (OS) treated with adjuvant chemo-therapy. *Proc. Am. Assoc. Clin. Res.*, **29**, 226.

Link, M.P., Shuster, J.J., Goorin, A.M. *et al.* (1988) Adjuvant chemotherapy in the treatment of osteosarcoma: Results of the Multi-Institutional Osteosarcoma Study, *Recent Concepts in Sarcoma Treatment.* Proceedings of the International Symposium on Sarcomas, (eds J.R. Ryan and L.H. Baker) Dordrecht, The Netherlands, Kluwer Academic Publishers.

Look, A.T., Hayes, A., Nitschke, R. *et al.* (1984) Cellular DNA content as a predictor of response to chemotherapy in infants with unresectable neuroblastoma. *N. Eng. J. Med.*, **311**, 231–5.

McArthur, J.W., Toll, G.D., Russfeld, A.B. *et al.* (1973) Sexual precocity attributable to ectopic gonadtropin secretion by hepatoblastoma. *Am. J. Med.*, **54**, 390–403.

McIntire, K.R., Waldmann, T.A., Moertel, C.G. and Go, V.L.W. (1975) Serum α–fetoprotein in patients with neoplasms of the gastrointestinal tract. *Cancer Res.*, **35**, 991–6.

Maeda, M., Tozuka, S., Kanayama, M. and Uchida, T. (1988) Hepatocellular carcinoma producing carcinoembryonic antigen. *Dig. Dis. Sci.*, **33**, 1629–31.

Mahour, G.H., Wogu, G.V., Siegal, S.E. and Isaacs, M. (1983) Improved survival in infants and children with primary malignant liver tumors. *Am. J. Surg.*, **146**, 236–40.

Maltz, C., Lightdale, C.J. and Winawer S.J. (1980) Hepatocellular carcinoma. New directions in etiology. *Am. J. Gastroenterol.*, **74**, 361–5.

Mann, J.R., Lakin, G.E., Leonard, J.C. *et al.* (1978) Clinical applications of serum carcinoembryonic antigen and alpha-fetoprotein levels in children with solid tumours. *Arch. Dis. Child.*, **53**, 366–74.

Masopust, J., Radl, J. and Houstek, J. (1970) Occurrence of alpha-1-fetoprotein in some infants suffering from hepatopathy. *Protides of the Biological Fluids.* **18**, 239–42.

Masseyeff, R., Gilli, J., Krebs, B *et al.* (1975) Evolution of α-fetoprotein serum levels throughout life in humans and rats, and during pregnancy in the rat. *Ann. N.Y. Acad. Sci.* **259**, 17.

Matsumoto, M., Anazawa, A., Zuzuki, K. *et al.* (1985) Urine mass screening for neuroblast-

oma by high performance liquid chromatography (HPLC). *Pediatr. Res.*, **19**, 625

Mautalen, C.A. (1970) Circadian rhythm of urinary total and free hydroxyproline excretion and its relation to creatinine excretion. *J. Lab. Clin. Med.*, **75**, 8–11.

Melia, W.M., Johnson, P.J., Carter, S. *et al.* (1981) Plasma carcinoembryonic antigen in the diagnosis and management of patients with hepatocellular carcinoma. *Cancer*, **48**, 1004–8.

Murthy, A.S.K., Vawter, G.F., Lee, A.B.H. *et al.* (1980) Hormonal bioassay of gonadotropin producing hepatoblastoma. *Arch. Pathol. Lab. Med.*, **104**, 513–7.

Muscettola, G., Wehr, T. and Goodwin, F.K. (1977) Effect of diet on urinary MHPG excretion in depressed patients and normal control subjects. *Am. J. Psychiatry*, **134**, 914–6.

Naito, H., Sasaki, M., Yamashiro, K. *et al.* (1990) Improvement in prognosis of neuroblastoma through mass population screening. *J. Pediatr. Surg.*, **25**, 245–8.

Nakagawara, A., Ikeda, K., Tsuneyoshi, M., Daimaru, Y. *et al.* (1985) Hepatoblastoma producing both alpha-fetoprotein and human chorionic gonadotropin. *Cancer*, **56**, 1636–42.

Nishi, S. (1970) Isolation and characterization of a human fetal α-globulin from the sera of fetuses and a hepatoma patient. *Cancer Res.*, **30**, 2507–13.

Nishi, M., Miyake, H., Takeda, T. *et al.* (1987) Effects of the mass screening of neuroblastoma in Sapporo City. *Cancer*, **60**, 433–6.

Odelstad, L., Pahlman, S., Lackgren, G. *et al.* (1982) Neurone-specific enolase: a marker for differential diagnosis of neuroblastoma and Wilms' tumour. *J. Pediatr. Surg.*, **17**, 381–5.

Ohaki, Y., Misugi, K., Sasaki, Y. and Tsunoda, A. (1983) Hepatitis B surface antigen positive hepatocellular carcinoma in children. Report of a case and review of the literature. *Cancer*, **51**, 822–8.

Packer, R.J., Sutton, L.N., Rorke, L.B. *et al.* (1984) Intracranial embryonal cell carcinoma. *Cancer*, **54**, 520–4.

Paradinas, F.J., Melia, W.M., Wilkinson, M.L. *et al.* (1982) High serum vitamin B_{12} binding capacity as a marker of the fibrolamellar variant of hepatocellular carcinoma. *Brit. Med. J.*, **285**, 840–2.

Pinkerton, C.R., Pritchard, J. and Spitz L. (1986) High complete response rate in children with

133

advanced germ cell tumours using cisplatin – containing combination chemotherapy. *J. Clin. Oncol.*, **4**, 194–9.

Pittaway, D.E. and Foyez, J.A. (1987) Serum CA-125 antigen levels increase during menses. *Am. J. Obstet. Gynecol.*, **156**, 75.

Potezny, N. and Rosenblatt, A.L. (1986) The effects of various dietary constituents on the urinary excretion of biogenic amines and their metabolites, in *The Clinical Biochemist*, (ed D.C. Sampson) A.A.C.B. Monogr, pp. 52–53.

Pratt, C.B., Rivera, G., Shanks, E. *et al.* (1977) Colorectal carcinoma in adolescents – implications regarding etiology. *Cancer*, **40** (Supp) 2464–72.

Pritchard, J., Barnes, J., Germond, S. *et al.* (1989) Stage and urinary catecholamine metabolite excretion in neuroblastoma. *Lancet*, **2**, 514–5.

Pui, C.-H., Ip, S.H., Iflah, S. *et al.* (1988) Serum interleukin-2 receptor levels in childhood acute lymphoblastic leukemia. *Blood*, **71**, 1135–7.

Pui, C.-H., Ip, S.H., Kung, P. *et al.* (1987) High serum interleukin-2 receptor levels are related to advanced disease and a poor outcome in childhood non-Hodgkin's lymphoma. *Blood*, **70**, 624–8.

Pui, C.-H., Ip, S.H., Thompson, E. *et al.* (1989) High serum interleukin-2 receptor levels correlate with a poor prognosis in children with Hodgkin's disease. *Leukemia*, **3**, 481–4.

Quin, J.J., Altman, A.J. and Frantz, C.N. (1980) Serum lactic dehydrogenase: an indicator of tumor activity in neuroblastoma. *J. Pediatr.*, **97**, 88–91.

Rao, B.N., Pratt, C.B., Fleming, I.D. *et al.* (1985) Colon carcinoma in children and adolescents: A review of thirty cases. *Cancer* **55**, 1322–6.

Rayfield, E.J., Cain, J.P., Casey M.P. *et al.* (1972) Influence of diet on urinary VMA excretion *J.A.M.A.*, **221**, 704–5.

Rosano, T.G. (1984) Liquid-chromatographic evaluation of age-related changes in the urinary excretion of free catecholamines in pediatric patients. *Clin. Chem.*, **30**, 301–3.

Rosen, S.W., Weintraub D.B., Vaitukaitis, J.L. *et al.* (1975) Placental proteins and their subunits as tumor markers. *Ann. Intern. Med.*, **82**, 71–83.

Ruibal, A., Encabo, G., Martinez-Miralles, E. *et al.* (1984) CA-125 serum levels in non-malignant pathologies. *Bull. Cancer* (Paris) **71**, 145–8.

Ruoslahti, E. and Seppälä (1979) α-Fetoprotein in cancer and fetal development. *Adv. Cancer Res.*, **29**, 275–346.

Sampson, D. (1987) Biochemical methods for diagnosis of carcinoid tumour: what should we really be measuring? *Clin. Biochem. Revs.*, **8**, 87–94.

Sawada, T., Kidowaki, T., Sakamoto, I. *et al.* (1984) Neuroblastoma. Mass screening for early detection and its prognosis. *Cancer*, **53**, 2731–5.

Sawada, T., Nakata, T., Takasugi, N. *et al.* (1984) Mass screening for neuroblastoma in infants in Japan. *Lancet*, **2**, 271–3.

Schuman, A.J., Alario, A.J. and Pitel, P.A. (1984) Occult gangioneuroma with diarrhoea: localization by venous catecholamines. *Med. Pediatr. Oncol.*, **12**, 93–6.

Sculier, J.P., Body, J.J., Jacobowitz, D. and Fruhling, J. (1987) Value of CEA determination in biological fluids and tissues. *Eur. J. Cancer Clin. Oncol.*, **23**, 1091–3.

Sharry, A., Janzer, R.C., Von Hochstelter, A.R. *et al.* (1985) Primary intracranial germ-cell tumours – A clinicopathologic study of 14 cases. *J. Neurosurg*, **62**, 826.

Soldin, S.J. and Hill, J.G. (1981) Liquid chromatographic analysis for urinary 4-hydroxy-3-methoxymandelic acid and 4-hydroxy-3-methoxyphenylacetic acid, and its use in the investigation of neural crest tumours. *Clin. Chem.*, **27**, 503–4.

Stenstrom, G., Sjogren, B. and Waldenstrom, J. (1983) Excretion of adrenalin, noradrenaline, vanilmandelic acid and metanephrins in 64 patients with phaeochromocytoma. *Acta. Med. Scand.*, **214**, 145–52.

Takashi, M., Haimoto, H., Tanaka, J. *et al.* (1989) Evaluation of gamma-enolase as a tumor marker for renal cell carcinoma. *J. Urol.*, **141**, 830–4.

Tatarinov, Y.S. (1964) Detection of embryospecific alpha-globulin in the blood sera of patients with primary liver tumours. *Vop. Med. Khim.*, **10**, 90–1.

Teilum, G. (1965) Classification of endodermal sinus tumour (mesoblastoma vitellinum) and so-called 'embryonal carcinoma' of the ovary. *Acta. Pathol. Microbiol. Scandinav.*, **64**, 407–29.

Tormey, D.C., Waalkes, T.P., Snyder, J.J. and Simon, R.M. (1977) Biological markers in breast carcinoma II. Clinical correlations with human chorionic gonadotrophin. *Cancer*, **39**, 2391–6.

Touitou, Y. and Bogdan, A. (1988) Tumor markers

in non-malignant diseases. *Eur. J. Cancer Clin. Oncol.*, **24**, 1083–91.

Touitou, Y. and Heshmati, H.M. (1988) Neurone-specific enolase in medullary thyroid carcinoma. *Clin. Chem.*, **34**, 2375–6.

Tuchman, M., Lemieux, B., Avray-Blias, C. *et al.* (1990) Screening for neuroblastoma at 3 weeks of age: Methods and preliminary results from the Quebec neuroblastoma screening project. *Pediatrics*, **86**, 765–73.

Tuchman. M., Morris, C.L., Ramnaraine, M.L. *et al.* (1985) Value of random urinary homovanillic acid and vanillylmandelic acid levels in the diagnosis and management of patients with neuroblastoma. Comparison with 24-hour urine collections. *Pediatrics*, **75**, 324–8.

Uctzelsen, C.L. and Bruninga G. (1968) Infantile choriocarcinoma: A characteristic syndrome. *J. Pediatr.*, **73**, 374–8.

Vaitukaitis, J.L., Braunstein, G.D., Ross, G.T. (1972) A radioimmunassay which specifically measures human chorionic gonadotrophin in the presence of human luteinizing hormone. *Am. J. Obstet. Gynecol.*, **113**, 751–8.

Vaitukaitis, J.L., Ross, G.T., Braunstein, G.D. and Rayford, P.L. (1976) Gonadotropins and their subunits: basic and clinical studies: *Recent Prog. Horm. Res.*, **32**, 289–331.

Von Eyben, F.E, Blaabjerg, O., Petersen, P.H. *et al.* (1988) Serum lactate dehydrogenase isoenzyme 1 as a marker of testicular germ cell tumor. *J. Urol.*, **140**, 986–90.

Wagner, D.K., Kiwanuka, J., Edwards B.K. *et al.* (1987) Soluble interleukin-2 receptor levels in patients with undifferentiated and lymphoblastic lymphomas: correlation with survival. *J. Clin. Oncol.*, **5**, 1262–74.

Walhof, C.M., Van Sonderen, L., Voûte, P.A. and

Delemarre, J.F.M. (1988) Half-life of alpha-fetoprotein in patients with a teratoma, endodermal sinus tumor or hepatoblastoma. *Pediatr. Hematol. Oncol.*, **5**, 217–27.

Waldmann, T.A. and McIntire, K.R. (1972) Serum AFP levels in patients with ataxia telangectasia. *Lancet*, **2** 1112–5.

Watcher, H., Hausen, A. and Grassmayr, K. (1979) Erhote Ausscheidung von neopterin im harn von patienten mit malignen tumoren und mit viruserkrankungen. Hoppe Seylers Z *Physiol. Chem.*, **360**, 1957–60.

Weetman, R.M., Rider, P.S., Oei, T.O. *et al.* (1976) Effect of diet on urinary excretion of VMA, HVA, metanephrine, and total free catecholamine in normal preschool children. *J. Pediatr.*, **88**, 46–50.

Weinberg, A.G. and Feinegold, M.J. (1983) Primary hepatic tumors in childhood. *Human Pathol.*, **14**, 512–37.

Wheeler, K., Pritchard, J., Luck, W. and Rossiter, M. (1986) Transcobalamin I as a 'marker' for fibrolamellar hepatoma. *Med. Pediatr. Oncol.*, **14**, 227–9.

Wilding, P., Senior, M.B., Innbushi, T. and Ludwick, M.L. (1988) Assessment of proton nuclear magnetic resonance spectroscopy for detection of malignancy. *Clin. Chem.*, **34**, 505–11.

Wu, J.T., Book, L. and Sudar, K (1981) Serum alpha fetoprotein (AFP) levels in normal infants. *Pediatr. Res.*, **15**, 50–2.

Zarate, A. and MacGregor, C. (1982) Beta subunit hCG and the control of trophoblastic disease. *Semin. Oncol.*, **9**, 187–90.

Zeltzer, P.M., Marangos, P.J., Evans, A.E. and Schneider, S.L. (1986) Serum neuron-specific enolase in children with neuroblastoma. Relationship to stage and disease course. *Cancer*, **57**, 1230–4.

Chapter 7

Tumour staging: an assessment of the roles of pre- and post-operative staging systems

H. EKERT

7.1 INTRODUCTION

The purpose of tumour staging is to describe accurately, comprehensively, and in an abbreviated form, the extent of local infiltration and distant spread of the cancer. The major benefits of tumour staging are that it permits national and international communication which in turn allows construction and evaluation of clinical studies. It also serves as a guide to prognosis by allowing statistical evaluation of the likelihood of response to treatment and duration of survival according to the extent of tumour spread. An accurate definition of the stage of the tumour can improve understanding of the basic nature of the cancer by defining relationships that may exist between biological markers of disease and its stage.

It should be noted that there are also some minor disadvantages to staging systems. Perhaps the most serious is the possibility of promoting an impersonal and mechanistic attitude to patient care by regarding the patient as one with a cancer of stage 'X' which requires under all circumstances the specified treatment for that stage. Another problem is related to the development of multiple institutional or national classification methods which may cause confusion when information is reported at international or national levels. Occasionally staging systems based on outdated approaches to treatment may lead to unnecessarily invasive investigations such as staging laparotomy in Hodgkin's disease. Staging systems based on operative findings have an inbuilt bias towards primary surgical treatment, an approach which may become superceded by advances in other treatment modalities.

Two major staging systems exist for the main solid tumours of childhood. The first is based on surgical findings and pathological examination of the operative specimens. The second is based on the definition of the anatomical extent of the disease defined by investigations undertaken before treatment. The tumour node metastases (TNM) classification and staging (see below) represents such a system; its basic principles are applicable to all sites regardless of treatment (Hermanek and Sobin, 1987).

7.2 OUTLINE OF THE TNM STAGING SYSTEM

In this system, three components are assessed:

1. T–The extent of the primary tumour. T0 indicates no primary tumour; T1–4 increasing size and/or local extent of the tumour;
2. N–The absence or presence and extent of regional lymph node metastasis: N0 denotes no metastasis, N1–3 increasing involvement of regional lymph nodes;
3. M–The absence or presence of distant metastasis: M0 represents no metastasis and M1 the presence of metastasis.

Details of the TNM classification are shown in Table 7.1. The classification makes no presuppositions on the value of different treatment modalities and relies heavily on the accuracy of pre-operative investigations. Improvements in imaging and nuclear medicine technology have greatly strengthened the accuracy of pre-operative investigations but detection of lymph node infiltration can be difficult despite these advances.

The surgical and pathological staging or grouping systems are based on the fact that many patients with solid tumours are initially admitted to surgical wards and that surgery prior to the use of all other modalities is, in this model, the treatment of choice in all the curable tumours. The weakness of the surgical staging systems is that they encourage initial major surgical intervention in all but widely disseminated tumours. This removes the option of the use of pre-operative chemotherapy or irradiation in an attempt to increase cure rates and decrease morbidity.

7.3 RELEVANCE OF THE TNM SYSTEM TO PAEDIATRICS

Only a minority of children with cancer have access to treatment facilities which give them a chance of cure. The majority live in parts of

Table 7.1 General principles of TNM classification

T-Primary Tumour	
TX	Primary tumour cannot be assessed
T0	No evidence of primary tumour
Tis	Carcinoma *in situ*
T1, T2, T3, T4	Increasing size and/or local extent of the primary tumour

N-Regional Lymph Nodes	
NX	Regional lymph nodes cannot be assessed
N0	No regional lymph node metastasis
N1, N2, N3	Increasing involvement of regional lymph nodes
Notes:	Direct extension of the primary tumour into lymph nodes is classified as a distant metastasis.
	Metastasis in any lymph node other than regional is classified as a distant metastasis.

M-Distant Metastasis	
MX	Presence of distant metastasis cannot be assessed
M0	No distant metastasis
M1	Distant Metastasis

Note: The category M1 may be further specified according to the following notation:

Pulmonary	PUL	Bone Marrow	MAR
Osseous	OSS	Pleura	PLE
Hepatic	HEP	Peritoneum	PER
Brain	BRA	Skin	SKI
Lymph nodes	LYM	Other	OTH

the world which simply cannot afford to spend money on cancer therapy, or where there is a gross maldistribution of health resources. In many such countries there is medical and nursing expertise of sufficient skill to develop cancer treatment centres but

137

there is inadequate financial support for investigative and therapeutic facilities. Often oncology is practised in an *'ad hoc'* fashion, or by following some treatment protocol developed in an industrialized nation with highly sophisticated cancer centres. It is possible that the adoption of an internationally accepted cancer staging system such as the UICC TNM classification, may help to promote the development of better treatment facilities by accrual of statistical information on death rates from cancer according to stage. These data can be presented to politicians and health administrators in order to convince them of the need to devote more resources to cancer treatment.

7.4 AN APPRAISAL OF PRESENT CLASSIFICATION SYSTEMS

In those parts of the world with well developed cancer treatment resources complex organizations undertake cooperative national and international clinical studies. In Europe the main cooperative group is La Société Internationale d'Oncologie Pédiatrique (SIOP). In North America the major cooperative groups are the Children's Cancer Study Group (CCSG) and the Pediatric Oncology Group (POG). Each of these major groups have defined their own staging systems and in many instances these differ substantially. The choice of therapy frequently depends on the stage of disease, and since these groups define stages differently, there can be confusion in communication of the results of treatment between the groups. In addition, clinical units which do not belong to one of these major groups tend to adopt a variety of staging systems and treatment protocols which span all three groups. This has resulted in quite serious misinterpretation of data and in confusion on the reporting of results of treatment.

Table 7.2 IRS clinical grouping classification

Group I	Localized disease, completely resected
A	Confined to organ or muscle or origin
B	Infiltration outside organ or muscle or origin; regional nodes not involved
Group II	Compromised or regional resections of three types including the following:
A	Grossly resected tumours with microscopic residual
B	Regional disease, completely resected, in which nodes may be involved and/or extension of tumour into an adjacent organ present
C	Regional disease with involved nodes, grossly resected, but with evidence of microscopic residual
Group III	Incomplete resection or biopsy with gross residual disease
Group IV	Distant metastases, present at onset

7.4.1 SOFT TISSUE SARCOMAS WITH SPECIAL REFERENCE TO RHABDOMYOSARCOMA

There are two main systems for staging of these particular tumours. The surgical/pathological one is the Intergroup Rhabdomyosarcoma Study (IRS) grouping (Maurer, 1975) shown in Table 7.2. It is based on whether or not surgical resection can be achieved. The pre-operative system used is the TNM classification with staging based on pre-operative investigative findings. The classification and staging system are shown in Tables 7.3 and 7.4. The TNM classification allows for operative findings by a reclassification after surgery using the prefix 'p'. The classification is therefore similar to the IRS one but places no time restraint on when surgery is undertaken. The IRS staging has established value in defining prognostic groups and evaluating post surgical modalities of treatment. The TNM classification,

Table 7.3 TNM classification of soft tissue sarcomas

T-Primary tumour

TX	Primary tumour cannot be assessed
TO	No evidence of primary tumour
T1	Tumour limited to organ or tissue of origin
	T1a Tumour 5 cm or less in greatest dimension
	T1b Tumour more than 5 cm in greatest dimension
T2	Tumour invades contiguous organ(s) or tissue(s) and/or with adjacent malignant effusion
	T2a Tumour 5 cm or less in greatest dimension
	T2b Tumour more than 5 cm in greatest dimension

Note: The categories T3 and T4 do not apply. The existence of more than one tumour is generally considered a primary tumour with distant metastasis.

N-Regional lymph nodes

NX	Regional lymph nodes cannot be assessed
NO	No regional lymph node metastasis
N1	Regional lymph node metastasis
M	Distant metastasis

Table 7.4 Clinical stage grouping (TNM, cTNM)

Stage I	T1a	NO	MO
	T1b	NO	MO
Stage II	T2a	NO	MO
	T2b	NO	MO
Stage III	Any T	N1	MO
Stage IV	Any T	Any N	M1

Note: When the regional lymph nodes cannot be assessed clinically or radiologically, NX should be considered NO in Stages I and II.

rarely used in this study. The TNM classification was used to define four stages as shown in Table 7.4. This resulted in the definition of three prognostic groups with Stage I consisting of 242 patients with 48 deaths and Stage IV of 103 with 80 deaths. Stages II and III could not be separated in terms of clinical outcome as clinical evidence of lymph node involvement was found in only 21 of 160 patients, who, on the basis of N status, may have fitted into either Stage II or III. Comparison of the TNM classification with the IRS showed that the TNM discriminated more significantly between groups I, and II and III combined. Clearly, the major weakness of the TNM system was assessment of regional lymph nodes. This poses the question of whether surgical exploration of regional lymph nodes should be considered as part of the TNM staging in this tumour type.

In a further attempt to develop a common staging system for rhabdomyosarcoma, SIOP organized an international workshop in 1987 (Rodary *et al.*, 1989) with the objective of developing a common definition of stage, relevant end points and standardized statistical methods of reporting results. Records of 100 children with rhabdomyosarcoma were reviewed by ten paediatric oncologists who were predominantly accustomed to either the TNM or IRS classifications. Other methods of classification (St. Judes, Royal Marsden and

although not yet utilized in USA prospective studies (Pedrick *et al.*, 1986) is well suited to clinical trials aimed at evaluating all therapeutic questions.

In a retrospective study, Lawrence and colleages (1987) analysed 505 eligible patients entered into IRS between 1978–82. In this study T and N status before surgery was determined from patient records. Local invasiveness was assessed from clinical description and available radiological examinations. Regional lymph node evaluation was clinical only. Lymphograms and CT scans were

139

Memorial Sloan Kettering) were considered to be similar to IRS and not included in this review. There has been good agreement between the reviewers using either system but it has varied for each category, being lowest for patients with Stage I and II disease. The greatest area of disagreement was in distinguishing between tumours with or without contiguous organ or tissue involvement, particularly in the pelvis, abdomen or orbit. Another source of disagreement was the assessment of regional lymph node involvement with confusion regarding the regional lymph node drainage areas. Added to this was the difficulty of imaging detection of lymph node involvement in difficult anatomical sites such as the peri-aortic, presacral and retropharyngeal lymph nodes. Overall there were significant differences in the distribution of patients in early stages and this carries with it therapeutic and prognostic implications. Using the TNM system, 31% of cases were Stage I whereas with the IRS only 12% were Stage I. The majority of patients, were either Stage II in the TNM system (47%) or group III in the IRS (55%). Classifying TNM Stage I patients with the IRS resulted in 'upstaging' two-thirds of patients to group II or III. Using the same procedure, two-thirds of IRS group III were 'downstaged' to TNM Stage II. The conclusion of the working party was that the TNM classification allowed better discrimination between apparently different prognostic groups and excluded the variable of the value or otherwise of early attempts at surgical resection of the tumour.

In recent years there have been continuing improvements in chemotherapeutic treatment of most solid tumours including rhabdomyosarcoma. Clinical experience of the ability of chemotherapy to markedly reduce tumour size is expanding. It can be expected that this will make complete tumour resection more frequent. In addition, pre-operative chemotherapy may reduce the need for irradiation in sites where the long-term mor-

bidity of irradiation has particularly severe consequences, e.g. in the pelvic area, and eliminates the need for mutilating surgery. The use of this approach to treatment strongly supports the TNM classification. By agreeing to its acceptibility international studies of the role of tumour size reduction prior to complete surgical removal of the tumour could be initiated and evaluated with the possibility of increased cure rates and reduction of treatment-related complications.

7.4.2 WILMS' TUMOUR

Major advances in the treatment of Wilms' tumour have occurred as a result of sequential group studies in the USA (the National Wilms' Tumour Studies [NWTS]) which investigated the role of adjuvant irradiation and chemotherapy. These were randomized, controlled studies which were aimed at improving cure rates and reducing the incidence of therapy-related complications. The staging system used by the NWTS is based on the premise that the first step in the treatment is surgical exploration and attempt at excision of the tumour. The staging system is therefore post-surgical (Table 7.5). If one adheres to the concept that early surgery is desirable in all patients with Wilms' tumour then there is little to be gained from adopting a pre-surgical staging such as the TNM classification.

European studies have investigated the role of pre-operative irradiation and chemotherapy in advanced or massive tumours (Lemerle *et al.*, 1978; Lemerle *et al.*, 1983). These studies have demonstrated that impressive tumour bulk reduction can occur, resulting in the conversion of non-operable to readily operable tumours, i.e. NWTS Stage III to Stage II. In Stage V tumours, pre-operative chemotherapy has reduced bulky tumours to such an extent that only partial nephrectomies have been possible with retention of function in both kidneys.

Table 7.5 NWTS staging system

	Stage
I	Tumour limited to kidney and completely excised.
	The surface of the renal capsule is intact. Tumour was not ruptured before or during removal. There is no residual tumour apparent beyond the margins of resection.
II	Tumour extends beyond the kidney but is completely removed.
	There is regional extension of the tumour i.e. penetration through the outer surface of the renal capsule into perirenal soft tissues. Vessels outside the kidney substance are infiltrated or contain tumour thrombus. The tumour may have been biopsied or there has been local spillage of tumour confined to the flank. There is no residual tumour apparent at or beyond the margins of excision.
III	Residual nonhaematogenous tumour confined to abdomen
	Any one or more of the following occur:
	a. Lymph nodes on biopsy are found to be involved in the hilus, the periaortic chains, or beyond.
	b. There has been diffuse peritoneal contamination by tumour such as by spillage of tumour beyond the flank before or during surgery, or by tumour growth that has penetrated through the peritoneal surface.
	c. Implants are found on the peritoneal surfaces.
	d. The tumour extends beyond the surgical margins either microscopically or grossly.
	e. The tumour is not completely resectable because of local infiltration into vital structure.
IV	Haematogenous metastases.
	Deposits beyond Stage III: e.g. lung, liver, bone and brain.
V	Bilateral renal involvement at diagnosis.
	An attempt should be made to stage each side according to the above criteria on the basis of extent of disease before biopsy.

Table 7.6 Wilms' tumour TNM classification

T-Primary tumour
TX   Primary tumour cannot be assessed
TO   No evidence of primary tumour
T1   Unilateral tumour 80 cm^2 or less in area (including kidney)
T2   Unilateral tumour more than 80 cm^2 in area (including kidney)
T3   Unilateral tumour rupture before treatment
T4   Bilateral tumours

N-Regional lymph nodes
NX   Regional lymph nodes cannot be assessed
NO   No regional lymph node metastasis
N1   Regional lymph node metastasis

M-Distant metastasis

These findings make it reasonable to consider the role of a pre-operative classification and staging in further group studies of Wilms' tumour aimed at reducing the morbidity of treatment. The TNM classification and staging as shown in Tables 7.6 and 7.7 are well suited to such studies. There has been debate on the need for pathological confirmation of the diagnosis prior to chemotherapy or irradiation. Needle biopsy under imaging control is possible in all cases but it must, in the author's opinion, be considered as breaching the tumour capsule and therefore constituting tumour spill. Fortunately, NWTS have shown that local spillage can be controlled using chemotherapy only and therefore needle biopsy is not an indication for tumour bed irradiation. There appears, therefore, to be no good reason against staging Wilms' tumours by the TNM system and designing studies which can investigate the optimum timing of surgery in relation to the other modalities of treatment.

Pre-surgical investigations, even with modern imaging techniques, are unable to distinguish between regional lymph node infiltration and reactive hyperplasia. If one were to use the treatment methods defined

141

Table 7.7 Wilms' tumour clinical stage grouping (TNM, cTNM)

Stage I	T1	NO	MO
Stage II	T2	NO	MO
Stage III	T1	N1	MO
	T2	N1	MO
	T3	Any N	MO
Stage IVA	T1	Any N	M1
	T2	Any N	M1
	T3	Any N	M1
Stage IVB	T4	Any N	Any M

Pathological stage grouping (pTNM)			
Stage I	pT1	pNO	pMO
Stage II	pT1	pN1a*	pMO
	pT2	pNO, pN1a*	pMO
Stage IIIA	pT3a	pNO, pN1a*	pMO
Stage IIIB	pT1	pN1b†	pMO
	pT2	pN1b†	pMO
	pT3a	pN1b†	pMO
	pT3b	Any pN	pMO
	pT3c	Any pN	pMO
Stage IVA	pT1	Any pN	pM1
	pT2	Any pN	pM1
	pT3a	Any pN	pM1
	pT3b	Any pN	pM1
	pT3c	Any pN	pM1
Stage IVB	pT4	Any pN	Any pM

* pN1a Regional lymph node metastasis completely resected.
† pN1b Regional lymph nodes metastasis incompletely resected.

by NWTS for patients staged by the TNM pre-operative system then there exists the possibility of 'downstaging' a NWTS Stage III patient to TNM Stage II (T2/N0/M0). If such patients are treated with pre-operative chemotherapy to reduce tumour bulk, and at operation there is no evidence of lymph node infiltration, then by the post-surgical TNM staging the patient remains at Stage II and post-operative irradiation is not required. However, had the patient been treated with initial surgery it may well have been found that there was lymph node infiltration and the patient would have been staged as Stage III and given post-operative irradiation. The question of whether such a patient has been under or over treated by one or other staging system is as yet unresolved. European experience of the good results of pre-operative chemotherapy for massive Wilms' tumours suggests that 'downstaging' with a TNM classification is unlikely to be harmful.

Both NWTS and TNM staging systems require allowance for histological features of the tumour. The three entities of clear cell sarcoma, rhabdoid tumours and anaplastic form of Wilms' are grouped as unfavourable histology (UH). Other histological appearances are grouped as favourable histology (FH) and the prefix FH or UH is added to the staging.

The TNM classification has a provision for pathological staging (Table 7.7) which is very similar to the NWTS system. Retrospective studies of NWTS data using the TNM systems should provide information on how often the TNM system would have 'downstaged' a NWTS Stage III patient to TNM Stage II. Comparison of European pre-operative chemotherapy results for TNM Stage II and III with NWTS Stage III results could indicate whether withholding of irradiation for pre-operative TNM Stage III but post-chemotherapy Stage II has detrimental effects.

7.4.3 NEUROBLASTOMA

The prognosis for advanced neuroblastoma remains poor despite attempts at radical treatment including allogeneic and autologous transplantation. Certain biological factors which are inter-related separate patients with an intrinsically good prognosis from those with a poor outlook. Age under 12–18 months and the absence of bone metastasis are associated with a better prognosis as are non-abdominal sites of disease and small

Table 7.8 Evans and D'Angio staging system for neuroblastoma

Stage I	Tumour confined to the organ or structure of origin.
Stage II	Tumour extending in continuity beyond the organ or structure of origin but not crossing the midline. Regional lymph nodes on the homolateral side may be involved.
Stage III	Tumours extending in continuity beyond the midline. Regional lymph nodes bilaterally may be involved.
Stage IV-S	Patients who would otherwise be Stage I or II but who have remote disease confined to one or more of the following sites: liver, skin, or bone marrow (without evidence of bone metastases).

Table 7.9 Neuroblastoma TNM clinical classification

T-Primary tumour

Because it is often impossible to differentiate between the primary tumour and the adjacent lymph nodes, the T assessment relates to the total mass. When there is doubt between multicentricity and metastasis, the latter is presumed.

Note: Size is estimated clinically and/or radiologically. For classification, the larger measurement should be used.

TX	Primary tumour cannot be assessed
TO	No evidence of primary tumour
T1	Single tumour 5 cm or less in greatest dimension
T2	Single tumour more than 5 cm but not more than 10 cm in greatest dimension
T3	Single tumour more than 10 cm in greatest dimension
T4	Multicentric tumours occurring simultaneously

N-Regional lymph nodes

NX	Regional lymph nodes cannot be assessed
NO	No regional lymph node metastasis
N1	Regional lymph node metastasis

M-Distant metastasis

primary tumours. Complete surgical excision of the primary tumour in patients with these favourable features has not been shown to be associated with a better chance of cure. In patients with unfavourable biological features there is dispute about the role of complete surgical excision. These unique features of neuroblastoma mitigate against a prognostically useful classification based on the assessment of tumour bulk and the extent of local infiltration.

There are two major systems of staging. The most widely used is the Evans and D'Angio staging system shown in Table 7.8. The TNM classification and staging are shown in Tables 7.9 and 7.10. While both systems fail to allow for essential biological features, the Evans and D'Angio classification defines a group of patients who have an intrinsically good prognosis, namely Stage IV-S. In the TNM system these patients would be classified as T4/NX/M1 with multiple subscripts for the sites of metastatic disease. This is an unsatisfactory system because it is cumbersome, assumes that the tumours are multi-centric,

and fails to take into account the size and extent of regional spread of the primary tumour. The Evans and D'Angio system therefore appears to be superior in this case because it clearly distinguishes between patients with disseminated disease who have a good prognosis and those with a poor prognosis. Prognostically, it fails to accurately separate in the other groups, since more than half the children older than one year with Stages I–III disease do not survive.

To try and distinguish prognostic groups in localized disease, the POG has developed a

Table 7.10 Neuroblastoma clinical stage grouping (TNM, cTNM)

Stage I	T1	NO	MO
Stage II	T2	NO	MO
Stage III	T1	N1	MO
	T2	N1	MO
	T3	Any N	MO
Stage IVA	T1	Any N	M1
	T2	Any N	M1
	T3	Any N	M1
Stage IVB	T4	Any N	Any M

Pathological stage grouping (pTNM)			
Stage I	pT1	pNO	pMO
Stage II	pT1	pN1a	pMO
Stage IIIA	pT3a	pNO, pN1a	pMO
Stage IIIB	pT1	pN1b	pMO
	pT3a	pN1b	pMO
	pT3b	Any pN	pMO
	pT3c	Any pN	pMO
Stage IVA	pT1	Any pN	pM1
	pT3a	Any pN	pM1
	pT3b	Any pN	pM1
	pT3c	Any pN	pM1
Stage IVB	pT4	Any pN	Any pM

Table 7.11 Paediatric oncology group (POG) staging for neuroblastoma

Stage A Complete gross excision of primary tumour, margins histologically negative or positive. Intracavitary lymph nodes not intimately adhered to and removed with resected tumour are histologically free of tumour. If primary is in abdomen (including pelvis), liver is histologically free of tumour.

Stage B Incomplete gross resection of primary. Lymph nodes and liver histologically free of tumour as in Stage A.

Stage C Complete or incomplete gross resection of primary. Intracavitary nodes histologically positive for tumour. Liver histologically free of tumour.

Stage D Disseminated disease beyond intra-cavitary nodes (i.e. bone marrow, bone, liver, skin, or lymph nodes beyond cavity containing primary tumour).

system based on surgical/pathological staging similar to the NWTS. This system is shown in Table 7.11. It is based on the finding of Hayes and co-workers (1983) of a 83% survival rate in patients without lymph node infiltration compared to 31% in those with lymph node disease, irrespective of whether total tumour clearance could be achieved. If one were to adopt the POG staging system for localized tumours then the definition of lymph node disease becomes critical. As previously discussed, imaging techniques are often ineffective in defining lymphatic spread and therefore many patients would require surgical exploration to define the stage of their disease. For this to be widely accepted it would have to be shown that different treatment intensity can be used safely for

POG stages A and B disease compared with stage C. At present such information is not available. In the absence of a totally satisfactory staging system and curative therapy, for the majority of patients with advanced disease, it seems desirable to continue with the Evans and D'Angio staging or preferably the modified (INSS) system – see Chapter 17.

7.4.4 LYMPHOMAS, BONE TUMOURS AND GERM CELL CARCINOMAS

To propose a TNM classification is not considered practical in Hodgkin's disease or non-Hodgkin's lymphoma. The TNM classification is also of little value in bone tumours or germ cell carcinomas where the key factors are the presence or absence of metastatic disease and the drug sensitivity of the tumour as demonstrated by response to pre-operative chemotherapy.

REFERENCES

Evans, A.E., D'Angio, G.J. and Randolph, J. (1971) A proposed staging for children with neuroblastoma. *Cancer*, **27**, 374–8.

Hayes, F.A., Green, A., Hutsu, H.O. and Kumar, M. (1983) Surgicopathologic staging of neuroblastoma: prognostic significance of lymph node metastasis. *J. Pediatr.*, **102**, 59–62.

Hermanek, P. and Sobin, L.H. (eds) (1987) *TNM Classification of Malignant Tumours*, Springer, Berlin.

Lawrence, W. Jr., Gehan, E.A., Hays, D.M. *et al.* (1987) Prognostic significance of staging factors of the UICC staging system in childhood rhabdomyosarcoma: A report from the intergroup rhabdomyosarcoma study (IRS-II) *J. Clin. Oncol.*, **5**, 46–54.

Lemerle, J., Voûte, P.A., Tournade, M.F. *et al.* (1978) Pre-operative versus post-operative radiotherapy, single versus multiple courses of Actinomycin D in the treatment of Wilms' tumour. *Cancer*, **38**, 647–54.

Lemerle, J., Voûte, P.A., Tournade, M.F. *et al.* (1983) Effectiveness of pre-operative chemotherapy in Wilms' tumour: results of an international society of Paediatric Oncology (SIOP) clinical trial. *J. Clin. Oncol.*, **1**, 604–9.

Maurer, H.M. (1975) The intergroup rhabdomyosarcoma study: objectives and clinical staging classification. *J. Pediatr. Surg.*, **10**, 977–8.

Pedrick, T.J., Donaldson, S.S. and Cox, R.S. (1986) Rhabdomyosarcoma: the Stanford experience using a TNM staging system. *J. Clin. Oncol.*, **4**, 370–8.

Rodary, C., Flamant, F. and Donaldson, S.S. (1989) An attempt to use a common staging system in rhabdomysarcoma: a report of an international workshop initiated by the International Society of Pediatric Oncology (SIOP). *Med. Pediatr. Oncol.*, **17**, 210–5.

Chapter 8

The role of the clinical trial

R.P. A'HERN

8.1 INTRODUCTION

Greater emphasis on the critical evaluation of new cancer treatments over the past few decades has led to the emergence of the clinical trial as a distinct discipline within medicine. Its use requires the expertize of clinicians, statisticians and data managers as part of a multi-disciplinary team. In some situations in oncology it is not possible to detect improvement clinically; the benefit of treatments can only be inferred statistically from clinical trials – adjuvant chemotherapy for early cancer provides such an example. Long-term monitoring of patients under the guidance of a defined trial protocol is necessary to adequately measure the outcome of such interventions.

   This chapter examines the role of clinical trials in paediatric oncology. The variation of response to the same treatment shown by different patients is perhaps one of the most noteworthy medical phenomena and is central to understanding the role of clinical trials. Part of medical statistics is the study of such variability and a brief introduction to this subject is therefore included in order to add to the understanding of the later contents of the chapter. Following this, the different types of clinical trials are examined beginning with the first tentative use of a compound in Phase I trials and ending with the combination of results from several randomized trials (overviews or meta-analyses), by which time a treatment may be in widespread use.

8.2 EFFECTIVENESS OF THE CLINICAL TRIAL MODEL

8.2.1 THE RANDOMIZED CONTROLLED TRIAL

Clinical trials provide the most efficient method of assessing the value of an intervention, the scientific rigor of randomized controlled trials (RCTs) in particular guarding against the types of bias which cannot be excluded when studies are carried out by other methods. The efficiency of clinical trials lies in the strength of evidence they yield relative to the number of patients treated. A therapy which is of value can therefore be recognized and introduced more rapidly into standard treatment programmes; equally, one which is of no value can be discarded having minimized the number of patients who have received it and with the minimum expense. Clinical trials are therefore preferable ethically since as few patients are exposed to risk as possible.

The role of RCTs in cancer research can be illustrated by considering the different types of study that are presented as evidence of the value of an intervention. Green and Byar (1984) place such studies in an eight-level pyramid: as the pyramid is descended, the weight of evidence presented by the study types increases. Beginning at the top, the first three levels are, in descending order of validity, anecdotal case reports, case series without controls, and series with literature controls. Case reports present isolated cases which may be highly selected but there is less likelihood of such a high degree of selection if a series is presented. Series with literature controls make an effort to present controls for comparative purposes. However, they do not come from the same institution(s) and hence any difference in outcome may represent differences in factors associated with the institutions and not the treatments. The next three levels of the pyramid include analyses using computer databases, 'case control' observational studies, and series based on historical control groups. These studies make greater attempts to compare patients given the intervention with similar groups, than simply to use literature controls. Though the evidence gained from these types of study is comparable, the order of each relative to the other will reflect the particular methodology used.

Analyses using computer databases may be inadequate because not all relevant features concerning choice of treatment have been recorded. Some factors may be impossible to record finely enough or may simply be impossible to record at all. Performance status, for example, can be an important prognostic factor which may have an impact on the choice of treatment. If it is not recorded on the database this association will be lost and differences in outcome due to performance status may be interpreted as a treatment

effect. 'Case control' observational studies may suffer from a similar weakness. Comparisons of series based on historical control groups are susceptible to changes over time; diagnostic techniques, for example, may change; unwary correction for presenting features may bias the comparison between treatment groups, as for example, reported by Feinstein *et al.* (1985).

The final two study types presented by Green and Byar consist of single and confirmed RCTs. RCTs decrease the chance of an important imbalance in prognostic factors (both known and unknown) between groups which may bias treatment comparisons. Since any patient is equally likely to be put into any of the study arms, the proportions of patients in particular prognostic groups should be the same in all arms. The larger the number of patients in the trial the less likely is such an imbalance to occur. The importance of the role of RCTs in clinical research is attributable to the fact that they offer a method of comparing treatments in which the only difference between the groups being compared should be the treatments themselves.

(a) Variability of response to treatment

Under ideal circumstances, the decision whether to give a patient a treatment would be based on knowledge of the outcome of the treatment in all similar past, present and, indeed, future patients. This is known statistically as the population of patients. Because this information is never available, the only method of assessing the treatment is to give it to a group of patients and measure its effectiveness: this group of patients constitutes a sample drawn from the population. From the results obtained in the sample, inferences are then made about the treatment's value in the population. It is important to ensure that the sample is unbiased, i.e. it represents the population accurately.

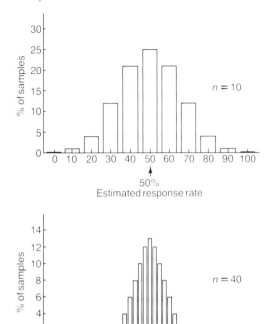

Fig. 8.1 The variation in estimated response rates shown with samples of size 10 and 40, given that the population from which they are drawn has a response rate of 50%. Note that the larger sample size shows less variation in the estimated response rate.

Suppose, for example, it was intended to investigate the effectiveness of a chemotherapeutic agent in a childhood cancer which has a response rate in the population of such children of 50%. This would mean that exactly half the patients who have been given it or are going to be given it will respond. If this chemotherapy were used in a group of ten patients then the most likely outcome would be that five would respond, but one could get any number of responders from zero to ten depending upon the sample of patients that one obtained. The probability

associated with each of these outcomes is shown in Fig. 8.1. Though the probability of getting 5 responders is greatest: 0.25 or 25%, all 11 possible outcomes corresponding to numbers of responders can occur. The total probability of all possible outcomes is one, or 100%. Note that if one were to get three responders one would conclude that the most likely population response rate was 30%, or if there were six responders one would conclude the most likely value was 60%, etc. Thus the estimate of the population response rate shows a variation, called the sampling variation. This variation decreases with increasing sample size; the larger the sample taken, the more information one has about the population value. Fig. 8.1 shows the sampling variation when a sample of 40 patients is studied: note that the range of estimates of the response rate is more tightly clustered around the true response rate of 50%.

If one were performing a comparative study such as a randomized controlled trial in which interest focused on the difference between, for example, response rates of two chemotherapy regimens there will be sampling variation in each of the two estimates of the response rates. The difference in these estimates will therefore show more variation than either of the single estimates. In fact, the variation shown by the difference is approximately 40% greater.

Two further hypothetical situations need to be considered: firstly, that there is in fact no difference in response rates, and, secondly, that a real difference does exist.

(b) No difference in response to treatment

If both regimens were equally effective it would be expected that the difference in response rates would be close to zero, with the variation about zero being determined by the number of patients in the trial (Fig. 8.2).

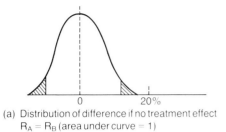

(a) Distribution of difference if no treatment effect
$R_A = R_B$ (area under curve = 1)

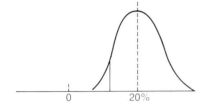

(b) Distribution of difference if treatment effect
$R_A > R_B$ $R_A - R_B = 20\%$

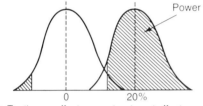

(c) Testing no effect versus treatment effect

Fig. 8.2 The variation in the difference (R_A–R_B) between the response rates in two arms of a trial (a) assuming there is no difference (R_A–R_B =0%); (b) assuming a 20% difference (R_A–R_B =20%); and (c) testing these two hypotheses against each other. The shaded area denotes the probability that it is concluded there is a treatment difference if the true difference is 20%. This is known as the statistical power.

The distribution of sample values is now denoted by a curve line rather than as a histogram as in Fig. 8.1, the area under the line is again one or 100%. One would be prepared to accept there was no difference in response rates if there was only a small difference; however, if the difference were large, a method of deciding whether a real difference exists is needed. In fact it is con-

cluded that a difference exists if it is unlikely that the difference observed would have occurred if there was no difference. This likelihood is the *p-value*. If this is small, conventionally 5% or less, than it is concluded that a real difference exists. Since it is still possible that there is really no difference, concluding that there is a difference may be incorrect; this kind of error is known as a Type I error. The probability of a Type I error should be kept as small as possible. The Type I error is shown in Fig. 8.2 as the small shaded areas in the two tails of the curve corresponding to the probability of large differences in the response rates. Each of these shaded areas equals 2.5%; combined, they represent a total probability of 5%.

(c) Difference in response to treatment

If a difference in response rates really existed and was, say, 20%, then the sampling variation of the difference would be similar, but this time the variation would be about this 20% value (Fig. 8.2b). If the two curves are combined (Fig. 8.2c), it can be seen that the probability that the hypothesis of no treatment difference is rejected; this is denoted by the shaded area under the second curve. Statistically, this is known as the *power* to reject the hypothesis of no treatment effect at the 5% significance level, given that a 20% difference exists. Note that the power varies with the number of patients in the comparison (Fig. 8.3). If there are only a small number of patients then it is unlikely that one would conclude there was a difference even if one existed; if there were only 100 patients in the study this power would be only 55%. It is therefore of prime importance that an adequate number of patients are entered into comparative trials.

Just as it is possible to conclude that a treatment difference exists when none in fact exists, it is also possible to conclude that there is no difference when one does exist.

149

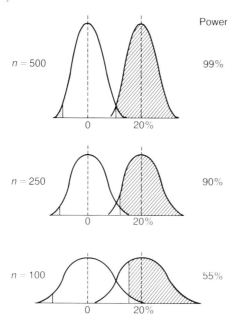

Fig. 8.3 The relationship between power and sample size. The larger the number of patients in a trial the greater the probability that a given difference is detected. The improvement in response used to illustrate this relationship has been assumed to be from 30% to 50%.

The probability of making such a Type II error should also be kept as low as possible.

Although this example has focused on the sampling variation of response rates one should note that an exactly analogous sampling distribution exists for variables which are continuous such as blood counts, biochemical parameters, etc. Similar distributions also exist for hazard ratios which are used to summarize differences between survival or similar curves used to compare the time to an event, although in this case it is the number of events (deaths, recurrence, etc.) which is important in determining power rather than the number of patients. Thus the power of a comparison can be calculated in all comparative situations.

8.3 PHASE I AND PHASE II CLINICAL TRIALS

For ease of presentation the application of Phase I and Phase II trials to the assessment of new drugs is presented below. Analogous methods can also be applied to the assessment of new surgical, radiotherapeutic or other interventions. A Phase II trial in surgery, for example, would consist of assessing a new surgical technique in patients with advanced disease in whom standard surgical procedures had failed. A Phase I trial of radiotherapy may consist of assessing the toxicity associated with differing fields, doses and schedules applied to treat a particular condition.

An important consideration in the setting up of clinical trials is the use of standardized criteria for reporting results of treatment; comparison of results with those of other series are therefore more meaningful (Miller *et al.*, 1981).

8.3.1 PHASE I TRIALS

The main aim of Phase I studies is to determine the maximum tolerated dose (MTD) of a new agent with the smallest number of patients and with the minimum risk to them. The MTD is usually defined as the highest safely tolerable dose (Carter, 1977), though this definition may vary among clinicians. Secondary aims are to establish whether the toxicity is reversible and predictable, and which organs are involved. Phase I trials also seek evidence of efficacy against the tumour. However, patients will have advanced, usually heavily pre-treated disease and may receive an inadequate dose of the drug, hence lack of antitumour activity should not influence whether or not a drug progresses on to Phase II trials.

Several criteria need to be satisfied before a drug is first used in man. Firstly a reliable assay for blood levels of the drug in the blood and other body fluids is required. Secondly, knowledge is needed of the pharmaco-kinetics derived from several animal species after a varying number of doses when the drug is given by the route to be employed in man. Thirdly, the drug levels at which toxicity was observed need to be known, together with drug levels at which activity against the tumour was seen. Lastly, information on the means by which the drug is eliminated and how it is distributed around the body is also required.

Patients entered into Phase I trials should not have received the drug before. It is important that each patient is given only one dose because it would then not be possible to determine whether any toxicity observed was due to a cumulative effect or the level of the last dose given.

The methods used for dose escalation in Phase I trials have been developed by trial and error. The most commonly used method, the Fibonacci search scheme, employs in-itially large dose increases with smaller incre-ments as toxic levels are approached. If the starting dose is D, the second dose is 2D (a 100% increase), the third dose is 3.3D (a 65% increase on the previous dose), the fourth 5D (a 50% increase) and the fifth 7D (a 40% increase). All subsequent doses are a 33% increase on the previous dose.

Three patients are given the drug at each dose level, the second and third patients being entered four weeks after the first patient if no toxicity is observed in this patient. The second and third patients can be entered one week apart. If no toxicity is observed in the four weeks after the third patient received the drug then patients are entered at the next dose level. As soon as any toxicity is observed six patients are entered at the corresponding dose level and at all fol-lowing dose levels up to the maximum toler-ated dose. Cumulative and chronic toxicity are observed by entering three additional patients at the maximum tolerated dose level

and maintaining them on therapy if tumour response is shown (Von Hoff *et al.*, 1984).

Although Phase I studies are designed to ascertain a single MTD, when interpreting Phase I studies it must be borne in mind that the MTD achieved will be related to the previous treatment that the patients have received. This must be considered when deciding on the dose to use in further clinical study.

8.3.2 PHASE II TRIALS

When the MTD has been determined in Phase I trials attention is then focused on determining whether a new agent shows meaningful anti-tumour activity. Phase II trials are carried out to determine whether a new drug is effective in a particular tumour type or types, the outcome of interest usually being the proportion of patients responding to treatment. Patients who are entered into Phase II trials normally have advanced dis-ease and have shown progressive disease after having received standard treatment. The expected response rate therefore has to reflect the treatment history of patients entered into trials. Entry of patients who are unlikely to respond may cause a worthwhile agent to be discarded. An example of the techniques used to identify such poor prog-nosis groups is provided by Blackledge *et al.* (1989).

(a) Phase II trial designs

In order to choose an appropriate design for a Phase II trial the minimum response rate that would indicate a drug is worthy of further study needs to be defined. Two other important factors are levels for the two types of error it is possible to make when under-taking such trials. These are the false positive and false negative errors. A false positive error occurs when a drug is incorrectly declared effective; under such circumstances

151

Table 8.1 Probability scores

Probability 1	1 patient does not respond	$= 0.80$
Probability 2	2 patients do not respond	$= 0.80 \times 0.80 = 0.80^2 = 0.64$
Probability 3	3 patients do not respond	$= 0.80^3 = 0.51$
	.	
	.	
	14 patients do not respond	$= 0.80^{14} = 0.04$

an ineffective drug may progress into Phase III trials and be given to a large number of patients. A false negative error occurs when a drug is declared to be of no value when it is effective; in this case a valuable agent may be missed. A false positive error constitutes a Type I error and false negative error a Type II error (see above). Definition of relevant (small) values for these two error rates allows an appropriate trial design to be chosen.

The minimum response rate of interest in a Phase II trial is typically between 20% and 30%. This value is used to calculate the false negative error rate associated with a given study design. Thus, for example, if the minimum response rate were 20%, the study might be stopped if there were no responders among 14 patients. The rationale for this is that there is a 5% probability (or 4.4% probability to be exact) of getting no responses in 14 patients if the response rate is 20%. The use of this number of patients can be understood by noting that if the probability a particular patient responds is 0.20 (0.20 equals 20%), then the probability they do not respond is 0.80 or 80% (Table 8.1).

The false positive error rate is calculated by defining a response rate which would indicate that a drug was highly ineffective. Suppose 5% was considered a suitable value and the design chosen was a two-stage design which consisted in entering 14 patients in the first stage and 11 in the second stage. If there was no response in the first 14, the trial would be stopped. If there were one or more responses then 11 more patients would be entered giving a total of 25 patients in the trial. If in total there were three or fewer total responses the agent would be declared ineffective. The false negative error rate for such a design can be calculated to be 3% (Table 8.2).

Thus, the probability that the drug will be rejected if the true response rate is 5% is 0.97, or 97%. Thus the probability the drug is erroneously not rejected is $1 - 0.97 = 3\%$.

There are a large number of potential designs for Phase II trials, investigators planning such a trial should consult a medical statistician for assistance in choosing the most appropriate method.

Table 8.2 Method of predicting whether drug will be rejected

No. of responders		
First 14	*Remaining 11*	*Probability of true response rate 5%*
0	–	0.49
1	0,1 or 2	0.36
2	0 or 1	0.11
3	0	0.01
		0.97

(b) Randomized Phase II trials

Randomization can play a role in some Phase II trials. Investigators may be more willing to enter patients into a randomized trial. It can be employed both to ensure patients who are likely to respond are entered into trials, and to reduce selection bias. Randomization between a new agent and a standard treatment may be considered ethical if the standard agent has a low response rate, or, alternatively, if patients treated with the new agent receive the standard agent afterwards without being seriously disadvantaged. Randomization between two new agents will help to ensure that patients with a better prognosis are not preferentially given one of the agents. A further benefit occurs if an agent is being tested in a number of cancer types and it is possible to perform a randomized controlled trial. In this case valuable information on the toxicity of the new agent relative to the standard agent can be obtained by combining toxicity data from patients in all cancer types.

8.4 PHASE III CLINICAL TRIALS

8.4.1 AIMS

Phase II trials do not provide sufficient evidence to justify the use of a new agent, they simply indicate whether an agent is effective. The place of the agent in current therapy is investigated in Phase III trials which are randomized and should include a control group. The inclusion of a control group ensures that the value of a new treatment is assessed against a standard therapy allowing decisions to be made about the benefits of replacing the standard therapy with the new therapy. In the situation in which no standard therapy exists the new treatment may be compared with a placebo arm.

Note:
The term 'treatment' is used in this section to mean treatment option, thus 'masterly inactivity' or no treatment is included under the term treatment.

A number of different types of endpoints

are used in Phase III trials. Response rates in trials of advanced cancer and survival and disease-free survival in both advanced and early cancer are used most frequently. Unfortunately, the definition of disease-free survival varies and this can complicate the interpretation of results from different studies. Definitions of endpoints used by the United Kingdom Children's Cancer Study Group are supplied in the Appendix; use of standard criteria such as these improves consistency across studies.

Phase III trials do not necessarily arise from Phase II trials; they may also be undertaken to assess new combinations, intensities, or scheduling of existing therapies. Some Phase III trials are also designed to assess whether treatments are equally effective in terms of major endpoints but have different toxicity profiles; in this case attention may focus on detecting differences in toxicity rather than more obvious outcome measures such as response rates or duration of survival.

8.5 STUDY DESIGN

8.5.1 RANDOMIZATION

Randomization serves a number of important purposes. It avoids selection bias; hence more reliable estimates of treatment differences are obtained. In addition, both known and unknown prognostic factors tend to be balanced across the arms of the trial, making the arms comparable. Prospective data collection according to a defined protocol is undertaken; the possibility of missing data is therefore less likely. Lastly, randomization assures the validity of statistical methods employed to analyse the results. Randomized trials compare two or more treatments which are considered to be of equal value, given the current stage of knowledge concerning their efficacy. It is thus ethically justifiable and their use should include seeking patients' or parents' informed consent.

The means used to carry out randomization vary according to circumstances. In multicentre trials, telephone randomization to a central co-ordinating office is the method of choice to ensure that randomization is properly performed. Randomization in this case can also include eligibility checks to ensure that the patients satisfy entry criteria. The use of sealed envelopes with the allocation recorded inside is open to abuse since more than one can be opened at once or they can be opened out of order. In single centre studies, every effort should be made to maintain the independence of the person performing randomization and the individual obtaining the randomization for treatment purposes. In this case, telephone randomization within the institution may be a useful option.

It is important to ensure that measurement of prognostic factors is not affected by the treatment allocation; patients in different arms should therefore have the same staging and diagnostic procedures. Examination of the association between prognostic factors and the treatment allocated can also be used to check that randomization has been properly carried out.

In many situations it is of value to perform randomization separately for different prognostic groups to make certain that similar numbers of patients within every group receive each treatment. Patients with different disease stages, for example, may be randomized separately. Since in multi-centre trials, centres may vary considerably in terms of factors such as referral patterns, diagnostic techniques and ancillary treatment, randomization is commonly performed independently for each centre to ensure that the number of patients given each treatment in a particular institution are similar.

Blocked randomization is commonly used in randomized trials. A block is simply a defined number of patients with an equal number of patients randomized to each arm; thus, after each block of patients has been entered into a trial, there are equal numbers of patients in each arm. Blocks of size six are commonly used; thus, if there were two arms, three patients would receive one treatment and three patients the other treatment. The advantage of blocked randomization is that if a small number of patients are entered by a particular investigator or centre in a multi-centre trial then there are still similar numbers of patients given each treatment. A disadvantage is that investigators may discover the block size; indeed, guessing the next allocation can become a favoured activity. A simple expedient is to vary the block size, e.g. to use random block sizes of four or six. A further consideration to be taken into account when deciding randomization procedures is that several sequential allocations to the same arm may be inconvenient and may cause participants concern. Randomization which excludes more than a given number of sequential allocations to the same arm can be employed to overcome this.

Minimization is a further useful technique, particularly if trial size is likely to be small. Minimization is used to try to ensure that patient characteristics do not differ markedly between the treatment groups. Patients are allocated to a treatment in order to minimize any existing prognostic differences between the treatment groups.

8.5.2 FACTORIAL DESIGNS

It is sometimes possible to address two or more questions simultaneously in one clinical trial by using a factorial design. This does not involve the loss of any statistical power. A prerequisite of such trials is that it is possible to give a patient any combination of treatments based on the allocation. The Medical Research Councils' UKALL X is an example of such a trial in which the two comparisons are early intensification therapy versus no

Table 8.3 Example of a randomized trial protocol

		Early therapy		
		None	*Early*	
Late therapy	*None*	A	B	
				A+B v C+D assesses the effect of late therapy
	Late	C	D	
		A+C v B+D assess the effect of early therapy		

early therapy and late therapy versus no late therapy; the design is shown schematically in Table 8.3; patients are allocated to options A, B, C or D.

The effect of early therapy is assessed by comparing patients in groups A and C with those in groups B and D; similarly, the effect of late therapy is assessed by comparing those in groups A and B with those in groups C and D. In evaluating early therapy half the patients who have received early therapy (B and D) will have received late therapy as well (group D), but this will also be true amongst the patients (A and C) who have not received early therapy; the patient treatment characteristics thus match in these two groups and the estimations of the effect of early therapy is not affected. Factorial designs are not employed for the purpose of comparing the single groups, e.g. A versus B; A versus C, etc. There are six possible such comparisons, leading to a high probability of a Type I error. The fact that there are a smaller number of patients in these groups also makes these comparisons less sensitive to treatment effects.

Phase III trials may employ designs which allow more patients to be randomized to one arm than another. There is little loss of power in allocations such as 2:1, investigators may adopt such a design if they wish to gain more experience of the new treatment (Pocock, 1983).

8.5.3 OPTIMUM SIZE FOR PHASE III TRIALS

The importance of obtaining large numbers of patients to carry out an adequate treatment comparison has been discussed above. If a trial is set up to compare response rates in two groups and the expected response rate in the control group was 50%, then 1040 patients would be needed to have a good chance (90% power) of detecting a 10% improvement in response rate to 60% (Machin *et al.*, 1987). Similar figures for a 20% and 30% improvement are 250 and 100 patients respectively. By implication, if such a trial were published with a total of 100 patients and a negative result then a true difference in response rates of 30% could not be ruled out. If the endpoint is survival and the five-year-survival rate in the control arm was 50%, 1020 patients would be needed to detect a 10% improvement and 260 patients would be needed to detect a 20% improvement. The number of patients required in this case depends on the number of events (deaths). The relationship between the event rate and the statistical power of a comparison means that studies in cancer types with a low event rate pose a particular problem. An example of this is the CCSG study of ALL (Miller *et al.*, 1989), which included an investigation of the role of three versus five years of continuing treatment. There were a total of 310 patients in this comparison and 7 years after randomization there were 28 events. In order to detect a halving in the risk of an event (the event rate was approximately 8%) then 125 events would have been needed. The authors' conclusion that prolongation of therapy beyond three years does not improve disease-free survival is not therefore justifiable. The assumption that if a significant difference is not found then a difference does not exist is a common mistake that is made in interpreting results, this is a Type II error; a method of countering this is to present the size of difference that the study could reliably detect.

The need for large trials implies that the smaller the number of arms a trial has the more likely it is to be able to accrue sufficient patients. It is therefore important to identify as few salient questions as possible (ideally only one) to be addressed by a trial. For similar reasons, factorial designs should be employed wherever possible if two questions are to be addressed.

8.5.4 MULTI-CENTRE TRIALS GROUPS

In many situations it is not possible to obtain sufficient patients from one centre to undertake a randomized trial; in such cases multi-centre trials offer a method of achieving appropriate trial sizes. Specialized administrative and data management skills are needed to undertake multi-centre trials; they are therefore best undertaken by co-ordinating centres which concentrate on the development of such expertise. Although superficially the extension of a trial from a single institution trial to becoming a multi-centre trial may appear simple, the effort required to maintain the quality of such a trial is greater than would be needed if such an extension were possible within the same institution. The importance of being able to deal with factors such as randomization, eligibility and compliance checks and patient follow-up, and the need for appropriate computing and data handling capabilities highlights the benefit of having such facilities in a single unit devoted to multi-centre trials. An example of the role that can be played by study groups participating in multi-centre trials addressing questions in paediatric cancer is given by the

Medical Research Council ALL trials (UKALL, 1986), a total of 2358 patients were entered into trials over the period 1972 to 1984.

Comparative trials are often undertaken to establish whether new treatments are of equal value to the standard treatment. This type of study is relevant when the new treatment is less toxic or invasive, but its efficacy relative to the standard treatment is unknown. In this case the traditional trial design which attempts to show that a difference exists can be misleading since the failure to find a difference is frequently interpreted as evidence that no difference exists. A method of dealing with this is to design the study to show that the two treatments are equivalent, this requires a definition of equivalence be agreed upon. In a trial of adjuvant chemotherapy, for example, it might be that the difference in five-year survival rates is no greater than 10%.

8.6 OVERVIEWS OR META-ANALYSES

Overviews provide a method of combining results from several randomized clinical trials addressing the same question, with an associated increase in the ability to detect treatment effects. An overall estimate of the treatment effect is obtained from all relevant studies together with a guide to the generalizability of results from variation between studies. Overviews also provide a 'state of the art' summary of current topics and therefore aid in planning new trials. In addition, the increase in patient numbers makes valid subgroup analyses possible (subgroup analyses are discussed below). Analysis of treatment effects in differing time periods during follow-up can also be performed where sufficient patients are at risk in the time periods of interest. A subject of special interest in childhood cancer would be whether treatments increase the risk of a second cancer occurring several years after treatment.

The existence of statistical techniques to

combine results from several studies has the effect that even if individual studies are unable to accrue sufficient patients, if similar trials addressing the same question exist, an overview of all studies may be adequate to provide an answer. This has led to the suggestion that parallel protocols should be adopted in different studies which are likely to accrue only a small number of patients (Freedman, 1989); these are particularly relevant in trials involving rare tumours.

In conclusion, four topics which need to be considered in setting up and analysing clinical trials will be mentioned briefly. These are also valuable points to bear in mind when reading medical literature since they often explain apparently contradictory results in different studies. These topics are multiple endpoints and comparisons, subgroup analyses, repeated analyses, and follow-up procedures.

8.6.1 MULTIPLE COMPARISONS AND ENDPOINTS

The most common type of study undertaken involves investigating whether there is a difference between two treatments. As mentioned above, the p-value is the probability there is no difference between treatments, if it is small then it is concluded that a difference does exist. The level of defining significance (Type I error rate) is usually set at $p=0.05$. This means one is prepared to accept there is a treatment difference if there is a one-in-twenty or lower chance that results observed which favour one treatment may have occurred if there was no treatment difference.

If two unrelated endpoints are examined in a study, then the probability that a Type I error is made increases. In fact the probability that a false positive error is made for one or both endpoints is approximately two chances in twenty. The more endpoints that are examined the greater the probability that one or more errors of this type occurs. Hence it is

important to examine as few endpoints as possible. If multiple endpoints are examined, the p-value used to determine significance should be reduced. The simplest method is to divide 5% by the number of endpoints and to use this value to define the critical level of significance; this is known as the Bonferoni correction.

For similar reasons, if more than two arms of a trial are compared this probability also increases; in this case due to multiple comparisons.

8.6.2 SUBGROUP ANALYSES

It is very common for analyses to be performed looking at the effect of treatments in differing subgroups of patients; these subgroup results are usually emphasized if there is no overall treatment effect. Subgroup analyses are another example of a situation in which the false positive error rate can be increased inadvertently. It can be shown that if there is a suggestion of an overall treatment effect in a trial, say with a p-value of 0.10, then if these patients are then divided into two equal groups there is a one-in-three chance that the treatment effect in one group will be 'significant' ($p=0.05$) and there will be no difference in the other group. This is purely a statistical phenomenon and is unrelated to the basis of the subdivision of the patients. The greater the number of subgroups that are examined the more likely it is that a spurious result will be found. The correct method of dealing with results such as these is to perform a statistical test for interaction.

8.6.3 REPEATED ANALYSES

A common temptation when undertaking a randomized trial is to look at the data at frequent intervals as the number of patients and the amount of follow-up increases. The more often the results are examined the more

157

likely one is to find a false difference because the difference between treatments will itself vary as the trial progresses. Examination of results should therefore be done infrequently and with caution. One way of approaching this problem is to define a stringent stopping criteria for these interim analyses (Pocock, 1982).

8.6.4 FOLLOW-UP PROCEDURES

It is not commonly realized that bias can be introduced into treatment comparisons by employing differing follow-up procedures in the arms of a clinical trial. If, for example, maintenance therapy was being compared with no maintenance therapy in a two-arm trial, patients in the arm receiving maintenance therapy may be seen more frequently because they have to attend hospital to receive the treatment. Disease recurrence would be detected sooner in these patients because their disease state is assessed more often than patients in the other arm, making it appear that patients in this arm recur earlier. It is possible to construct theoretical examples showing a significant difference between two arms of a trial in which the difference is explicable solely in terms of differing follow-up patterns.

8.7 APPENDIX

The definition of endpoints used by the United Kingdom Children's Cancer Study Group is as follows:

Survival
Time to death from any cause. For surviving patients, survival is censored at the date of last follow-up.

Disease-free survival
Time to relapse. If the patient has not relapsed and is disease-free at death or last follow-up, DFS is censored at death or last follow-up respectively. Patients who died

without remitting are considered to have relapsed at time 0. For surviving patients who have not remitted, DFS is censored at time 1 day. (Most of the latter will still be on treatment.)

Event-free survival
For patients who have relapsed, EFS is the time to relapse. For patients who have died but not relapsed, EFS is the time to death. For all other patients, EFS is censored at the last follow-up.

REFERENCES

Blackledge, G., Lawton, F., Redman, C. and Kelly, K. (1989). Response of patients in phase II studies of chemotherapy in ovarian cancer: implications for patient treatment and the design of phase II trials. *Br. J. Cancer*, **59**, 650–3.

Buyse, M.E., Staquet, M.J. and Sylvester, R.J. (1984) *Cancer Clinical Trials, Methods and Practice*. Oxford University Press.

Carter, S.K. (1977) Clinical trials in cancer chemotherapy. *Cancer*, **40**, 544–57.

Feinstein, A.R., Sosin, D.M. and Wells, C.K. (1985) The Will Rogers phenomenon: Stage migration and new diagnostic techniques as a source of misleading statistics for survival in cancer. *N. Eng. J. Med.*, **312**, 1604–8.

Freedman, L.S. (1989) The size of clinical trials in cancer research – what are the current needs? *Br. J. Cancer*, **59**, 396–400.

Glantz, S.A. (1977) *Primer of Biostatistics*. McGraw-Hill.

Green, S.B. and Byar, D.P. (1984) Using observational data from registries to compare treatments: the fallacy of omnimetrics. *Statistics in Medicine*, **3**, 361–70.

Machin, M., Campbell, M.J. (1987). *Statistical Tables for the Design of Clinical Trials*. Blackwell Scientific.

Miller, A.B., Hoogstraten, B., Staquet, M. and Winkler, A. (1981) Reporting results of cancer treatment. *Cancer*, **47**, 207–14.

Miller, D.R., Leikin, S.L., Albo, V.C. *et al.* (1989) Three versus five years of maintenance therapy are equivalent in childhood acute lymphoblastic leukaemia: a report from the children's cancer study group. *J. Clin. Oncol.* **7**, No. 3 316–25.

Peto, R. (1982) Statistical aspects of cancer trials, in *Treatment of Cancer*, Ed Halman.

Peto, R., Pike, M.C., Armitage, N.E. *et al.* (1976) Design and analysis of randomised clinical trials requiring prolonged observation of each patient. I Introduction and Design. *Br. J. Cancer* (1976) **34**, 585–610; II Analysis and examples. *Br. J. Cancer* (1977) **35**, 1–39.

Pocock, S.J. (1982) Interim analyses for randomised clinical trials: The group sequential approach. *Biometrics*, **38**, 153–62.

Pocock, S.J. (1983) *Clinical Trials*, John Wiley, Chichester.

UKALL. (1986) Improvement in treatment for children with acute lymphoblastic leukaemia. The Medical Research Council UKALL Trials 1972–1984. *Lancet*, **i**, 408–11.

Von Hoff, D.D., Kuhn, J. and Clark, G.M. (1984) Design and conduct of Phase I trials, in *Cancer Clinical Trials, Methods and Practice*, 210–20. Oxford University Press.

FURTHER READING

Hauck, W.W., Anderson, S.A. (1986) A proposal for interpreting and reporting negative studies. *Stats in Med.*, **5**, 203–209.

Gardner, M.J., Altman, D.G. (1986) Confidence intervals rather than P values: estimation rather than hypothesis testing. *BMJ*, **292**, 746–50.

Gardner, M.J., Machin, D., Campbell, M.J. (1986) Use of check lists in assessing the statistical content of medical studies. *BMJ*, **292**, 810–12.

Part Two

Diagnosis and Management
of Individual Cancers

Chapter 9

Acute myeloblastic leukaemia (AML)

H.G. PRENTICE and I.M. HANN

9.1 INTRODUCTION

Acute myeloblastic leukaemia (AML) is more frequent in adults than in children, with two-thirds of all cases occurring beyond the age of 40; it is, however, also a significant malignancy in children, accounting for approximately one in five cases of childhood leukaemia. Unlike the situation in acute lymphoblastic leukaemia (ALL), much of what we have learned of the management of AML in children is attributable to studies done in adults. Significant developments in the treatment of this disease were first seen in the 1960s with the introduction of the drugs which even today remain the mainstay of treatment, that is: cytarabine and the anthracyclines. During the past two decades there has been some further progress, attributable, in the main, to three developments, (1) the application of high dose (HD) therapy (e.g. HD cytarabine) in first complete remission (1st CR), or ablative regimens (e.g. high dose busulphan plus cyclophosphamide) with rescue by autologous bone marrow transplantation (ABMT), (2) the identification of the importance of the major histocompatibility complex leading to the successful application of allogeneic bone marrow transplantation

(BMT) and its safe use in the early stages of the disease, (3) the recognition of the important role of infection and the development of prophylaxis for the prevention of potentially lethal Gram-negative infection along with current progress against cytomegalovirus (CMV). Between about a third to a half of children with AML who are treated by current intensive chemotherapy are permanently cured, although we still lack the ability to accurately predict which they will be. Of those who have an HLA-matched sibling donor and have a BMT in 1st CR, more than 70% are cured although some will not have required this risky procedure.

Epidemiological studies show that some constitutional chromosomal abnormalities including Down's syndrome (trisomy 21) and Klinefelter's syndrome are associated with an increased risk of AML. In Down's syndrome there is a preponderance of the megakaryoblastic subtype (French-American-British [FAB] type M7). Those who have DNA repair disorders or fragile chromosomes also have an increased susceptibility to acute leukaemia, such as Fanconi's anaemia, ataxia telangiectasia and Bloom's syndrome (Linet, 1985). Twin studies show increased concordance for leukaemia among monzygotic twins; this may result either from a common intrauterine cause or transfer between circulations (Hartley and Sainsbury, 1981). Paternal exposure to hydrocarbons or radiation may be important but remains unproven as a cause of AML. Case-control studies are being done to investigate an apparent increased risk of childhood leukaemia associated with exposure to irradiation, electromagnetism or infections. None of these associations are likely to be direct causes of AML but most probably increase the risk because of an increased rate of DNA breaks and faulty repair by inappropriate rearrangement. North American studies suggest a slightly higher rate of AML in black children (Gordis *et al.*, 1981).

It is not the purpose of this chapter to review the rare myelodysplastic syndromes (MDS) of childhood and for these the reader is referred to a recent review by Chessells (1991). It can be said, however, that refractory anaemia with or without sideroblasts is rarely seen, but refractory anaemia with excess of blast cells (RAEB) is relatively common and usually progresses rapidly to frank AML. Thus this condition is usually treated as if it is AML from the outset. Monosomy 7 can present with a myeloproliferative picture or, less frequently, myelodysplasia with excess blast cells or frank AML. Those without acute leukaemia usually progress rapidly to that state (Baranger *et al.*, 1990). It can, however, run a more chronic course. Juvenile chronic myeloid leukaemia is the childhood equivalent of chronic myelomonocytic leukaemia and the preferred therapy is with BMT from a matched sibling or matched unrelated donor if the former is not available (Hann, 1990).

9.2 BIOLOGY AND CLINICAL FEATURES OF AML

AML is a clonal disease; this has been demonstrated employing X-linked enzyme markers in female heterozygotes or by studying DNA polymorphisms (Jacobsen, 1984;

Fearon, 1986). A high proportion of samples from patients with AML show a clonal chromosomal abnormality which can reasonably be assumed to play a central role in the block in differentiation of that clone.

With some exceptions, the chromosomal findings are similar in children and adults, the most frequent abnormalities being t(8;21), -7, t(15;17), inv16, 5q-, +8. Three haematopoietic growth factors (GM-CSF, M-CSF and Interleukin 3) are encoded by genes found on chromosome number 5 (q20-q30) which also encodes for the M-CSF receptor which is identical to the oncogene c-*fms*. Chromosome 5q- predominates in therapy-related myelodysplasia (MDS) and acute leukaemia (Nimer and Golde, 1987). These observations must be viewed with caution since the G-CSF gene is located at 17 (q11), close to the breakpoint t(15;17) found in acute promyelocytic leukaemia (FAB M3) but is not in fact involved (Tanaka *et al.*, 1990). The three *ras* genes H-, N- and K-*ras* encode membrane-associated GTP- and GDP-binding proteins. Point mutations in these genes create proteins that may contribute to leukaemic transformation. Recently, a quarter of a series of childhood AML cases were found to contain *ras* mutations, predominantly N-*ras*, as with adult AML (Farr *et al.*, 1991). Although proof is lacking, it seems reasonable to associate many of these observations with causality.

The principle clinical manifestations of AML are the result of bone marrow failure, the features of which are almost uniform at diagnosis. Anaemia with pallor and lethargy are usual. Thrombocytopenia leads to petechial haemorrhages seen in the skin, especially around the ankles, the palate, and in sites where capillaries can be directly visualized – for example, the retinae. Overt bleeding from the nose and gums is also seen but major haemorrhage is only seen in association with lesions such as mycotic aneurysms. Bleeding may occur in other sites such as the lung where it is associated with leukostasis due to very high white cell counts and certain morphological subvarieties (see below). Life-threatening haemorrhage is frequent only in FAB M3 AML (promyelocytic) where disseminated intravascular coagulation (DIC) adds another dimension to the coagulation defect. Many patients present with bacterial or fungal oropharyngeal or respiratory tract infection. Bone pain is seen in only a minority of patients at presentation. Those with the FAB M4 and M5 subtypes (myelomonoblastic and pure monoblastic) have more extramedullary disease including skin, perianal region and gum infiltration and more CNS involvement with cranial nerve palsies causing diplopia and headache (Chessells *et al.*, 1986; Pui *et al.*, 1985). Monoblastic leukaemias are prominent in younger children (<2 years). Because of the characteristics of this cell type and high cell count, leukostasis is frequent (Odom *et al.*, 1990). Other rare distinctive findings are myeloblastic chloromas which are solid tumours found around the orbits, spinal cord or cranium and occasionally the gut. Testicular involvement is very rare although meningeal involvement affects about one in six children with AML at diagnosis. Liver and spleen enlargement are seen less frequently than in ALL, and lymphadenopathy is unusual other than in monoblastic cases (M4 and M5).

9.3 CLASSIFICATION OF AML

9.3.1 MORPHOLOGY

The FAB classification (Bennett *et al.*, 1985) is based on morphology using Romanowsky stains, Sudan Black and the combined esterases (special stains).

(a) M1 (Acute myeloid leukaemia–undifferentiated)

Granulation is not prominent and there is little if any differentiation. The cytoplasm is more abundant than that in ALL and Sudan Black and chloroacetate esterase staining is seen in a proportion of cells.

(b) M2 (Acute myeloid leukaemia with differentiation)

Cytoplasmic granulation and occasional Auer rods are seen.

(c) M3 (Acute promyelocytic leukaemia)

Granulation is prominent and the granules are often more coarse than normal. Multiple Auer rods with strong Sudan Black positivity are sometimes present. In occasional 'atypical' cases the granulation can be less prominent and the nucleus is folded or 'cottage-loaf' in shape.

(d) M4 (Acute myelomonocytic leukaemia)

This shows a mix of monoblasts and myeloblasts often with some differentiation. Other myeloid cells are intermixed with the cytochemical stains showing positivity for myeloid (Sudan Black and chloroacetate esterase) and monocytic (non-specific esterase) cells.

(e) M5 (Acute monoblastic M5a and monocytic M5b)

Monoblasts show grey/blue cytoplasm which may include some fine azurophilic granules and vacuolation. Non-specific esterase stains are positive. In addition the stain for acid phosphatase is often positive with a diffuse pattern.

(f) M6 (Erythroleukaemia)

Megaloblastic erythropoiesis predominates with a minor population of myeloblasts. Multinucleated forms are the best clue to the diagnosis. A characteristic PAS positivity (Malkin and Freeman, 1989) is seen in some but not all cases.

(g) M7 (Acute megakaryocytic leukaemia)

Marrow aspiration is often difficult because of a marked marrow fibrosis in most cases. The cells are mainly undifferentiated but cytoplasmic blebs are sometimes seen along with some more mature yet abnormal megakaryocites. PAS and acid phosphatase are often positive. Non-specific esterase is strongly positive but alpha-naphthol butyrate esterase negative.

9.3.2 IMMUNOLOGY

Immunophenotyping is of assistance in M1, M6 and M7. The undifferentiated cases can usually be distinguished from ALL by their lack of B and T cell markers and terminal deoxynucleotidyl transferase (TdT) negativity but up to 10% of AML cases can be positive for TdT and some for other lymphoid markers such as CD10 (common ALL). These features can be referred to as showing 'lineage infidelity' (Greaves *et al.*, 1986). The M6 erythroleukaemia cases are positive for markers detecting spectrin and glycophorin; M7 for antibodies to platelet glycoproteins, IIb/IIIa and CD51. CD34 is a 'stem cell' marker present in a high proportion of AML cases. CD15 stains AML cells with granulocytic differentiation and the normal granulocytic lineage from promyelocytes onwards; CD13 recognizes AML with granulocyte or monocyte differentiation; CD11c and CD14 recognize monocytes and CD33 is positive in most AML cases. (CD13 and CD33 are also present in some cases of ALL.) Recently Van der Schoot *et al.* (1990) have described an anti-myeloperoxidase (MPO) which appears more specific for myeloid cells than some of the other older monoclonal antibodies.

9.3.3 CYTOGENETICS

There have been a large number of studies of chromosomal abnormalities in children and adults with acute myeloid leukaemia. A comprehensive study of 155 children treated at St. Jude's Hospital between 1980 and 1987 was undertaken (Kalwinsky *et al.*, 1990). Adequate banding was achieved in 120. Of these, 20% of metaphases were classified as normal, 30% had miscellaneous clonal abnormalities. The others showed (by decreasing frequency): Inv(16)/del(16q) n=15, t(8;21) n=14, t(15;17) n=9, t(9;11) n=9, t(11;v)/del(11q) n=7, and -7/del(7q) n=6. The inv(16)/del (16q)–positive AML cases frequently had central nervous system (CNS) disease at diagnosis or experienced initial relapse at this site. There was no predilection for any FAB subtype. The infants with M5 disease and t(9;11) did significantly better than others within the M5 group who had higher counts, coagulation problems and short survival.

Children with monosomy 7 had resistant leukaemia with only 17% entering remission. Those with t(15;17) had M3 disease and some, because of DIC, died before or during therapy from haemorrhage. Recent developments with the use of all-trans retinoic acid (ATRA) should circumvent this problem in a group who otherwise have a better chance of cure than those with other FAB types. Treatment with ATRA is further discussed below.

9.4 MANAGEMENT

9.4.1 SUPPORTIVE CARE

Right atrial (Hickman) catheter insertion is now mandatory to provide proper supportive care. Partial correction of thrombocytopenia to maintain a platelet count $>20 \times 10^9/l$ considerably reduces the risk of haemorrhage. The management of DIC remains controversial but if significant fibrinogen consumption is seen cautious anticoagulation with heparin may be necessary combined with coagulation factor replacement, although in the majority, evidence suggests that intensive product support without heparinization (Goldberg *et al.*, 1986; Cunningham *et al.*, 1988) is appropriate. This problem is likely to be correctable by the use of ATRA.

(a) Tumour lysis syndrome

The use of allopurinol (in all cases) along with forced diuresis in those at risk of tumour lysis syndrome can be life saving (O'Connor *et al.*, 1989). Temporary dialysis may be required if renal impairment is significant.

(b) Leukostasis

Hyperleukocytosis leukostasis in a minority of patients is associated with cerebral and lung dysfunction and secondary haemorrhage at those sites. Transfusion must proceed cautiously in this group otherwise these complications can be precipitated. This problem is seen most frequently in the monoblastic leukaemias. Chemotherapy reduces the counts rapidly and is much more successful than leukaphoresis.

(c) Emesis and nutrition

The recent introduction of $5HT_3$ receptor blockers has transformed the quality of life of patients undergoing highly emetic therapies (Hunter *et al.*, 1991). Good nutritional support, including parenteral nutrition when required, and maintained activity (e.g. exercise bicycle) have also played a part in improving patient outcome.

9.4.2 INFECTION PREVENTION AND TREATMENT

Prentice (1984) and Rubin and Young (1987) have reviewed this important topic exten-

sively. As a general rule, prevention is now considered far more important than interventional therapy. The following manoeuvres are therefore considered mandatory in patients expected to have periods of neutropenia exceeding 10–14 days:

1. High efficiency particulate air (HEPA) filtration with frequent air changes in a single room can almost totally prevent the acquisition of aspergillus and mucor infection. Laminar air flow systems are very expensive and probably add no more in terms of protection.
2. Patients seropositive for Herpes simplex virus (HSV) can be protected against recrudescence following intensive chemotherapy or bone marrow transplantation (BMT) by prophylactic acyclovir 5 mg/kg b.d. IV or oral acyclovir at higher doses (10 mg/kg 4–5 times daily). Partial protection from CMV infection, including pneumonitis by high dose acyclovir, is claimed from one North American study (Meyers *et al.*, 1988). This study, which showed a significant reduction in mortality, is the subject of a European confirmatory trial. Ganciclovir which has been used successfully in treatment (with immunoglobulin) has been shown to be of benefit in BMT and early fears of significant marrow toxicity seem unwarranted (Schmidt *et al.*, 1991).
3. Co-trimoxazole 480 mg/m² twice daily three times a week prevents *Pneumocystis carinii* pneumonia following BMT. Inhaled aerosolyzed pentamidine every 2–4 weeks may have the same effect, although we have seen occasional failures, probably because smaller children are unable to use the equipment properly.
4. The gastrointestinal (GI) tract is a major reservoir for the more dangerous opportunistic pathogens, particularly Gram-negative organisms. Studies in adults have now proven conclusively that when com-

bined with a clean (i.e. near sterile) diet, GI decontamination is beneficial in reducing the risk of Gram negative sepsis (to near zero) and of some Gram positive infections (mainly those due to *Staphylococcus aureus*). The recently introduced quinolones ciprofloxacin and norfloxacin are responsible for this breakthrough (Nazareth *et al.*, 1989; Karp *et al.*, 1987) and are proven to be superior to conventional non-absorbable antibiotics. Unfortunately, at the present time, these agents are not licensed for use in children because of preclinical studies which showed problems in developing cartilage. Compassionate use in children has not revealed any problem to date and it is likely that this situation will be revised shortly. In studies at the Royal Free Hospital ciprofloxacin was combined with oral colistin in an attempt to reduce the theoretical risk of emergence of resistant strains, an approach which appears to be successful.

Selective or total GI decontamination increases the risk from fungal overgrowth and should therefore be accompanied by antifungal measures. Fluconazole is effective against a broad range of *Candida* species and has proved useful in clinical practice (Brammer *et al.*, 1990). At the Royal Free Hospital, the practice is to combine fluconazole with amphotericin B suspension. Although this combination is theoretically antagonistic the fluconazole is well absorbed in the upper GI tract, and provides systemic protection; it is also separated from the non-absorbed amphotericin which treats the lower GI tract. The spectrum of activity of this combination is broader and in non-randomized trials appears superior (Prentice *et al.*, unpublished).

5. *Skin and orifice decontamination*
Reduction of the skin flora and scrupulous care of catheter entry sites is man-

datory. Antiseptics such as chlorhexidine or iodine-containing preparations are preferred. Similar care should be taken of orifices and dental hygiene requires expert assistance.

6. *Myeloid growth factors*
The recently available myeloid growth factors G and GM-CSF certainly shorten the period of neutropenia after chemotherapy or BMT (Ohno *et al.*, 1990, Powles *et al.*, 1990). Studies have also shown a reduced infection rate and antibiotic usage. Larger studies are required to determine the effect on mortality. G-CSF is now licensed in both the USA and Europe (Amgen/Roche). Use in AML is not yet clearly established as being safe because of the theoretical risk of proliferation of clonogenic leukaemia cells (Griffin *et al.*, 1986).

9.4.3 PROPHYLAXIS

The Royal Free Hospital (RFH) protocol for infection prophylaxis is detailed in Table 9.1. As has been emphasized, the quinolones are not yet licensed for use in children.

(a) Management of febrile episodes in the neutropenic child

Empirical treatment: the best tested and most effective initial empirical antibiotic regimen for treating febrile neutropenic patients is the combination of an aminoglycoside and a ureidopenicillin (Sage *et al.*, 1988) or an aminoglycoside and ceftazidine (EORTC, 1987). But it should be noted that this is the appropriate approach where Gram-negative sepsis (and potential rapid lethality) is a high risk. Where the risk of Gram-negative sepsis is minimal then an empirical approach targeted to include Gram-positive infection (i.e. including vancomycin and teicoplanin) may well be more appropriate.

It should be emphasized that in the neutropenic ($<0.5 \times 10^9$/l) patient empirical anti-

Table 9.1 Royal Free Hospital regimen for antimicrobial prophylaxis in neutropenic leukaemia post BMT

Prophylaxis	Agent	Dosage	Duration
Antibacterial	Ciprofloxacin[c]	500 mg 12 hourly	During period of neutropenia
	Colistin	1.5 MU 12 hourly	During period of neutropenia
Antituberculous	Isoniazid	5 mg/kg/day	During period of neutropenia 6 months post BMT
Antifungal	Fluconazole	100 mg once daily	During period of neutropenia 6 months post BMT
	Amphotericin B suspension	500 mg 6-hourly	During period of neutropenia 6 months post BMT
Pneumocystis carinii	Cotrimoxazole	960 mg 12-hourly 3 times/week	6 months post BMT
	(Nebulized pentamidine in adults)	(300 mg fortnightly)	During period of neutropenia
[a]*Herpes simplex*	Acyclovir	400–800 mg (oral) 4–5 times/day	During period of neutropenia Long term where clinically indicated
[b]*Cytomegalovirus*	Acyclovir	High dose (trial)	
	Ganciclovir		Under consideration

Note: These regimens should be used in conjunction with a protected environment, sterile diet and mucocutaneous antisepsis.
[a] Sero-positive patients
[b] BMT patients only
[c] Not yet licensed for use in children

biotics must be instituted urgently. The usual recommendation is for investigation by blood culture (via catheter and vein), throat, urine and sputum samples and chest x-ray followed by immediate institution of the locally determined broad spectrum antibiotic cover. Action should be taken where a single fever of 39°C or two of 38°C one hour apart is recorded in the absence of any other obvious cause (e.g. blood transfusion reaction). We also recommend institution of appropriate antibiotics for proven mucosal colonization by dangerous pathogens such as *Pseudomonas aeruginosa* because of high subsequent rates of infection with considerable mortality (unpublished observations). We believe that the use of double beta lactam combinations and monotherapy are not justified until they have been subjected to large randomized trials although preliminary studies do suggest equivalence (Kibbler *et al.*, 1989).

Patients receiving an aminoglycoside, particularly if given with a ureidopenicillin and amphotericin B, are very susceptible to renal tubular leaks of potassium, magnesium and calcium. The most important of these metabolites is potassium and severe hypokalaemia is sometimes seen. This problem can be largely abrogated by supplementation and the use of the potassium-sparing diuretics amiloride or spironolactone. Calcium and magnesium supplements may also be required. The oto- and nephro-toxicity of the regimens used can be contained at a low level (Sage *et al.*, 1988) with careful monitoring of aminoglycoside and vancomycin levels.

The evidence suggests that the antibiotic course should last at least 7 days and certainly 4–5 days after resolution of fever. There is no evidence that continuing antibiotics during the full period of neutropenia is beneficial and this practice is likely to increase the risk of fungal super-infection.

Patients who fail to respond by 72 hours should have their treatment modified to cover organisms not covered by the initial empirical therapy, e.g. by adding vancomycin/teicoplanin where appropriate. Non-response at 96 hours is best managed by the empirical addition of IV amphotericin B since the EORTC trials have shown that this group of patients have a high mortality associated in a significant number with fungal infection found at postmortem. The toxic side effects are best ameliorated by pethidine (by slow IV infusion), but the recently introduced liposomal preparations of amphotericin B almost totally abolish side effects (Meunier *et al.*, 1991; Ringden, 1991) and can be obtained commercially (AmBisome/Vestar Inc).

Herpes group viral infections: Herpes simplex lesions, including those clinically suspected, such as ulcerated lesions of the tongue and oropharynx, require treatment with acyclovir preferably by the IV route). Varicella-zoster virus (VZV) requires patient isolation and nursing by immune staff and treatment by IV acyclovir 10 mg/kg t.d.s. for at least one week.

CMV infection (including pneumonitis) is now treatable in about 60% of patients by the combined use of ganciclovir and CMV hyper-immune globulin (Reed *et al.*, 1988, Schmidt *et al.*, 1991). Lethal infections are still seen and successful treatment is often followed by recurrent infection in BMT patients such that long-term survival after this complication, regrettably, remains poor (Ljungman *et al.*, in preparation).

(b) Febrile patient with respiratory symptoms or signs

An aggressive approach to investigation is mandatory. The lung is the most frequent target for lethal infection in patients on chemotherapy and especially on BMT. The context is critical. In BMT, CMV and *Pneumocystis carinii* (PC) are frequent pathogens where a diffuse radiological lesion is seen and the onset rapid with hypoxia. CMV is uncommon in patients receiving chemotherapy where, in addition to the usual bacterial causes, the major pathogens are PC, measles, mycoplasma, legionella and the respiratory viruses. We would recommend bronchoalveolar lavage (BAL) as an immediate diagnostic manoeuvre where no sputum is available. At the same time treatment to cover the above causes is instituted with high dose co-trimoxazole, ganciclovir plus CMV hyper-immune globulin (BMT only) and erythromycin to cover legionella and mycoplasia with the addition of broad spectrum antibiotics to cover bacterial pneumonias.

Aspergillus infection of the lung often shows a cavitating lesion (mycotic lung sequestrum) mimicking aspergilloma. This lesion is well detected by CT scanning and we would recommend this where other studies have been negative. Immediate institution of amphotericin B or liposomal entrapped amphotericin B as well as surgery is recommended (Kibbler *et al.*, 1988), since these lesions are avascular and successful treatment using drugs alone is only 30–50%.

White cell transfusions are of limited value in the management of infection and increase the risk of transmission of latent viral infection such as CMV. Persistent destructive local infection, such as perineal pseudomonas lesions, may be targets for this treatment in a patient likely to remain neutropenic for more than seven days. An outline approach to 'planned progressive therapy' for fever of unknown origin (FUO) in the neutropenic patient is given in Table 9.2.

9.4.4 THE SUPPORT TEAM FOR OPTIMAL CARE

In addition to the clinical haematology and expert nursing teams the support team needed to provide optimal patient care

Table 9.2 Planned progressive therapy for fever of unknown origin in the neutropenic phase

1.	Initiation of therapy	Pyrexia >38°C for >2 hours or >39°C
	Sample:	Blood (catheter and peripheral veins)
		Throat and urine culture
		Review surveillance data
	Start:	Aminoglycoside + ureidopenicillin or ceftazidime
		or vancomycin + ceftazidime (if good Gram-negative prophylaxis, e.g. quinolone)

2.   Review after 48 hours (or earlier if deterioration)
     (a) If positive isolate – appropriate therapy
     (b) Otherwise where no response: add/substitute Gram-positive cover (e.g. vancomycin/teicoplanin) or improve Gram-negative cover
     (c) Improving: continue to 7 days (or at least 4 days afebrile)

3.   Review 72–96 hours
     Where no response, add IV amphotericin B (or liposomal amphotericin B)

should include: microbiologist, chemical pathologist/endocrinologist, psychologist, social worker, dietitian, occupational therapist, liaison health visitor, play therapist and physiotherapist.

9.5 TREATMENT

9.5.1 INDUCTION THERAPY

Modern intensive chemotherapy in its many different guises yields high remission rates in children (>80%) and a variable proportion of cures (20–50%). The detailed discussion of remission induction regimens is in our view now less critical than that of the post-remission induction treatment options, a review of which follows.

The mainstay of current induction chemotherapy is a combination of cytarabine (for 7–10 days in standard 100–200 mg/m²/d dose) and an anthracycline for three days. Daunorubicin is the best studied anthracycline but recent trials of idarubicin in adults show an apparent marginal superiority (Berman *et al.*, 1989). There is evidence that infusions can reduce early and late cardiac toxicity which is a particular worry in children (Lipshultz *et*

al., 1991). Very large MRC studies show a higher CR rate than most US studies, and suggest that the addition of a third agent (thioguanine or epipodophyllotoxin) may add somewhat to the result (Rees *et al.*, 1986). MRC AML 9 also showed a higher rate of CR for DAT 3+10 than the less intensive DAT 1+5. Overall, an 85% CR (up to age 40) was seen, 75% of whom achieved CR with the first course. Time to remission was faster and the more intensive therapy also reduced the need for supportive care (Rees *et al.*, 1989). In the current MRC AML 10 trial, the CR rate is 91% in children, with 85% of remitters achieving CR after a single course of intensive three-drug chemotherapy. Only 4% failed to achieve CR because of resistant disease (Stevens, 1991).

All patients should have an early diagnostic/therapeutic lumbar puncture and at least those with monoblastic subtypes, with a higher risk of CNS disease (Pui *et al.*, 1985), should have intrathecal therapy during the six-month therapy course.

About 5% of childhood AML is currently refractory to modern chemotherapy; a further 5% of children succumb to infection and a small number to haemorrhage during remission induction. Recent studies with all-trans retinoic acid (ALTRA) from China and France (Huang *et al.*, 1988; Castaigne *et al.*, 1990) show a dramatic biological effect. This vitamin will induce remission through differentiation in FAB M3 AML. Of 22 mainly relapsed patients in the French confirmatory study, 14 treated with ALTRA alone have achieved CR. Remarkably, the coagulopathy reverses rapidly in two to three days but a rising WBC carries a risk of leukostasis; this can, however, be halted by institution of chemotherapy. This development appears to be a remarkable advance in this otherwise dangerous setting. Overexpression of P-glycoprotein in AML blast cells is correlated with multidrug resistance (Ma *et al.*, 1987). The problem is likely to be of significance in relapsed or secondary AML. Studies with clonogenic cells from children with AML have demonstrated that the sensitivity of these cells in culture to daunorubicin and cytarabine correlates with treatment outcome. Further studies are required to determine whether these assays can be used in deciding therapeutic options (Dow *et al.*, 1986).

9.5.2 POST-REMISSION THERAPY IN AML

It is reasonable to assume that children, like adults, should receive at least one further course of 'reinduction/consolidation' chemotherapy in CR prior to any further therapy designed to eliminate clonogenic cells assumed to remain and detectable as 'minimal residual disease' (MRD) by immunological or combined immunological and culture methods (Campana *et al.*, 1990; Gerhartz and Schmetzer, 1990). Two further courses are probably optimal with the possible exception of the more intensive regimens such as timed sequential therapy (Geller *et al.*, 1990). Details of the outcome of treatment for several published studies of chemotherapy are given in Table 9.3.

Further therapy options to eradicate MRD are:

Table 9.3 Results of recent therapeutic studies of AML in childhood

Study	(1) BFM-78	(2) St Jude's 80	(3) AIEOP 82043	(4) BFM-83	(5) VAPA	(6) Boston 80–035	(7) USCCSG 251	(8) UK Joint Trial	(9) UK MRC 10
Era	1978–82	1980–83	1982–86	1983–86	1976–80	1980–84	1979–83	1982–85	1990–
Patient number	151	87	133	143	61	64	508	66	118
Induction deaths	19	16	13	18	16	19	161	6	5
Resistant disease	13	6	13	21					6
Complete response rate	80%	75%	80%	79%	74%	70%	68%	91%	91%
Event-free survival (excluding BMT)	49%	20%	33%	52%	33%	29%	25%	42%	N/A

References: (1) Creutzig *et al.* (1987) *Am. J. Paediatr. Hematol. Oncol.*, **9**, 324–30.
(2) Dahl *et al.* (1987) *Acute Leukaemias*, Springer pp. 83–7.
(3) Amadori *et al.* (1987) *J. Clin. Oncol.*, **5**, 1356–63.
(4) Creutzig *et al.* (1987) 4th Int. Symp on Acute Leukaemia, Rome, 220.
(5) Weinstein *et al.* (1983) *Blood*, **62**, 315–19.
(6) Weinstein *et al.* (1987) *Acute Leukaemias*, Springer pp. 88–92.
(7) Nesbit *et al.* (1987) *Proc. Am. Clin. Oncol.*, **6**, 163.
(8) Marcus *et al.*, (1987) *Acute Leukaemias*, Springer 346–51.
(9) Stevens, R. (1991) *Bailliere's Clinical Haematology*, **42**, p. 2.
Data adapted from Lie, S. (1989) with permission of the editor of *Eur. J. Paediatr.*

1. Further cycles of therapy

These can be similar to (or variants of) the remission induction therapy. But additional courses showed no benefit in at least one study in adults (Rohatiner *et al.*, 1988).

2. Intensive (but not ablative) treatment

This includes regimens such as high dose cytarabine containing combinations (Wolff *et al.*, 1987). The long-term disease-free survival (DFS) with this approach in adults yields results similar to that of many published reports of BMT. The appropriate randomized controlled comparisons are not yet underway, however, and could prove difficult to plan.

3. Continuing low dose therapy

This appears to have no important role to play in AML, unlike in ALL (Bloomfield, 1985). But this approach may be beneficial in

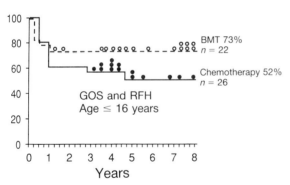

GOS = Hospital for Sick Children, Great Ormond Street, London

RFH = Bone Marrow Transplant Programme, Royal Free Hospital, London

Fig. 9.1 The results of intensive chemotherapy in children with AML are improving and approach those achieved with HLA matched sibling donor BMT in 1st CR. (With thanks to Professor J. Chessells, Dr M. Phillips and Dr M. Hann for data analysis.)

children where the prior therapy is sub-optimal (Woods *et al.*, 1990).

4. Myeloablative therapy followed by bone marrow rescue

BMT may be carried out using the allogeneic or autologous grafts:

(a) Allogeneic BMT: there is no doubt that ablative therapy by high dose cyclophosphamide (120 mg/kg) and total body irradiation (TBI) followed by rescue with HLA matched marrow (usually a sibling) donor has a dramatic impact on the relapse risk, reducing this from about 50% to 10–15% (Fig. 9.1). Despite this benefit the survival advantage is less dramatic because of the considerable risks from graft versus host disease (GvHD) and infection (especially CMV interstitial pneumonitis). Nevertheless 60–80% of children become long-term disease-free survivors. Considerable progress against GvHD by T-cell depletion (TCD) (Prentice, 1991), cyclosporin A plus short-term methotrexate (Storb *et al.*, 1989), and in the treatment and prophylaxis of CMV infection (see above) has been made recently. Better GvH prevention requires better 'conditioning' since it is now clear that it is the graft versus leukaemia (GvL) effect which imparts the benefit of BMT since the immune advantage must be derived from the donor marrow (Prentice, 1991). The conditioning *per se* has little impact on the disease as has been made clear in studies where TCD was employed without adjustment to the conditioning regimens (Pollard *et al.*, 1986; Maraninchi *et al.*, 1987; Atkinson *et al.*, 1988) and experience in identical twin transplants. But conditioning must be adjusted to counterbalance the partial loss of antileukaemic activity of the donor marrow (GvL) where better GvHD prevention is used.

The major outstanding problem remains that of donor availability (approximately 30%). While progress is being made, the results using non-HLA matched relatives or unrelated HLA identical donors do not yet justify this approach in 1st CR of AML in children (Beatty *et al.*, 1985; Beatty *et al.*, 1989).

(b) Autologous BMT: logic would suggest that ABMT should add little to the cure of AML since a GvL effect is not expected. Two lines of evidence suggest that this might not be the case. First, ABMT in 2nd CR of AML can rescue 20–40% of children (Yeager *et al.*, 1986; Yeager *et al.*, 1990). 'Purging' of the marrow with the cyclophosphamide congener 4-hydroxy-peroxycyclophosphamide (4HC) or mafosfamide (Yeager *et al.*, 1986; Gorin *et al.*, 1989) may add to the benefit although this could be through an effect on immune reconstitution (Rizzoli *et al.*, 1991), discussed below. Secondly, we have identified a dysregulated cellular immune pattern after ABMT identical to that seen in BMT. Activated large granular lymphocytes (LGLs) circulate in increased numbers for several weeks (Reittie *et al.*, 1989). These have antileukaemic (AML) activity *in vitro* and secrete both gamma interferon (IFN) and tumour necrosis factor (TNF) (Heslop *et al.*, 1989) both of which we have also shown to have synergistic antileukaemic activity. Thus, the immune microenvironment is hostile to the residual leukaemia population.

Randomized controlled trials in adults suggest a benefit for ABMT in 1st CR but this is not as great as that of allogeneic BMT (Lowenberg *et al.*, 1990; Reiffers *et al.*, 1991) but both appear superior to chemotherapy. A major current UK randomized study (MRC AML 10) should answer these questions.

The issue of chemotherapy alone versus TBI protocols, e.g. busulphan/cyclophosphamide (Bu/Cy) is unresolved, but evidence to date favours TBI (Maraninchi, personal communication). Unfortunately TBI is certain to be a problem in young (<5 years) children with consequence both to their growth and intellect (Sanders *et al.*, 1988).

5. Immunotherapy in the setting of MRD in childhood AML

Many historical studies have attempted immunotherapy, e.g. with BCG or killed leukaemic cells. Much work has been done by Matthe in France and Powles in the UK. A biological effect was always demonstrable but no impact on the cure rate was seen.

Studies in BMT/ABMT have revealed the GvL effectors as:

(a) cytotoxic T lymphocytes (CTLs);
(b) activated killers (AK) or lymphokine activated cells (LAK);
(c) γINT + TNF;
(d) monocytes/macrophages (by analogy with solid tumour).

Modern immunotherapy should allow us to reproduce these effects without recourse to BMT. Our own studies with interleukin 2 (IL2) have shown that application of this cytokine can produce a cellular pattern and secondary cytokines similar to those seen in BMT (Gottlieb *et al.*, 1989b).

A recent review of European experience with IL2 in AML shows encouraging results (Prentice, 1991). While occasional dramatic benefit in relapsed disease is reported (Foa *et al.*, 1991), the greatest benefit appears to be as post-induction therapy in 1st CR. Patients with an antecedent haematological disorder (AHD) do not appear to benefit but those with primary AML do. The best results are seen in patients treated after ABMT but benefit may also be seen after consolidation chemotherapy (Prentice, 1991; Blaise *et al.*,

171

1991). Some AML samples express IL2 receptors, particularly those with monoblastic features (Carron and Cawley, 1989) – thus caution is required, but in the setting of MRD it seems likely that such target cells may not proliferate and effectors will outnumber target cells and benefit of treatment will be seen (Foa *et al.*, 1990). European randomized controlled trials are now underway in AML (and ALL) in adults to determine the extent of this benefit.

IL2 is a cytokine with considerable toxicity but continuous infusion studies have shown that this can be reduced to tolerable levels (Gottlieb *et al.*, 1989b). All studies note that toxicity is rapidly reversed with cessation of therapy. An alternative drug, linomide, which has similar biological effects and can be taken by mouth is now also under study. Very preliminary data suggest limited toxicity (unpublished company data, Pharmacia Leo Therapeutics, AB). Immunotherapy appears promising and has the potential for benefit to all patients. It is most likely to be of value in MRD such as 1st CR of AML after ABMT where the effectors are already primed (Prentice, 1991).

9.5.3 TREATMENT BEYOND 1ST CR IN CHILDHOOD AML

In early relapse or 2nd remission chemotherapy-induced CR, a small fraction of children can be rescued by BMT. In this setting, an unrelated (HLA-matched) donor or a minor mismatched relative may be an option, but the results of ABMT in 2nd CR are currently equivalent. The application of immunotherapy is less likely to be of benefit in this setting but deserves study.

9.6 LATE TOXIC EFFECTS OF THERAPY

Little information is available on the long-term consequences of the treatments detailed above but some facts are indisputable. The risk of second malignancy appears so far to be small. Persisting oto- and nephrotoxicity in patients who have been heavily treated with aminoglycoside antibiotics is a serious problem in a few patients. There is reason for concern that long-term cardiac toxicity could lead to premature deaths in patients exposed to high doses of anthracyclines.

Much is known about the late effects of allogeneic BMT with TBI (Hann, 1990). It would seem that the introduction of fractionated radiotherapy has reduced immediate and late problems, particularly cataracts, but has not completely eradicated them. International Bone Marrow Transplant Registry (IBMTR) data suggest that in the setting of T-cell depletion (TCD), BMT single fraction deep x-ray therapy (DXT) might be preferred since it appears to be more immunosuppressive – as is fast dose rate. Delayed effects on growth and endocrine function are being seen in long-term follow-up studies. One-third of children treated with cyclophosphamide/TBI develop a compensated hypothyroidism with elevated TSH and normal T_4. About 8% develop overt hypothyroidism requiring replacement therapy. The risk of thyroid malignancy has not been quantified, but in one series, two of 116 children developed a neoplasm 4 and 8 years after BMT. At least two-thirds of patients develop growth hormone deficiency and the response to recombinant growth hormone is still being evaluated. Gonadal dysfunction is clearly defined. Two-thirds of pre-pubertal boys have delayed onset of secondary sexual characteristics and many require androgen therapy. Two-thirds of pre-pubertal girls experience delayed puberty and many require replacement therapy. Most of the post-pubertal boys and girls develop gonadal failure. All of the girls develop amenorrhoea; one-third recover but some may have recurrence of ovarian failure. All post-pubertal boys studied exhibit azoospermia.

9.7 CONCLUSION AND CURRENT CONTROVERSIES

Real progress in the treatment of AML in childhood has been made over the last two decades (Phillips *et al.*, 1991). Allogeneic BMT offers the best antileukaemic activity thus far and studies have revealed some of the mechanisms responsible for this effect. We believe that the application of modern immunotherapy early in the course of treatment shows great promise for the near future.

9.7.1 DO CLINICALLY RELEVANT PROGNOSTIC SUBGROUPS EXIST?

In adults, because of the poor overall outcome in AML, treatment is rarely stratified on the basis of risk factors. In children, where the cure rate is higher, it is possible that, as in the case of ALL, treatment could ultimately be based on biological characteristics at diagnosis. Previous reviews of clinical prognostic factors have shown little of significance other than age and white cell count (Buckley *et al.*, 1989; Grier *et al.*, 1987). As has been the case in ALL, improved results with more intensive chemotherapy have now abolished some of the earlier prognostic features such as age and FAB subtype (Phillips *et al.*, 1991; Pui, 1988). Now that more sophisticated immunocytochemistry and cytogenetics of blast cells are becoming standard practice in large series, new prognostic factors are beginning to emerge (Kalwinsky *et al.*, 1990; Schwarzinger *et al.*, 1990; Benedetto *et al.*, 1986).

These factors could become important in decisions regarding the need for aggressive CNS-directed therapy. In adult practice this is often excluded with the exception of patients with monoblastic subtypes. In paediatric practice it is only comparatively recently that the German BFM group has omitted cranial irradiation from their protocol

and it remains standard practice in most paediatric protocols to include several injections of intrathecal methotrexate. Accurate subdivision of patients on the basis of probable prognosis could also avoid the late sequelae of allogeneic bone marrow transplantation or high dose chemo-radiotherapy as these may not be necessary for cure in all cases. Conversely, patients with bad risk features would be candidates for procedures that are still at the experimental stage such as matched unrelated donor allograft.

9.7.2 HOW MUCH CONSOLIDATION THERAPY IS REQUIRED FOLLOWING ATTAINMENT OF REMISSION?

This decision is influenced by what treatment option follows complete remission. In cases where a matched allogeneic donor is available, it is likely that little, if any, further consolidation is required prior to allograft (Parikh *et al.*, 1990; Lobo *et al.*, 1991). It is rarely practical to proceed this rapidly into a transplant and therefore at least one further course of consolidation is generally given. The required intensity of this is debatable and in some centres this may consist of comparatively non-myelosuppressive combinations of cytarabine and 6-thioguanine (Krischer *et al.*, 1989). It should be added that to continue with a number of high morbidity regimens is likely to increase the risk of complications following allograft and may add little to the outcome. Where high dose chemo-radiotherapy and autologous bone marrow rescue is planned, further cytoreduction is necessary; the number of courses, however, must be balanced against normal marrow stem cell toxicity. This will impair the quality of subsequent bone marrow harvest and may result in prolonged delay or even failure of engraftment. Where no high dose procedure is planned it is possible that the prolongation of continuing treatment recommended by the

BFM group may be desirable, although this has never been demonstrated in a randomized study.

9.7.3 WHAT TYPE OF TRANSPLANT AND WHEN?

There is little doubt that elective matched allogeneic transplantation in first complete remission in childhood AML results in the best relapse-free survival. It is argued, however, that if allograft can rescue a significant proportion of patients at time of relapse, then this procedure, with its attendant high early and late morbidity, could be kept until second CR. Whilst published data suggest that the result of allograft is little different in first or second CR these data are derived from patients who had relapsed after non-intensive initial chemotherapy regimens, and in whom salvage therapy was more intensive and consequently effective. In patients relapsing after present-day multi-agent regimens it is not only more difficult to achieve a second CR but the toxicity of aggressive second line therapy is considerable and may influence the morbidity of subsequent allograft.

For the majority of patients who do not have a donor, autologous bone marrow rescue following high dose chemo-radiotherapy remains of unproven benefit in childhood and the outcome of the MRC AML X trial will shed light on this. The benefits of bone marrow purging remains a contentious issue. The conclusions of Gorin *et al.* (1989) are based on non-randomized comparative data. Decisions regarding purging and the methods used remain empirical thus far and lack any firm scientific backing (Yeager *et al.*, 1986; Michel *et al.*, 1988; Burnett *et al.*, 1984).

Although total body irradiation remains a conventional component of most high dose therapy its late sequelae make it desirable to design alternative drug-based regimens. If the benefit of megatherapy is demonstrated in current randomized studies, an important next step would be to randomize total body irradiation versus non-TBI regimens. Likely candidates would be busulphan and cyclosphosphamide or busulphan and melphalan (Kanfer and McCarthy, 1989; Aurer and Gale, 1991; Beelen *et al.*, 1989; Meloni *et al.*, 1990; Geller *et al.*, 1989).

9.7.4 FUTURE TREATMENT OPTIONS

The benefits of the graft versus leukaemia effect, whatever its precise mechanism, has led to the use of matched unrelated donors. Although early studies in adults that used this approach were disappointing due to unacceptably high incidences of fatal graft-versus-host disease and graft failure, improved immunological manipulation including pre- and post-transplant treatment with T cell modifying agents and the use of partially T cell depleted bone marrow may improve the outcome (Casper, 1990).

Attempts to induce a graft versus leukaemia affect using cyclosporin have been reported (Jones *et al.*, 1989) and there is considerable current interest in other methods of immune modulation post transplantation (Prentice, 1991).

In the case of induction drug regimens, it seems likely that there is little scope for improvement although some optimization of drug scheduling is feasible. Further steps forward in the treatment of AML will depend upon either increasing the number for whom allogeneic transplantation is an option or on the instigation of completely novel strategies.

C.R.P.

REFERENCES

Amadori, S., Ceci, A., Cornelli, A., Madon, E. *et al.* (1987) Treatment of acute myelogenous leukemia in children: results of the Italian Cooperative Study AIEOP/LAM 8204. *J. Clin. Oncol.*, **5**(9), 1356–63.

Atkinson, K., Downs, K., Biggs, J. *et al.* (1988) High

incidence of early relapse in patients given cyclosporin and T-cell depleted HLA-identical sibling marrow transplants for acute leukemia in first remission. *Aust. N.Z. J. Med.*, **18**, 587–00.

Aurer, I. and Gale R.P. (1991) Are new conditioning regimens for transplants in acute myelogenous leukemia better? *Bone Marrow Transpl.*, **7**, 255–61.

Avvisati, G., Tencate, J.W., Buller, H.R. and Mandelli, F. (1989) Tranexamic acid for control of haemorrhage in acute promyelocytic leukaemia. *Lancet*, **ii**, 122–4.

Baranger, L., Baruchel, A., Leverger, G. *et al.* (1990) Monosomy-7 in childhood hemopoietic disorders. *Leukaemia*, **4**, 345–9.

Beatty, P.G., Ash, R., Hows, J.M. and McGlave, P.B. (1989) The use of unrelated bone marrow donors in the treatment of patients with chronic myeloid leukaemia: Experiences of four marrow transplant centres. *Bone Marrow Transplant.*, **4**, 287–90.

Beatty, P.G., Clift, R.A., Mickelson, E.M. *et al.* (1985) Marrow transplantation from related donors other than HLA-identical siblings. *N. Engl. J. Med.*, **313**, 765–71.

Beelen, D.W., Quabeck, K., Graeven, U. *et al.* (1989) Acute toxicity and first clinical results of intensive postinduction therapy using a modified busulfan and cyclophosphamide regimen with autologous bone marrow rescue in first remission of acute myeloid leukemia. *Blood*, **74**, (5) 1507–16.

Benedetto, P., Mertelsmann, R., Szatrowski, T.H. *et al.* (1986) Prognostic significance of terminal deoxynucleotidyl transferase activity in acute nonlymphoblastic leukemia. *J. Clin. Oncol.*, **4**, 489–95.

Bennett, J.M., Catovsky, D., Daniel, M-T. *et al.* (1985) Criteria for the diagnosis of acute leukaemia of megakaryocytic lineage (M7). *Ann. Intern. Med.*, **103**, 460–2.

Berman, E., Raymond, V., Gee, T. *et al.* (1989) Idarubicin in acute leukaemia: Results of studies at Memorial Sloan-Kettering Cancer Center. *Sem. Oncol.*, **16**, (Suppl 2) 30–4.

Blaise, D., Stopa, A.M., Olive, D. *et al.* (1991) Use of recombinant IL-2 (RU 49637) after autologous bone marrow transplantation (BMT) in patients with haematological neoplasms: A phase I study. *Bone Marrow Transplant.*, **7**, (Suppl 2) 146.

Bloomfield, C.D. (1985) Post-remission therapy in AML. *J. Clin. Oncol.*, **3**, 1570–2.

Brammer, K.W. (1990) Management of fungal infection in neutropenic patients with fluconazole. *Haematol. Bluttransfus.*, **33**, 546–50.

Buckley, J.D., Chard, R.L., Robert, L. *et al.* (1989) Improvement in outcome for children with acute nonlymphocytic leukaemia. *Cancer*, **63**, 1457–65.

Burnett, A.K., Goldman, A.H., Gray, R.G. *et al.* on behalf of the MRC Adult and Childhood Leukaemia Working Parties (1990) Medical Research Council's 10th AML TRIAL, *Brit. J. Haematol.*, **74**, Suppl 1, 4.

Burnett, A.K., Watkins, R., Maharaj, D. *et al.* (1984) Transplantation of unpurged autologous bone marrow in acute myeloid leukaemia in first remission. *Lancet*, **ii**, 1068–70.

Campana, D., Coustan-Smith, E. and Janossy, G. (1990) The immunologic detection of minimal residual disease in acute leukemia. *Blood*, **76**, 163–71.

Capizzi, R.L., Poole, M., Cooper, R. *et al.* (1984) Treatment of poor risk acute leukaemia with sequential high dose Ara-C and asparaginase. *Blood*, **63**, 694–700.

Carron, J.A. and Cawley, J.C. (1989) IL2 and myelopoiesis: IL2 induces blast cell proliferation in some cases of acute myeloid leukaemia. *Brit. J. Haematol.*, **73**, 168–72.

Casper, J.T., Bunin, N., Truitt, R. *et al.* (1990) Pediatric bone marrow transplantation utilizing unrelated donors. in *Bone Marrow Transplantation in Children*. (eds F.L. Johnson and C. Pochedly) New York, pp. 301–25.

Castaigne, S., Chomienne, C., Danel, M.T. *et al.* (1990) All-trans retinoic acid has a differentiation therapy for acute promyelocytic leukemia. I. Clinical Results. *Blood*, **76**, 1704–9.

Chessells, J.M. (1991) Myelodysplasia in childhood, in *Paediatric Haematology*, (eds J.S. Veyman and I.M. Hann) Baillière Tindall.

Chessells, J.M., O'Callaghan, U. and Hardisty, R.M. (1986) Acute myeloid leukaemia in childhood: clinical features and prognosis. *Brit. J. Haematol.*, **63**, 555–64.

Creutzig, U., Ritter, J., Riehm, H. *et al.* (1987) The childhood AML studies BFM 78 and 83: Treatment results and risk factor analysis, in *Haema-*

tology and Blood Transfusion (eds T. Buchner, G. Schellong and W. Hiddemann) Berlin, **30**, 71–5.

Cunningham, I., Gee, T.S., Reich, L.M. *et al.* (1988) Acute promyelocytic leukaemia: treatment results during a decade at Memorial Hospital. *Blood*, **73**, 1116–22.

Dahl, G.V., Kalwinsky, D.K. and Mirro, J. (1987) A comparison of cytokinetically based versus intensive chemotherapy for childhood acute myelogenous leukaemia, in *Acute Leukaemias. Haematology and Blood Transfusion* (eds T. Buchner, G. Schellong and W. Hiddemann) Springer, Berlin, pp. 87–8.

Dow, L.W., Dahl, G.V., Kalwinsky, D.K. *et al*, (1986) Correlation of drug sensitivity *in vitro* with clinical responses in childhood AML. *Blood*, **68**, 400–5.

EORTC International Antimicrobial Therapy Co-operative Group (1987) Ceftazidine combined with a short or long course of amikacin for empirical therapy of Gram-negative bacteraemia in cancer patients with granulocytopenia. *N. Engl. J. Med.*, **317**, 1692–8.

Farr, C., Gill, R., Katz, F. *et al.* (1991) Analysis of *ras* gene mutations in childhood myeloid leukaemia. *Brit. J. Haematol.*, **77**, 323–7.

Fearon, E., Burke, P., Schiffer, C. *et al*, (1986) Differentiation of leukaemic cells to polymorphonuclear leukocytes in patients with AML. *N. Engl. J. Med.*, **315**, 15–24.

Foa, R., Caretto, P., Fierro, M.T. *et al.* (1990) Interleukin 2 does not promote the *in vitro* and *in vivo* proliferation and growth of human acute leukaemia cells of myeloid and lymphoid origin. *Brit. J. Haematol.*, **75**, 34–40.

Foa, R., Meloni, G., Tosti, S. *et al.* (1991) Treatment of acute myeloid leukaemia patients with recombinant Interleukin 2: a pilot study. *Brit. J. Haematol.*, **77**, 491–6.

Geller, R.B., Saral, R., Karp, J. *et al.* (1990) Cure of acute myelocytic leukaemia in adults: A Reality. *Leukaemia*, **4**, 313–15.

Geller, R.B., Saral, R. Piantadosi, S. *et al.* (1989) Allogeneic bone marrow transplantation after high-dose busulfan and cyclophosphamide in patients with acute nonlymphocytic leukemia. *Blood*, **73**, (8) 2209–18.

Gerhartz, H.H. and Schmetzer, H. (1990) Detection of minimal residual disease in acute myeloid leukemia. *Leukemia*, **4**, (7) 508–16.

Goldberg, M.A., Ginsburg, D., Mayer, R.J. *et al.* (1986) Is heparin administration necessary during induction chemotherapy for patients with acute promyelocytic leukaemia? *Blood*, **69**, 187–91.

Gordis, L., Szkli, M., Thompson, B. *et al.* (1981) An apparent increase in the incidence of AML in black children. *Cancer*, **47**, 2763–8.

Gorin, N.C., Aegerter, P. and Auvert, B. (1989) Autologous bone marrow transplantation (ABMT) for acute leukaemia in remission: Fifth European Survey. Evidence in favour of marrow purging. *Bone Marrow Transplant.*, **4**, 206.

Gottlieb, D.J., Brenner, M.K., Heslop, H.E. *et al.* (1989a) A Phase I clinical trial of recombinant interleukin 2 following high dose chemo-radiotherapy for haematological malignancy: Applicability to the elimination of minimal residual disease. *Br. J. Cancer*, **60**, 610–15.

Gottlieb, D.J., Prentice, H.G., Heslop, H.E. *et al.* (1989b) Effects of recombinant Interleukin 2 administration on cytotoxic function following high dose chemo-radiotherapy for haematological malignancy. *Blood*, **74**, 2335–42.

Greaves, M.F., Chan, L.C. Furley, A.W. and Moolgaard, M.V. (1986) Lineage promiscuity in hemopoietic differentiation and leukemia. *Blood*, **67**, 1–11.

Grier, H., Gelber, R.D., Cammitta, B.M. *et al.* (1987) Prognostic factors in childhood AML. *J. Clin. Oncol.*, **5**, 1026–32.

Griffin, J.D., Young, D., Wiper, H.D. *et al.* (1986) Effects of recombinant human GM-CSF on proliferation of clonogenic cells in SML. *Blood* **67**, 1448–53.

Hann, I.M. (1988) Infections in immunosuppressed children. *Current Opinion in Infectious Diseases*, **1**, 607–9.

Hann, I.M., (1990) Bone marrow transplantation. *Current Opinion in Paediatrics*, **2**, 143–50.

Hartley, S.E. and Sainsbury, C. (1981) Acute leukaemia and the same chromosome abnormality in monzygote twins. *Hum. Genet.*, **58**, 408–10.

Heslop, H.E., Gottlieb, D.J., Reittie, J.E. *et al.* (1989) Spontaneous and Interleukin 2 induced secretion of tumour necrosis factor and gamma interferon following autologous marrow transplantation or chemotherapy. *Brit. J. Haematol.*, **72**, 122.

Huang, M-E., Ye, H-C., Chen, S-R. *et al.* (1988)

Use of all-trans retinoic acid in the treatment of acute promyelocytic leukaemia. *Blood*, **72**, 567–72.

Hunter, A., Prentice, H.G., Pothercary, K. *et al.* (1991) Granisetron, a selective 5HT3 receptor antagonist, for the prevention of radiation induced emesis during total body irradiation. *Bone Marrow Transplant.* (in press).

Jacobsen, R.J., Temple, M.J., Singer, J.W. *et al.* (1984) A clonal complete remission in a patient with AML originating in a multipotent stem cell. *N. Engl. J. Med.*, **310**, 1513–17.

Jones, R.J., Hess, A.D., Mann, R.B. *et al.* (1989) Induction of graft-versus-host disease after autologous bone marrow transplantation. *Lancet*, 754–6.

Kalwinsky, D.K., Mirro J. Jr., Schell, M. *et al.* (1988) Early intensification of chemotherapy for childhood acute nonlymphoblastic leukemia: Improved remission induction with a five-drug regimen including etoposide. *J. Clin. Oncol.*, **6**, (7), 1134–43.

Kalwinsky, D.K., Raimondi, S.C., Schell, M.J. *et al.* (1990) Prognostic importance of cytogenetic subgroups in De Novo pediatric acute nonlymphocytic leukemia. *J. Clin. Oncol.*, **8**, (1), 75–83.

Kanfer, E.J. and McCarthy, D.M. (1989) Cytoreductive preparation for bone marrow transplantation in leukaemia: To irradiate or not? *Br. J. Haematol.*, **71**, 447–50.

Karp, J.E., Merz, W.G., Hendricksen, C. *et al.* (1987) Oral Norfloxacin for prevention of gram negative bacterial infections in patients with acute leukaemia and granulocytopenia. *Ann. Intern. Med.*, **106**, 1–7.

Kibbler, C.C., Milkins, S.R., Bhamra, A. *et al.* (1988) Apparent pulmonary mycetoma following invasive aspergillosis in neutropenic patients. *Thorax*, **43**, 108–12.

Kibbler, C.C., Prentice, H.G., Sage, R.J. *et al.* (1989) A comparison of double beta-lactam combinations with netilmicin/ureidopenicillin regimens in the empirical therapy of febrile neutropenic patients. *J. Antimicrob. Chemother.*, **23**, 759–71.

Krischer, J.P., Steuber, C.P., Vietti, T.J. *et al.* (1989) Long-term results in the treatment of acute nonlymphocytic leukemia: A pediatric oncology group study. *Med. Ped. Oncol.*, **17**, 401–8.

Lie, S.O. (1989) Acute myelogenous leukaemia in children. *Eur. J. Paediatr.*, **148**, 382–8.

Linet, M.S. (1985) The Leukaemias: epidemiological aspects, in *Monographs in Epidemiology and Biostatistics.* (ed A.M. Lilienfield) Oxford University Press pp. 1–293.

Lipshultz, S.E., Steven, D.C., Gelber, R.D. *et al.* (1991) Late cardiac effects of doxorubicin therapy for acute lymphoblastic leukemia in childhood. *N. Engl. J. Med.*, **324**, 808–14.

Ljungman, P., Engelhard, D., Link, H. *et al.* (in preparation) Cytomegalovirus interstitial pneumonitis; treatment with Ganciclovir and intravenous immune globulin. EBMT experience.

Lobo, P.J., Powles, R.L., Hanrahan, A. and Reynolds, D.K. (1991) Acute myeloblastic leukaemia – a model for assessing value for money for new treatment programmes. *Br. Med. J.*, **302**, 323–6.

Lowenberg, B., Verdonck, L.J., Dekker, A.W. *et al.* (1990) Autologous bone marrow transplantation in acute myeloid leukaemia in first complete remission: Results of a Dutch prospective study. *J. Clin. Oncol.*, **8**, 287–94.

Ma., D.D.F., Davey, R.A., Harman, D.H. *et al.* (1987) Detection of a multidrug resistant phenotype in AML. *Lancet*, **i**, 135–7.

Malkin, D. and Freeman, M.H. (1989) Childhood erythroleukaemia: Review of clinical and biological features. *Am. J. Pediatr. Haematol. Oncol.*, **11**, 348–59.

Maraninchi, D. (1987) Impact of T cell depletion on outcome of allogeneic bone-marrow transplantation for standard risk leukaemias. *Lancet*, **ii**, 175–8.

Marcus, R.E., Catovsky, D., Prentice, H.G. *et al.* (1987) Intensive induction and consolidation chemotherapy for adults and children with AML. Joint AML Trial 1982–1985. Haematology and Blood Transfusion, Vol. 30, *Acute Leukaemias*, Springer, Berlin, pp. 346–51.

Meloni, G., De Fabritiis, P., Carella, A.M. *et al.* (1990) Autologous bone marrow transplantation in patients with AML in first complete remission. Results of two different conditioning regimens after the same induction and consolidation therapy. *Bone Marrow Transpl.*, **5**, 29–32.

Meunier, F., Prentice, H.G. and Ringden, O. (1991) Liposomal amphotericin B (AmBisome):

safety data from a phase II/III clinical trial. *J. Antimicrob. Chemother.* (in press).

Meyers, J.D., Reed, E.G., Shepp, D.H. *et al.* (1988) Acyclovir for prevention of cytomegalovirus infection and disease after allogeneic marrow transplantation. *N. Engl. J. Med.*, **318**, 70–5.

Michel, G., Maraninchi, D., Demeocq, F. *et al.* (1988) Repeated courses of high dose melphalan and unpurged autologous bone marrow transplantation in children with acute non-lymphoblastic leukemia in first complete remission. *Bone Marrow Transpl.*, **3**, 105–11.

Nazareth, B., Prentice, H.G., Bhamra, A. *et al.* (1989) A comparison of oral ciprofloxacin and colistin versus neomycin and colistin for antibacterial prophylaxis in neutropenic patients. Abstract No. 60. 16th International Congress of Chemotherapy, Jerusalem.

Nieuwenhuis, H.K. and Sixma, J.J. (1985) Treatment of disseminated intravascular coagulation in APML with low molecular weight heparinoid Org. 10172. *Cancer*, **58**, 761–4.

Nimer, S.D. and Golde, D.W. (1987) The 5q-abnormality. *Blood*, **70**, 1705–12.

O'Connor, N.T.J., Prentice, H.G. and Hoffbrand, A.V. (1989) Prevention of urate nephropathy in the tumour lysis syndrome. *Clin. Lab. Haematol.*, **11**, 97–100.

Odom, L.F., Lampkin, B.C., Tannous, R. *et al.* (1990) Acute monoblastic leukaemia – a review from the CCSG. *Leukaemia Res.*, **14**, 1–10.

Ohno, R., Tomonaga, M., Kobayashi, T. *et al.* (1990) The effect of G-CSF after intensive induction therapy in relapsed or refractory acute leukaemia. *N. Engl. J. Med.*, **323**, 871–7.

Parikh, P., Powles, R., Treleaven, J. *et al.* (1990) High-dose cytosine arabinoside plus etoposide as initial treatment for acute myeloid leukaemia: a single centre study. *Br. J. Cancer*, **62**, 830–3.

Phillips, M., Richards, S. and Chessells, J. (1991) Acute myeloid leukaemia in childhood: the costs and benefits of intensive treatment. *Br. J. Haematol.*, **77**, 473–7.

Pollard, C.M., Powles, R.L. and Millar, J.L. (1986) Leukaemic relapse following CAMPATH-2 treated marrow transplantation for leukaemia. *Lancet*, **ii**, 1343.

Powles, R., Smith, C., Milikan, S. *et al.* (1990) Human recombinant GM-CSF in allogeneic bone marrow transplantation for leukaemia: double blind placebo controlled trial. *Lancet*, **336**, 1417–20.

Prentice H.G. (ed) (1984) Infections in Haematology, in *Clinics in Haematology*, **13**, W.B. Saunders, London, p. 3.

Prentice, H.G. (1991) How do BMTs cure leukaemia? – New directions. *Bone Marrow Transplant.* **7**, (Suppl 2) 11–13.

Prentice, H.G., Blacklock, H.A., Janossy, G. *et al.* (1984) Depletion of T lymphocytes in donor marrow prevents significant graft versus host disease in matched allogeneic leukaemic marrow transplant recipients. *Lancet*, **i**, 472–6.

Prentice, H.G. and Hann, I.M. (1985) The prophylaxis and treatment of infections in patients with bone marrow failure, in *Recent Advances in Haematology* (ed. A.V. Hoffbrand), **4**, Churchill Livingstone, Edinburgh, pp. 119–219.

Pui, C-H., Dahl, G.V., Kalwinsky, D.K. *et al.* (1985) CNS leukaemia in children with acute non-lymphoblastic leukaemia. *Blood*, **66**, 1062–7.

Pui, C-H., Kalwinsky, D.K., Schell, M.J. *et al.* (1988) Acute nonlymphoblastic leukemia in infants: Clinical presentation and outcome. *J. Clin. Oncol.*, **6**, 1008–13.

Reed, E.C., Bowden, R.A., Dandiker, P.S. *et al.* (1988) Treatment of cytomegalovirus pneumonia with ganciclovir and intravenous cytomegalovirus immunoglobulin in patients with marrow transplants. *Ann. Intern. Med.*, **109**, 783–8.

Rees, J.K. (1989) Chemotherapy of acute myeloid leukaemia (AML) in U.K. Past, present and future. *Bone Marrow Transplant.*, **4**(Suppl 1), 110–13.

Rees, J.K.H., Gray, R.G., Swirsky, D. and Hayhoe, F.G.S. (1986) Principal results of the MRC 8th AML Trial. *Lancet*, **ii**, 1236–41.

Reiffers, J., Stoppa, A.M., Rigal-Huguet, F. *et al.* (1991) Allogeneic versus autologous bone marrow transplantation versus chemotherapy for treatment of acute myeloid leukaemia in first complete remission (BGM 84 and BGMT 87 studies). *Bone Marrow Transplant.*, **7** (Suppl 2), 36.

Reittie, J., Gottlieb, D., Heslop, H.E. *et al.* (1989) Endogenously generated activated killer cells circulate after autologous and allogeneic marrow transplantation but not after chemotherapy. *Blood*, **73**, 1351–8.

Ringden, O., Meunier, F., Tollemar, J. *et al.*

(1991) Efficacy of amphotericin B encapsulated in liposomes (AmBisome) in the treatment of invasive fungal infections in immunocompromized patients. *J. Antimicrob. Chemother.* (in press).

Ritter, J., Vormoor, J., Creutzig, U. and Schellong, G. (1989) Prognostic significance of Auer rods in childhood acute myelogenous leukaemia. The childhood AML studies BFM 78 and 83: Treatment results and risk factor analysis in *Haematology and Blood Transfusion* (eds T. Buchner, G. Schellong and W. Hiddemann), Springer, Berlin.

Rizzoli, V., Mangoni, L., Carlo-Stella, C. *et al.* (1991) Autologous marrow transplantation in first remission acute myeloid leukaemia using marrow purged with Mafosfamide. *Bone Marrow Transplant.*, **7** (Suppl 2), 37.

Rohatiner, A.Z.S., Gregory, W.M., Bassan, R. *et al.* (1988) Short term therapy for acute myelogenous leukaemia. *J. Clin. Oncol.*, **6**, 218–26.

Rubin, R.H. and Young, L.S. (1987) *Clinical Approach to Infection in the Compromised Host.* 2nd edn, Plenum, New York.

Sage, R., Hann, I., Prentice, H.G. *et al.* (1988) A randomised trial of empirical antibiotic therapy with one of four β-lactam antibiotics in combination with netilmicin in febrile neutropenic patients. *J. Antimicrob. Chemother.*, **22**, 237–47.

Sanders, J.E., Buckner, C.D., Sullivan, K.M. *et al.* (1988) Growth and development in children after bone marrow transplantation. *HOPM Res.*, **30**, 92–7.

Schmidt, G.M., Horak, D.A., Niland, J.C. *et al.* (1991) A randomised controlled trial of prophylactic ganciclovir for cytomegalovirus pulmonary infection in recipients of allogeneic bone marrow transplants. *N. Engl. J. Med.*, **324**, 1005–11.

Schwarzinger, I., Valent, P., Koller, U. *et al.* (1990) Prognostic significance of surface marker expression on blasts of patients with De Novo acute myeloblastic leukemia. *J. Clin. Oncol.*, **8**, (3) 423–30.

Stevens, R.F. (1991) Acute leukaemias, in *Baillière's Clinical Haematology*, **4**, (2) p. 2, Baillière Tindall, London.

Storb, R., Deeg, H.J. and Pepe, M. (1989) Methotrexate and cyclosporine versus cyclosporine alone for prophylaxis of graft-versus-host disease in patients given HLA-identical marrow grafts for leukemia. Long-term follow up of a controlled trial. *Blood*, **73**, 1729–34.

Swirsky, D.M., de Bastos, M., Parish, S.E. *et al.* (1986) Features affecting outcome during remission induction of AML in 619 adult patients. *Brit. J. Haematol.*, **64**, 435–53.

Tanaka, S., Nishigaki, H., Misawa, S. *et al.* (1990) Lack of involvement of the G-CSF gene by chromosomal translocation 6(15;17) in acute promyelocytic leukaemia. *Leukemia*, **4**, 494–6.

United States OHRST, National Centre for Health Statistics (1981) Vital Statistics of the US Vol. II Mortality Part A. Washington DC, US Government Printing Office.

Van der Schoot, C.E., Daams, G.M., Pinkster, J. *et al.* (1990) Monoclonal antibodies against myeloperoxidase are valuable immunological reagents for the diagnosis of AML. *Brit. J. Haematol.*, **74**, 173–8.

Verdegier, A., Fernandez, J.M., Esquembre, C. *et al.* (1990) Hepatosplenic candidiasis in children with acute leukaemia. *Cancer*, **65**, 874–7.

Weinstein, H., Grier, H., Gelber, R. *et al.* (1987) Post-remission induction intensive sequential chemotherapy for children with AML – treatment results and prognostic factors. *Haematol. Bluttransfus.*, **30**, 88–92.

Wolff, S.N., Herzig, R.H., Phillips, G.L. *et al.* (1987) High dose cytosine arabinoside and daunorubicin as consolidation therapy for acute non-lymphocytic leukemia in first remission: An update. *Sem. Oncol.*, **14**, 12–17.

Woods, W.G., Ruymann, F.B., Lampkin, B.C. *et al.* (1990) The role of timing of high-dose cytosine arabinoside intensification and of maintenance therapy in the treatment of children with acute nonlymphocytic leukemia. *Cancer*, **66**(67), 1106–13.

Yeager, A.M., Kaizer, H., Santos, G.W. *et al.* (1986) Autologous bone marrow transplantation in patients with acute nonlymphocytic leukaemia, using *ex vivo* marrow treatment with 4-hydroperoxycyclophosphamide. *N. Engl. J. Med.*, **315**, (3) 141–7.

Yeager, A.M., Rowley, S.D., Kaizer, H. and Santos, G.W. (1990) Ex-vivo chemo-purging of autologous marrow with 4-hydroxyperoxycyclophosphamide to eliminate occult leukemic cells. *Amer. J. Pediatr. Haematol. Oncol.*, **12**(3), 245–56.

Chapter 10

Acute lymphoblastic leukaemia

F. LAMPERT, U. BERTRAM and H. RIEHM

10.1 INTRODUCTION

Acute lymphoblastic leukaemia (ALL) can be defined (Van der Does *et al.*, 1990) as a malignant clonal proliferation of lymphoid precursor cells, with unknown aetiology, leading to replacement of normal haematopoiesis by lymphoblasts, comprising 25% or more of bone marrow cells, and to infiltration of lymph nodes, spleen, liver or other organs. Malignant transformation may occur at any stage of early (immature) B- or T-cell differentiation, which explains the heterogeneity of ALL.

For the purposes of therapy, ALL and non-Hodgkin's lymphoma are considered and treated as the same entity if blast cell infiltration in the bone marrow exceeds 25% of cells. Dramatic improvements in treatment over the past 25 years mean that ALL has changed from being a uniformly fatal disease to one which can be completely cured in the majority of children.

10.2 PROFILE OF ALL

10.2.1 AETIOLOGY

There is probably no decisive single cause of ALL. As ALL can now be considered as a heterogeneous group of entities, different events in sequence during the course of lymphoid cell maturation could lead to a differentiation block and subsequent clonal proliferation.

The chances for DNA-errors are, of course, much higher in cell populations with an increased proliferation rate and in conditions of chromosomal instability. Thus, it has been known for many years that patients with congenital chromosomal breakage syndromes and a reduced DNA-repair mechanism (Ataxia telangiectasia, Fanconi aplastic anaemia; Bloom's syndrome) have a much higher risk of leukaemia and lymphoma, estimated at about 1:10.

Patients with Down's syndrome (DS) (where the additional chromosome 21 in all somatic cells is responsible for the numerical aneuploidy), have a 10- to 20-fold higher risk, estimated at about 1:80, to develop leukaemia (Fong and Brodeur, 1987). As to the type of leukaemias found in patients with Down's syndrome, an acute non-lymphoblastic leukaemia (ANLL) is more common below the age of three years, and megakaryoblastic leukaemia or, in a weaker form as transient myeloproliferative disorder (TMD), is characteristic for the newborn. Common-ALL, however, is the predominant type of leukaemia in DS patients above the age of three years (Lampert *et al.*, 1991).

The highest possible risk (about 1:5) for developing leukaemia occurs in the identical twin of a child with leukaemia during infancy. Of possible environmental factors, the significance of ionizing radiation at a much higher than normal exposure dose (e.g. to the survivor of an atomic bomb explosion or atomic reactor incident) has been documented, with an estimated risk for developing leukaemia of about 1:60, and leading predominantly to ALL in children in contrast to ANLL in adults. There is also increasing evidence that not only radiotherapy but also intensive chemotherapy (alkylating agents) for a primary tumour increases the risk for developing a secondary leukaemia 5 to 20 years later in at least 5% of the patients.

The role of viruses and whether they play a direct part in causing human childhood leukaemias or, as in Epstein-Barr virus infections, probably act as stimulators for proliferation of a certain lymphocyte population, is still not known.

10.2.2 EPIDEMIOLOGY

ALL is the most common of the childhood malignancies, comprising about 30% of all paediatric neoplasms, with an annual incidence of 3.5 per 100 000 children under 15 years of age as documented in over 10 000 cases of childhood cancer during 1980–88 in western Germany (previously FRG) (Kaatsch and Michaelis, 1989). Every year, there are up to 2000 new cases of childhood ALL in the USA, and 300 to 400 in western Germany. The highest incidence of ALL is found in patients between two and six years of age (7 per 100 000/year). There is a slightly higher incidence in males (ratio 1.2 to 1.0).

Although some variation of incidence rates might be influenced by race (e.g. higher inci-dence of ALL in Costa Rica or of ANLL in New Zealand Maoris) and gender throughout the world (Parkin *et al.*, 1988) the occurrence rates for ALL, if one assumes correct diagnosis and recording, have remained remarkably stable in the industrialized nations within the last 30 years.

10.2.3 CLINICAL PRESENTATION

In the majority of patients with ALL there is pallor, tiredness, irritability, often accompanied by fever, bone (and/or abdominal) pain, and bruising, increasing over a period of weeks, sometimes even months. The symptoms depend on the degree of lymphoblast infiltration into medullary or extramedullary organs.

Physical examination at diagnosis as has been summarized in over 1600 children with ALL revealed hepatomegaly in over 80%, splenomegaly in almost 70%, a mediastinal mass in 10% and CNS involvement (leukaemic blast cells in the cerebrospinal fluid) in less than 5% of the patients (Riehm *et al.*, 1986).

Blood examination showed erythro-, thrombo- and granulocytopaenia, but leukocytosis over 25.000/μl in only 30% of the patients. Haemoglobin below 10 g/dl was found in almost 80% , and thrombocytes below 100 × 10^9/litre also in almost 80% of the patients at diagnosis (Riehm *et al.*, 1986).

10.2.4 DIAGNOSIS

In all cases of ALL the diagnosis must be confirmed by a bone marrow aspirate. In about 90% of cases the diagnosis is simple. In the remaining 10% of patients diagnosis has to be established beyond any doubt by repeated punctures, by Jamshidi needle biopsy or by observing the natural course for another 1–3 weeks. Bone marrow aspirates should be taken from the posterior iliac crest or, in infants, from the tibia.

Cytomorphologic classification according

Table 10.1   Non-random occurrence of cytogenetic abnormalities in ALL-subtypes*

Karyotypic abnormality	Incidence (in % of all patients)	Immunophenotypes†				
		c/pB (75%)	B (3%)	pT/T (15%)	ppB/0 (5%)	Mixed (2%)
Diploid normal	20–30%	+	(+)	+	(+)	(+)
Hyperdiploid (>50)	25–30%	+	–	–	–	–
t(1;19)/*der*1q23	2–5 %	+	–	–	–	–
t(4;11)/*der*11q23	4–5 %	–	–	–	+	+
t(8;14)/*der*8q24	2–3 %	–	+	–	–	–
t(9;22)/*der*22q11	3–5 %	+	–	–	–	–
t(11;14)/*der*14q11	2–4 %	–	–	+	–	–
del(6q)	3–5 %	+	–	+	–	–
der(9p)	3–5 %	+	–	(+)	–	–
der(12p)	2–3 %	+	–	(+)	–	–
Others	20%	+	–	+	+	–

* Data based on both chromosomal analysis of leukaemia karyotypes in 792 children with ALL (Lampert, *et al.*, 1991) and on the literature.

† ALL-Immunophenotypes as defined by clusters of differentiation (CD) (over 20% positive leukaemic blast cells):

    c (common):   CD19, CD10, HLA-DR, TdT
    pB (pre-B):   CD19, CD10, Cytμ, HLA-DR, TdT
    ppB/0 (pre-pre-B): CD19, CD24, HLA-DR, TdT
    B: CD19+/−, SIgM+, Kappa/lambda, HLA-DR
    pT/T(pre-T/T):   CD7, CyD3, TdT.

to the FAB-criteria should be done in May Grünwald Giemsa or Wright stained smears: L_1 = small lymphoblasts with scanty cytoplasm, indistinct nucleoli; 85% of cases. L_2 = larger and more heterogeneous lymphoblasts, retiform nuclear membrane, more cytoplasm, prominent nucleoli; 10–15% of cases. L_3 = large lymphoblasts with deep basophilic cytoplasm, prominent vacuolation, one or more nucleoli; 1–3% of cases. Except for the L_3B– ALL association, FAB types do not correlate exclusively to defined immunophenotypes. For cytochemical differentiation from acute non-lymphoblastic leukaemia (ANLL) the myeloperoxidase (POX) or the Sudan Black (SB) reaction should also be carried out. In ALL, the POX- and/or SB reaction is negative, or only slightly positive (under 3% positive blast cells).

Immunophenotyping and cytogenetic studies (in samples of heparinized bone marrow and blood) are nowadays regarded as an absolute requirement for establishing the proper subtypes of ALL. Correlation of specific chromosomal aberrations with ALL-immunophenotypes underlining the heterogeneity of ALL are summarized in Table 10.1.

There are lineage-specific cell markers only to be found in ALL (as compared to ANLL) such as E-rosettes, membrane-bound or cytoplasmic immunoglobulins, chromosomal aberrations involving t(8;14), t(1;19), *der*(14q11) and rearrangement of IgH and IgL κ/λ. On the other hand, there are lineage-associated markers besides cell morphology for ALL such as CD10, CD2/4/5/7, CD19/CD20/CD24, TdT and gene loci rearrangements for IgH-, T-cell receptor (TCR) β-, γ-, δ-chains.

The largest subgroup is common-ALL, which is only to be distinguished from the pre-B type by the absence of cytoplasmatic heavy chain (μ). In this group, there are about

30% of the patients, whose leukaemic karyotypes are characterized by a hyperdiploidy with 50 or more chromosomes per nucleus, peaking at about 54 chromosomes. In this same (pre-B/c-ALL) group, however, not only a specific numerical but also a structural aberration, namely the Philadelphia-translocation t(9;22), considered to bear a very bad prognostic risk, can be found in up to 5% of the children (as compared to adult-ALL, where it can be detected in up to 20% of the patients).

Another translocation of the same frequency and also specific for *pre*-B ALL is t(1;19) where part of the long arm of chromosome 1 is transferred to the short arm of chromosome 19, to the site of the insulin receptor.

In *pre*-T and mature T-ALL's, comprising 10–15% of all patients, normal diploidy is common. In one-third of the patients, however, breakpoint 14q11 is involved, at the site of the α/δ T-cell-receptor.

In B-ALL, the classical translocation is t(8;14) transferring the proto-oncogene c-*myc* from chromosome 8 to the distal end of chromosome 14, to the gene locus of the immunoglobulin heavy chains.

Chromosomal breakpoints in the ALL-karyotype probably pinpoint the location where decisive gene rearrangements during lymphocyte differentiation take place and where mistakes can occur.

Due to immunophenotyping by monoclonal antibodies in large series of patients it has become clear that about 5% of patients with ALL also demonstrate myeloid antigen (CD13, CD55, CDw65 in over 20% of blast cells) expression (Ludwig *et al.*, 1988). The majority of these patients with acute hybrid or 'mixed lineage' leukaemia (or *My*-positive ALL) had characteristic clinical (age under one year, high initial leukocyte count, CNS-disease, high risk for relapse) and cellular features with CD10-negative pre-pre-B-ALL phenotype and chromosomal translocations involving breakpoint 11q23, such as, for example, t(4;11) (Lampert *et al.*, 1987).

10.3 ALL IN INFANTS AND ADOLESCENTS

ALL arising in the age group of patients <1 and >10 years generally has a poorer prognosis compared to ALL in patients in the age group 1–9 years. This difference in outcome may partially be explained by the adverse clinical and cellular factors which are more frequently encountered.

Infant's ALL (Van Wering and Kamps, 1986; Pui *et al.*, 1987; Stark *et al.*, 1989; Bucsky *et al.*, 1990) is characterized by more extensive disease at diagnosis, i.e. hyperleukocytosis and CNS-infiltration, and unfavourable blast cell cytogenetic and immunophenotypical features. The infant's leukaemic karyotype lacks hyperdiploidy with over 50 chromosomes but instead exhibits pseudodiploidy. Structural chromosome aberrations are common. Typical translocations are t(4;11), t(11;19) and others, mainly with involvement of chromosome region 11q23. The CD19-positive blast cell immunophenotype lacks the common ALL antigen (CALLA; CD10) and sometimes also expresses myeloid antigen. A progenitor of B-cell lineage is considered to be the main target cell for this vigorous clonal growth of ALL in infants.

Adolescent's ALL (Santana *et al.*, 1990) also is characterized by more frequently adverse prognostic features, including higher initial leukocyte count, T-cell phenotype, and ploidy other than hyperdiploidy >50. In the age group of patients ≥16 years, outcome with only about 20% survival rate is even worse compared to patients aged 10–15 years.

10.3.1 EXTENSION OF DISEASE ('STAGING')

ALL is always a widespread disease, causing

haematopoietic symptoms at a tumour burden of 10^{11} to 10^{12} cells (about 1 kg) in the patient's body.

The extension of the disease at diagnosis or at relapse, however, is important for the choice of treatment and the detection of sanctuaries for residual disease. The amount of leukaemic cell mass can be estimated by the absolute number of blast cells in the peripheral blood and by the size of liver and spleen (Langermann *et al.*, 1982). Involvement of lymph nodes, testicles, cranial nerves, skin and fundi oculi should also be noted. The examination of the cerebrospinal fluid in a cytospin preparation is absolutely mandatory. CNS leukaemia is diagnosed by the presence of more than five cells per μl cerebrospinal fluid and blast cell morphology.

10.3.2 DIFFERENTIAL DIAGNOSIS

There are a number of more common non-malignant diseases in children which may mimic leukaemia. In all cases of doubt a bone marrow aspiration should clarify the diagnosis. Nonmalignant and malignant diseases include the following:

(a) Infectious mononucleosis, because of hepatosplenomegaly, lymph node enlargement and increased lymphomonocytic cell count in the peripheral blood, can be confused with acute leukaemia.

(b) Idiopathic thrombocytopenic purpura with the alarming symptoms of bruising, nose bleeding, petechiae and anaemia (in case of blood loss, or accompanying immune-haemolytic [Evans-] syndrome) may require a bone marrow aspiration.

(c) Juvenile rheumatoid arthritis is often suspected instead of leukaemia because of bone pains, low grade fever and organ involvement and should require a diagnostic bone marrow examination.

(d) Kala Azar (Leishmaniasis); this de-velops over months in young children returning from holidays in Mediterranean countries and may mimic leukaemia by hepatosplenomegaly, pancytopenia and fever.

(e) Aplastic anaemia is probably the most important condition that has to be considered in differential diagnosis of ALL and needs bone marrow histology in all cases.

(f) Metastatic neuroblastoma and, more rarely, metastatic alveolar rhabdomyosarcoma or metastatic Ewing's sarcoma are the classical malignant conditions in which leukaemia can often only be distinguished by cytogenetic and immune-histologic work-up of the bone marrow sample.

(g) Myeloproliferative syndromes, in particular during the newborn and infant period, often pose a difficult diagnostic problem, even for the experienced haemato-cytologist.

(h) Persistent viral infections (e.g. EBV) with (phagocytic) lymphohistiocytosis causing pancytopaenia in the peripheral blood, can be difficult to distinguish from ALL.

10.4 TREATMENT PROTOCOLS

10.4.1 CHEMOTHERAPY AND PROGNOSIS

As the symptoms of ALL arise by the massive accumulation of proliferating undifferentiated cells, the principle of therapy is simple: eradication of all leukaemic cells in all body compartments (by cell kill or permanent cell division arrest).

Chemotherapy with drugs which act against DNA to prevent cell division in lymphoblasts were developed in the 50s and 60s: methotrexate (MTX), corticosteroids (PRED), 6-mercapto-purine (6-MP), vincristine (VCR), cyclophosphamide (CP), cytarabine (ARA-C), daunorubicine (DR), adriamycin (ADR) and L-asparaginase (L-ASP). With more and more knowledge of side effects and dose intensification, combination chemotherapy up to the maximal tolerance of the host, evolved and was then combined with irradiation to the hidden sites of leukaemic cell proliferation such as the brain and meninges. (The latter might today possibly be replaced by intrathecal chemotherapy in the majority of patients.)

Improvements in supportive care – mainly in preventing infections – has helped to decrease the non-leukaemic fatality rate from over 10% to less than 5% of patients. Thus, survival in ALL has improved from 1% in 1965 (Burchenal and Murphy, 1965) to 50% in the mid-70s (Pinkel, 1979) and up to 70% in the mid-80s (Riehm *et al.*, 1986; Clavell *et al.*, 1986; Steinherz *et al.*, 1986).

Due to more effective and risk-adapted chemotherapy prognostic factors ('probabilities for risk of relapse') such as mediastinal mass, T-cell features, high initial white blood count, even some specific chromosome translocations in the leukaemic karyotype (Fletcher *et al.*, 1989) lost their significance. Chemotherapy will be tailored more and more to the individual patient as subtypes of ALL can now be precisely defined by pretherapeutic immunophenotyping and cytogenetics.

The length of the risk period is determined by the proliferative behaviour of the leukaemic cell clone. Relapses in T-, B- or 0-ALL usually occur within a year as compared to common-ALL (with a very low mitotic index in the leukaemic bone marrow) where relapses can appear as late as 2–4 years after cessation of leukaemia therapy. Maintenance or continuation therapy with antimetabolites for about two to three years is therefore particularly necessary in c-ALL.

10.4.2 INDUCTION THERAPY AND REINDUCTION

It has been the experience of many study groups in the USA and Europe (Niemeyer *et al.*, 1985), but in particular by the German BFM study group for almost 20 years, that an intensified and prolonged induction therapy regimen, adjusted for the patient's tolerance, is the most important factor in overcoming the leukaemic cell's resistance and thus improving cure rates. In all patients with non-B-cell ALL, regardless of risk, an 8-drug, 8-week induction regimen (Riehm *et al.*, 1980) had been successfully applied. Of course, complete remissions with lowering of the leukaemic cell burden to less than 5% in the bone marrow can surely be achieved with fewer drugs and lesser time but the 'quality of remission' (Simone, 1976) will need this more intensive approach. This induction protocol I is still the cornerstone of the BFM-ALL-90 protocol, and only minor modifications such as a prephase with Prednisone monotherapy, omission of one cyclophosphamide dose and no cranial irradiation in induction phase 2 had been made to ease applicability (Fig. 10.1). In experienced hands, this protocol can be realized in all patients, i.e. 100% of dosage given within the time schedule.

Furthermore, initial steroid monotherapy not only helps to reduce side effects due to rapid cell destruction, but also serves to define a biological risk factor. Inadequate response to steroid exposure, i.e. over 1000 leukaemic blast cells per μl in the blood smear at day 8, will already select a small group of patients with an unfavourable outcome in the majority of cases.

Patients with an increased risk of relapse have been shown to benefit from a shortened reinduction protocol administered three months after protocol I. This 6-week course (Protocol II; Fig. 10.2) was introduced in 1976 and was followed by an improved cure rate of at least 20% (Henze *et al.*, 1981). This intensified reinduction would probably improve the outcome even in patients with no obvious features that predict higher risk of relapse.

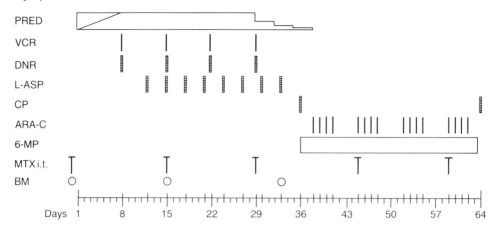

Fig. 10.1 Induction therapy in ALL (BFM 1990) for patients (standard and medium risk group) with non-B-ALL (protocol I). Therapy starts with steriod monotherapy for 7 days in increasing concentrations, as reduction of tumour volume indicates. PRED (Prednisone) p.o. 60 mg/m²/day; VCR (vincristine) i.v. 1.5 mg/m²/day (maximum single dose 2 mg); DNR (daunorubicin) p.i. (1 h) 30 mg/day; L-ASP (L-asparaginase) p.i. (1 h) 10.000 units/m²/day; CP (cyclosphosphamide) p.i. (1 h) 1000 mg/m²/day (with MESNA); ARA-C (cytosine arabinoside) i.v. 75 mg/m²/day; 6-MP (6-mercaptopurine) p.o. 60 mg/m²/day; MTX (methotrexate) i.th., dosages age dependent, <year 6 mg, 1 and <2 years 8 mg, 2 and <3 years 10 mg, >3 years 12 mg. Patients with initial CNS-involvement receive in addition 2 more MTX i.th. on day 8 and 22.
BM = bone marrow aspiration (p.i. = infusion; i.th. = intrathecal).

10.4.3 CONTINUATION THERAPY

In slowly proliferating malignancies such as non-B and non-T ALL's, daily cytotoxic treatment for about two to three years, preferably with antimetabolites, is absolutely necessary to maintain complete continuous remission and eradicate remaining, dormant leukaemic cells. Individual dosages of 6-mercaptopurine or 6-thioguanine (daily) and methotrexate (weekly) are adjusted to the leukocyte count of the patient which should not be raised over 3000/μl or fall below 1000/μl. The more total the dose of chemotherapy that can be applied in a patient the better are the chances for eradicating leukaemia. Good patient care on an ambulatory basis with routine visits at about two-week intervals is also very important. In severe lymphocytopaenia (lympho-cytes below 100/μl) opportunistic infections, the most dangerous one being *Pneumocystis carinii* pneumonia, and in severe granulo-cytopenia (granulocytes below 500/μl) bacterial infections and septicaemia might develop and require hospitalization.

After discontinuation of therapy, the relapse rate will still be 10 to 20%, regardless of the total duration of maintenance therapy. Most of the relapses will occur within the first year after therapy stops. Generally, the more aggressive the therapy and the more rapidly dividing the leukaemic cell population, the shorter the risk period for relapse. In the BFM studies, the risk for relapse dropped to almost zero at the end of the sixth year after diagnosis.

There is no need to perform routine bone marrow or lumbar punctures during or after

186

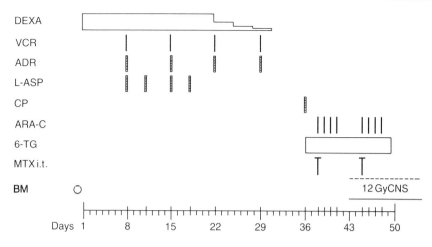

Fig. 10.2 Reinduction therapy in ALL (BFM 1990) for patients (standard and medium risk group) with non-B-ALL (protocol II), to be applied in early remission. DEXA (dexamethasone) p.o. 10 mg/m²/day; VCR (vincristine) i.v. 1.5 mg/m²/day (maximum single dose 2 mg); ADR (adriamycin) p.i. (1h) 30 mg/m²/day; L-ASP (L-asparaginase) p.i. (1h) 10 000 units/m²/day; CP (cyclophosphamide) p.i. (1h) 1000 mg/m²/day; (with MESNA); ARA-C (cytosine arabinoside) i.v. 75 mg/m²/day; 6-TG (6-thioguanine) p.o. 60 mg/m²/day; MTX (methotrexate) i.th., dependent on age from 6 to 12 mg as in Fig. 10.1. CNS (cranial) irradiation 12 Gy (medium risk group only; no irradiation in patients <1 year). Patients with initial CNS-involvement: <1 year 0 Gy; >1 year and <2 years 18 Gy >2 years 24 Gy.

discontinuation of therapy. However, one should not hesitate to go ahead with these procedures if suspicious blood findings (pancytopaenia, presence of undifferentiated cells or symptoms of CNS-leukaemia [headache, vomiting]) arise.

10.4.4 BONE MARROW TRANSPLANTATION

Bone marrow ablation and allogeneic transplantation (BMT) from a compatible donor (sibling) is now a routine procedure and is indicated in CML patients during the chronic phase and in some ANLL patients in first remission. In ALL patients, BMT should only be considered in second or subsequent remission(s).

BMT in ALL patients in first complete remission is still controversial and should be restricted only to certain very poor, prognostic features, for example, chromosomal aberrations such as t(9;22) or −5/5q⁻ or late responders to induction therapy.

Data from the nationwide German ALL-relapse trials indicated that in controlled studies BMT was not more curative than modern combination chemotherapy (Henze, personal communication). In addition, BMT may be followed by growth failure, graft versus host disease, endocrinopathies, and serious pulmonary and renal disorders. However, in desperate situations and with the availability of a compatible donor BMT should be carried out; this still provides a realistic chance of cure in up to one-third of these patients. Generally speaking, however, with regard to the majority of patients, BMT appears to have only a minor place in the treatment of children with ALL.

187

10.4.5 THERAPY OF B-CELL ALL:

ALL arising from B-lymphocytes is a rare (about 3% of all ALL cases) and biologically distinct entity with very high proliferative capacity and therefore should be treated differently. Clinically, CNS disease and abdominal tumour can be present at diagnosis, and, often, bone marrow replacement is not complete.

Cytologically, blast cells have bluish, vacuolated cytoplasm (FABL$_3$ morphology) with detectable immunoglobulins on the cell surface (seen by immunophenotyping) and translocation t(8;14) on chromosome analysis. Mitotic index in the leukaemic cell population is high, thus shortening the risk period for relapse to less than one year.

Outcome in those patients to whom specific therapy is applied has changed dramatically in the last four years. A combination of high-dose methotrexate, cyclophosphamide (ifosphamide), prednisone, cytarabine, etoposide and adriamycin (Fig. 10.3), given in alternating 5- to 7-day courses over several months without continuation therapy (BFM-protocol 86), achieved cures in over half of the patients (Reiter *et al.*, 1989).

10.5 MANAGEMENT OF RELAPSE IN PATIENTS

Relapse (as defined by re-occurrence of evident leukaemia) is the most serious threat confronting the patient and the family. Prospects for cure are then greatly diminished. For prognostic reasons, one has to differentiate the site from the time after treatment at which relapse occurs. On the basis of site, there are three types: medullary (bone marrow only), extramedullary (outside the bone marrow only, e.g. CNS, testes, iris), and those which are medullary and extramedullary. On the basis of time, there are two types: early relapse, i.e. during treatment or

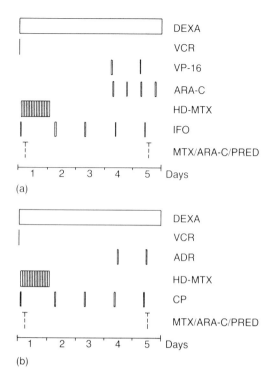

Fig. 10.3 (a) Cytotoxic cycle AA for therapy in B-ALL (to be applied after a 5 day prephase with prednisone p.o. 30 mg/m^2/day and cyclophosphamide p.i (1h) 200 mg/m^2/d): Dexamethasone (DEXA) p.o. 10 mg/m^2/d; Vincristine i.v. 1.5 mg/m^2 (maximum single dose 2 mg); Etoposide (VP-16) p.i. (1h) 100 mg/m^2/d; cytarabine (ARA-C) p.i. (1h) 150 mg/m^2 × 4; high-dose methotrexate (HD-MTX) p.i. (24h) 5 g/m^2 (with CF-rescue); Ifosphamide (IFO) p.i. (1h, with MESNA) 800 mg/m^2/d; Methotrexate/cytarabine/prednisone (MTX/ARA-C/PRED) i.th. <1 year: 3/8/2 mg, 1 and <2 years 4/10/3 mg) 2 and <3 years 5/13/4 mg, >3 years 6/15/5 mg. (b) Cytotoxic cycle BB for therapy in B-ALL (following cycle AA): Dexamethasone (DEXA) p.o. 10 mg/m^2/d; Vincristine i.v. 1.5 mg/m^2 (maximum single dose 2 mg); adriamycin (ADR) p.i. (1h) 25 mg/m^2/d; high-dose methotrexate (HD-MTX) p.i. (24 h) 5 g/m^2 (with CF-rescue); cyclophosphamide (CP) p.i. (1h, with MESNA) 200 mg/m^2/d; Methotrexate/cytarabine/prednisone (MTX/ARA-C/PRED) i.th. <1 year: 3/8/2 mg, 1 and <2 years 4/10/3 mg) 2 and <3 years 5/13/4 mg, >3 years 6/15/5 mg.

within six months after cessation of treatment, and late relapse, i.e. occurring more than six months after cessation of treatment. With extramedullary relapses and late relapses there is still a chance of total cure.

Newer laboratory methods such as the polymerase chain reaction will certainly help to detect minimal residual disease or very early relapse. However, whether early treatment of relapse really will improve the outcome remains to be seen.

10.5.1 EARLY BONE MARROW RELAPSE

This is the most serious complication in leukaemia management. Prognosis is very poor, and cures by chemotherapy are very rare. However, on the basis of new protocols with short-term alternating cycles of very cytotoxic combination chemotherapy, a 40% event-free survival probability after two years was reported for early, non-T-ALL relapse, but only 7% in very early or T-ALL relapse (Henze *et al.*, 1990). It might be possible that bone marrow transplantation by a compatible sibling could improve the results slightly.

10.5.2 LATE BONE MARROW RELAPSE

A remission rate is possible in about 90% of patients, and an event-free survival probability at two years of around 50% was reported in 57 children with late, non-T-ALL (Henze *et al.*, 1990). Due to the complications of bone marrow transplantation, the preferred option in this condition where there is no compatible donor would be new and aggressive chemotherapy employing infusions of high dose methotrexate and cytarabine.

10.5.3 CENTRAL NERVOUS SYSTEM RELAPSE

This extramedullary relapse usually occurs, even after adequate CNS treatment, in 3–8%

of patients within 18 to 24 months after the start of front-line treatment, and the same pattern of relapse can be observed in second remission after isolated marrow relapse. Thus, treatment for subclinical CNS leukaemia is also required in all late marrow relapses (Rivera *et al.*, 1983). Local therapy to the meninges by intrathecal chemotherapy combined with systemic chemotherapy together with CNS-irradiation in nonirradiated children will cure about 40% of patients.

10.5.4 TESTICULAR RELAPSE

This extramedullary relapse usually manifests itself 3–4 months after cessation of maintenance therapy and because of possible systemic spread needs systemic treatment. Up to 10% of the boys could be affected. Clinically, a painless testicular enlargement, usually unilateral, is the presenting feature. The Prader orchidometer will help in defining the testicular volume and, in suspicious cases, allows precise observation over several weeks. For confirmation of the diagnosis, a biopsy would still be recommended. A biopsy in the contralateral, asymptomatic testis can usually be omitted.

The prognosis of isolated late testicular relapse is favourable (Fengler *et al.*, 1982) with a cure rate of up to 70%, and certainly this condition will need no life-threatening procedures such as bone marrow transplantation. A single involved testis should probably be removed, and in bilateral involvement local irradiation with 20 Gy should be applied. Systemic chemotherapy should also include maintenance therapy for at least one year.

10.5.5 COMBINED RELAPSES

This condition, often seen quite early in the course of patients with rapidly proliferating T-ALL, most frequently involves bone marrow and CNS. The prognosis is as unfavourable as with early medullary relapse, and transplantation probably provides the only chance, if any, for cure.

10.5.6 SUPPORTIVE CARE AND THERAPY COMPLICATIONS

Proper supportive care to prevent infections (including adequate caloric and protein intake) is very important to enable the carrying through of intensive cytotoxic therapy protocols. This means during the induction period routine prophylactic cotrimoxazol for prevention of *Pneumocystis carinii* pneumonia and antimycotic treatment of mucous membranes and broad-spectrum antibiotics in case of suspected or established septicaemia. Almost all intravenous chemotherapy should be accompanied by pre- and post-hydration. Good blood banking facilities are important to give erythrocyte and thrombocyte concentrations at any time in sufficient quantities if anaemia (haemoglobin below 8 g/dl) or severe thrombocytopaenia develop. The value of granulocyte infusions is still a debated issue.

Pediatric oncologic emergencies include septicaemia, antibiotic-resistant fever, obstruction or paralysis of the bowel (e.g. after Vinca alkaloids), toxic enterocolitis (e.g. after methotrexate), intracranial or gastrointestinal haemorrhage, renal, hepatic and cardiac failure (e.g. after fluid overload or anthracyclines, even many years afterwards), ketoacidosis and electrolyte disturbances and acute brain oedema with convulsions. The use of portocaths or Hickman catheters, although they make intravenous therapy much more tolerable for the child, can be complicated by obstruction and infection.

Of special concern is a complication arising in the initial treatment period: namely, hyperuricaemia due to rapid cell destruction leading to renal failure. This can be prevented by forced fluid uptake, urine alkaliniz-ation, allopurinol and, of course, mild cytotoxic treatment in the first days.

Viral infections still remain a problem, although acyclovir in varicella-zoster and gancyclovir in cytomegalo-virus are effective drugs to reduce virus replication. To combat hepatitis B virus infection, screening and passive/active immunization is considered to be mandatory for all new patients (and persons) on hospital wards.

Protective isolation of hospital patients is not necessary. More important are well trained specialized nurses in sufficient numbers (at least one nurse per patient). Hand washing before and after touching patients is obligatory for all persons involved in the care of patients, i.e. physicians, nurses, relatives and visitors.

Psychosocial care for the patient and the family by social workers, occupational therapists, psychotherapists, etc. plays a major role in making the hardship of treatment periods more bearable. Accommodation for housing parents near to the hospital should be available at all treatment centres.

Due to advanced supportive care, death due to non-leukaemic cause has decreased at experienced treatment centres to less than 5%.

Death due to bone marrow failure resulting from leukaemic relapse is usually caused by overwhelming infection or gastrointestinal respiratory or cranial bleeding. These young children in their terminal phase of life should be given all our support including liberal intake of analgesics, and the wish whether to die in the hospital or preferably at home should be respected.

10.5.7 OUTCOME

By 1970 it had become possible to cure approximately one half of all children with ALL by chemotherapy or chemotherapy combined with irradiation (Aur *et al.*, 1971). These results have been reproduced or even improved throughout the world in many thousands of children. In the USA, five-year relative survival of patients with leukaemia increased from 15% in the 1967–73 period to 51% in the 1973–81 period (Young *et al.*, 1986). In western Germany (population approximately 60 million) there are now over 2000 persons who have been cured of childhood ALL.

Cure in ALL means continuous complete (not only haematological) remission five years after cessation of therapy. This goal can now be achieved in almost 70% of all patients. At present, it seems quite difficult to overcome this 'magic' cure rate by current therapeutic means. We can strive, however, towards simplifying curative treatment, reducing side effects, and making the availability of proper treatment facilities more widespread.

10.6 LATE SEQUELAE

As a result of treatment, the cure rate in children with ALL has increased dramatically since 1970. Now, in the 1990s, there are many thousands of cured patients. Careful monitoring for late effects of antileukaemic therapy, however, becomes more and more important, and the 'quality of cure', will be measured against the full integration of these patients into a normal working and family life.

Of major concern are malignancies arising 2 to 20 years after cytotoxic treatment for a primary tumour. It is still uncertain if the total accumulated rate will be below or around 5% or even 10% in the patients after cure of the primary disease.

10.6.1 SECOND MALIGNANCIES

Irradiation and chemotherapy, alkylating agents in particular, can produce chromosomal damage in normal cells. The risk of developing a second malignant tumour 5 to 20 years after therapy is thus increased in otherwise cured patients. In western Germany, among 100 patients developing a second malignancy (most frequently osteosarcomas, ANLLs, CNS tumours and thyroid cancers) after treatment for a childhood cancer in the years 1967–88, the predominant primary malignancy (30 patients) was found to be ALL (Gutjahr, 1990). As many as 7% of second malignancies, mostly acute non-lymphoblastic leukaemias, were observed in Great Britain occurring within seven years of intensive combination chemotherapy of children with non-Hodgkin's lymphomas and T-cell leukaemias (Ingram *et al.*, 1987). Interestingly, not only deletions of chromosomes 5 or 7, as known from adults, have then been detected in the karyotype of secondary leukaemias after treatment for ALL but also the most common breakpoint in childhood leukaemias was involved, namely chromosome region 11q23 (Pui, *et al.*, 1989).

In spite of all concern for curing the patient the clinician will more and more in the future have to consider the nature and dose of cytotoxic drugs in respect to second malignancies.

10.6.2 CENTRAL NERVOUS SYSTEM

Despite concern about exposing the brains of children to ionizing radiation, the introduction of cranial irradiation was a decisive step in the prevention of CNS leukaemia, thus achieving more cures in ALL. Retro- and prospective studies, however, have now revealed abnormal CT-scans and a slight impairment of psychomotor skills (Harten *et al.*, 1984) and attention deficits (Browers and Poplack, 1990) after cranial irradiation, particularly in children under two years of age (Dowell *et al.*, 1987). Patients who experienced a somnolence syndrome – a reversible, 'harmless' disorder appearing 6–8 weeks after cranial irradiation – were also more likely to develop neuropsychological dysfunction some years later (Chien *et al.*, 1980).

Although the dose of cranial irradiation seems to be important, a reduction from 24 Gy to 18 Gy did not show a difference in the incidence of abnormalities on computed tomography, fits, or changes in IQs in two groups of carefully observed children (Chessells *et al.*, 1990). Present treatment protocols tend more and more to replace cranial irradiation by intrathecal or high-dose chemotherapy and this can be presumed to have a lower risk for brain damage.

10.6.3 REPRODUCTIVE AND ENDOCRINOLOGIC FUNCTION

Next to intellectual performance, fertility is of major concern once cure can be expected. So far, the available reports are optimistic, although adolescent males may be at risk for spermatogenic dysfunction following cyclophosphamide. Successful parenthood in long-term survivors has been reported, and there has been no excess of congenital abnormalities or childhood cancer in the offspring (Moe, 1984; Hawkins *et al.*, 1987; Green *et al.*, 1989). As to growth and development, some minor alterations have been reported (Meadows *et al.*, 1986).

10.6.4 CARDIAC, PULMONARY AND RENAL DYSFUNCTION

Cardiotoxicity of anthracyclines after cumulative dosage of over 450 mg/m², increased by local irradiation, is well known and may lead to progressive lethal heart insufficiency. Careful cardiac monitoring (echocardiography) now has revealed that decreased diastolic function and increased endsystolic mural tension can even occur after cumulative doses of only 360 mg m² (Hausdorf *et al.*, 1988).

There are still relatively few studies on pulmonary function in childhood leukaemia survivors (Shaw *et al.*, 1989). Drugs which potentially effect the lungs (causing intestial pneumonitis) are busulfan, bleomycin, chlor-

ambucil and methotrexate. Pulmonary fibrosis may develop in about 5% of patients after pneumonitis.

As to the kidney, besides acute renal toxicity after ifosphamide, there is also the possibility of developing tubular damage, i.e. Fanconi-syndrome with vitamin D-resistant rickets (Smeitirik *et al.*, 1988).

10.7 CURRENT CONTROVERSIES

10.7.1 CLUES TOWARDS AETIOLOGY

Recent studies of clustering in cases of ALL have failed to demonstrate convincingly any associations with nuclear power installations or high tension electricity systems, although there is evidence that paternal exposure to radiation may be a factor (Gardner *et al*, 1990). There is increasing evidence, however, that a viral aetiology may be relevant, involving the introduction of a viral pathogen into an isolated community not previously exposed to it (Alexander *et al*, 1990; Lancet editorial, 1990). Another hypothesis is that the immune system of the infant is particularly susceptible to spontaneous mutation following viral exposure, resulting in the eventual appearance of a malignant clone (Greaves, 1986).

10.7.2 PHENOTYPE-GENOTYPE-SPECIFIC CHEMOTHERAPY

'Species-specific' therapy (Pinkel, 1989) has been increasingly demonstrated over the last two decades to be the best therapeutic approach in leukaemia. Using cell morphology alone, it became clear that effective drugs and schedules are different for acute lymphoblastic leukaemia (ALL) versus acute non-lymphoblastic leukaemia (ANLL). With immunophenotyping it is apparent that treatment results improve if different drug combinations are used in mature B-cell ALL versus T-cell or non-T, non-B. With routine karyotyping of ALL it is becoming clear that chromosomal abnormalities are of prognostic significance. Common-ALL with no structural abnormalities and >50 chromosomes is curable in the majority of patients, whereas common-ALL with the Philadelphia t(9;22) will need more aggressive treatment, perhaps including BMT (Ribeiro, 1987). It is disappointing that to date there is no specific leukaemia subtype which can be eradicated in 100% of patients. Even in the hyperdiploid subgroup, late relapses occur, lowering the cure rate to <80%. Conversely, many structural abnormalities hitherto thought to be a bad prognostic sign can be overcome by intensive chemotherapy.

The issue of whether pre-B ALL should be treated more aggressively remains unclear (Crist *et al.*, 1989; Lilleyman *et al.*, 1989). It is possible that within the pre B patients only the subgroup with pseudodiploid karyotype will do badly (Pui *et al.*, 1986), but further prospective evaluation of these patients is required.

10.7.3 CAN CRANIAL IRRADIATION AS EARLY CNS-DIRECTED THERAPY BE OMITTED IN ALL PATIENTS?

Due to the late effects of ionizing radiation on a child's brain there is a general tendency to replace cranial irradiation by intravenous and intrathecal chemotherapy. The Norwegian group (Moe *et al.*, 1986), using the latter strategy in all risk groups of patients, claim to have as low a CNS relapse rate as was achieved with radiation-containing regimens. A number of prospective randomized studies have demonstrated the comparable effectiveness of chemotherapy-only protocols in low and standard risk patients (Freeman *et al.*, 1983; Green *et al.*, 1980). However, there is doubt whether this approach is adequate for high risk patients, particularly boys presenting with a high white cell count. In prospec-

tive BFM trials (Riehm, *et al.*, 1990) intermediate dose methotrexate was not as effective as irradiation, even in standard risk patients. An alternative approach may be to reduce the dose of cranial irradiation to 12 Gy. Randomized studies have demonstrated that reduction from 24 to 18 Gy was not associated with any reduced efficacy (Chessells, *et al.*, 1990; Nesbit *et al.*, 1981).

10.7.4 CAN RISK FACTORS BE USED TO ALLOCATE TREATMENT?

With over two-thirds of all childhood ALL now being curable, it has become important to distinguish between patients in whom treatment intensity may be reduced and those in whom further intensification is necessary for cure. Traditional risk factors, such as organomegaly, presenting haemoglobin, platelet count, mediastinal mass, extensive lymphadenopathy and a number of other clinical characteristics, have disappeared with the use of more intensive front line chemotherapy (Miller, 1988; Sather *et al.*, 1981). In order to identify patients with a poor prognosis on the basis of initial response, evaluation of bone marrow on day 8 or day 15 after conventional induction therapy, or disappearance of initial circulating blast cells after a short course of steroid therapy have been used (Miller *et al.*, 1989). However, there is little consensus at present amongst international groups as to which ALL patients do sufficiently badly to warrant extreme dose escalation or bone marrow transplantation as part of initial therapy (Bordigoni, 1989; Wingard *et al.*, 1990).

Despite dose intensification it appears that high white cell count over $200 \times 10^9/l$, younger age, and certain translocations do distinguish patients, and alternative procedures are currently under evaluation in this respect.

It is of note that after one year of treatment virtually all initially presenting prognostic features disappear, with the possible exception of age.

10.7.5 INFANTS WITH LEUKAEMIA

The poor prognosis for infants presenting under a year of age is associated with a higher incidence of high white cell count at presentation (Leiper and Chessells, 1986; Crist *et al.*, 1986), CNS disease and CNS relapse, and chromosomal translocations. Alternative strategies for this group have included further dose intensification, particularly with drugs aimed at treating the central nervous system (Reaman *et al.*, 1989). Traditional methods of CNS irradiation are inappropriate, due to potential severe sequelae in terms of growth and intellect. High dose methotrexate, cytarabine and etoposide have been used for this purpose, along with intensified triple intrathecal therapy (methotrexate, cytarabine and hydrocortisone). The use of non-TBI-based high dose regimens with autologous or allogeneic bone marrow rescue has thus far been disappointing but continues to be evaluated (Bordigoni, 1990).

10.7.6 WHAT IS THE ROLE OF HIGH DOSE THERAPY WITH BONE MARROW RESCUE?

High dose therapy in first remission patients is currently reserved for those presenting with a very high white cell count or certain chromosome translocations, non-responders to steroid monotherapy, and patients slow to achieve complete remission with conventional chemotherapy. There is no single series large enough to establish the advantage of transplantation in such patients, although pilot studies of allogeneic transplantation in high count ALL have been encouraging, with disease-free survival of over 70% in some small series (Bordigoni *et al.*, 1989).

In the relapsed patient, an allograft provides the best chance of cure. In the absence of a suitable donor, purged or non-purged autologous bone marrow can be used (Kersey, *et al.*, 1987; Sallan *et al.*, 1989; Schroeder *et al.*, 1990). Results are very disappointing where there is early recurrence on treatment, i.e. less than 18 months from diagnosis, and these patients are probably incurable in the absence of an allograft (Rivera *et al.*, 1986). In these cases innovative regimens, for example, the use of matched unrelated donors, are under evaluation. However, alternative therapies, such as immune modulation post autograft, need to be evaluated. Conventional but more intensive alternative chemotherapy may induce prolonged second remissions in patients who relapse late, and this strategy requires randomized assessment against autologous bone marrow transplantation in this patient group.

REFERENCES

Alexander, F.E., McKinney, P.A., Ricketts, T.J. and Cartwright, R.A. (1990). Community lifestyle characteristics and risk of acute lymphoblastic leukaemia in children. *Lancet*, **336**, 1461–5.

Aur, R.J.A., Simone, J., Hustu, H.O. *et al.* (1971) Central nervous system therapy and combination chemotherapy in childhood lymphocytic leukemia. *Blood*, **37**, 272–81.

Bordigoni, P. (1990) Bone marrow transplantation following busulfan cyclophosphamide and high dose cytosine-arabinoside as treatment for infants with translocation (4;11) acute leukaemia. *Br. J. Haematol.*, **72**, 293–4.

Bordigoni, P., Vernant, J.P., Souillet, G. *et al.* (1989) Allogeneic bone marrow transplantation for children with acute lymphoblastic leukemia in first remission: a cooperative study of the groupe d'Etude de la Greffe de Moelle Osseuse. *J. Clin. Oncol.*, **7**, 747–53.

Browers, P. and Poplack, D. (1990) Memory and learning sequelae in long-term survivors of acute lymphoblastic leukemia: association with attention deficits. *Am. J. Ped. Hem. Onc.*, **12**, 174–81.

Bucsky, P., Sauter, S., Dopfer, R. *et al.* (1990)

Acute lymphoblastic leukemia in infants: Clinical characteristics and response to therapy in the multicenter therapy studies ALL-BFM 70/76/79/81/83/86, in *Cancer in the First Year of Life* (eds F. Lampert *et al.*) Karger, Basel, pp. 18–29.

Burchenal, J.H. and Murphy, M.L. (1965) Long-term survivors in acute leukemia. *Cancer Res.*, **25**, 1491–4.

Chessells, J.M., Cox, T.C.S., Kendall, B. *et al.* (1990) Neurotoxicity in lymphoblastic leukaemia: comparison of oral and intramuscular methotrexate and two doses of radiation. *Arch. Dis. Child.*, **65**, 416–22.

Chien, L.T., Aur, R.J.A., Stagner, S. *et al.* (1980) Long-term neurological implications of somnolence syndrome in children with acute lymphocytic leukemia. *Am. Neurol.*, **8**, 273–7.

Clavell, L.A., Gelber, R.D., Cohen, H.J. *et al.*, (1986) Four-agent induction and intensive asparaginase therapy for treatment of childhood acute lymphoblastic leukemia. *N. Engl. J. Med.*, **315**, 657–63.

Crist, W., Boyett, J., Jackson, J., Vietti, T. *et al.* (1989) Prognostic importance of the pre-B-cell immunophenotype and other presenting features in B-lineage childhood acute lymphoblastic leukemia: A Pediatric Oncology Group study, *Blood*, **74**, 1252–9.

Crist, W. Pullin, J. Boyett, J. *et al.* (1986) Clinical and biologic features predict a poor prognosis in acute lymphoid leukemias in infants: A Pediatric Oncology Group study. *Blood*, **67**, 135–40.

Dowell, R.E. and Copeland D.R. (1987) Cerebral pathology and neuropsychological effects. Differential effects of cranial radiation as a function of age. *Am. J. Pediat. Hematol. Oncol.*, **9**, 68–72.

Fengler, R., Henze, G., Langermann, H.-J. *et al.* (1982) Häufigkeit und Behandlungsergebnisse testikulärer Rezidive bei der akuten lymphoblastischen Leukämie im Kindesalter. *Klin. Pädiatr.*, **194**, 204–8.

Fletcher, J.A., Kimball, V.M., Lynch, E. *et al.* (1989) Prognostic implications of cytogenetic studies in an intensively treated group of children with acute lymphoblastic leukemia. *Blood*, **74**, 2130–5.

Fong, C.T. and Brodeur, G.M. (1987) Down's syndrome and leukemia: epidemiology, genetics, cytogenetics and mechanism of leukemogenesis. *Cancer Genet. Cytogenet.*, **28**, 55–76.

Freeman, A.I., Weinberg, V., Brecher, M.L. *et al.* (1983) Comparison of intermediate-dose methotrexate with cranial irradiation for the post induction treatment of acute lymphocytic leukaemia in childhood. *N. Engl. J. Med.*, **308**, 477–84.

Gardner, M.J., Snee, M.P., Hall, A.J. *et al.* (1990) Results of a case-control study of leukaemia and lymphoma among young people near Sellafield nuclear plant in West Cumbria. *Br. Med. J.*, **300**, 423–9.

Greaves, M.F. (1986) Is spontaneous mutation the major 'cause' of childhood acute lymphoblastic leukaemia? *Br. J. Haematol.*, **64**, 1–13.

Green, D.M. *et al.* (1980) Comparison of three methods of central nervous system prophylaxis in childhood acute lymphoblastic leukaemia. *Lancet*, **i**, 1398–402.

Green, D.M., Hall, B. and Zevon, M.A. (1989) Pregnancy outcome after treatment for acute lymphoblastic leukemia during childhood or adolescence. *Cancer*, **64**, 2335–9.

Gutjahr, P. (1990) Das Risiko zweiter bösartiger Neubildungen nach erfolgreicher onkologischer Behandlung im Kindesalter. *Pädiat. Prax.*, **40**, 213–26.

Harten, G., Stephanie, U., Henze, G. *et al.* (1984) Slight impairment of psychomotor skills in children after treatment of acute lymphoblastic leukemia. *Eur. J. Pediatr.*, **142**, 189–97.

Hausdorf, G., Morf, G., Beron, G. *et al.* (1988) Long-term doxorubicin cardiotoxicity in childhood: non-invasive evaluation of the contractile state and diastolic filling. *Br. Heart J.*, **60**, 309–15.

Hawkins, M.M., Draper, G.J. and Kingston, J.E. (1987) Incidence of second primary tumours among childhood cancer survivors. *Br. J. Cancer*, **56**, 339–47.

Henze, G., Langermann, H.-J., Ritter, J. *et al.* (1981) Treatment strategy for different risk groups in childhood acute lymphoblastic leukemia: A report from the BFM study group. *Haematol. Blood Transfus.*, **26**, 87–93.

Henze, G., Fengler, R., Hartmann, R. *et al.* (1990) BFM group treatment results in relapsed childhood acute lymphoblastic leukemia. *Haematol. Blood Transfus.*, **33**, 619–26.

Ingram, L., Mott, M.G., Mann, J.R. *et al.* (1987) Second malignancies in children treated for non-

Hodgkin's lymphoma and T-cell leukemia with the UKCCSG regimens. *Br. J. Cancer*, **55**, 463–6.

Kaatsch, P. and Michaelis, J. (1989) Jahresbericht 1988 des Kinderkrebsregisters Mainz.

Kersey, J.H., Weisdorf, D. Nesbit, M.E. *et al.* (1987) Comparison of autologous and allogeneic bone marrow transplantation for treatment of high-risk refractory acute lymphoblastic leukemia. *N. Engl. J. Med.*, **317**, 461–7.

Lampert, F., Harbott, J., Ludwig, W.-D. *et al.* (1987) Acute leukemia with chromosome location (4;11): 7 new patients and analysis of 71 cases. *Blut*, **54**, 325–35.

Lampert, F., Harbott, J. and Ritterbach, J. (1991) Chromosomenaberrationen bei akuten Leukämien im Kindesalter. Analyse von 1009 Patienten. *Klin. Pädiatr.*, **203**, 311–18.

Lancet Editorial (1990) Childhood leukaemia: an infectious disease? *Lancet*, **336**, 1477–8.

Langermann, H.-J., Henze, G., Wulf, M. and Riehm, H. (1982) Abschätzung der Tumorzellmasse bei der akuten lymphoblastischen Leukämie im Kindesalter. Prognostische Bedeutung und praktische Anwendung. *Klin. Pädiatr.*, **194**, 209–13.

Leiper, A.D., Chessells, J. (1986) Acute lymphoblastic leukaemia under 2 years. *Arch. Dis. Child.*, **61**, 1007–12.

Lilleyman, J.S., Hinchliffe, R.F. (1989) Pre-B and 'common' lymphoblastic leukaemia of childhood compared. *Br. J. Haematol.*, **71**, 227–31.

Ludwig, W.D., Bartram, C.R., Ritter, J. *et al.* (1988) Ambiguous phenotypes and genotypes in 16 children with acute leukemia as characterized by multiparameter analysis. *Blood*, **71**, 1518–38.

Meadows, A.T. and Silber, J. (1986) Delayed consequences of therapy, in *Cancer in Children*, (eds P.A. Voûte, *et al.*) 2nd edn, Springer, Berlin, pp. 70–81.

Miller, D.R. (1988) Childhood acute lymphoblastic leukemia: 1. Biological features and their use in predicting outcome of treatment. *Am. J. Pediatr. Hematol./Oncol.*, **10**, 163–73.

Miller, D.R., Coccia, P.F., Bleyer, W.A. *et al.* (1989) Early response to induction therapy as a predictor of disease-free survival and late recurrence of childhood acute lymphoblastic leukemia: a report from the Children's Cancer Study Group. *J. Clin. Oncol.*, **7**, 1807–15.

Moe, P.J. (1984) Recent advances in the management of acute lymphocytic leukemia. *Eur. Paediatr. Haematol. Oncol.*, **1**, 19–28.

Moe, P.J., Wesenberg, F., Kolmannskog, S. (1986) Methotrexate infusions in poor prognosis acute lymphoblastic leukemia. II. High-dose methotrexate (HDM) in acute lymphoblastic leukemia in childhood. *Med. Ped. Oncol.*, **14**, 189–90.

Nesbit, Jr. M.E. *et al.* (1981) Presymptomatic central nervous system therapy in previously untreated childhood acute lymphoblastic leukaemia: comparison of 1800 RAD and 2400 RAD. A report from Children's Cancer Study Group. *Lancet*, **i**, 461–5.

Niemeyer, C.M., Hitchcock-Bryan, S. and Sallan, S.E. (1985) Comparative analysis of treatment programs for childhood acute lymphoblastic leukemia. *Sem. Oncol.*, **12**, 122–30.

Parkin, D.M., Stiller, C.A., Draper, G.J. and Bieber, C.A. (1988) The international incidence of childhood cancer. *Int. J. Cancer*, **42**, 511–20.

Pinkel, D. (1979) The Ninth Annual David Karnofsky Lecture: Treatment of acute lymphocytic leukemia. *Cancer*, **43**, 1128–37.

Pinkel, D. (1989) Species-specific therapy of acute lymphoid leukemia, in *Modern Trends in Human Leukemia VIII*, (eds. R.D. Neth *et al.*) Springer, Berlin, pp. 27–35.

Pui, C.H., Behm, F.G., Raimondi, S.C. *et al.* (1989) Secondary acute myeloid leukemia in children treated for acute lymphoid leukemia. *N. Engl. J. Med.*, **321**, 136–42.

Pui, C.H., Raimondi, S.C., Murphy, S.B. *et al.* (1987) An analysis of leukemic cell chromosomal features in infants. *Blood*, **69**, 1289–93.

Pui, C.H., Williams, D.L., Kalwinsky, D.K. *et al.* (1986) Cytogenetic features and serum lactic dehydrogenase level predict a poor treatment outcome for children with pre-B-cell leukemia. *Blood*, **67**, 1688–92.

Reaman, G., Lange, B., Feusner, L. *et al.* (1989) Intensive systemic and intrathecal chemotherapy improves the outcome for infants with acute lymphoblastic leukemia (ALL). Proceedings ASCO, 8.

Reiter, A., Sauter, S., Kabisch, H. *et al.* (1989) Probability for cure as related to therapy in childhood B-type acute lymphoblastic leukaemia (B-ALL) in consecutive BFM-trials. *Med. Ped. Oncol.*, **17**, 321.

Ribeiro, R.C., Abromowitch, M. Raimondi, S.C. *et*

al. (1987) Clinical and biologic hallmarks of the Philadelphia chromosome in childhood acute lymphoblastic leukemia. *Blood*, **70**, 948–53.

Riehm, H., Gadner, H., Henze, G. *et al.* (1980) The Berlin childhood acute lymphoblastic leukemia therapy study, 1970–1976. *Am. J. Paediatr. Haematol. Oncol.*, **2**, 299–306.

Riehm, H., Gadner, H., Henze, G. *et al.* (1990) Results and significance of six randomized trials in four consecutive ALL-BFM studies, in *Haematology and Blood Transfusion* 33, Acute Leukemias II, (eds T. Buchner, G. Schellong and W. Hiddemann) Springer, Berlin, pp. 439–50.

Riehm, H., Feickert, H.-J. and Lampert, F. (1986) Acute lymphoblastic leukaemia, in *Cancer in Children*, (eds P.A. Voûte *et al.*) 2nd edn, Springer, Berlin, pp. 101–18.

Rivera, G.K., Buchanan, G., Boyett, J.M. *et al.* (1986) Intensive retreatment of childhood acute lymphoblastic leukemia in first bone marrow relapse: A Pediatric Oncology Group study. *N. Engl. J. Med.*, **315**, 273–8.

Rivera, G., George, S.L., Bowman, W.P. *et al.* (1983) Second central nervous system prophylaxis in children with acute lymphoblastic leukemia who relapse after elective cessation of therapy. *J. Clin. Oncol.*, **1**, 471–6.

Sallan, S.E., Niemeyer, C.M., Billett, A.L. *et al.* (1989) Autologous bone marrow transplantation for acute lymphoblastic leukemia. *J. Clin. Oncol.*, **7**, 1594–601.

Santana, V.M., Dodge, R.K., Christ, W.M. *et al.* (1990) Presenting features and treatment outcome of adolescents with acute lymphoblastic leukemia. *Leukemia*, **4**, 87–90.

Sather, H., Coccia, P., Nesbit, M. *et al.* (1981) Disappearance of the predictive value of prognostic variables in childhood acute lymphocytic leukemia. *Cancer*, **48**, 370–6.

Schroeder, H., Pinkerton, C.R., Powles, R.L. *et al.* (1991) High dose melphalan and total body irradiation with autologous marrow rescue in childhood acute lymphoblastic leukaemia after relapse. *Bone Marrow Transplant.*, **7**, 11–15.

Shaw, N.J., Pivedale, P.M. and Eden, O.B. (1989) Pulmonary function in childhood leukaemia survivors. *Med. Pediatr. Oncol.*, **17**, 149–54.

Simone, J.V. (1976) Annotation: Factors that influence haematological remission duration in acute lymphocyte leukaemia. *Brit. J. Haematol.*, **32**, 465–72.

Smeitirik, J., Verrenssel, M., Schröder, C. and Lippens, R. (1988) Nephrotoxicity associated with ifosfamide. *Eur. J. Pediatr.*, **148**, 164–6.

Stark, B., Vogel, R., Cohen, I.J. *et al.* (1989) Biologic and cytogenetic characteristics of leukemia in infants. *Cancer*, **63**, 117–25.

Steinherz, P.G., Gaynon, P. Miller, D.R. *et al.* (1986) Improved disease-free survival of children with acute lymphoblastic leukemia at high risk for early relapse with the New York regimen – A new intensive therapy protocol: A report from the children's cancer study group. *J. Clin. Oncol.*, **4**, 744–52.

Van der Does-van der Berg, A., Bartram, C.R., Basso, G. *et al.* (submitted) Minimal demands for the diagnosis, the classification and the evaluation of treatment results of childhood acute lymphoblastic leukemia (ALL) in the 'BFM-family' co-operative group.

Van Wering, E.R. and Kamps, W. (1986) Acute leukemia in infants. A unique pattern of acute nonlymphocytic leukemia. *Am. J. Pediatr. Hematol. Oncol.*, **8**, 220–4.

Wingard, J.R., Piantadosi, S., Santos, G.W. *et al.* (1990) Allogeneic bone marrow transplantation for patients with high-risk acute lymphoblastic leukemia. *J. Clin. Oncol.*, **8**, 820–30.

Young, Jr., J.L., Ries, L.G., Silverberg, E. *et al.* (1986) Cancer incidence, survival, and mortality for children younger than age 15 years. *Cancer*, **58**, 598–602.

Chapter 11

Childhood non-Hodgkin's lymphoma

C. PATTE

11.1 INTRODUCTION

The term non-Hodgkin's lymphoma (NHL) has been adopted to describe the heterogeneous malignant proliferations of lymphoid tissue. Childhood NHL differs in a number of ways from that of the adult:

1. almost invariably diffuse, high grade histology;
2. clinical presentation is predominated by the presence of extra nodal disease with very rapid tumoral growth and dissemination which is not contiguous, and in particular involves the bone marrow and central nervous system;
3. proliferation of immature lymphoid cells belonging to either B or T cell lineage.

Recent biological and immunological studies have greatly contributed to a better classification of NHL. The prognosis for a child with widespread disease has also changed in the last 20 years as a result of better understanding of the pathological process and better use of intensive chemotherapeutic regimens.

11.2 EPIDEMIOLOGY

NHL has a peak incidence between the ages of seven and ten years, being uncommon before two years of age. A male predominance is evident with a sex ratio of 2.5:1 to 3:1 (Patte *et al.*, 1981a; Murphy *et al.*, 1989). An annual incidence of approximately seven cases per million children, makes it the third most common childhood malignancy (Young and Miller, 1975).

A few familial cases have been described; certain individuals with an increased risk of developing NHL have also been identified. These include heritable conditions associated with immunodeficiency such as ataxia telangiectasia, Wiskott-Aldrich syndrome, and conditions where immunodeficiency has been acquired as in post organ transplantation or acquired immunodeficiency syndrome (AIDS). Purtillo has also described an X-linked syndrome characterized by a particular sensibility to Epstein-Barr virus (EBV) and the occurrence of malignant lymphomas, especially of the Burkitt's type, and fatal infectious mononucleosis (Grierson and Purtillo, 1987). Specific geographical areas are also recognized for particular types of lymphoma, such as the 'Mediterranean' or Heavy Chain lymphoma (Tabbane *et al.*, 1976), and the 'African' Burkitt's lymphoma (Lenoir *et al.*, 1985).

Aetiology has been linked particularly with

EBV, after it was noted that EBV particles were present in the nucleus of malignant cells in endemic Burkitt's lymphomas (Lenoir *et al.*, 1985). Human T-cell leukaemia/lymphoma virus, (HTLV-1), is also thought to play a role in the genesis of adult T-cell malignancy in Japan. Although these viruses are known to have transforming and immortalizing properties on B and T cells *in vitro*, and are inferred as having a role in the oncogenic process, other events are also needed to establish a malignant state (see Chapter 2). Furthermore, primary evidence of viral participation in oncogenesis is rare, EBV being found in only 20% of non endemic Burkitt's lymphoma, and to date no viral particles have been found in childhood T-cell lymphomas.

11.3 BIOLOGY

11.3.1 HISTOLOGY

On account of the difficulty of classifying the histology of NHL, various systems have been used. Because of their different groupings, however, this has made intercorrelation difficult (Falcon and Isaacson, 1990). The modified Rappaport (R) classification (Nathamani *et al.*, 1978) and now, for clinical use, the Working Formulation (WF) (National Cancer

Institute-sponsored study, 1982) are most widely used in America, while in Europe the Kiel (K) classification (Lennert, 1981; Stansfeld *et al.*, 1988) is preferred (Table 11.1). It should be noted that the term 'lymphoblastic' is used in a more restrictive way by the R and WF classification; in the K classification, it applies to most of the paediatric NHL.

Childhood NHL are virtually all diffuse and are generally limited to three major histological types: (1) the lymphoblastic Burkitt's (K) or small non cleaved (WF); (2) the lymphoblastic (WF) non Burkitt's (K); (3) the immunoblastic and centroblastic (K) or large cell (WF). The first two groups represent 70% to 90% of the diagnosis, while the third is more heterogeneous and diversely recognized with variable separation from the first two depending on the classification used and the pathologist involved.

Alternatively, as the pattern of disease is always diffuse, a diagnosis may be made by cytological studies. L_1 and L_2 morphology using the FAB classification correspond with T-lymphoblastic disease, and L_3 with B-lymphoblastic.

11.3.2 IMMUNOPHENOTYPING

Immunophenotyping (Bernard *et al.*, 1979) more than histopathology has advanced our

Table 11.1 Histopathological classification of childhood non-Hodgkin's lymphoma

Kiel classification	Rappaport classification	Working formulation
High grade Lymphoblastic Burkitt's and other B-lymphoblastic	Diffuse undifferentiated (Burkitt's/non Burkitt's)	**High grade** Small non cleaved cell
Lymphoblastic convoluted Lymphoblastic unclassified	Diffuse lymphoblastic (Convoluted/non convoluted)	Lymphoblastic
Immunoblastic Centroblastic	Diffuse histiocytic	Large cell immunoblastic **Intermediate grade** Diffuse large cell

understanding of NHL, especially with the advent of monoclonal antibodies which allow identification of lymphoid cell surface antigen characteristics of T or B cell lineage and also of cell maturation stage. These antibodies are grouped in 'clusters of differentiation' (CD), and although each CD is typical of a certain cell lineage, it is not entirely specific and can be encountered in a subgroup of another lineage. Immunotyping must therefore include a parallel of antibodies. It must be said that although some abnormalities are in favour of a malignant clone of cells, immunophenotyping of a cell population cannot confirm the malignancy.

As has been said, childhood NHL can be divided into three groups: (1) B-cell proliferation, characterized by the presence of monoclonal immunoglobulins on their surface; (2) T-cell proliferation; and (3) non T-non B proliferations, which are in fact immature cells already committed to B cell lineage (pre-B; pre pre-B and CALLA+).

These three groups are identical to those found in acute lymphoblastic leukaemia (ALL), but with a different frequency. In ALL, about 80% are non T-non B-derived neoplasms; 20% are T-cell-derived and less than 2% are B-cell-derived. Conversely, non T- non B lymphomas are very rare – less than 10%.

The most reliable immunological results are obtained using a suspension of fresh cells, but as sufficient cells are often difficult to obtain, this is not always possible. Immunohistochemistry can also be done using frozen sections; these give a more reliable result than using paraffin block material, the techniques of which are still being developed.

11.3.3 CYTOGENETICS AND MOLECULAR BIOLOGY

Cytogenetic and molecular biological studies have contributed to our knowledge of the fundamental processes in NHL, but have not yet contributed to therapy. In Burkitt's lymphoma, tumour cells are characterized by a translocation involving the long arm of chromosome 8, region q23-q24, whilst the majority of cases exhibit a translocation of t(8;14) (q24; q32). Variant translocations include t(2;8) (p12; q24) and t(8;22) (q24; q11) (Lenoir *et al.*, 1985). In the translocation t(8;14), the oncogene c-*myc* moves from its normal position on chromosome 8 and is rearranged with the gene for heavy chain immunoglobulin. In the variant translocations, c-*myc* remains on chromosome 8, but the kappa and lambda immunoglobulin light chain genes translocate from their normal positions on chromosomes 2 and 22 respectively, to a region distal to the c-*myc* oncogene. Transcriptional deregulation of the c-*myc* gene results and this leads to elevated expression; something that is thought to play a crucial role in the genesis and/or maintenance of this malignancy (Croce and Nowell, 1985).

In T-cell tumours, chromosomal abnormalities are more heterogeneous. They can involve chromosome 14 where is the locus of the gene for the alpha-chain of the T-cell receptor, or chromosome 7 where is the locus of the gene for the beta chain of the T-cell receptor (Hecht *et al.*, 1985).

11.4 CLINICAL FEATURES

11.4.1 ABDOMEN

The abdomen is the most frequent primary site (30–45%) (Patte *et al.*, 1981a; Murphy *et al.*, 1989), but its distribution may differ according to geographical area: abdominal NHL are more common in Southern Europe than in Northern Europe. Intussusception leading to the discovery of a small excisable abdominal tumour is a rare presentation, the more frequent clinical picture is that of a large and rapidly growing abdominal mass often associated with ascites. Ultrasonographic scanning objectively assesses the intraperitoneal mass and defines precisely any intrabdominal spread. Laparotomy should be avoided, except in the event of an abdominal emergency and the diagnosis made by cytological examination of ascites or percutaneous needle biopsy. Surface markers invariably show B-cell phenotype and histology lymphoblastic Burkitt's lymphoma.

11.4.2 MEDIASTINUM

Mediastinal tumours (25–35%) are, typically, T-cell lymphoblastic lymphomas. Mediastinal compression and/or cervical or axillary lymphadenopathy clarify the diagnosis. Chest x-ray shows a localized thymic mass often associated with pleural or pericardial effusions. Patients are at particular risk of developing respiratory distress, provoked by general anaesthesia. Diagnosis should therefore be done using cytological examination of effusions or bone marrow smears. If a tumour biopsy is needed, then this should be done by percutaneous needle biopsy, or by mediastinoscopy.

11.4.3 OTHER SITES

The third most frequent site is that of the head and neck (Bergeron *et al.*, 1989) including Waldeyer's ring and the facial bones (10–20%), followed by the superficial lymph nodes (5–10%). The remaining 5–10% includes tumours that arise from less common sites such as bone, skin, thyroid, orbit, eyelid, kidney, and epidural space. Diagnosis is confirmed by tissue biopsy with immunophenotyping since no particular type of lymphoma is associated with these sites. Bone lymphoma can be localized, but can be also generalized and is often associated with hypercalcaemia (Coppes *et al.*, 1991). Kidney lymphoma can be confused with nephroblastoma, but suspicion should be aroused where the tumour

is bilateral, the infiltration multinodular or diffuse, or when renal failure is present. (Sub)cutaneous lymphoma occurs particularly in young children less than two years of age, and is of non T- non B phenotype (Bernard *et al.*, 1982).

11.5 INITIAL WORK-UP AND STAGING

Once the diagnosis of NHL has been made, a speedy assessment of classification, staging and general evaluation must be done in order that appropriate treatment can be commenced as soon as possible.

11.5.1 DIAGNOSIS AND CLASSIFICATION

Diagnosis can be obtained utilising biopsy material, cytological examination of effusion fluids, or bone marrow smears; also recommended are accompanying immunological and cytogenetic studies. For practical purposes, in order to decide therapy, a tumour must be classified. There are two main clinical groups: B-lymphoblastic and T-lymphoblastic. Criteria for each group are:

A. B-lymphoblastic:
   (1) positivity and monoclonality of B-cell surface immunoglobulins and other B-cell markers (e.g. CD 19–24);
   (2) translocation (8;14), t(2;8) or t(8;22);
   (3) histology: Burkitt's and B-lymphoblastic (K) (or undifferentiated (R) or small non cleaved (W);
   (4) L_3 morphology in FAB classification;
   (5) abdominal primary.
B. T-lymphoblastic:
   (1) positivity of T-cell markers (e.g. CD 3, 5–8);
   (2) histology: lymphoblastic;
   (3) L_1 or L_2 morphology in FAB classification;
   (4) focal positivity of acid phosphatase reaction;
   (5) thymic primary.

Table 11.2 St Jude's staging

Stage I	A single tumour (extranodal) or single anatomical area (nodal) with the exclusion of the mediastinum or abdomen
Stage II	A single tumour (extranodal) with regional node involvement
	Two or more nodal areas on the same side of the diaphragm
	Two single (extranodal) tumours with or without regional node involvement on the same side of the diaphragm
	A primary gastrointestinal tract tumour, usually in the ileocaecal area, with or without involvement of associated mesenteric nodes only, grossly completely resected
Stage III	Two single tumours (extranodal) on opposite sides of the diaphragm
	Two or more nodal areas above and below the diaphragm
	All the primary intrathoracic tumours (mediastinal, pleural, thymic)
	All extensive primary intra-abdominal disease, unresectable.
	All paraspinal or epidural tumours, regardless of other tumour site(s)
Stage IV	Any of the above with initial CNS and/or bone marrow involvement.

Non-B and non-T cell lymphomas (i.e. absence of SIg and T-cell markers, but with CD9 and CD10 positivity and occasionally the presence of intracellular immunoglobulins), are grouped separately unless they originate in the abdomen or have B-cell morphology.

Due to the predominance of extra nodal primaries and the unpredictable pattern of spread, the Ann Arbor Classification is un-adaptable to childhood NHL. Several classifications have been proposed (Wollner *et al.*, 1976; Murphy, 1980; Janus *et al.*, 1984) and the most commonly used system is that of Murphy (Table 11.2). Certain problems still remain with these systems: the size and number of tumours and the fact that the histopathological and immunohistological characteristics are not taken into account. Within the same stage, there may be a different prognosis depending on the localization or previous excision; in Stage I, orbital or Waldeyer's ring tumours appear to have a worse prognosis than excised local nodal disease. In Stage II, abdominal tumours have a better prognosis than a large nasopharyngeal tumour invading the base of the skull.

The traditional boundary between leukaemia and lymphoma has been arbitrarily defined by more or less than 25% blast cells in the bone marrow, but this does not correspond to either clinical or biological differences (Bernard *et al.*, 1986).

CNS involvement is defined on the basis of unequivocal malignant cells in a cytocentri-

Table 11.3 Initial work-up

Mandatory:
Physical examination
Chest and nasopharyngeal x-rays
Abdominal ultrasonography
Two bone marrow aspirations
CSF examination
Complete blood count
LDH, serum electrolytes, BUN, creatinine, uric acid levels

Optional, depending on clinical circumstances:
Bone scan and skeletal survey
Local CT scan (head and neck tumours)
MRI (CNS disease)

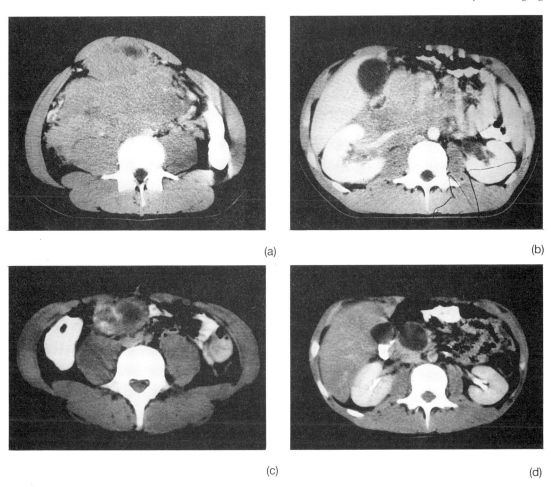

(a)

(b)

(c)

(d)

Fig. 11.1 Large abdominal tumour (a) with extension in retroperitoneum (b). After the first 3 induction courses, residual masses were removed surgically and examined histologically: the abdominal mass (c) still contained tumour, while the pancreatic region mass (d) was necrotic.

fuged specimen of spinal fluid, and/or the presence of obvious neurological deficits, such as cranial nerve palsies.

Staging procedures are outlined in Table 11.3. Abdominal ultrasonography is adequate for abdominal disease; CT scanning is not necessary in the primary investigations of abdominal and mediastinal disease.

11.5.2 GENERAL EVALUATION

Patients often have other complications, such as malnutrition, infection, post-surgical problems and respiratory and metabolic abnormalities; these may be life threatening or compromise the onset of therapy. Hypercalcaemia which is not always related to bone marrow involvement requires treatment as a separate entity (Leblanc *et al.*, 1984). The tumour lysis syndrome may be present prior to treatment or develop during treatment. Preventive measures must always therefore be instituted. Definition of the mechanisms causing renal failure must also be established (uric acid nephropathy; tumour infiltration or urinary obstruction), in order that prompt, appropriate and adequate treatment can be started; this may include dialysis or transcutaneous pyelostomy.

In order to minimize these complications, both the French and German protocols commence with low-dose therapy which produces a tumour regression; this is then followed a week later by a more intensive regimen.

11.6 TREATMENT

Up until the 70s, childhood NHL had a poor prognosis, with only a few localized tumours being cured by surgery and radiotherapy. The majority of children died within weeks of diagnosis of local progression, or if local control was achieved, from marrow or CNS disease. Considerable therapeutic improvements have been achieved in the last 15 years as a result of increased knowledge of the disease and better use of chemotherapy.

11.6.1 SURGERY

Indications for elective surgery are very few (Wakim *et al.*, 1989). A small localized tumour may be completely excised. In the case of abdominal tumours, diagnosis will often be a fortuitous event as a result of surgery for intestinal intussusception or acute appendicitis when lymphoma is unexpectedly discovered. Primary surgical excision or debulking of abdominal, head and neck, and mediastinal tumours should not be attempted; there have been some reports of a better prognosis after tumour excision (Janus *et al.*, 1984; Fleming *et al.*, 1990), but this probably relates more to the localized nature of the tumour. Extensive surgery is uselessly mutilating, is often followed by tumoral regrowth and it delays and may complicate chemotherapy.

Rarely, abdominal surgery may be needed during treatment for complications such as intestinal perforation. If this occurs during a neutropaenic period, mortality is high. Only at the time of remission evaluation should a residual mass be removed or widely biopsied for careful pathological excision before determining whether a complete or partial remission has been obtained. In the French experience, less than one-third of residual masses contain viable malignant cells (Helardot *et al.*, 1989).

11.6.2 RADIOTHERAPY

Radiotherapy can be highly efficacious in lymphoma, but it is a local therapy and NHL should always be regarded as a potentially generalized disease. In cases of extensive disease, radiotherapy is not necessary and adds both immediate and long-term toxicity to the treatment.

In France, commencing with the advanced stages, radiotherapy has been totally withdrawn from the treatment protocols since 1977 (Patte *et al.*, 1981b). Recent published reports of randomized studies (Link *et al.*, 1990), for example, have confirmed that combined chemotherapy and radiotherapy gives no advantage over chemotherapy alone. In a British study for mediastinal tumours, however, additional radiotherapy showed a significantly better survival (Mott *et al.*, 1984). However, the equivalent outcome can be achieved by changing the chemotherapy regimen alone.

In conclusion, indications for radiotherapy are few, but it may be warranted in emergency situations although chemotherapy is often as effective. Localized residual tumours may, however, benefit from radiotherapy.

11.6.3 CHEMOTHERAPY

Chemotherapy is the treatment of choice in childhood NHL which should be considered to be a systemic disease, even in the presence of apparently local disease. The conclusions from protocols carried out in the 70s (Patte *et al.*, 1981b; Janus *et al.*, 1984; Mott *et al.*, 1984; Muller-Weihrich *et al.*, 1985; Lemerle *et al.*, 1986) were:

1. complete remission was obtained in 85–95% of all patients;
2. survival rates were improved, but were disappointing in advanced stages, being 30–50%;
3. despite CNS treatment with intrathecal therapy, often accompanied by cranial radiotherapy, CNS relapses were frequent (10–20%);
4. treatment for all histological types was the same, but, contrary to the findings of Wollner, results were different for B-cell and T-cell derived lymphomas, even for the same stage (Anderson *et al.*, 1983; Muller-Weihrich *et al.*, 1985; Lemerle *et al.*, 1986). B-cell lymphomas benefit from intensive short pulse chemotherapy such as COMP (Anderson *et al.*, 1983) or COPAD (Lemerle *et al.*, 1986), whereas T-cell and non-T non-B disease benefit from a 'leukaemic' regimen, i.e. continuous and prolonged chemotherapy as in LSA2L2 (Wollner *et al.*, 1979; Anderson *et al.*, 1983) or in the BFM protocols (Muller-Weihrich *et al.*, 1985);
   also been been defined, being in the first year in B-cell lymphoma, and generally within the first two years but up until four years in T-lymphoblastic disease;
6. Phase II studies have shown the efficacy of high-dose methotrexate (MTX), not only on systemic disease, but especially in CNS disease, with a response rate of 60% in the study carried out at the Institut Gustave-Roussy (Patte *et al.*, 1986a);
7. relapses could be salvaged by high-dose chemotherapy with bone marrow transplantation (Philip *et al.*, 1983; Hartmann *et al.*, 1984).

11.7 ADVANCED STAGE B-CELL LYMPHOMAS

Most present protocols are based on fractionated cyclophosphamide (CPM), intermediate (ID) or high dose (HD) methotrexate (MTX), cytosine arabinoside (Ara-C), vincristine (VCR), adriamycin (ADR), and prednisone (Pred), administered in various combinations but usually as short-pulse courses.

Since 1981, the largest studies have taken place in Europe, both in France (LMB protocols) and Germany (BFM protocols), and as a result of these well organized multicentre studies, considerable improvement in outcome has resulted over the last 8 years.

11.7.1 LMB PROTOCOL

The general scheme of the LMB protocols is a cytoreductive phase (COP course) with low doses of VCR, CPM, Pred the week before the intensive induction based on HD MTX, fractionated CPM (two courses of COPAD M), followed by a consolidation phase based on Ara-C in continuous infusion. CNS directed therapy is given with HD MTX and IT MTX. SFOP (the French Pediatric Oncology Society) have conducted several successive multi-centre (French, Belgian, Dutch) studies (0181, 0281, 84). Reported improvements were: reduction of total treatment duration from 12 to 4 months, and the decrease of toxicity, especially of toxic death rates, parallel to the investigator's experience (Patte *et al.*, 1986b; 1988; 1991b). The pertinent points of these studies are:

1. Stage III and IV CNS (-) NHL have reached a 75–80% EFS. Bone marrow involvement is not a factor of poor prognosis value;
2. CNS therapy by HD MTX and IT TMTX is efficient (CNS relapse rate <3%);
3. partial remission at the end of induction

205

can be cured by treatment intensification and high dose therapy with autologous bone marrow transplantation (Philip *et al.*, 1988). Residual tumour has to be documented histologically since two-thirds of masses are entirely necrotic (Helardot *et al.*, 1989);

4. the absence of tumour reduction after the COP appears to be a factor indicative of a poor prognosis (Patte *et al.*, 1988).

For patients with initial CNS involvement whose EFS was only 19% in the LMB 0281 protocol (Patte *et al.*, 1986b), and for those B-ALL without abdominal primaries, the LMB 86 protocol was initiated in November 1985. It was based on higher dose of MTX (8 g/m² in 4 hr), triple IT and a consolidation with continuous infusion and HD Ara-C and VP16 (CYVE courses [Gentet *et al.*, 1990]). The EFS improved to 82% for 11 B-ALL CNS, and 75% for 25 B-NHL and B-ALL CNS + (Patte *et al.*, 1990).

11.7.2 BFM PROTOCOL

The BFM group also began multi-centre studies for B-cell neoplasis in 1981. The BFM

protocols consisted of four (study 81) or three (study 83) cycles of alternating courses: CPM, ID MTX and IT MTX were administered at each course, and ADR was alternated with Ara-C and VM26. This was preceded by a cytoreductive phase with Pred and CPM. Cranial irradiation was given. During the 81–83 period, the EFS was 73% for 75 Stage III, 57% for 15 Stage IV and 45% for 46 B-ALL patients (Muller-Weihrich *et al.*, 1987).

In study 86, vincristine was added, ifosfamide partially replaced cyclophosphamide, cranial irradiation was withdrawn, and for Stage IV and B-ALL, HD MTX was given at the dosage of 5 g/m² in 24-hour infusions. With these modifications, the EFS of 45 patients (only 3 with CNS involvement) with Stage IV and B-ALL improved to 81% (Reiter *et al.*, 1989).

11.7.3 UKCCSG PROTOCOL

In Great Britain, the UKCCSG have developed the MACHO protocol, a short intensive multi-agent regimen based on HD fractionated CPM, HD Ara-C and MTX for patients

(a)   (b)

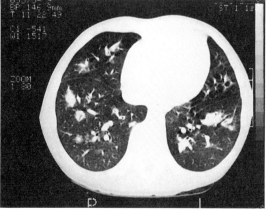

Fig. 11.2   B-ALL in a 5-year-old boy presenting with lung (a), liver, bone (particularly vertebrae), soft tissue (b), and CNS involvement. Cure was obtained after treatment according to LMB 86 protocol.

with B-ALL. The EFS of 11 patients was 62%; patients with bulky abdominal disease, however, did not fare so well (Hann *et al.*, 1988).

11.7.4 INSTITUTO NAZIONALE TUMORI (MILAN) PROTOCOL

In Italy there is no national study for childhood NHL. The Instituto Nazionale Tumori of Milan has developed its own protocol, based on VCR, CPM, HD MTX, ADR, and a consolidation with Ara-C 6 g/m² and CDDP 80 mg/m² in 96-hr continuous infusion. The EFS of 22 patients (1 Stage I, 13 Stage III and 8 Stage IV) was 66% (Gasparini *et al.*, 1987). Other centres have adopted protocols such as the BFM, the St. Jude's (Murphy *et al.*, 1986) or the LMB protocols.

11.7.5 OTHER PROTOCOLS

In North America, several small series have been published showing interesting results for Stage III lymphomas; however, results for Stage IV and B-ALL remain disappointing (Sullivan and Ramirez, 1985; Murphy *et al.*, 1986). The recent Pediatric Oncology Group (POG) study appears promising although results have remained poorer than those of the SFOP and BFM studies (Bowman *et al.*, 1990).

In countries with limited resources where Burkitt's lymphoma is common, therapeutic improvements have also been achieved thanks to the adaptation of therapy to the local environmental and to better management of the initial, especially the metabolic, problems (Ladjaj *et al.*, 1984; Sullivan *et al.*, 1985; Rivera-Luna *et al.*, 1986; Al-Attar *et al.*, 1989).

11.8 ADVANCED STAGE NON B-CELL LYMPHOMAS

These patients with T-cell or non-B non-T lymphoma should be treated with a pro-

tocol similar or identical to those of high-risk forms of acute lymphoblastic leukaemia.

11.8.1 BFM AND DERIVED PROTOCOLS

Since 1976, non B-type lymphomas have received the same protocol as acute lymphoblastic leukaemias (Muller-Weihrich *et al.*, 1985). The induction (protocol I) and the reinduction (protocol III) were subject to very few modifications during the studies (76, 81, 83) and are followed by continuing treatment with daily 6-MP and weekly MTX. In study 86, 4 HD MTX (5 g/m² in 24-hr infusion) was introduced to replace cranial irradiation for CNS directed therapy. Since 1976, the results are about the same since regimens have been similar in the successive studies: EFS was 78% for 42 Stage III and IV patients treated in study 76 and 79% for 33 patients treated in studies 81–83 (Muller-Weihrich *et al.*, 1985).

Several European groups and centres who have now adopted the BFM protocol or slightly modified protocols for treatment of leukaemias use the same protocol to treat non-B lymphomas.

11.8.2 LSA2L2 PROTOCOL AND DERIVED PROTOCOLS

The LSA2L2 protocol, a 2- or 3-year 10-drug intensive regimen, delivering drugs five days a week during consolidation and every two weeks during continuing treatment, was developed by Wollner (Wollner *et al.*, 1979). As shown by the CCSG randomized trial (Anderson *et al.*, 1983), it appeared effective on mediastinal (Pullen *et al.*, 1982; Sullivan *et al.*, 1985), but not in abdominal lymphomas (Otten *et al.*, 1981; Pullen *et al.*, 1982; Pichler *et al.*, 1982; Sullivan *et al.*, 1985; Dluzniewska *et al.*, 1985). With CNS therapy based on IT MTX, isolated CNS relapse rate was 8–15%.

Vecchi in Italy has reported a series of patients for whom CNS direct therapy was improved by the addition of cranial irradiation (Vecchi, *et al.*, 1981).

At the Institut Gustave-Roussy, in France, the original protocol was modified by the addition of 10 HD MTX (3 g/m² in 3-hr infusions). The EFS was 79% for 33 Stage III patients and 72% for 43 Stage IV patients (24 of these had more than 25% bone marrow involvement). Only one isolated CNS relapse occurred among the 69 patients, without CNS involvement (Patte *et al.*, 1991a).

11.8.3 OTHER PROTOCOLS

In France, the centres who registered their patients with leukaemia in the FRALLE study (conducted by the St. Louis Hospital) treated their patients with non-B NHL with the same regimen (Benz-Lemoine *et al.*, 1988).

In 1985, the Memphis group published a series of 22 patients with Stage III and IV lymphoblastic lymphomas, the results of a protocol based on early and intermittent reinductions with VM26 and Ara-C in addition to VCR, Pred, Asparaginase, triple IT and continuing treatment with allopurinol and MTX. The EFS was 73% with a regimen containing no CPM and no anthracyclines (Dahl *et al.*, 1985). These results have not so far been confirmed on a larger series of patients. In the UK, T-NHL is treated according to the MRC-UKALL protocols (Wheeler *et al.*, 1990).

11.9 LOCALIZED NHL

These require less intensive treatment than non-localized lymphomas and CNS directed therapy can be avoided in Stage I and abdominal Stage II (Murphy, 1980). In the US, localized NHL is treated with the same protocol whatever the histology (Meadows *et al.*, 1989; Link *et al.*, 1990), except in the case of a CCSG study where the T-cell disease excluded (Jenkin *et al.*, 1984). These studies have decreased the intensity and the duration

of treatment, keeping EFS > 85%. Radiotherapy appeared not to be beneficial.

In Europe, treatment is adapted to histology and immunophenotype as in the advanced stage. In the BFM studies, Stages I and II (with B-NHL, only Stage II resected) have been treated with the same scheme as the other stages, but for only half the duration for B-NHL, and without reinductions for non B-NHL. Cranial irradiation was not performed, but ID MTX and IT MTX were given. Local irradiation was withdrawn in 1983. Survival was above 80% (Muller-Weihrich *et al.*, 1985).

In France, no national registration for localized disease was done until 1989. Generally, B-cell Stage I and abdominal Stage II were treated according to the COPAD protocol without CNS prophylaxis with 100% EFS in the Institut Gustave-Roussy (personal data). Non-B Stage I had a protocol similar to the other non B-NHL but shorter and without HD MTX or cranial irradiation. The other Stage II patients were treated as for the advanced stages. No local irradiation has been performed since 1977.

11.9.1 INDICATIONS FOR HIGH-DOSE CHEMOTHERAPY AND BONE MARROW TRANSPLANTATION

The need for HD chemotherapy with BMT has greatly diminished in parallel with the improvement in survival using intensive conventional regimens. Two indications are now recognized: partial remissions (histologically documented) after an intensive induction, and relapses which respond to a second line chemotherapy. However, relapses which have occurred under the present protocols are more 'resistant' than those previously, and to find a second line chemotherapy has become a challenge (Gentet *et al.*, 1990). The choice of the high dose regimen is a decision made within the centres undertaking the treatment and will not therefore be discussed.

11.10 CURRENT CONTROVERSIES

11.10.1 THE ROLE FOR SURGERY AND RADIOTHERAPY

With the exception of the rare localized primary tumour which is amenable to complete resection, surgery has little role beyond biopsy taking for a histological diagnosis. There is no place for debulking surgery in extensive thoracic or abdominal disease (Al-Attar *et al.*, 1989). In the case of abdominal B cell disease where there is a residual mass post chemotherapy, a second look laparatomy is of importance: if there is residual disease at this time, the patient may still be cured by dose escalation and bone marrow rescue (Patte *et al.*, 1986b; Philip *et al.*, 1988). Similarly, the only indication for radiotherapy is refractory localized disease, or as consolidation of second remission following local recurrence. Cranial irradiation is still generally used where there is initial lymphoma of the central nervous system, but not as part of routine early CNS-directed therapy. Testis and bone irradiation are still used where these are initial sites of disease. This is unneccessary in most cases.

11.10.2 CAN CNS THERAPY BE IMPROVED?

CNS therapy has been improved by the use of HD MTX which has advantageously replaced cranial irradiation whose neurological and endocrinal damage is well known. Questions remain as to the optimal dosage of HD MTX, infusion duration, number of courses and modality of folinic rescue, and the usefulness or otherwise of combined intrathecal injections (Borsi and Moe, 1987; Lippens and Winograd, 1988; Vassal *et al.*, 1990).

CNS involvement especially in B-cell NHL is usually regarded as a very bad prognostic indicator. The reported French study LMB 86 has shown that this is curable with intensive chemotherapy and without bone marrow transplantation (Patte *et al.*, 1990). HD MTX and HD Ara-C are the drugs of choice along with triple intrathecal injections. Could CNS irradiation therefore be avoided?

11.10.3 ARE THERE PROGNOSTIC FACTORS WITHIN MURPHY STAGES III AND IV PATIENTS TO INDICATE THOSE WHO REQUIRE MORE/LESS TREATMENT?

Since relatively high survival rates have now been reached, the question posed is how to decrease treatment intensity without jeopardizing survival rates. To do so, it is necessary to find new prognostic factors; these prove more and more difficult to find, however, as they change depending on the therapeutic regimens employed.

Will biological features emerge as prognostically independent factors, i.e. ploidy, proliferation index, associated chromosome abnormalities, resistance genes? The absence of tumour regression one week after COP appeared to be a factor for bad prognosis in the reported French study (Patte *et al.*, 1988), and this is taken into account in order to justify intensifying earlier chemotherapy.

Controversies regarding localized tumours are readily found. Treating these lymphomas with the same protocol whatever their histology and phenotype does not seem adequate in the view of European investigators, nor is the equal treatment of Stages I and II whatever the localization, tumour size and previous excision. On the other hand, treatment intensity could be further decreased for some patients. This is being done for B-cell resected Stage I and abdominal Stage II which are treated in the French LMB 89 study by only two courses of COPAD. However, when treatment is thought not to have immediate life-threatening consequences nor long-term sequelae, the rationale behind a further decrease in therapy is debatable.

Within the advanced stages, it is necessary to find prognostic subgroups to try and decrease therapy for the better prognostic types noting that prognostic factors identified in one study might not be relevant in another. For example in abdominal tumours, extra abdominal extension as defined by Ziegler (Stage C or Stage D) was not prognostic in the French studies LMB 81+84. Within the abdominal Stage III, a subclassification has been proposed by Philip and Pinkerton which differentiates Stage III A: limited but unresectable tumour, often a large tumour with ascites, from Stage III B with extensive abdominal multi-organ involvement or with any extra abdominal disease (Philip *et al.*, 1987). Stage III B was a significant unfavourable prognostic factor in 250 patients treated in the LMB 81+84 studies, but this was not significant in the LMB 84 study alone. Bone marrow involvement was not a prognostic factor in the LMB studies, whereas in most of the other studies it was (Muller-Weihrich *et al.*, 1985; Murphy *et al.*, 1986). A variety of prognostic factors are being evaluated prospectively in Stage III and IV patients in the current cooperative SFOP–UKCCSG study.

One of the aims of decreasing treatment is to decrease long-term sequelae such as infertility, especially in boys. Cyclophosphamide given above a cumulative dose of 9 g/m² produces male sterility (Aubier *et al.*, 1989), so reaching this dosage should be avoided, at least for patients who have no bad prognostic factors. In fact, it would be preferable not to exceed 5 g/m² for there are individual susceptibilities, and factors such as age at treatment or modality of drug administration remain undetermined. Some protocols no longer use cyclophosphamide – as in the current UKCC-SG 90 study for B-cell Stage I and II – but others prefer to give a low dose (3 g/m²) as in the French study already discussed, in order to avoid the risk of relapse. The POG group, conversely, have opted to omit doxorubicin because of potential cardiotoxicity.

11.10.4 HOW SHOULD POST TRANSPLANT B CELL NON-HODGKIN'S LYMPHOMA BE MANAGED?

With the increasing use of organ transplantation, there is an awareness of both polyclonal and monoclonal B cell lymphomas developing in patients profoundly immunosuppressed by high dose cyclosporin. Such patients, usually recipients of cardiac or renal transplants, will develop 'high grade' tumours which are histologically indistinguishable from true malignant disease (Swinnen *et al.*, 1990). In some patients there may be a clear viral pathogen, such as EBV, in which case a polyclonal tumour may be demonstrable.

The outcome of these tumours is generally good, and with reduction or cessation of cyclosporin they often resolve spontaneously (Starzyl *et al.*, 1984). However, in a number of patients the disease will be more aggressive and may require therapy.

11.10.5 IS THERE A ROLE FOR TUMOUR-SPECIFIC TARGETED THERAPY IN B CELL NON-HODGKIN'S LYMPHOMA?

Monoclonal antibody targeted therapy for B cell lymphomas in adults has produced encouraging results with significant cytoreduction in chemoresistant patients (Press *et al.*, 1989; Scheinberg *et al.*, 1990). This has not yet been extensively evaluated in paediatric practice but may well have a role. An innovative approach is the use of the antisense oligonucleotides to inhibit c-*myc* oncogene amplification (Lancet, 1990).

C.R.P.

REFERENCES

Al-Attar, A., Attra, A., Al-Bagdadi, R. *et al.* (1989) 'Debulking' surgery is unnecessary in advanced abdominal Burkitt's lymphoma in Iraq. *Br. J. Cancer*, **59**, 610–12.

Anderson, J.R., Wilson, J.F., Jenkin, D.T. *et al.* (1983) Childhood non Hodgkin's lymphoma:

results of a randomised therapeutic trial comparing a 4 drug regimen (COMP) to a 10 drug regimen (LSA2L2). *N. Engl. J. Med.*, **308**, 559–65.

Aubier, F., Flamant, F., Brauner, R. *et al.* (1989) Male gonadal function after chemotherapy for solid tumors in children. *J. Clin. Oncol.*, **7**, 304–9.

Benz-Lemoine, E., Leverger, G., Bancillon, A. *et al.* (1988) Treatment of thoracic lymphoblastic lymphoma and acute lymphoblastic leukemia (ALL) with mediastinal mass. Results of 'high-risk FRALLE 83 protocol in 67 children. *Med. Ped. Oncol.*, (16): 386 (abstract).

Bergeron, C., Patte, C., Caillaud, J.M. *et al.* (1989) Aspects cliniques, anatomo-pathologiques et résultats thérapeutiques de 63 lymphomes malins non Hodgkiniens ORL de l'enfant. *Arch. Fr. Pediatr.*, **46**, 583–7.

Bernard, A., Boumsell, L., Bayle, C. *et al.*, (1979) Subsets of malignant lymphomas in children related to the cell phenotype. *Blood*, **54**, 1058–68.

Bernard, A., Boumsell, L., Patte, C. and Lemerle, J. (1986) Leukemia versus lymphoma in children. A worthless question? *Med. Ped. Oncol.*, **14**, 148–57.

Bernard, A., Murphy, S., Melvin, S. *et al.* (1982) Non-T non-B lymphomas are rare in children and associated with cutaneous tumors. *Blood*, **59**, 549–54.

Borsi, J.D. and Moe, P.J. (1987) A comparative study on the pharmacokinetics of methotrexate in a dose range of 0.5 g to 33.6 g/m² in children with acute lymphoblastic leukemia. *Cancer*, **60**, 5–13.

Bowman, W.P., Shuster, J., Cook, B. *et al.* (1990) Results of treatment for advanced stage (IV) diffuse small non-cleaved cell non-Hodgkins (NHL) lymphomas and B(SIg+) cell acute lymphoblastic leukemia (ALL): The Pediatric Oncology Group (POG) Experience, 1986–89. Fourth International Conference on Malignant Lymphoma. Lugano (abstract).

Coppes, M.J., Patte, C., Couanet, D. *et al.* (1991) Childhood malignant lymphoma of bone. *Med. Ped. Oncol.*, **19**, 22–7.

Croce, C.M. and Nowell, P.C. (1985) Molecular basis of human B-cell neoplasia. *Blood*, **65**, 1.

Dahl, G.V., Rivera, G., Pui, C.H. *et al.* (1985) A novel treatment of childhood lymphoblastic non-Hodgkin's lymphoma: early and intermittent use of teniposide plus cytarabine. *Blood*, **66**, 110–14.

Dluzniewska, A., Depowska, T. and Armata, J. (1985) 'Smouldering' and symptomatic forms of central nervous system involvement in the course of non-Hodgkin's lymphoma in children. *Folia Haematol.*, Leipzig, **112**, 241–7.

Falcon, M. and Isaacson, P.G. (1990) Histological classification of the Non-Hodgkin's lymphoma. *Blood Review*, **4**, 111–15.

Finlay, J.L., Trigg, M.E., Link, M.P. and Friedrich, S. (1989) Poor risk non-lymphoblastic lymphoma of childhood. Results of an intensive pilot study. *Med. Pediatr. Oncol.*, **17**, 29–38.

Fleming, I.D., Turk, P.S., Murphy, S.B. *et al.* (1990) Surgical implications of primary gastrointestinal lymphoma of childhood. *Arch. Surg.*, **125**(2), 252–6.

Gad-El-Mawla, N., Hussein, M.H., Abdel-Hadi, S. *et al.* (1989) Childhood non-Hodgkin's lymphoma in Egypt: preliminary results of treatment with a new ifosfamide-containing regimen. *Cancer Chemother. Pharmacol.*, **24** (Suppl), 520–523.

Gasparini, M., Rottoli, L., Gianni, C. *et al.* (1987) Intensive short-term chemotherapy for advanced childhood Burkitt-type non-Hodgkin's lymphoma (B-NHL). Proceedings of the Third International Conference on Malignant Lymphoma, Lugano, abstract No.47, p. 44.

Gentet, J.C., Patte, C., Quintana, E. *et al.* (1990) Phase II study of cytarabine and etoposide in children with refractory or relapsed non-Hodgkin's lymphoma: a study of the French Society of Pediatric Oncology. *J. Clin. Oncol.*, **8**, 661–5.

Grierson, H. and Purtillo, D.T. (1987) Epstein-Barr virus infections in males with the X-linked lymphoproliferative syndrome. *Ann. Int. Med.*, **106**, 538–45.

Hann, I.M., Eden, O.B., Barnes, J. and Pinkerton, C.R. (1988) MACHO chemotherapy for Stage IV B cell lymphoma and B cell acute lymphoblastic leukemia of childhood. *Br. J. Haem.*, **76**, 359–64.

Hartmann, O., Pein, F., Beaujean, F. *et al.* (1984) High dose polychemotherapy with autologous bone marrow transplantation in children with relapsed lymphomas. *J. Clin. Oncol.*, **2**, 979–85.

Hecht, F., Morgan, R., Gemmill, R.M. *et al.* (1985) Translocations in T-cell leukemia and lymphoma. *N. Engl. J. Med.*, **313**, 758.

Helardot, P.G., Wakim, A., Kalifa, C. *et al.* (1989)
The place of surgery in the remission assessment of childhood abdominal malignant non Hodgkin's lymphoma (NHL). *Med. Ped. Oncol.,* **17**, 322 (abstract).

Janus, C., Edwards, B.K., Sariban, E. and Magrath, I.T. (1984) Surgical resection and limited chemotherapy for abdominal undifferentiated lymphomas. *Cancer Treat. Rep.,* **68**, 599–605.

Jenkin, R.D.T., Anderson, J.R., Chilcote, R.R. *et al.* (1984) The treatment of localized non-Hodgkin's lymphoma in children: a report from the children's cancer study group. *J. Clin. Oncol.,* **2**, 88–97.

Ladjaj, Y., Philip, T., Lenoir, G.M. *et al.* (1984) Abdominal Burkitt-type lymphomas in Algeria (a report of 49 cases). *Brit. J. Cancer,* **49**, 503–12.

Leblanc, A., Caillaud, J.M., Hartmann, O. *et al.* (1984) Hypercalcemia preferentially occurs in unusual forms of childhood non-Hodgkin's lymphoma, rhabdomyosarcoma, and Wilms' tumor. *Cancer,* **54**, 2132–6.

Lemerle, J., Bernard, A., Patte, C. and Plo, J.K. (1986) Malignant B cell lymphoma of childhood, in *Cancer in Children, Clinical Management 2nd edn.* (eds A. Barrett, H.J.G. Bloom, J. Lemerle *et al.*) UICC Handbook, Springer, Berlin pp. 137–51.

Lennert, K. (1981) Lymphomas of high-grade malignancy, in *Histopathology on Non Hodgkin's Lymphomas.* Springer, Berlin, pp. 72–102.

Lenoir, G. O'Connor, G. and Olweny, C.L.M. (1985) Burkitt's lymphoma. A human cancer model. Lyon, *IARC* Scientific Publications No.60.

Link, M.P., Donaldson, S.S., Berard, C.W. *et al.* (1990) Results of treatment of childhood localized non-Hodgkin's lymphoma with combination chemotherapy with or without radiotherapy. *N. Engl. J. Med.,* **322**, 1769–74.

Lippens, R.J. and Winograd, B. (1988) Methotrexate concentration levels in the cerebrospinal fluid during high dose methotrexate infusions: an unreliable prediction. *Ped. Hemat. Oncol.,* **5**, 1145.

Meadows, A.T., Sposto, R., Jenkin, R.D.T. *et al.* (1989) Similar efficacy of 6 and 18 months of therapy with four drugs (COMP) for localized non-Hodgkin's lymphoma of children: A report

from the Children Cancer Study Group. *J. Clin. Oncol.,* **7**, 92–9.

Mott, M.G., Eden, O.B. and Palmer, M.K. (1984) Adjuvant low dose radiation in childhood non-Hodgkin's lymphoma. *Br. J. Cancer,* **50**, 463–9.

Muller-Weihrich, S.E., Henze, G., Odenwald, E. and Riehm, H. (1985) BFM trials for childhood non-Hodgkin's lymphoma, in *Malignant Lymphomas and Hodgkin's Disease* (eds F. Cavalli, G. Bonadonna and G. Rosencwei) Experimental and therapeutic advances. Martinus Nijhoff, Boston, pp. 633–42.

Muller-Weihrich, S.T., Ludwig, R., Reiter, A. *et al.* (1987) B-type non Hodgkin's lymphomas and leukemia: the BFM study group experience. Lugano, Proceedings of the Conference on Malignant Lymphoma, 42.

Murphy, S.B. (1980) Classification, staging and end results of treatment of childhood non-Hodgkin's lymphoma: Dissimilarities from lymphomas in adults. *Semin. Oncol.,* **7**, 332–9.

Murphy, S.B., Bowman, W.P., Abromowitch, M. *et al.* (1986) Results of treatment of advanced-stage Burkitt's lymphoma and B cell (SIg+) acute lymphoblastic leukemia with high-dose fractionated cyclophosphamide and coordinated high-dose methotrexate and cytarabine. *J. Clin. Oncol.,* **4**, 1732–9.

Murphy, S.B., Fairclough, D.L., Hutchison, R.E. and Berard, C.W. (1989) Non-Hodgkin's lymphomas of childhood: an analysis of the histology, staging, and response to treatment of 338 cases at a single institution. *J. Clin. Oncol.,* **7**, 186–93.

Nathamani, B.N., Kim, H., Rappaport, H. *et al.* (1978) Non Hodgkin's lymphoma: a clinicopathologic study comparing two classifications. *Cancer,* **41**, 303–25.

National Cancer Institute sponsored study of classification of non-Hodgkin's lymphomas: summary and description of a working formulation for clinical usage. (1982) *Cancer,* **49**, 2112–35.

Otten, J., Benoit, Y., Casteels-Vandaele, M. *et al.* (1981) Non-Hodgkin's lymphoma in children. A preliminary report of a study by the Belgian Cooperative Group for the treatment of solid tumours in children. *Acta. Pediatr. Belg.,* **34**, 157–64.

Patte, C., Bernard, A., Hartmann, O. *et al.* (1986a) High dose methotrexate and continuous infusion Ara-C in children's non Hodgkin's lymphoma. *Pediatr. Hematol. Oncol.* **3**, 11–18.

Patte, C., Gerard-Marchant, R., Caillou, B. *et al.* (1981a) Les lymphomes malins non hodgkiniens de l'enfant. Aspects pratiques. *Arch. Fr. Pediatr.* **28**, 359–67.

Patte, C., Kalifa, C., Flamant, F. *et al.* (1991a) Results of the LMT81 protocol, a modified LSA2L2 protocol with high dose methotrexate, on 84 children with non B-cell lymphoma. (In press).

Patte, C., Leverger, G., Perel, Y. *et al.* (for the SFOP) (1990) Updated results of the LMB 86 protocol of the French Pediatric Oncology Society (SFOP) for B-cell non Hodgkin's lymphoma (B-NHL) with CNS involvement (CNS+) and B-ALL. *Med. Ped. Oncol.*, **18**, 397.

Patte, C., Philip, T., Rodary, C. *et al.* (1986b) Improved survival rate in children with stage III and IV B-cell non Hodgkin's lymphoma and leukemia using a multiagent chemotherapy: results of a study of 114 children from the French Pediatric Oncology Society. *J. Clin. Oncol.*, **4**, 1219–29.

Patte, C., Philip, T., Rodary, C. *et al.* (for the SFOP) (1988) Updated results of the protocol LMB 84 of the French Pediatric Oncology Society (SFOP): randomized study to shorten duration of treatment of advanced stage B-cell non-Hodgkin's lymphoma (NHL) without CNS involvement. *Med. Ped. Oncol.*, **16**, 406 (abstract).

Patte, C., Philip, T., Rodary, C. *et al.* (1991b) High survival rate in advanced stage B-cell lymphomas and leukemias without CNS involvement with a short intensive polychemotherapy. Results of a randomized trial from the French Pediatric Oncology Society (SFOP) on 216 children. *J. Clin. Oncol.*, **9**, 123–32.

Patte, C., Rodary, C., Sarrazin, D. *et al.* (1981b) Résultats du traitement de 178 lymphomes malins non hodgkiniens de l'enfant de 1973 à 1978. *Arch. Fr. Ped.*, **38**, 321–7.

Philip, T., Biron, P. and Herve, P. (1983) Massive BACT therapy with autologous bone marrow transplantation in 17 cases of non Hodgkin's lymphomas with a very bad prognosis. *Eur. J. Cancer*, **19**, 1379–83.

Philip, T., Hartmann, O., Biron, P. *et al.* (1988) High-dose therapy and autologous bone marrow transplantation in partial remission after first-line induction therapy for diffuse non-Hodgkin's lymphoma. *J. Clin. Oncol.*, **6**, 1118–24.

Philip, T., Pinkerton, R., Biron, P. *et al.* (1987) Effective multiagent chemotherapy in children with advanced B-cell lymphoma: Who remains the high risk patient? *Brit. J. Haematol.*, **65**, 159–64.

Philip, T., Pinkerton, R., Hartmann, O. *et al.* (1986) The role of massive therapy with autologous bone marrow transplantation in Burkitt's lymphoma. *Clinics in Haematol.*, **15**(1), 205–17.

Pichler, E., Jurgensen, O., Radaskiewicz, T. *et al.* (1982) Results of LSA2L2 therapy in 26 children with non-Hodgkin's lymphoma. *Cancer*, **50**, 2740–6.

Press, O.W., Eary, J.F., Badger, C.C. *et al.* (1989) Treatment of refractory non-Hodgkin's lymphoma with radiolabelled MB-1 (anti-CD37) antibody. *J. Clin. Oncol.*, **7**(8), 1027–38.

Pullen, D.J., Sullivan, M.P., Falletta, J.M. *et al.* (1982) Modified LSA2L2 treatment in 53 children with E-rosette positive T-cell leukemia: results and prognostic factors (a pediatric oncology group study). *Blood*, **60**, 1159–68.

Reiter, A., Sauter, S., Kabisch, H. *et al.* (1989) Probability for cure as related to therapy in childhood B-type acute lymphoblastic leukemia (B-ALL) in three consecutive BFM trials. *Med. Ped. Oncol.*, **17**, 321 (abstract SIOP).

Rivera-Luna, R., Martinez-Guerra, G., Borrego-Roman, R. and Rivera-Marquez, H. (1986) Burkitt's lymphoma. Experience at the Instituto Nacional de Pediatria. Mexico City. *Am. J. Pediatr. Hermatol. Oncol.*, **8**(3), 183–90.

Rodary, C., Philip, T., Pinkerton, R. *et al.* (for the SFOP) (1988) B-cell non-Hodgkin's lymphoma with abdominal involvement: prognostic value of stage IIIA and IIIB in the SFOP series. *Med. Ped. Oncol.*, SIOP (16): 6 (abstract).

Scheinberg, D.A., Straus, D.J., Yeh, S.D. *et al.* (1990) A Phase I toxicity, pharmacology, and dosimetry trial of monoclonal antibody OKB7 in patients with non-Hodgkin's lymphoma: effects of tumor burden and antigen expression. *J. Clin. Oncol.*, **8**(5), 792–803.

Stansfeld, A.G., Diebold, J., Kapanci, Y. *et al.* (1988) Updated Kiel classification for lymphomas. *Lancet*, **1**, 293–4.

Starzyl, T.E., Porter, K.A., Iwatsuki, S. *et al.* (1984) Reversibility of lymphomas and lymphoproliferative lesions developing under cyclosporin-steroid therapy. *Lancet*, **1**, 583.

Sullivan, M., Boyett, J., Pullen, J. *et al.* (1985)

Pediatric oncology group experience with modified LSA2L2 therapy in 107 children with non Hodgkin's lymphoma (Burkitt's lymphoma excluded). *Cancer*, **55**, 323–36.

Sullivan, M.P. and Ramirez, I. (1985) Curability of Burkitt's lymphoma with high-dose cyclophosphamide – high-dose methotrexate therapy and intrathecal chemoprophylaxis. *J. Clin. Oncol.*, **3**, 627–35.

Swinnen, L.J., Costanzo-Nordin, M.R., Fisher, S.G. *et al.* (1990) Increased incidence of lymphoproliferative disorder after immunosuppression with the monoclonal antibody OKT3 in cardiactransplant recipients. *N. Engl. J. Med.*, **323**, 1723–8.

Tabbane, S., Tabbanz, F., Cammoun, H. and Mourali, N. (1976) Mediterranean lymphomas with heavy chain monoclonal gammapathy. *Cancer*, **38**, 1989–96.

Vassal, G., Valteau, D., Bonnay, M. *et al.* (1990) Cerebrospinal fluid and plasma methotrexate levels following high-dose regimen given as a 3-hour intravenous infusion in children with non Hodgkin's lymphoma. *Pediatr. Hematol. Oncol.*, **7**, 71–7.

Vecchi, V., Pession, A., Serra, L. *et al.* (1981) Non-Hodgkin's lymphoma in children: results of treatment with the modified LSA2L2 protocol. *Med. Ped. Oncol.*, **9**, 483–91.

Wakim, A., Helardot, P.G. and Sapin, E. (1989) The surgeon facing malignant non-Hodgkin's lymphoma of the abdomen in children. *Chir. Pediatr.*, **30**(5), 197–200.

Wheeler, K. and Chessells, J.M. (1990) UKALL X – an effective treatment for Stage III mediastinal non-Hodgkin's lymphoma. *Arch. Dis. Child.*, **65**, 252–4.

Wollner, N., Burchenal, J.H., Lieberman, P.H. *et al.* (1976) Non Hodgkin's lymphoma in children, a comparative study of two modalities of therapy. *Cancer*, **37**, 123–34.

Wollner, N., Exelby, P.R. and Lieberman, P.H. (1979) Non Hodgkin's lymphoma in children. A progress report on the original patients treated with the LSA2L2 protocol. *Cancer*, **44**, 1990–9.

Young, J.L. and Miller, R.W. (1975) Incidence of malignant tumors in US children. *J. Pediatr.*, **86**, 254–8.

(1990) Molecular targets for cancer therapy. *Lancet*, **1**, 826.

Chapter 12

Hodgkin's disease

O. OBERLIN and H.P. McDOWELL

12.1 AETIOLOGY AND EPIDEMIOLOGY

Despite the advances in molecular and cellular biology which have yielded increasing information concerning Hodgkin's disease, the cell of origin of this disease remains unclear, as does its aetiology.

The true nature of Hodgkin's disease may still be obscure but its neoplastic behaviour was finally demonstrated by cytogenetic studies which exhibited the aneuploidy and the clonality of the giant cells, Reed Sternberg and Hodgkin cells, which are now accepted as the tumoral population in Hodgkin's lymphoma.

The possible progenitor for these cells is still unknown and there is in fact no cell lineage in the haematolymphoid system that has not been suggested as being the nonmalignant precursor of these malignant cells (T- or B-cells, macrophage/histiocytes, interdigitating cells, dendritic cells, antigen-presenting cells, granulocytic cells). However, the majority agree with the view that Hodgkin and Reed Sternberg cells are lymphocytic in origin and may be related to either T-or B-cells, are phenotypically heterogeneous, and resemble activated T- or B-cells in a differentiated stage (Stein *et al.*, 1989).

The cause of Hodgkin's disease (or perhaps we should say, causes) remains unknown; reports of case clustering among relatives of patients or student groups suggests an environmental or infectious aetiology (Alexander *et al.*, 1989). There are several arguments for a role for Epstein-Barr virus (EBV) infection: in advanced socioeconomic countries, Hodgkin's disease is more prevalent in patients with a preceding history of infectious mononucleosis and antibody titres against various antigens of the Epstein-Barr virus are found to be elevated in the serum from these patients (Levine *et al.*, 1971). There is now evidence that Reed Sternberg cells harbour the EBV genome in more than 50% of cases (Stein, 1990).

The present hypothesis for the pathogenesis of Hodgkin's disease is that of a chronic antigen stimulation and EBV seems to be involved in a significant number of cases (Mueller, 1990). The gene rearrangement occurring secondarily to chronic stimulation may result in the expression or amplification of normal genes controlling the production of cytokines which are responsible for the presence of non malignant cells around Hodgkin and Reed Sternberg cells.

Although Hodgkin's disease is less common than non-Hodgkin's lymphoma (NHL) among patients with congenital or acquired immunodeficiencies, in recent years there have been four cases in children with ataxia-

Table 12.1 Age and sex distribution of 220 children with Hodgkin's disease included in the first French cooperative study

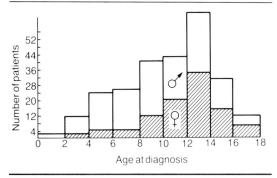

telangiectasia reported to the registration office of the French study for paediatric Hodgkin's disease.

No clear relation exists between Hodgkin's disease and particular distribution of HLA histocompatibility antigens HLA A1, B5 and B15 (Svejgraad *et al.*, 1975). There are some data indicating an increased risk of developing the disease for parents and siblings in the same family which could indicate either environmental or genetic influence (Grufferman *et al.*, 1979).

Reported annual incidences of Hodgkin's disease in one British and one US registry are 3.6 and 5.7 per million children (Young and Miller, 1975; Birch *et al.*, 1980). The age-specific incidence curve is bi-modal with one peak in young adults 15–30 years, and the

second at 45–55 years. Paediatric cases represent the beginning of the first peak and explain the increased incidence with advancing age through childhood. The disease is uncommon before five years and very rare under two years of age (Table 12.1).

In underdeveloped countries, the pattern of incidence is somewhat different in that Hodgkin's disease occurs more frequently among young children less than 10 years, and gives further support to the theory that an infective agent has an aetiological role in this disease.

With progressing age, the sex ratio male: female incidence changes, being 10:1 under 7 years of age, with the male preponderance falling as low as 1.1 after the age of 12 years (Table 12.2).

12.2 PATHOLOGY

A correct diagnosis is only possible with adequate tissue samples from an open surgical nodal biopsy. Needle biopsies and frozen section material are not suitable for the examination of lymph node architecture and the stromal cellular elements.

Central to the diagnosis of Hodgkin's disease is the identification of the characteristic Reed Sternberg cell: large multinucleated giant cells with inclusion-like nucleoli surrounded by a clear halo. Variants of the Reed Sternberg cell may exist such as the mononuclear Hodgkin's cell or a lacunar Reed Sternberg cell, the latter one being character-

Table 12.2 Sex ratio, stages, mediastinal involvement and histology by age group in HD

	Total	<7 years	8–11 years	>12 years
No.	220	39	74	107
Sex ratio m:f	2	10	2.6	1.1
Stages I and II	72%	77%	75%	69%
Mediastinal involvement	56%	39%	46%	70%
Histology:				
nodular sclerosis	35.5%	16%	29%	47%
mixed cellularity	45.5%	64%	49%	36%

istic of nodular sclerosing Hodgkin's disease. The presence of these cells alone, although necessary for diagnosis, is not sufficient for a histological diagnosis of Hodgkin's disease since cells of similar appearance may also be found in reactive processes, infectious mononucleosis, phenytoin-induced 'pseudolymphoma', rubeola, graft versus host reactions and even NHL.

The lymph node architecture is usually disorganized by the accumulation of reactive cells: lymphocytes of various sizes, histiocytes, eosinophils, plasma cells and fibroblasts. Collagen bands or diffuse fibrosis are the two different types of connective tissue proliferation. The relative proportions of Reed Sternberg cells, lymphocytes, and both sclerosis and fibrosis are taken into account when using the Rye histopathological classification (Lukes *et al.*, 1966).

The frequency of the different histological subtypes varies according to different paediatric series. These discrepancies may be due in part to the lack of comparability with respect to age and sex distribution but may also be due to disagreement concerning histopathologic interpretation among the various pathologists concerned (Table 12.3).

Certain patterns of disease are consistent with their histological subtype. The lymphocytic type is often associated with localized cervical or inguinal disease, whilst nodular sclerosis commonly presents with mediastinal involvement in the adolescent age group. Mixed cellularity and the rare cases of lymphocyte depletion may be associated with a more diffuse disease occurring above and below the diaphragm.

The introduction of an effective multimodal therapy in the treatment of Hodgkin's disease has erased the previous prognostic difference between the two more frequent types: nodular sclerosis and mixed cellularity. However, clinical and pathological experience over the past two decades suggests that the two original subtypes of lymphocyte (nodular and diffuse) predominant forms proposed by Lukes and Butler (1966) should be distinguished, as the nodular form presents at a single nodal site, and even without therapy progresses extremely slowly over a period of many years. A proportion of these patients may later develop either another type of Hodgkin's disease, or large cell non-Hodgkin's lymphoma, even if untreated (Trudel *et al.*, 1987).

Cytogenetic studies have so far failed to identify a constant change of karyotype although a number of chromosomes, including 1, 2, 7, 11, 14, 15 and 21, have exhibited alterations which are considered to be nonrandom. Two of these chromosomes, 7 and 11, have also been observed to be abnormal in secondary leukaemias and the question arises whether a genetically determined chromosome instability is inherent in

Table 12.3 Distribution of various histologic subtypes in children with Hodgkin's disease

Series	No. of patients	Lymphocytic predominance %	Nodular sclerosis %	Mixed cellularity %	Lymphocyte depletion %	Unclassified %
Stanford	55	9	62	20	2	7
Australia	53	11	68	17	4	–
Memphis	88	12.5	33	34	20.5	–
Turkey	40	7.5	17.5	67.5	7.5	–
France	220	10.5	35.5	45.5	0.5	8

Data from Donaldson and Link, 1987; Ekert *et al.*, 1988; Smith and Rivera, 1976; Cavdar *et al.*, 1977; French unpublished study.

patients with Hodgkin's disease (Fonatsch *et al.*, 1989).

12.3 CLINICAL PRESENTATION AND STAGING MODES

Painless cervical lymphadenopathy is the most frequent presenting symptom (in 80% of children), often with a pain-free and fluctuating course which causes a delay in diagnosis. About 60% have concomitant mostly asymptomatic involvement of the mediastinum; disease limited to the mediastinum, however, is very rare (1%), as confirmed in our French series.

An evaluation of constitutional symptoms such as those described in Table 12.4 should be made. The presence of one of these symptoms is of prognostic significance and confers a disease classification 'B' in the staging procedure. B symptoms were noted in 32% of the children registered in the French study. Their frequency increases with advanced stages of the disease (5% in Stage I, 28% in Stage II, 64% in Stage III and 81% in Stage IV). In terms of diagnosis, isolated splenomegaly, hepatomegaly or symptoms relating to lung or pleural involvement often pose the most difficult challenges.

12.3.1 CLINICAL STAGING PROCEDURES

On the basis of past experience, the goal of a detailed staging procedure at diagnosis is to tailor treatment to the extent of the disease.

Table 12.4 Constitutional symptoms in the Ann Arbor classification

Presence of unexplained fever
Night sweats
Unexplained loss of 10% or more of body weight in the 6 months before admission
No constitutional symptoms = A; one or more of these = B

(a) Initial physical examination

This should include careful evaluation of all peripheral nodal areas. Doubtful nodes should be explored by cytology or even biopsy if disease in that site leads to a change of stage and/or therapy. Evaluation of the liver and spleen can be difficult as they are often normally palpable in young children. However, abnormal clinical findings for the most part are in concordance with those ascertained using imaging techniques.

(b) Thoracic imaging

Mediastinal involvement is present in around 60% of cases but this incidence varies with age from 40% before eight years to 70% after 12 years (Table 12.2). Posteroanterior and lateral chest x-rays evaluate mediastinal involvement, but CT scan has replaced conventional tomography and is now essential for recognizing lymphatic spread to the diaphragmatic region, and extralymphatic extension to the pericardium, pleura or pulmonary parenchyma. To evaluate the response to therapy, serial CTs are also used; the impact of this procedure, however, still has to be evaluated.

CT scanning now detects previously unevaluated mediastinal disease and this may result in some patients receiving mediastinal irradiation when, in the past, no mediastinal irradiation gave the same outcome.

Gallium scanning has been readopted as an imaging tool to delineate mediastinal involvement. Comparison with CT scanning shows it to have a lower false positive rate and despite the possibility of false negativity either at diagnosis or at relapse it is useful in assessing response to treatment (Drossman *et al.*, 1990). The role of radiolabelled monoclonal antibody imaging and magnetic resonance imaging are still awaiting definition.

Both clinical and radiological examination

are required to exclude nasopharyngeal and oropharyngeal disease. Any suspicious areas should be biopsied to confirm the diagnosis, especially as disease involving Waldeyer's ring is exceptionally uncommon (only one case out of 220 children in our series).

(c) Abdominal investigation

Discussion concerning the most efficacious way of abdominal lymph node imaging in children continues. Correlation between the results of lymphography and of histological examination is excellent with a 95% accuracy rate (Dunnick *et al.*, 1977). In centres with expertise in lymphangiography, the success rate is similar to that with adults. General anaesthesia is necessary for the procedure to be carried out in very young children and patients with massive mediastinal and pulmonary involvement should be excluded from this procedure because of a high risk of morbidity.

Abdomino-pelvic CT scans in children are an easier and less invasive procedure than lymphangiography but results of studies comparing lymphangiography with CT scan in surgically staged children are still awaited. Only lymphangiography can evaluate both the size and abnormal architecture of pelvic and para-aortic lymph nodes. In the presence of enlargement, the abnormalities in architecture may be the only means to differentiate Hodgkin's disease from reactive hyperplasia: 'foamy' reticular pattern filling defects correlate with histological lymphomatous infiltration. Pathological nodes of normal size, missed by CT scan, may be detected using lymphangiography. CT scan would appear to be complementary to lymphangiography since it can visualize the enlarged nodes of the coeliac axis, porta hepatis, splenic pedicle and mesenteric nodes. In some rare cases, with negative lymphangiography, abdominal involvement can be detected only by CT scan.

Ultrasonic imaging is also non-invasive, relatively simple to carry out, inexpensive, and, in expert hands, reliable. Visualization of the same nodal areas as seen on CT scan can be carried out, but in addition a high degree of accuracy in the determination of splenic size and intrahepatic masses can be obtained. It remains a useful tool in the follow-up of patients provided that a baseline investigation is done at diagnosis.

12.3.2 SURGICAL STAGING PROCEDURES

Should surgery play a role in staging at all? Advocates for surgery argue that accurate anatomical verification of disease extent is obtained that is unavailable by the investigations described above; this can alter the clinical stage of approximately one-third of the patients with localized disease IA-IIA with the finding of occult subdiaphragmatic involvement (Andrieu *et al.*, 1981; Russell *et al.*, 1984). Historically, surgery was essential in order to calculate radiation fields when radiotherapy was the only mode of therapy and in itself this improved the relapse-free survival rate of children (Russell *et al.*, 1984).

Laparotomy is, however, a major surgical procedure, requiring the assessment of all the lymph node region of the abdomen. It is painful, costly, and delays the beginning of the treatment. Moreover, all surgical procedures are not without risk to the patient. Although perioperative mortality or severe morbidity, in experienced hands, is minimal, there is the late post-operative complication of intestinal obstruction: a 1 to 10% incidence as reviewed by Jenkin and Berry (1980).

Serious regard should also be given to the risk of overwhelming postsplenectomy sepsis. A review of the data from four large series of patients splenectomized for Hodgkin's disease and lymphoma reveals an incidence rate of serious bacterial infection ranging from 1 to 10%, with a mortality from 0 to 5% (Desser and Ultmann, 1972; Rosenstock *et al.*, 1974;

Chilcote *et al.*, 1976; Donaldson *et al.*, 1978). In the Stanford experience, the rate of bacterial infection was related to the intensity of treatment and significantly increased when chemotherapy was given compared to radiotherapy alone (Donaldson *et al.*, 1978). Acquisition of antibody response following pneumococcal vaccination is variable, particularly in view of haste often needed to make a diagnosis and commence treatment (Siber *et al.*, 1978). Consequently, lifelong antibiotic prophylaxis against *Streptococcus pneumoniae* has been recommended for these patients. The exact role of vaccination against *Haemophilus influenzae* remains unclear; efficacious prophylaxis already exists in the form of rifampicin given after close contact.

The decision regarding the use of laparotomy relates directly to treatment options. When treatment with radiation alone is to be considered, laparotomy may be indicated but this option applies to a very limited group of children. On the other hand, if chemotherapy alone is used, an accurate evaluation of subdiaphragmatic disease may not be essential, and laparotomy has been avoided in an Australian study and by the UK group (Ekert *et al.*, 1988; Martin and Radford, 1989). Many investigators now recommend combined-modality treatment. In such programmes, comparison of the two staging strategies (clinical only or clinical plus surgical) before similar treatment (4–6 cycles of multiagent chemotherapy plus involved field radiotherapy) does not show any superiority of surgical staging versus clinical staging (Loeffler *et al.*, 1989).

The use of laparotomy has been abandoned in France since 1975. Although there is a risk of failing to detect subdiaphragmatic disease, the incidence of abdominal relapses in patients clinically staged IA-IIA and treated by chemotherapy before involved field radiation therapy is very low: 4.4% in an adult series (Andrieu *et al.*, 1981), 0% for 37 children treated with the MOPP regimen before involved field

radiotherapy (Oberlin *et al.*, 1985), 2% in a recent French cooperative study (Leverger *et al.*, 1990). Chemotherapy has thus cured radiologically non-apparent disease in the majority of this group of patients.

The Italian national group observed similarly good results in clinically staged patients (Vecchi *et al.*, 1988). Three consecutive German paediatric studies have, in a step by step fashion, reduced the indications of laparotomy and splenectomy. In the last study, indications were restricted to patients with abnormal abdominal imaging or enlargement of pulmonary hilar nodes (Brämswig *et al.*, 1990).

At Stanford, the previously routinely performed pathological staging during earlier paediatric studies is now omitted for patients: Stage IA with high cervical nodes of lymphocytic predominant histology, patients with positive lymphangiogram or with isolated mediastinal involvement or with Stage IV disease (Mefferd *et al.*, 1979). In the UK, irradiation alone is used for clinically staged high cervical Stage IA patients. Virtually all those with undetected disease are cured with subsequent chemotherapy (UKCCSG unpublished data).

The necessity to perform oophoropexy in girls before pelvic irradiation does not warrant systematic laparotomy and is not always necessary since iliac node involvement is rare (less than 10% of cases). If required, this procedure can be performed prior to radiation therapy in those who are to receive pelvic radiation.

(a) Search for extranodal involvement

In children, the differential diagnosis of multiple pulmonary parenchymal nodular lesions is seldom difficult although infection and Hodgkin's disease may coexist. Most commonly lung involvement is associated with mediastinal and hilar lymph adenopathies and a nodular sclerosing pathology.

In the presence of hepatomegaly, where distinct intrahepatic nodules are present, needle biopsy can be undertaken using radiographic guidance. However, unless atypical, these lesions can be clinically considered as lymphoma. In the case of diffuse hepatic enlargement, in accordance with the SIOP Study Group, a 'mini' laparotomy is adequate in order to inspect the organ, define the most likely regions involved, and to take an adequate biopsy. Possible microscopic involvement of the liver can remain undetected in patients clinically staged who have an apparently normal hepatic size. However, the now very rare liver relapses after combined treatment demonstrate the efficacy of chemotherapy to sterilize occult involvement.

In children, bone marrow involvement is infrequent: 3% in the French study. These patients were found to differ significantly from those without marrow involvement with regard to B symptoms, clinical stage, haemoglobin level and erythrocyte sedimentation rate. Bone marrow biopsies should therefore always be performed in the presence of advanced disease, systemic symptoms, abnormal blood count or local bone involvement. In the rare cases of bone involvement at diagnosis, lesions are usually located in the spine and the pelvis. Marrow involvement may be the single site of extranodal involvement and MRI seems to be a valuable non-invasive procedure to evaluate this (Schicha *et al.*, 1989). The initial status of the bone marrow should be assessed in order to pinpoint the potential cases who, in the event of relapse, may be candidates for high-dose chemotherapy with bone marrow rescue. Involvement of other extranodal sites (kidney, skin and central nervous system, for example) is seldom present at diagnosis.

Table 12.5 Recommendations for diagnostic work-up of children with Hodgkin's disease

---

1. Mandatory procedures
   Surgical biopsy reviewed by pathologist
   History with special attention to fever, sweating and weight loss
   Physical examination with cytology or biopsy of doubtful nodes
   Complete blood count and erythrocyte sedimentation rate
   Chest x-ray (postero-anterior and lateral views)
   Lymphangiogram or CT scan in the younger child

2. Required procedures under certain conditions
   Chest CT scan if mediastinal, hilar or pulmonary involvement is present or suspected
   Abdominal ultrasound or CT scan if lymphangiogram is equivocal
       or if the child has hepatomegaly
       or if he has splenomegaly or systemic symptoms with normal lymphangiogram
   Post nasal space x-ray if cervical nodes are involved
   Bone marrow biopsy if systemic symptoms are associated with Stage II-IV
   Liver biopsy if hepatomegaly is homogeneous
   Radioisotopic bone scan if Stage IV
   Pleural cytology if there is a pleural effusion

3. Promising research procedures
   Mediastinal Gallium 67 scan
   Mediastinal magnetic resonance imaging
   Interleukin-2 receptor and CD8 serum dosages

Table 12.6 Ann Arbor staging classification (Carbone *et al.* [1971] with the permission of the editor of *Cancer Research [Baltimore]*)

Stage I:	Involvement of a single lymph node region (I) or a single extralymphatic organ or site (IE)
Stage II:	Involvement of two or more lymph node regions on the same side of the diaphragm (II) or solitary involvement of an extralymphatic organ or site and of one or more lymph node regions on the same side of the diaphragm (IIE)
Stage III:	Involvement of lymph nodes regions on both sides of the diaphragm (III) which may be accompanied by localized involvement of extralymphatic organ or site (IIIE) or by involvement of the spleen (IIIS) or both (IIISE)
Stage IV:	Diffuse or disseminated involvement of one or more extralymphatic organs or tissues with or without associated lymph node enlargement

Table 12.5 summarizes the procedures for diagnostic work-up of children with HD. On completion of these diagnostic investigations, the stage of the disease can be assigned as shown in Table 12.6 according to the 'Ann Arbor Classification' (Carbone *et al.*, 1971).

The modality of staging influences the stage distribution of the patients and this is shown in Table 12.7. If staging is only clinical, the incidence of localized Stages (I and II) reaches 70%. When investigations include laparotomy, half of the children are in Stages I and II and one-third are Stage III. This distribution should be taken into account when comparing the intensity of treatment in children treated by a protocol stratified according to stage.

(b) Laboratory studies

Laboratory studies must include a complete blood count and measurement of erythrocyte sedimentation rate (ESR). Neutrophilia is frequently found and eosinophilia occurs in 15% of patients. Lymphopenia is a sign of advanced disease. An elevated ESR is closely related with stage and the presence of systemic symptoms; its prognostic importance was recognized early and highlighted in multivariate analysis (Tubiana *et al.*, 1984). However, the introduction of chemotherapy to many paediatric protocols and adaptation of treatment to stage and systemic symptoms has eliminated this prognostic tool.

Elevated serum copper levels have been

Table 12.7 Stage distribution according to the staging modality

Series	Staging	N	I	II	I+II	III	IV
Stanford	Pathological	55	15%	35%	50%	40%	11%
Memorial Hospital	Pathological	110	29%	33%	56%	32%	12%
German group	Pathological	170	24%	29%	53%	39%	8%
	Selective lap.	207	24%	36%	60%	31%	9%
Australia	Clinical	53	32%	40%	72%	19%	9%
France	Clinical	220	29%	43%	72%	18%	10%

Data from Donaldson and Link, 1987; Tan *et al.*, 1983; Brämswig *et al.*, 1990; Ekert *et al.*, 1988; personal data described (in adults) as a non-specific bio-chemical indicator, predominantly useful as a predictive indicator of relapse (Hrgovcic *et al.*, 1973).

Recent studies have shown that increased serum levels of interleukin-2 receptors and of CD8 antigen (a surface membrane component of suppressor/cytotoxic T cells) correlate with a poor prognosis. They are significantly higher in patients with advanced disease and with B symptoms but appear to be very important predictors even in multivariate analysis (Pui *et al.*, 1989).

12.4 TREATMENT METHODS

There is universal agreement that the cure for this disease should be attained utilizing the minimum amount of therapy. Progress in this respect is due to a review of past clinical experience. Appropriate treatment depends both on the extent of the disease and the age of the patient since despite the similarity of the disease between adults and children it is now obvious that the sequelae of therapy, and especially those of radiotherapy, are of paramount importance in children. The therapeutic regimens that will enable this goal to be attained remain the subject of hot debate.

12.4.1 RADIOTHERAPY

Kaplan (1970) was the first to point out that a radiation dose ranging from 40 Gy to 44 Gy was the optimal tumoricidal dose to cure Hodgkin's lymphoma. He also described the definition of the fields to treat multiple lymph node chains in continuity thus avoiding junctions within the field and the risk of overlapping in that plane. The 'mantle field' includes all the main lymph node chains above the diaphragm: the two cervical and supraclavicular areas, the two axillar areas and the mediastinum with lung hilus. The 'inverted Y field' encompasses all the major abdominal

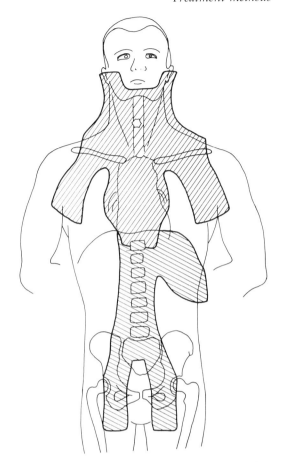

Fig. 12.1 Total nodal irradiation – mantle field and inverted Y.

lymph nodal chains: para-aortic, iliac and inguinal lymph nodes, spleen extension often being added. These two fields require a single junction and represent the so-called TNI (total nodal irradiation) method (Fig. 12.1).

Extended field radiotherapy covers the treatment of apparently uninvolved lymphatic regions and the extent of the field varies greatly from study to study and from stage to stage. For a cervical Stage II, for example, it may encompass the ipsilateral axillary areas or a complete mantle or even a complete mantle and a lumbosplenic field (Fig. 12.2).

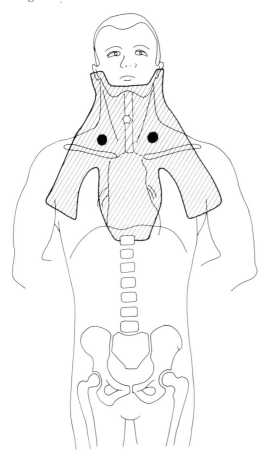

Fig. 12.2 An example of an extended field for cervical Stage II.

'Involved fields' should be employed only for treatment limited to the involved lymph node chain. However, the definition of 'involved' field varies from one group of workers to another: our group, for example, do not consider that the axillary area constitutes an anatomic continuity to be irradiated if only cervical nodes are involved (Figs. 12.3a and 12.4a); this is contrary to that defined at the Rye symposium which concluded that if cervical, infraclavicular or axillar nodes are involved, all three regions should be treated (Figs. 12.3b and 12.4b). We consider bilateral radiation of the neck in unilateral disease

only indicated to avoid later cosmetic problems of asymmetry. In the French study, the limited fields employed also varied in single node disease (Fig. 12.5).

The late effects of high-dose radiotherapy are now well recognized as a result of the increasing number of cured patients and the longer follow-up times. These effects correlate closely to the dose, the fields irradiated, and the age at the time of treatment, being more detrimental when delivered to younger patients. Radiation induces soft-tissue and skeletal growth impairment that may result in abnormally short sitting heights and standing heights (Donaldson *et al.*, 1988). A mantle field results in a thin chin and neck, a narrow chest with short clavicles and high spinal kyphosis (Fig. 12.6). These so-called cosmetic deficits severely impair the quality of life of these children when they have grown into young adults.

The most frequent radiation-induced thyroid dysfunction, occurring in two-thirds of children, is compensated chemical hypothyroidism with elevated thyroid-stimulating hormone (TSH) and normal free thyroxine (T4). Depressed thyroxine values are less frequent (less than 20%) (Kaplan *et al.*, 1983). Controversies still exist concerning the role of lymphangiography on the incidence of hypothyroidism: some studies have demonstrated that preirradiation lymphangiography significantly increases the incidence of hypothyroidism (Smith *et al.*, 1981), contrasting with the series from Green showing a protective effect of lymphangiogram (Green *et al.*, 1984).

The treatment of these abnormalities is also the subject of some debate. Low levels of thyroxine obviously require thyroid replacement therapy. Animal studies show that there is a predisposition to thyroid adenoma or carcinoma by chronic stimulation of thyroid by high level of TSH and this is an argument to treat those patients even with compensated hypothyroidism. However, the incidence of thyroid carcinoma after irradiation for Hodg-

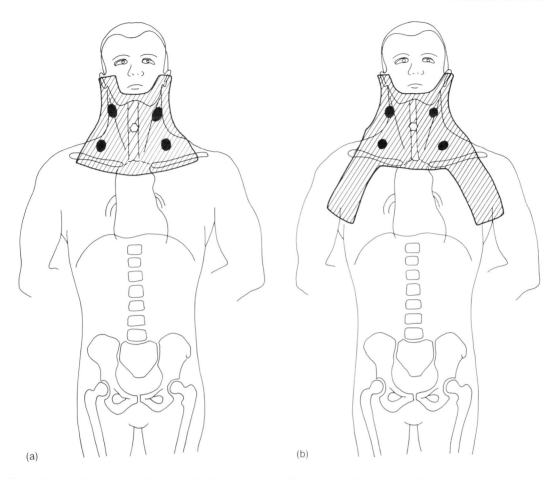

Fig. 12.3a Limited involved field for cervical Stage II.

Fig. 12.3b Limited field according to the Rye symposium for same stage.

kin's disease is very low: four cases among 979 children with two to 29 years follow-up (Meadows *et al.*, 1989). The long latency of these tumours does however impede any prospective randomized study to fully answer this question in children.

High-dose radiation may induce late pleural or pericardial effusion (Fig. 12.7). In long-term survivors, we have observed constrictive pericarditis occurring more than ten years after the treatment. An increased incidence of coronary artery disease has also been shown by recent data from the Institut Gustave Roussy (Cosset *et al.*, 1990). In the same study, late functional pulmonary involvement was related to the total dose of radiation and a fraction size greater than 200 rads. Green found also a high incidence of asymptomatic pericardial thickening on echocardiogram in long-term survivors after childhood Hodgkin's disease (Green *et al.*, 1985). The clinical significance of these findings remains to be assessed with longer follow-up.

The risk of chronic radiation enteritis with sub-acute obstruction and malabsorption are increased by staging laparotomy and exten-

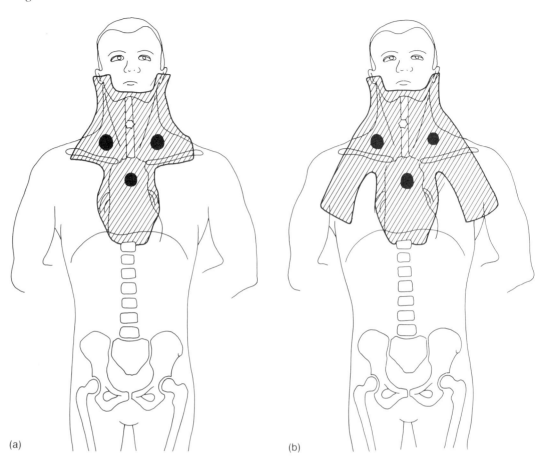

Fig. 12.4a Limited involved field with mediastinal involvement.

Fig. 12.4b Limited involved field with mediastinal involvement as defined by the Rye symposium.

sive intra-operative investigation. Soft-tissue fibrosis may also induce limb lymphoedema or retroperitoneal fibrosis with ureteric obstruction. As a final point, oophoropexy should be performed in all girls receiving pelvic irradiation in order to protect ovarian function. A lateral transposition technique reduces the scattered dose received by the ovaries.

12.4.2 CHEMOTHERAPY

The MOPP regimen was first described by Carbone in 1967. It consists of a combination of drugs (nitrogen mustard, oncovin, procarbazine and prednisone (Table 12.8). It has achieved dramatic results in advanced disease previously not curable (De Vita *et al.*, 1970). Several modifications have been made to the MOPP programme, vinblastine being substituted for vincristine or/and cyclophosphamide, or chlorambucil being substituted for mechlorethamine. However, none of these combinations has proven to be significantly better than the MOPP regime. A new four-drug combination (ABVD) was devel-

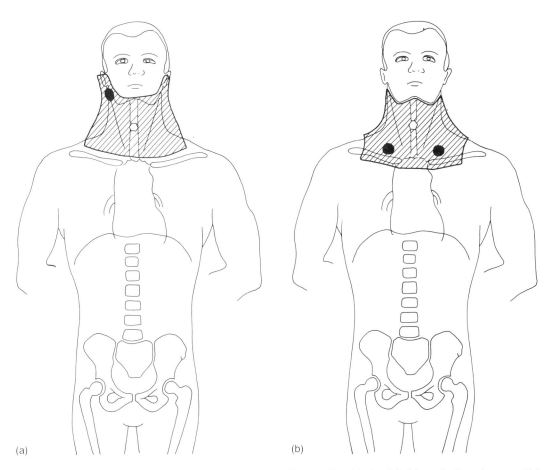

Fig. 12.5a Limited field, excluding the clavicles, for a single upper cervical node.

Fig. 12.5b Limited field, excluding the mandible, for single supraclavicular nodes.

oped in 1974 with components that are totally different from those included in the MOPP combination; adriamycin, bleomycin, vinblastine and DTIC (Table 12.8). The efficacy of ABVD has been tested in randomized studies versus MOPP and the usefulness of alternating non-cross-resistant regimens is still being discussed (Bonadonna *et al.*, 1989).

Chemotherapy also has side effects. Gonadal injury is now clearly defined. All boys develop normal puberty after MOPP, even if they are azoospermic. Recent data regarding male fertility after chemotherapy did not confirm that prepubertal testes are less sensitive to alkylating agents than adult testes: as in adults, six cycles of MOPP will result in azoospermia; however, azoospermia was also observed in two boys who received two and three cycles of MOPP respectively. The toxic dose of procarbazine and mechlorethamine still requires assessment (Aubier *et al.*, 1989). In the same study, elevated follicle-stimulating hormone (FSH) was well correlated with azoospermia. The German paediatric data show a relationship between the FSH level and the dose of procarbazine (Brämswig *et al.*, 1990). The significance of these findings still has to be assessed with

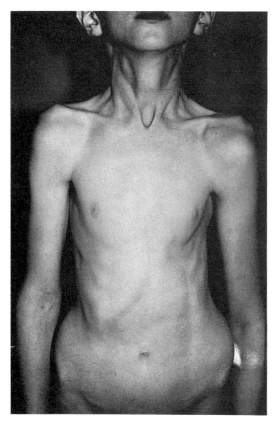

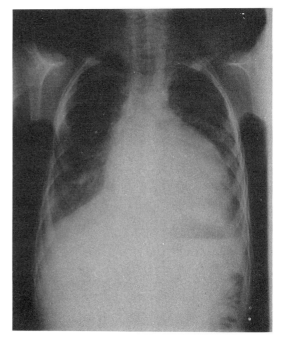

Fig. 12.7 Pericarditis that occurred 11 years after a 40 Gy mantle field received at the age of 15 years.

Fig. 12.6 Thoracic and abdominal musculo-skeletal abnormalities in a boy who received 40 Gy in a mantle field and lumbo-splenic field at age of four years.

longer follow-up since we, for example, have seen patients with normal FSH despite azoo-spermia. In contrast, the Milan studies showed a preservation of fertility in most of the men who received ABVD chemotherapy as adults (Bonadonna *et al.*, 1989). MOPP chemotherapy may also induce ovarian damage but young age at the time of treatment is associated with less gonadal damage even if the incidence of premature ovarian ageing is not well known (Donaldson and Kaplan, 1982).

Pulmonary function tests have been sequentially evaluated in patients treated as adults with high-dose mantle irradiation and six cycles of either ABVD or MOPP combination. The mean vital capacity at the end of treatment was statistically lower in the ABVD group with incomplete recovery at two years

Table 12.8 MOPP and ABVD chemotherapy regimens

	MOPP		
Mechloretamine	6 mg/m^2	I.V.	day 1 and day 8
Vincristine	1.5 mg/m^2	I.V.	day 1 and day 8
Procarbazine	100 mg/m^2	P.O.	day 1 to day 14
Prednisone	40 mg/m^2	P.O.	day 1 to day 14
	ABVD		
Adriamycin	25 mg/m^2	I.V.	day 1 and day 15
Bleomycin	10 mg/m^2	I.V.	day 1 and day 15
Vinblastine	6 mg/m^2	I.V.	day 1 and day 15
DTIC	375 mg/m^2	I.V.	day 1 and day 15

(Cosset *et al.*, 1989). The paediatric experience of three ABVD alternating with three MOPP in conjunction with low dose radiation show that with a 27.5 months mean follow-up, out of 20 patients, 40% had abnormal lung volumetric measures. Out of 11 patients, six had a low value of carbon monoxide diffusion capacity (DLCO) (Mefferd *et al.*, 1979). In the same study, two out of 14 asymptomatic patients were considered as having abnormal cardiac nuclear gated angiogram (Mcfferd *et al.*, 1979). These results, which are rather concerning, need to be confirmed in a larger group of patients and with a longer follow-up.

The American Late Effects Study Group have reported the incidence of second neoplasms in a large series of nearly 1000 children, followed for a median of seven years (Meadows *et al.*, 1989). The actuarial risk is 4% at 10 years and rises to 18% at 20 years. The number of leukaemias or non-Hodgkin's lymphomas and the number of solid tumours are similar; the median delay of leukaemias, however, is five years, with no risk after 10 years, whereas the median delay of solid tumours is 12 years with a still increasing risk at 20 years. All the solid tumours occurred in an irradiated area; set against this, however, there is a strong relationship between leukaemias and alkylating doses. These above data confirm studies carried out in adults. Experience in children treated with ABVD is relatively recent, however; in adults the leukaemia risk seems to be very small or even absent after ABVD therapy (Valagussa *et al.*, 1986).

The potential sequelae and mechanisms discussed above have been taken into account in designing the paediatric protocols since the late 1970s. Since both radiotherapy and chemotherapy are characterized by their well-known efficacy and late effects, the problem is to retain the former while avoiding the latter. In discussing the strategies for decreasing treatment, experience differs from one team or group to another; this is summarized in Table 12.9.

12.5 EXPERIENCES IN REDUCING THERAPY

12.5.1 CLINICAL STAGING

As has been said, we now assume laparotomy and splenectomy to be unnecessary procedures taking into consideration cost and the efficacy of chemotherapy to treat occult infra-diaphragmatic disease.

12.5.2 THE REDUCTION OF RADIATION FIELDS

The introduction of effective primary chemotherapy has allowed limitation of the volume of irradiation. The first study by the 'Intergroup' Hodgkin's disease for pathological Stage I and II compared in a randomized three-arm study, involved field radiotherapy versus extended field radiotherapy versus involved field radiation given with six MOPP. There was no significant difference in survival; however, the disease-free survival in the MOPP arm was excellent (93%) at five years, contrasting with 67% for the first arm and 41% for the involved field radiation therapy (Gehan *et al.*, 1990).

In the first paediatric Institute Gustave Roussy study, 60 children were treated by involved field radiation after six or three courses of MOPP. In the group of 60 patients, the five-year survival is 93% and disease-free survival is 86% with only two relapses outside the irradiated area (Oberlin *et al.*, 1985).

12.5.3 THE REDUCTION OF RADIATION DOSES

This was first proposed both by the Stanford group and the Toronto team. In Stanford, after systematic splenectomy, 54 children

Table 12.9 Experiences in reducing therapy

Institution	No. of patients	Dates	Staging	Therapy	Results 5 years S	FFS
Series with high-dose involved field radiotherapy + chemotherapy						
Intergroup Hodgkin's disease study	279	75–81	PS I-II	IF RT EF RT IF RT + 6 MOPP	93%	41% 67% 95%
France Villejuif	60	75–80	CS I-IV	6 MOPP + IF RT	93%	86%
Series with low-dose radiotherapy + MOPP or procarbazine containing chemotherapy						
Stanford	55	70–83	PS I-II PS III-IV	6 MOPP + modif IF + EF	100% 78%	96% 84%
Toronto	57	73–79	CS I-III CS IV	6 MOPP + EF RT	92% 85%	88% 65%
France SFOP	62 73 21	82–87	CSIA-IIA CS IB-IIB-III CS IV	2 MOPP + 2 ABVD + 20 Gy IF 3 MOPP + 3 ABVD + 20 Gy IF	95% 94% 73%	90% 86% 62%
Italy	87	83–87	CS IIA (M/T>0.33) CS III CS IIIB-IV	3 MOPP + 3 ABVD + 20/25 Gy EF 5 MOPP + 5 ABVD + 20/25 Gy EF	94%	86%
Germany HD82	207	82–84	Selective Splen. CS I-IIA CS IIB-III CS III-IV	2 OPPA + 35 Gy IF 2 OPPA + 2 COPP + 30 Gy IF 2 OPPA + 4 COPP + 20 Gy IF	95%	98% 94% 86%
Series with radiotherapy + chemotherapy without alkylating agents						
France SFOP	66	82–87	CS IA-IIA	4 ABVD + 20 Gy IF	100%	91%
Italy Milan	57 39	83–87 79–85	CS IA-IIA (M/T<0.33) CS IA-IIA CS IB-IIB-III	3 ABVD + 20/25 Gy IF 3 ABVD + 30/35 Gy EF 6 ABVD + 30/35 Gy EF	97%	97%
Germany HD85	98	85–86	Selective lap. CS I-IIA2 CS IIB-IIIA CS IIIB-IV	OPA + 35 Gy IF 2 OPA + 2 COMP + 30 Gy IF 2 OPA + 4 COMP + 25 Gy IF	99%	86% 57% 54%

Table 12.9 Experiences in reducing therapy

Institution	No. of patients	Dates	Staging	Therapy	Results 5 years S	FFS
Series with chemotherapy alone						
Holland	21	75–84	CS I-III (<4 cm)	6–12 MOPP	100%	90%
UKCCSG	282	82–84	CS I-IV	6–8 ChlVPP (+RT large med.)	91%	73%
Australia	53	78–	CS I-IV	4–12 ChlVPP or MOPP	94%	92%

CS = clinically staged; PS = pathologically staged; RT = radiotherapy; M/T = mediastinum thoracic ratio;
MOPP = mechlorethamine + oncovin + procarbazine + prednisone; ABVD = adriamycin + bleomycin + vinblastine + DTIC;
OPPA = oncovin + procarbazine + prednisone + adriamycin; COPP = cyclophosphamide + oncovin + procarbazine + prednisone

IF = involved fields; EF = extended field
modif IF = for IA-IIA: IF 'according to Rye symposium', for IB-IIB-III = Total lymphoid RT

S = overall survival; FFS = failure-free survival

OPA = oncovin + prednisone + adriamycin
COMP = cyclophosphamide + oncovin + methotrexate + prednisone
ChlVPP = chlorambucil + vinblastine + procarbazine + prednisone

Data from Gehan et al., 1990; Oberlin et al., 1985; Donaldson and Link, 1987; Jenkin et al., 1982; Leverger et al., 1990; Vecchi et al., 1988; Brämswig et al., 1990; Leverger et al., 1990; Vecchi et al., 1990; Fossati-Bellani et al., 1985; Behrendt et al., 1987; Radford et al. 1991; Ekert et al., 1988.

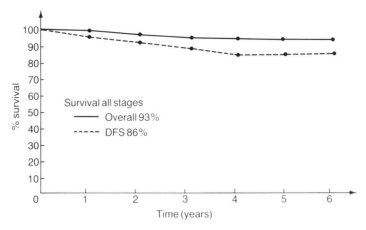

Fig. 12.8 Survival and disease-free survival (DFS) for the 220 children included in the French study.

were given six MOPP; radiation doses were then decided according to the age (ranging from 1500 to 2500 rads) and the response to treatment, with boosts often being added. Radiation ports were determined by the pathological staging: involved field irradiation was given in Stages IA-IIA; fields were more extended for patients with extranodal extension, and total nodal irradiation was given to children with B symptoms or Stage III disease (Donaldson and Link, 1987). In the Canadian series reported by Jenkin, radiation was given in extended fields with six MOPP (Jenkin *et al.*, 1982). Both these series had the same good results as those using high-dose radiotherapy.

Other national studies in Italy and France, on larger groups of patients, have confirmed the efficacy of low dose radiation. In these studies, radiation doses were tailored according to the response to primary chemotherapy. As it is now known, residual mass does not

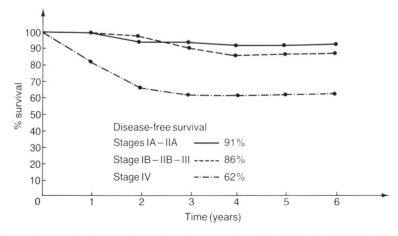

Fig. 12.9 Relapse-free survival according to the stage for the 220 children included in the French study.

always indicate active disease; a dose of 20 Gy was given if complete remission was achieved or if the mass reduction was estimated to be at least 70% of the initial mass. In the French study, radiation volume was limited to the strictly involved areas in Stages IA-IIA-III and IV but also encompassed a lumbo-splenic field in Stages IB-IIB (Table 12.9). With a median follow-up ranging from one to 7.5 years (median four years) the updated results show that at five years, overall survival is 93% and disease-free survival is 86.5% (Fig. 12.8). According to stages, the disease-free survival is 91% for Stages IA-IIA, 86% for Stages IB-IIB and III, 62% for Stages IV (Fig. 12.9). In the Italian protocol, involved fields are used only in Stages I and IIA with non massive mediastinal involvement. After a median observation time of 21 months, freedom from progression at four years was 88% and overall survival 94% (Vecchi et al., 1988).

In the German studies HD 82 and HD 85, radiation doses depended on the extent of the preceding chemotherapy: 35 Gy in Stages I-IIA after two cycles, 30 Gy in Stages IIB-IIIA after four cycles, and 25 Gy after six cycles – these gave similar excellent results (Brämswig et al., 1990).

All these studies clearly demonstrate that low-dose radiotherapy can be safely used to cure patients after effective primary chemotherapy. The French study also gives a clear indication that chemotherapy can be limited to four cycles rather than six in an attempt to minimize the drug-related sequelae (Leverger et al., 1990).

Again in the French study, age, histology and size of the mediastinum predicted patient outcome. Response to primary chemotherapy appeared to be a very strong prognostic indicator in terms of survival and disease-free survival. Among the 209 'good responders' (who exhibited >70% regression) 92% are long-term disease-free survivors, whereas this is the case in only 18% of the 11 'bad responders' (unpublished data). Stage IV have a lower disease-free survival than the other stages. However, after dose adjustment on response to chemotherapy, the fact that there is extra-nodal involvement is no longer predictive of outcome.

12.5.4 THE USE OF NONTOXIC CHEMOTHERAPY

The next challenge in the treatment of children with Hodgkin's disease, in order to minimize the late effects of sterility and acute leukaemias, was to reduce exposure to the MOPP combination. The results first reported by Milan are now confirmed by many groups. The first randomized French study demonstrated that four ABVD are equivalent to two MOPP plus two ABVD in localized stages (Leverger et al., 1990). The national Italian group and the Milan paediatric team have confirmed the efficacy of ABVD in a non random study (Fossati-Bellani et al., 1985; Vecchi et al., 1988).

One of the aims of the German study, begun in 1985, was to eliminate procarbazine from the chemotherapy. One result was that the OPPA regimen became OPA, and methotrexate replaced the procarbazine in the COPP combination resulting in the COMP regimen. Progression and relapse were significantly higher than in the preceding study (HD82) in Stages IE, IIE-IIIA and the study was prematurely stopped, highlighting the need for an effective drug to replace procarbazine (Brämswig et al., 1990).

Very few drugs are both non toxic (or have acceptable toxicity) and are active in Hodgkin's disease. Single-drug phase II studies are difficult to carry out because of the small number of relapsing patients and the existing concept which is to give combination chemotherapy as a salvage regimen. However, preliminary data indicate that etoposide might have a role to play (Taylor et al., 1982). In a pilot study, we studied a novel drug combination based on etoposide, vinblastine, bleomycin and prednisone (Oberlin *et al.*, 1990). Its encouraging efficacy led us to use it in our current study.

12.5.5 THE USE OF THE CHEMOTHERAPY ALONE OPTION

The option of treating children without the use of radiotherapy at all has been taken up by some teams. These studies have included six cycles of chemotherapy. In the Dutch study on a small group of patients, additional radiation therapy was given to large lymph node tumours (>4 cm) (Behrendt *et al.*, 1987). In the Australian study, there was no additional irradiation (Ekert *et al.*, 1988). In the British study, patients with a large mediastinum received 35 Gy after chemotherapy (Martin and Radford, 1989). Long-term follow-up for this study is lacking. All these series are based on alkylating and procarbazine-containing chemotherapy with their unacceptable late sterility and risk of secondary leukaemia. Another question of concern about such strategies is the proportion of relapsing patients who will be cured after heavy salvage therapy and the sequelae of their whole treatment.

12.6 TREATMENT OF ADVANCED, RESISTANT AND RELAPSING CASES

In the French study, disease-free survival for Stage IV is 62% at five years, disappointing even if rather better than those in adult series. The best paediatric results have been reported by the German study, 31 patients with an 81% event-free survival (Schellong *et al.*, 1987). A European cooperative study is being carried out by the SIOP (International Society of Pediatric Oncology) to confirm these excellent results on a larger group of patients, limiting the radiation dose to 20 Gy for good responders. The preliminary results are encouraging with no progression or relapse for the 19 patients included so far (Schellong *et al.*, 1990).

Patients who fail to achieve complete remission or who relapse after an initial response to chemotherapy have a poor prognosis. The complete remission rate with further chemotherapy is around 50% whatever the combination of non cross-resistant drugs given. However, this second remission has a short duration and with conventional salvage therapy, the cure rate is low. Therapeutic approaches with high-dose chemotherapy with bone marrow rescue show good results in adults, with little toxicity in patients who are treated early (Armitage *et al.*, 1989). We have reported similar results in a French paediatric study (Bessa *et al.*, 1990). However, it is now becoming necessary to define more precisely those subgroups of patients who will benefit from this regimen and the schedule of such therapy.

There are divided opinions regarding management of children with Hodgkin's disease to attain the universal goal: the maximal cure rate with the maximal quality of life. The combined modality therapy with low-dose radiation is the current treatment of choice for low-stage Hodgkin's disease. Obviously, advanced stages have benefited from effective chemotherapy.

However, some questions warrant further consideration: is there an effective nontoxic chemotherapy? Will the de-escalating therapy uncover new prognostic indicators? What is the best management for patients with a currently bad prognosis; an advanced stage of disease; who have failed primary treatment?

12.7 CURRENT CONTROVERSIES

12.7.1 PROGNOSTIC FACTORS

There are now data to suggest that the nodular sclerosis group of Hodgkin's disease patients can be split into 'better' and 'less good' prognostic subgroups (Haybittle *et al.*, 1985).

12.7.2 WHAT IS THE OPTIMAL MANAGEMENT OF EARLY STAGE DISEASE?

Two large centres have recently reviewed their treatment policies, comparing pathological staging and extended field radiotherapy with clinical staging and involved field radiotherapy. As would be predicted, there was a perceptibly higher relapse rate in Stage I patients treated by clinical staging and involved field radiotherapy; the critical point, however, was that the overall survival of both groups was the same (Donaldson *et al.*, 1990).

In an editorial that accompanies the above cited paper, Leventhal (1990) comes to her own conclusion that a combination of alkylating agent chemotherapy and low dose involved field radiotherapy constitutes optimal therapy (after clinical staging) thus providing clinicians with the full breadth of the debate around the current controversies.

12.7.3 WHEN IS RADIOTHERAPY INDICATED IN SUPRADIAPHRAGMATIC STAGE II DISEASE?

It has been suggested that there is a good case for post-chemotherapy radiotherapy for patients presenting with large mediastinal masses (Doreen *et al.*, 1984). Radiation portals of less than a full mantle may be advantageous (Glynne-Jones *et al.*, 1990). Ekert *et al.* (1988) have produced good relapse-free survival data using chemotherapy alone in this situation. After such treatment, a residual chest x-ray mediastinal abnormality is not necessarily indicative of persistent disease (Radford *et al.*, 1990).

12.7.4 THE MOVE AGAINST ALKYLATING AGENT CHEMOTHERAPY

In a recent report from the United States Children's Cancer Study Group (USCCSG), 64 children with advanced Hodgkin's disease were treated with ABVD (12 courses) followed by low dose regional radiotherapy. The event-free survival and overall survival was 87% at three years (Fryer *et al.*, 1990) – a very high remission rate, obtained with a pulmonary toxicity rate of 9% sequel that may be reduced by using less bleomycin. The controversy therefore must be: why are the USCCSG now studying a hybrid regimen of MOPP/ABVD when they have such excellent results with a non-alkylating agent regimen? Is it the fear of late cardiotoxicity that is making them 'hedge their bets' and return to the (adult) Bonadonna hybrid regimen? Is it a fear that salvageability after ABVD failure with MOPP therapy may be less than expected?

Also relevant here is the use of etoposide in front-line Hodgkin's chemotherapy regimens. It is included in VEEP (vincristine, epirubicin, etoposide, prednisolone) which for five years has been the first-line chemotherapy regimen of the London-based Children's Solid Tumour Group. Worrying for this group must be a few anecdotal reports of late acute myeloblastic leukaemia following etoposide therapy, and a slightly higher relapse rate now being seen.

12.7.5 THE DOSE OF RADIOTHERAPY AND THE PLACE OF RADIOTHERAPY IN ADVANCED DISEASE

A radical dose of radiotherapy for childhood Hodgkin's disease would be 3000 cGy over three weeks, conventionally fractionated to 3500 cGy to bulk disease. There is, however, accumulating evidence that lower doses are effective when used after 'chemotherapeutic debulking' (Donaldson and Link, 1987). Whether such low dose radiotherapy has a routine role in the management of patients presenting with advanced disease and bulky presentation sites is open to question but some groups do this routinely (Fryer *et al.*, 1990).

12.7.6 THE ROLE OF MEGATHERAPY AND BONE MARROW TRANSPLANTATION IN RELAPSE

Following relapse after primary chemotherapy where remission is achieved by further chemotherapy (chemosensitive disease) and in patients failing to achieve remission with primary chemotherapy (primarily chemorefractory disease), there is currently great interest in high dose therapy (Jones *et al.*, 1990; Wheeler *et al.*, 1990). The exact role of megatherapy and its timing are controversies that remain to be ironed out in the next decade.

P.N.P.

REFERENCES

Alexander, F.E., Williams, J., McKinney, P.A. *et al.*, (1989) A specialist leukaemia/lymphoma registry in the UK. Part 2: Clustering of Hodgkin's disease. *Br. J. Cancer*, **60**, 948–52.

Andrieu, J.M., Asselain, B., Bayle, Ch. *et al.* (1981) La séquence polychimiothérapie MOPP-irradiation ganglionnaire sélective dans le traitement de la maladie de Hodgkin, stades cliniques IA-IIIB. Bull. *Cancer*, 68, 190–9.

Armitage, J.O., Barnett, M.J., Carella, A.M. *et al.* (1989) Bone marrow transplantation in the treatment of Hodgkin's lymphoma: problems, remaining challenges and future prospects. in *New Aspects in the Diagnosis and Treatment of Hodgkin's Disease*. (eds V. Dielh, M. Pfreundschuh and M. Loeffler) Springer, Berlin pp. 1246–53.

Aubier, F., Flamant, F., Brauner, R. *et al.* (1989) Male gonadal function after chemotherapy for solid tumours in childhood. *J. Clin. Oncol.*, **7**, 304–9.

Behrendt, H., Van Bunningen, B. and Van Leeuwen, E.F. (1987) Treatment of HD in children without radiotherapy. *Cancer*, **59**, 1870–3.

Bessa, E., Oberlin, O., Hartmann, O. *et al.* (1990) High-dose combination chemotherapy for childhood Hodgkin's disease. The French Pediatric Oncology Society Experience. (Abstract 33) Fourth International conference on malignant lymphoma, Lugano.

Birch, J.M., Marsden, H.B. and Swindell, R. (1980) Incidence of malignant disease in childhood. A 24 year review of the Manchester children tumour registry data. *Br. J. Cancer*, **42**, 215–23.

Bonadonna, G., Valagussa, P., Santoro, A. *et al.* (1989) Hodgkin's disease: the Milan experience with MOPP and AVBD. in *New Aspects in the Diagnosis and Treatment of Hodgkin's Disease*. (eds V. Dielh, M. Pfreundschuh and M. Loeffler) Springer, Berlin 169–74.

Brämswig, J.H., Hörnig-Franz, I., Reipenhausen, M. and Schellong, G. (1990) The challenge of pediatric Hodgkin's disease: where is the balance between cure and long-term toxicity? *Leukemia and Lymphoma*, **3**, 183–93.

Carbone, P.P., Kaplan, H.S., Musshof, K. *et al.* (1971) Report of the committee on Hodgkin's disease staging. *Cancer Res.*, **31**, 1860–1.

Cavdar, A.O., Tacoy, A., Babacan, E. *et al.* (1977) Hodgkin's disease in Turkish children: a clinical and histopathological analysis. *J. Natl. Cancer Inst.*, **58**, 479–781.

Chilcote, R.R., Baehner, R.L., Hammond, D. and Children's Cancer Study Group (1976) Septicemia and meningitis in children splenectomized for Hodgkin's disease. *N. Engl. J. Med.*, **295**, 798–800.

Cosset, J.M., Henry-Amar, M. and Meerwaldt, J.H. (1990) Long-term toxicity of Hodgkin's disease treatment. (Abstract 12) Fourth International conference on malignant lymphoma. Lugano.

Cosset, J.M., Henry-Amar, M. Thomas, J. *et al.* (1989) Increased pulmonary toxicity in the ABVD arm of the EORTC H6-U Trial. *Proc. Am. Soc. Clin. Oncol.*, **8**, 985.

De Vita, V.T., Serpick, A. and Carbone, P.P. (1970) Combination chemotherapy in the treatment of advanced HD. *Ann. Int. Med.*, **73**, 881–95.

Desser, R.K. and Ultmann, J.E. (1972) Risk of severe infection in patients with Hodgkin's disease or lymphoma after diagnostic laparotomy and splenectomy. *Ann. Intern. Med.*, **77**, 143–6.

Donaldson, S.S. and Kaplan, H.S. (1982) Complications of treatment of Hodgkin's disease in children. *Cancer Treat. Rep.*, **66**, 977–89.

Donaldson, S.S., Glatestein, E. and Vosti, K.L. (1978) Bacterial infection in pediatric Hodgkin's disease: relationship to radiotherapy, chemotherapy and splenectomy. *Cancer*, **41**, 1949–58.

Donaldson, S.S. and Link, M.P. (1987) Combined modality treatment with low dose radiation and MOPP chemotherapy for children with Hodgkin's disease. *J. Clin. Oncol.*, **5**, 742–9.

Donaldson, S., Kleeberg, P. and Cox, R. (1988) Growth abnormalities with radiation in children with HD. *Proc. Am. Soc. Clin. Oncol.*, **7**, 864.

Donaldson, S.S., Whitaker, S.J., Plowman, P.N. *et al.* (1990) Stage I-II pediatric Hodgkin's disease: long term follow-up demonstrates equivalent survival rates following different management schemes. *J. Clin. Oncol.*, **8**, 1128–37.

Doreen, M.S., Wrigley, P.F.M., Laidlow, J.M. *et al.* (1984) The management of stage II supradiaphragmatic Hodgkin's disease at St. Bartholomew's Hospital. *Cancer*, **54**, 2882–8.

Drossman, S.R., Schiff, R.G., Kronfeld, G.D. *et al.* (1990) Lymphoma of the mediastinum and neck: evaluation with Ga-67 imaging and CT correlation. *Radiology*, **174**, 171–5.

Dunninck, N.R., Parker, B.R. and Castellino, R.A. (1977) Pediatric lymphography: performance, interpretation and accuracy in 193 consecutive children *Am. J. Rad.*, **129**, 639–745.

Ekert, H., Waters, K.D., Smith, P.J. *et al.* (1988) Treatment with MOPP or ChlVPP chemotherapy only for all stages of childhood Hodgkin's disease. *J. Clin. Oncol.*, **6**, 1845–50.

Fonatsch, C., Gradel, G. and Rademacher, J. (1989) Genetics of Hodgkin's lymphoma, in *New Aspects in the Diagnosis and Treatment of Hodgkin's Disease.* (eds V. Dielh, M. Pfreundschuh and M. Loeffler) Springer, Berlin, pp. 35–9.

Fossati-Bellani, F., Gasparini, M. Kenda, A. *et al.* (1985) Limited field and low-dose radiotherapy + ABVD chemotherapy for childhood Hodgkin's disease. Abstract XVIIth SIOP meeting, Venice 1985, 323–4.

Fryer, C.J., Hutchinson, R.J., Krailo, M. *et al.* (1990) Efficacy and toxicity of 12 courses of ABVD chemotherapy followed by low dose regional radiation in advanced Hodgkin's disease in children: a report from the Children's Cancer Study Group. *J. Clin. Oncol.*, **8**, 1971–80.

Gehan, E.A., Sullivan, M.P., Fuller, L.M. *et al.* (1990) The intergroup HD in children. A study of stages I and II. *Cancer*, **65**, 1429–37.

Glynne-Jones, R., Whitaker, S.J. and Plowman, P.N. (1990) The 'urn' portal; an alternative to the mantle portal in the chemoradiotherapy of paediatric Hodgkin's disease. *Clin. Oncol.*, **2**, 235–40.

Green, D., Gingell, R., Pearce, J. *et al.* (1985) Evaluation of cardiac function in patients treated with mediastinal irradiation during childhood and adolescence for HD. *Proc. Am. Soc. Clin. Oncol.*, **4**, C-818.

Green, D.M., Brecher, M.L., Yakar, D. *et al.* (1984) Thyroid function in pediatric patients after neck irradiation for HD. *Med. Pediatr. Oncol.*, **8**, 127–36.

Grufferman, S., Cole, P., Smith, P. and Lukes, R.J. (1979) Hodgkin's disease in siblings. *N. Engl. J. Med.*, **300**, 1006–11.

Haybittle, J.L., Bennett, M.H. *et al.* (1985) Review of the British National Lymphoma Investigation studies of Hodgkin's disease and development of prognostic index. *Lancet*, **i**, 967–72.

Hrgovcic, M., Tessmer, C.F., Thomas, F.B. *et al.* (1973) Significance of serum copper in adult patients with Hodgkin's disease. *Cancer*, **31**, 1337–45.

Jenkin, R.D., Chan, H. Freeman, M. *et al.* (1982) Hodgkin's disease in children: treatment results with MOPP and low-dose, extended field irradiation. *Cancer Treat. Rep.*, **66**, 949–59.

Jenkin, R.D. and Berry, M.P. (1980) Hodgkin's disease in children. *Semin. Oncol.*, **7**, 202–11.

Jones, R.J., Piantadosi, S., Mann, R.B. *et al.* (1990) High dose cytotoxic therapy and bone marrow transplantation for relapsed Hodgkin's disease. *J. Clin. Oncol.*, **8**, 527–39.

Kaplan, H.S. (1970) On the natural history, treatment and prognosis of HD. in *Harvey Lectures, 1968–1969.* Academic Press, New York pp. 251–9.

Kaplan, M.M., Garnick, M.B., Gelber, R. *et al.* (1983) Risk factors for thyroid abnormalities after neck irradiation for childhood cancer. *Am. J. Med.*, **74**, 272.

Leventhal, B.G. (1990) Management of Stage I-II Hodgkin's disease in children. *J. Clin. Oncol.*, **8**, 1123–4.

Leverger, G., Oberlin, O., Quintana, E. *et al.* (1990) ABVD vs MOPP/ABVD before low-dose radiotherapy in CS IA-IIA childhood Hodgkin's disease: a prospective randomized trial from the

French Society of Pediatric Oncology. *Proc. Am. Soc. Clin. Oncol.*, **9**, 1060.

Levine, P.H., Ablashi, D.V., Berard, C.W. *et al.* (1971) Elevated antibody titers to Epstein Barr virus in Hodgkin's disease. *Cancer*, **27**, 416–21.

Loeffler, M. Pfreundschuh, M., Rühl, U. *et al.* (1989) Risk factor adapted treatment of Hodgkin's lymphoma: strategies and perspectives. in *New Aspects in the Diagnosis and Treatment of Hodgkin's Disease.* (eds V. Dielh, M. Pfreundschuh and M. Loeffler) Springer, Berlin pp. 142–62.

Lukes, R.J. and Butler, J.J. (1966) The pathology and nomenclature of Hodgkin's disease. *Cancer Res.*, **26**, 1063–81.

Lukes, R.J., Craver, L.F., Hall, T.C. *et al.*, (1966) Report of the nomenclature committee. *Cancer Res.*, **26**, 1311.

Martin, J. and Radford, M. (1989) Current practice in Hodgkin's disease. The United Kingdom Children's Cancer Study Group, in *Hodgkin's Disease in Children: Controversies and Current Practice.* (eds W.A. Kampo, G.B. Humphrey and S. Poppema) Kluwer Academic, Boston pp. 263–75.

Meadows, A., Obringer, A., Marrero, O. *et al.* (1989) Second malignant neoplasms following childhood Hodgkin's disease: treatment and splenectomy as risk factors. *Med. Ped. Oncol.*, **17**, 477–84.

Mefferd, J.M., Donaldson, S.S. and Link, M.P. (1979) Pediatric HD: pulmonary, cardiac and thyroid function following combined modality therapy. *Int. J. Radiat. Oncol.*, **16**, 679–85.

Mueller, N.E. (1990) An epidemiologic view of the new cytogenic findings in Hodgkin's disease. (Abstract 3) Fourth International conference on malignant lymphoma, Lugano.

Oberlin, O., Paquement, H., Baruchel, A. *et al.* (1990) Vinblastine, etoposide, bleomycin, prednisone in CS IA-IIA Hodgkin's disease: A pilot study by the French Society of Pediatric Oncology. *Proc. Am. Soc. Clin. Oncol.*, **9**, 1067.

Oberlin, O., Boilletot, A., Leverger, G. *et al.* (1985) Clinical staging, primary chemotherapy and involved field radiotherapy in childhood Hodgkin's disease. *Eur. Paediatr. Hematol. Oncol.*, **2**, 65–70.

Pui, C.H., Ip, S.H., Thompson, E. *et al.* (1989) Increased serum CD8 antigen level in childhood Hodgkin's disease relates to advanced stage and poor treatment outcome. *Blood*, **73**, 209–13.

Radford, J.A., Cowan, R.A., Flanagan, M. *et al.* (1988) The significance of residual mediastinal abnormality on the chest radiograph following treatment for Hodgkin's disease. *J. Clin. Oncol.*, **6**, 940–6.

Radford, M., Barrett, A., Martin, J. and Cotterill, S. (1991) Treatment of Hodgkin's disease in children. Study HDI. *Med. Ped. Oncol.*, **19**, 400.

Rosenstock, J.G., D'Angio, G.J. and Kiesewetter, W.B. (1974) The incidence of complications following staging laparotomy for Hodgkin's disease in children. *Radiology*, **120**, 531–5.

Russell, K.R., Donaldson, S.S., Cox, R.S. and Kaplan, H.S. (1984) Childhood Hodgkin's disease: patterns of relapse. *J. Clin. Oncol.*, **2**, 80–7.

Schellong, G., Hörnig-Franz, I. and Muller, R.P. (1990) Preliminary report on the SIOP study on stage IV HD (SIOP HD IV 87). Abstract, *Med. Pediatr. Oncol.*, **18**, 426.

Schellong, G., Hörnig, I., Brämswig, J.H. *et al.* (1987) Favourable outcome of childhood Stage IV HD with OPPA/COPP chemotherapy and additional radiotherapy. Abstract XIXth SIOP meeting, Jerusalem, 132.

Schicha, H., Franke, M., Smolorz, J. *et al.* (1989) Diagnostic strategies and staging procedure for Hodgkin's lymphoma: bone marrow scintigraphy and magnetic resonance imaging. in *New Aspects in the Diagnosis and Treatment of Hodgkin's Disease.* (eds V. Dielh, M. Pfreundschuh and M. Loeffler) Springer, Berlin pp. 112–19.

Siber, G.R., Weitzman, S.A., Aisenberg, A.C. *et al.* (1978) Impaired antibody response to pneumococcal vaccine after treatment for Hodgkin's disease. *N. Engl. J. Med.*, **299**, 442–8.

Smith, K.L. and Rivera, G. (1976) Comparison of clinical course of Hodgkin's disease in children and adolescents. *Med. Pediatr. Oncol.*, **2**, 361–70.

Smith, R.E., Adler, R.A., Clark, P. *et al.* (1981) Thyroid function after mantle irradiation in HD. *JAMA*, **245**, 46–9.

Stein, H. (1990) Nature of Sternberg Reed cells and other biological problems (Abstract 1) Fourth International conference on malignant lymphoma, Lugano.

Stein, H., Schwarting, R., Dallenbach, F. and Dienemann, D. (1989) Immunology of Hodgkin's and Reed Sternberg cells. in *New Aspects in the Diagnosis and Treatment of Hodgkin's Disease.* (eds

V. Dielh, M. Pfreundschuh and M. Loeffler) Springer, Berlin pp. 14–26.

Svejgraad, A., Platz, P., Ryder, L.P. *et al.* (1975) HLA and disease association. A survey. *Transplant Rep.*, **22**, 3–73.

Tan, C., Jereb, B., Chan, K.W. *et al.* (1983) Hodgkin's disease in children. Results of management between 1970–82. *Cancer*, **51**, 1720–5.

Taylor, R.E., McElwain, T.J., Barrett, A. and Peckham, M.J. (1982) Etoposide as a single agent in relapsed advanced lymphomas. A phase II study. *Cancer Chemother. Pharmacol.*, **7**, 175–77.

Trudel, M.A., Krikorian, J.G. and Neiman, R.S. (1987) Lymphocytic predominance Hodgkin's disease: a clinicopathologic reassessment. *Cancer*, **59**, 99–106.

Tubiana, M., Henry-Amar, M., Burgers, M.V. *et al.* (1984) Prognostic significance of ESR in clinical stages I and II Hodgkin's disease. *J. Clin. Oncol.*, **2**, 194–200.

Valagussa, P., Santoro, A., Fossati-Bellani, F. and Bonadonna, G. (1986) Second acute leukemia and other malignancies following treatment of Hodgkin's disease. *J. Clin. Oncol.*, **4**, 830–7.

Vecchi, V., Comelli, A., Meloni, G. *et al.* (1988) Updated results of protocol MH83 of the Italian Association of Pediatric Hematology and Oncology for Childhood Hodgkin's disease. (Abstract 155) International Society of Pediatric Oncology.

Wheeler, C., Antin, J.H. and Hallowell, A.W. (1990) Cyclophosphamide, carmustine and etoposide with autologous bone marrow transplantation in refractory Hodgkin's disease and non-Hodgkin's lymphoma: a dose-finding study. *J. Clin. Oncol.*, **8**, 648–56.

Young, J. and Miller, R. (1975) Incidence of malignant tumours in US children. *J. Pediatr.*, **86**, 254–8.

Chapter 13

Tumours of the central nervous system

P.N. PLOWMAN

13.1 INTRODUCTION

The subject of paediatric brain tumour management has always been an important one since these tumours are the commonest malignant solid tumours in childhood and because they may cause extreme distress to the child and family during their often protracted natural history. They are of great academic clinical interest because they largely present a local control problem – and in an organ which is so sensitive to late treatment morbidity.

In the last decade improved imaging, neurosurgical techniques, radiobiological knowledge of central nervous system radiation tolerance and, recently, important advances in chemotherapy, have all made an impact on the currently recommended treatment strategies and on improved survival. Equally, however, within the last decade, the appraisal of late sequelae of brain tumour treatment has been more thorough and critical, such that cognitive, neuroendocrine and neuropsychological damage may now be quantified better than before. Future treatments must aim at improving the 'therapeutic ratio' of improved survival/ reduced sequelae.

13.2 CLASSIFICATION AND DISTRIBUTION

Although the posterior fossa contains the minority of the brain volume, approximately half paediatric brain tumours arise in that site, these being mainly medulloblastoma, cerebellar and brainstem astrocytomas and IVth ventricular ependymomas. Half of all paediatric brain tumours are gliomas with ependymomas and well differentiated astrocytomas being more frequent than high grade astrocytomas. The classic paediatric cerebellar and optic nerve gliomas represent good examples of low grade tumours. High grade astrocytomas account for 25% of the total (50% supratentorially, 37% in the brainstem) but are proportionately far less common than in adults. The histochemical stain for glial fibrillary acidic protein (GFAP) has proved an important marker for tumours of glial cell lineage (although glial cell reactions in tumours may give an apparent false positive result) (Bonnin and Rubinstein 1984).

The cerebellar medulloblastoma was never satisfactorily classified with gliomas and in recent years its morphological similarity to cerebral neuroblastoma/peripheral neurecto-

Table 13.1 Classification of paediatric CNS tumours

Glial tumours

Astrocytoma – Well differentiated   cystic cerebellar with mural nodule
                                             protoplasmic/fibrillary/pilocytic/gemistocytic
              – Intermediate
              – Anaplastic →(Glioblastoma multiforme)

Ependymoma – Well differentiated
            – Intermediate to poorly differentiated

Oligodendroglioma – Well differentiated
                  – Intermediate to poorly differentiated

Mixed gliomas – (these may include areas with neurectodermal features)

Neurectodermal tumours

            Medulloblastoma   (Medulloepithelioma)
            Other CNS neurectodermal tumours (peripheral neurectodermal tumours [PNET])

Pineal tumours

            Pineoblastoma
            Pineocytoma   Pineal glioma

            Pineal germ cell tumours – germinoma
                                      – teratoma
                                      (with subtypes)

Germ cell tumours

            Other primary CNS germ cell tumours (other sites usually midline IIIrd-IVth
               ventricles)

Neurinomas –   Optic nerve glioma
            Others (particularly in association nwith neurofibromatosis)

Craniopharyngioma
Pituitary tumour
Choroid plexus tumours (cyst/papilloma/undifferentiated or carcinoma)
Meningioma
Others

dermal tumour, pineoblastoma and retinoblastoma together with the sharing of common surface antigens by all these tumour types (e.g. as picked up by monoclonal antibody: UJ13A), have led to the classification of all these tumours into a distinct neuroectodermal tumour category (Rorke, 1983). The stain for neurone specific enolase has not proved to be as useful as predicted.

Not only do paediatric tumours differ from adult brain tumours in their tendency to be better differentiated and occupy the posterior fossa, but also in tumour types. Meningiomas and acoustic neuromas are rare and pituitary adenomas uncommon in children; craniopharyngiomas and pineal tumours on the other hand are proportionately much more common – particularly in the Far East.

Germ cell tumours which occur in the midline (pineal, IIIrd and IVth ventricle regions) are also commoner in the young.

The distribution of brain tumours in infants has been analysed by Deutsch (1982) who found that amongst 30 children under two years at presentation, 10 had medulloblastoma, five ependymoma, five midline/IIIrd ventricular tumours, three brainstem glioma, and seven miscellaneous (including choroid plexus tumours). The overall classification of paediatric brain tumours is shown in Table 13.1.

13.2.1 CEREBELLAR ASTROCYTOMA

The classic cerebellar astrocytoma occurs in the first decade of life, is slightly commoner in boys, and presents with midline cerebellar signs. The CT and operative findings are of a cystic tumour with a mural nodule. This pilocytic variety is usually curable by neurosurgical resection. However, in perhaps 15% of cases, a diffuse astrocytoma can be observed histologically and this correlates with a more solid form of tumour that is less easily completely excised, a fact that is of relevance to prognosis and the need for post-operative radiotherapy. Diffuse histology, incomplete resection, and brainstem invasion are poor prognostic features. A fully resected cystic, pilocytic astrocytoma has a better than 90% survival rate with no adjunctive radiotherapy, while an incompletely excised diffuse astrocytoma has only a 50–60% survival despite post-operative radiotherapy (Matson, 1956; Geissinger and Bucy, 1971).

13.2.2 SUPRATENTORIAL ASTROCYTOMAS

Approximately 35% of paediatric brain tumours are supratentorial astrocytomas and these are twice as common in boys. Approximately half arise in the cerebrum and half are deep seated – paraventricular, diencephalic, thalamic or basal ganglia in origin.

The Kernohan grading system I-IV is an oversimplification and liable to subjective variations: grade I and grade IV (glioblastoma multiforme) tumours, for example, are easily recognized, while the tumours in between are hard to reproducibly grade.

Several subtypes of well differentiated astrocytomas are recognized: pilocytic, fibrillary, protoplasmic and gemistocytic. Pilocytic tumours are more common in the paraventricular sites in contrast to the fibrillary tumours which are more often in the hemispheres (Russell and Rubinstein, 1977).

Anaplastic astrocytomas are histologically diagnosed by more frequent mitoses, cellular pleomorphism and general cellularity of the tumour. When areas of necrosis occur and the cells adopt bizarre forms and often large sizes, the term glioblastoma multiforme is appropriate – and carries with it a fatal prognosis. Such anaplastic astrocytomas are more likely to have a marked CT enhancing periphery and a non-enhancing (necrotic) centre than low grade astrocytomas; however, the growing edge of high grade tumours is considerably (perhaps 2 cm) beyond the CT enhancing rim. It is still unclear as to whether MRI will more exactly define the tumour volume from the surrounding oedematous brain. High grade astrocytomas are more commonly found in the cerebrum.

Diagnosis and first therapy is usually achieved with neurosurgery and complete removal is the aim in non-vital brain areas. The routine availability of stereotactic and microsurgical techniques is vital to a modern paediatric neurooncology unit. Post-operative wide field local radiotherapy is indicated for all children except those severely debilitated by high grade gliomas and (at the other end of the spectrum) children who have had full resection of pilocytic tumours. The overall prognosis varies widely from a five-year survival of 2% for glioblastomas to 80% for pilocytic astrocytomas after optimal surgery (Bloom, 1986), see also Fig. 13.1.

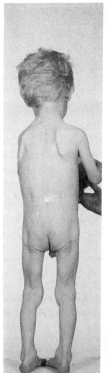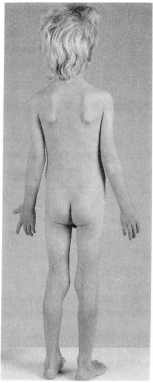

Fig. 13.1 Posterior-view photograph of a 3-year-old boy with a biopsy-proven low grade astrocytoma causing the classic wasting 'diencephalic syndrome'. A stereotactic needle biopsy and radiotherapy were administered. (Left panel: before radiotherapy; right panel: 2½ years later).

13.2.3 BRAINSTEM GLIOMA

Brainstem gliomas occur predominantly in children and young adults and, overall, they comprise 15–20% of paediatric CNS tumours. The sex incidence is equal and the commonest presenting age range is 5–10 years. Although half brainstem gliomas are low grade, these tumours are usually of diffuse fibrillary histology which, when infiltrating the brainstem, rules out surgical resection. When, however, a cystic, pilocytic brainstem glioma grows exophytically into the IVth ventricle, neurosurgical resection is more often achieved and prognosis improved – but such cases are less than 10% of the total. Clinical presentation is often due to obstructive hydrocephalus or progressing brainstem signs. The introduction of CT and MRI has helped to firmly differentiate these tumours from other brainstem disease. The advent of stereotactic biopsy has allowed a greater proportion of the endophytic tumours to be diagnosed histologically and their grading assessed, a fact that is of prognostic value. Radiotherapy is the definitive treatment and adjuvant chemotherapy studies have not been found to improve survival. Trials of a regime of two fractions per day radiotherapy have not shown promise.

Prognosis can be related to several factors. Patients with hypodense tumours on CT scan are more likely to have high grade/poor prognosis tumours, although stereotactic biopsy, where safe, is preferred for both certain diagnosis and histological grading. Patients with multiple cranial nerve palsies have extensive tumours within the brainstem and, not surprisingly, a poorer prognosis, (Cohen *et al.*, 1986; Shibamoto *et al.*, 1989).

There seems to be a variation in the histology of brainstem gliomas by site with a concentration of high grade tumours in the medulla oblongata and a higher proportion of lower grade tumours in the midbrain and diencephalon (Eifel *et al.*, 1987). The pons (the commonest site for brainstem gliomas) has an equal representation of the different histological varieties.

Despite radiotherapy, the use of which is restricted by the radiation tolerance of the paediatric brainstem, the vast majority of these patients will die from their disease. Virtually all patients with high grade brainstem gliomas will die within three years whereas perhaps 20–30% of low grade histology patients may survive long term. Series which have included unusually high numbers of diencephalic tumours have been reported with better survival figures.

13.2.4 EPENDYMOMAS

As expected from consideration of their cell of origin, ependymomas usually arise in paraventricular locations and make up 7% of paediatric brain tumours and 25% of paediatric spinal cord tumours. The age range of maximum incidence for intracranial ependymomas is the first decade whereas spinal ependymomas tend to present a little later in life. Two-thirds of intracranial ependymomas occur in the posterior fossa.

Ependymomas present clinically as space occupying masses with clinical features appropriate for their site of origin. Obstructive hydrocephalus is common at presentation. Their CT/MRI imaging features are non-diagnostic and appropriate neurosurgical biopsy and/or maximal debulking is the first line of therapy – as for any glioma. Histologically, good prognostic ependymomas must be distinguished from high grade tumours, with regards both to appropriate treatment and prognosis.

Ependymomas are both locally infiltrative and have a proclivity for CSF dissemination. CSF seeding occurs more frequently with infratentorial and high grade ependymomas. Although estimates of CSF seeding rates vary in the literature, the risk is probably considerably below 10% for supratentorial low grade tumours in contrast to greater than 20% risk for high grade infratentorial tumours (Cohen and Duffner, 1984). Neuraxis staging and radiation prophylaxis is indicated for all except low grade supratentorial ependymomas.

Although prognostically more favourable than solid astrocytomas, the majority of patients with high grade ependymomas (especially ependymoblastoma) die. However, the prognosis of five-year survival for low grade ependymomas may be as good as 50%

(Salazar *et al.*, 1983; Garret and Simpson, 1983; Cohen and Duffner, 1984).

13.2.5 SPINAL CORD TUMOURS

Primary intramedullary spinal cord tumours account for 5% of paediatric CNS tumours. Approximately two-thirds are astrocytomas and one-third ependymomas. Other intramedullary tumours occur but are unusual, and extramedullary meningiomas, schwannomas and metastases (especially neuroblastoma) must be distinguished. The MRI has revolutionized spinal cord imaging but surgical biopsy and maximal debulking is required as primary treatment. Indeed, with the current sophistication of ultrasonic surgical aspirators and lasers, maximal debulking is now more readily achieved and this is important prognostically.

Spinal cord gliomas tend to be of low grade histology and, with careful post-operative radiotherapy, the survival at five and ten years is above 50% and higher for low grade ependymomas (Reimer and Onofrio, 1985; Peschel *et al.*, 1983). Chemotherapy has no role.

13.2.6 OPTIC NERVE GLIOMA

Histologically, these tumours are low grade fibrillary or pilocytic astrocytomas. They account for 5% of all paediatric CNS tumours, approximately half of these patients also suffering from von Recklinghausen's disease. The peak incidence is in the first five years of life and 75% have clinically presented by ten years of age (and 90% by 20 years). Although progressive visual loss is a major consequence, clinical presentation in the young child is rarely due to this, but rather because of strabismus, nystagmus or developmental difficulties. In primarily intra-orbital cases, proptosis may be a feature.

CT scanning, supplemented by plain x-ray views of the optic canal, delineates these

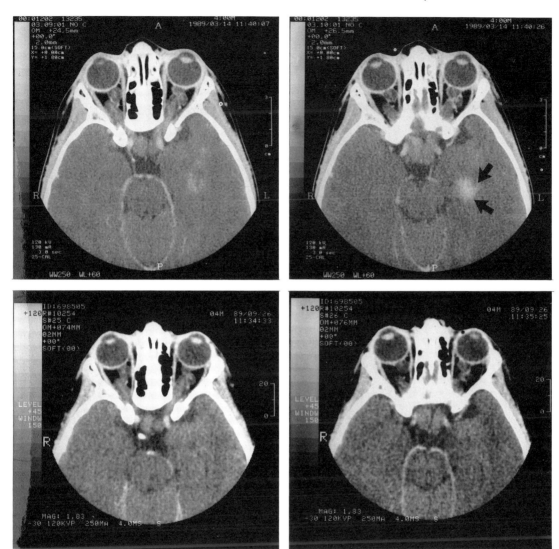

Fig. 13.2 Transaxial, enhanced CT scans (top pair, before radiotherapy; bottom pair, 9 months after radiotherapy) of a 5-year-old boy with neurofibromatosis, an extensive optic nerve glioma extending to both optic nerves through the chiasm. A separate enhancing glioma (arrowed, top right) was present in the left optic tract.

tumours well and allows the primarily intra-orbital cases to be distinguished from lesions involving an extension back to the chiasm. Some posterior/chiasmal tumours may be enormous at presentation, extending to involve pituitary or hypothalamus or ob-structing the ventricles. Presenting clinical features may consequently be as varied as diencephalic syndrome, endocrine presentations and internal hydrocephalus.

Stereotactic biopsy is often recommended to establish the diagnosis from that of other tumours although in children with neuro-fibromatosis, and given the diagnostic excellence of modern CT scanning, the clinical diagnosis may be considered so overwhelming as to render the invasive procedure redundant.

Intervention is often not immediately necessary. In the absence of rapidly deteriorating vision or CNS complications, a period of observation (with detailed and serial visual fields, visual acuities, VER studies and CT scanning) is indicated owing to the fact that some tumours appear to stabilize for long periods. This fact may delay radiotherapy for an important few years in the young child. However, large or extensive tumours, progressive visual deterioration, or growing tumours require treatment.

Optic nerve tumours when confined to the orbit are cured by radical surgery. For extensive intracranial tumours, radical transfrontal surgery is never complete and is often (if not usually) attended by worsening in the patient's condition; it is not therefore usually recommended. Occasional large semicystic tumours may first be safely and usefully debulked neurosurgically. However, accumulating clinical data suggest that conventional external beam radiotherapy is effective in at least preventing progression in the vast majority of cases, and carefully fractionated courses are the treatment of choice (Fig. 13.2); (Danoff *et al.*, 1980). Bloom reported a series of 29 advanced cases treated by radiotherapy with 100% five-year and 93% 15-year survival following radiotherapy (Horwich and Bloom, 1985).

13.2.7 MEDULLOBLASTOMA AND PERIPHERAL NEUROECTODERMAL TUMOURS

These account for 20% of paediatric CNS tumours. The classic paediatric cerebellar medulloblastoma is a vermis tumour that has its peak incidence in five-year-olds and 85% of cases have presented by the age of 15 years. There is a slight male predominance, M:F 1.3:1. (In young adults the tumour more often appears to arise in the cerebellar hemispheres.)

Medulloblastoma is now regarded as arising from primitive neuroepithelial cells that are present in embryological development in subependymal regions. In support of this concept, medulloblastoma shares certain morphological and surface antigen characteristics with other tumours arising from this lineage (e.g. retinoblastoma, neuroblastoma, pineoblastoma). Furthermore, tumours identical to medulloblastoma, which have previously been called 'cerebral neuroblastoma', occur in other brain areas in childhood. These tumours, often in the cerebrum, are now more properly classified as peripheral neurectodermal tumours (PNET) (Rorke, 1983). Microscopically, both medulloblastoma and PNET cells are made up of small round cells, with disproportionately large hyperchromatic nuclei; the cells are often clustered into rosettes. The more lateral, cerebellar hemisphere tumours, seen generally in older patients, have a more conspicuous stromal component – the desmoplastic medulloblastoma.

Both medulloblastomas and PNET tend to invade locally and also have the tendency to metastasize into the subarachnoid space, and disseminate via CSF carriage to other neuraxis sites. The incidence of CSF seeding at diagnosis ranges in different reports from 10–40%, but the risk is always substantial and myelography (preferable to MRI scanning) and CSF cytology are now *de rigueur* staging investigations for macroscopic and microscopic 'drop metastases' (Deutsch, 1984), while the diagnostic CT/MR scan of the head will search for other intracranial disease. In untreated cases of medulloblastoma, the incidence of neuraxis seeding at autopsy is at least 90%. Furthermore, medulloblastoma is the brain tumour *par excellence* that occasionally disseminates outside the CNS (5–15% of cases depending on reporting groups). Radio-

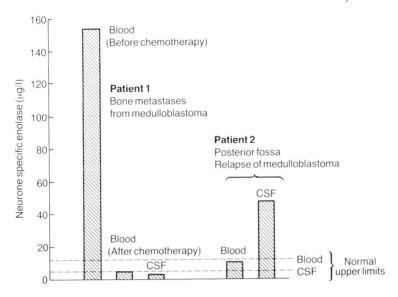

Fig. 13.3 Neurone specific enolase (NSE) levels in serum and CSF in patients with systemic/bone metastases (Patient 1) and posterior fossa relapse only (Patient 2) from medulloblastoma. It should be noted that following a complete response to chemotherapy in Patient 1, the serum NSE levels fell back to the normal range, supporting evidence that NSE is a useful marker for this disease.

logically sclerotic bone metastases are the commonest metastatic site. Interestingly, in our own and many other series, this propensity to seed outside the CNS does *not* appear to be correlated with the neurosurgical insertion of a ventriculo-peritoneal shunt. Serum neurone specific enolase levels provide an accurate marker of systemic relapse (Plowman, 1990) and CSF neurone specific enolase is elevated in neuraxis relapse (Fig. 13.3).

Clinically, children with medulloblastoma more commonly present with features of raised intracranial pressure than with cerebellar signs due to the common compression of the IVth ventricle. CT scanning demonstrates an often well-defined and homogeneously enhancing cerebellar tumour; brainstem invasion may be better delineated by current MR techniques.

Initial management is posterior craniectomy with maximal debulking, although shunt placement for obstructive hydrocephalus

may first be necessary. With modern neurosurgical techniques more complete excision is now possible than previously and this is prognostically useful.

What should follow neurosurgical resection and the staging procedures outlined above, is controversial. Classically, neuraxis radiotherapy followed by a posterior fossa boost is practised. Two trials in the 1980s both demonstrated that CCNU and vincristine based chemotherapy (delivered after the radiotherapy) prolonged disease-free survival (review, Allen *et al.*, 1986) and this generated much interest in adjuvant chemotherapy. However, given (1) the difficulty in administering cytotoxic chemotherapy so soon after the myelosuppressive effects of neuraxis radiotherapy; (2) the conceptual advantages of pre-radiation chemotherapy, and (3) improved drugs (see below), there is now a very great interest in delivering two cycles of chemotherapy (platinum-based), prior to radiotherapy. In infants, for whom the sequelae of neuraxis radiotherapy are considerable, longer periods of chemotherapy have been successfully used but in older children long-delayed neuraxis radiation has resulted in a high relapse rate.

Poor prognostic factors include brainstem invasion and incomplete macroscopic resection (which often go together) and evidence of dissemination (positive CSF cytology or, worse still, evidence of macroscopic neuraxis deposits). Younger children also have a worse prognosis. However, modern series have a 50% five-year survival overall, although relapses at 5–10 years are still encountered. Taking patients presenting without adverse prognostic features, the cure rate is considerably above 50% and it is hoped that the advent of improved chemotherapy will add to the survival figures for all patients.

The posterior fossa remains one of the commonest sites of relapse (approximately 40% of relapses occur here), and it may be that the failure to deliver 50 Gy to young children because of limited radiation tolerance contributes to the finding that young children have a worse outlook (Silverman and Simpson, 1982; Bloom, 1982). A dose of 50–55 Gy to the primary tumour bed is required in older children (but a dose of only 50 Gy to the whole brainstem).

13.2.8 CRANIOPHARYNGIOMAS

Craniopharyngiomas account for 8% of childhood brain tumours (2% in the adult) with a median age at clinical presentation of 8 years. Usually occurring in the midline suprasellar region, they may also appear intrasellar or, rarely, in adjacent sites. Derived from Rathke's pouch remnants, approximately 55% of the tumours are almost entirely cystic, 15% almost entirely solid, and the rest mixed solid-cystic masses. The cyst content is usually thick cholesterol-crystal-laden fluid,

escape of which into the CSF causes chemical meningitis. The surrounding tumour contains squamous epithelium. The capsule of the craniopharyngioma adheres tightly to adjacent brain tissue making complete surgical resection difficult and sometimes hazardous (see below).

Modes of presentation vary but raised intracranial pressure, visual changes, pituitary dysfunction and mental abnormalities are most common. Very young children tend to present with signs of hydrocephalus. Older children usually develop endocrinopathies with failure to thrive, growth failure or diabetes insipidus. Adolescents and young adults more commonly have visual field problems as their presenting complaint.

Modern radiological imaging techniques help to distinguish these tumours from other parasellar tumours. The plain x-ray will usually show an abnormal pituitary fossa and, importantly, calcification within the tumour is visible on this plain film in two-thirds of cases. CT scanning demonstrates a low density contrast-enhancing mass lesion with calcification and a variable sized cystic component. MRI scanning is most valuable at delineating the limits of the tumour.

A pre-operative neuroendocrine and ophthalmic work-up is essential. There is no question that neurosurgery is the most important initial management (preceded by a shunt if necessary). There is persisting controversy as to whether the neurosurgeon should attempt radical resection (with its often higher risk of morbidity), whether the neurosurgeon can ever reliably say he or she has 'completely' excised the lesion, and over the role of trans-sphenoidal surgery. For example, although Matson championed radical resection, late follow-up of his series showed a 27% relapse rate amongst 'complete' excision cases (Katz, 1975). Despite the introduction of improved neurosurgical techniques (the operating microscope, dexamethasone cover, improved neuroanaesthesia, etc.), the operative mortality of attempted complete resection of craniopharyngioma remains at 5–7%. The relapse rate (usually within the first four post-operative years) is not less than 25% – and cannot be accurately predicted by the surgeon. Furthermore, surgeons vary in the 'complete' resection rate and one highly experienced surgical team (Baskin and Wilson, 1986) considered that, using all modern techniques, they had only 'completely' removed 10% of 74 consecutive craniopharyngiomas. The foregoing is not in any way intended to detract from the viewpoint that 'complete' resection is a desirable objective and, providing the neurosurgeon does not risk major morbidity (e.g. by traction on tenacious capsule tethered to sensitive optic apparatus or hypothalamus), such an operation is recommended. In pooled data on 111 subtotally excised craniopharyngioma cases, Amacher (1980) found that 75% of these cases regrew and required retreatment.

The clinical place of post-operative radiotherapy has been questioned but data now available are overwhelmingly in favour of its routine use: in 1974, Kramer published a small series of ten patients with long-term follow-up after post-operative radiotherapy; six of six children and three of four adults remained disease free. More recently, Sung *et al*. (1980), reported on 109 patients: 74 patients had been treated by surgery alone and the five and ten year survival rates were 63% and 48% respectively. For 32 patients treated at the same institution by combined surgery and radiotherapy, however, the survival rates were 82% and 71% respectively, being particularly good for children. Manaka *et al*. (1985) reported on 125 patients of whom 80 had neurosurgery alone and 45 had post-operative radiotherapy. The five- and ten-year survival rates were 35% and 27% (surgery alone) versus 89% and 76% (surgery plus radiotherapy). The case for routine post-operative radiotherapy (irrespective of the neurosurgeon's impression of completeness

of excision) is overwhelming. All patients (over the age of four years) receive postoperative radiotherapy; younger patients are individually assessed.

Patients who relapse despite neurosurgical resection and external beam radiotherapy require individualized retreatment. However, those with cystic recurrences are now usually successfully treated by intracystic radioisotope installation. The Great Ormond Street/ St. Bartholomew's Paediatric Brain Tumour Unit favours ^{90}yttrium installation, and following Backlund's guidelines (Backlund, 1972), delivers 200 Gy to the cyst's surface secretory epithelium. Due to the physical properties of the beta emission, the optic apparatus and other adjacent sensitive structures do not receive a significant dose.

For those patients with semi-solid, semi-cystic recurrences, a mixed ^{90}yttrium installation (for the cystic component) and stereotactic multiple arc external beam radiotherapy/ radiosurgery technique (for the solid component) is employed.

13.2.9 PINEAL TUMOURS

The pineal gland arises embryologically as an evagination in the back of the ectoderm of the forebrain and it is therefore not surprising that neurectodermal tumours arise from it (the pineoblastoma and the pineocytoma). Histologically, the pineoblastoma exactly resembles the medulloblastoma and retinoblastoma and a pineoblastoma may arise as part of familial retinoblastoma (Kingston *et al*., 1985). Although the pineocytoma may be similar, the cells are larger and without the rosette formation, resembling more closely the normal gland. Germ cell tumours of the pineal gland (from germinoma through choriocarcinoma to mature teratoma) are more common and may also occur in other sites within the IIIrd ventricle (particularly anteriorly).

In a compilation of 278 histologically verified tumours collected from 12 published series,

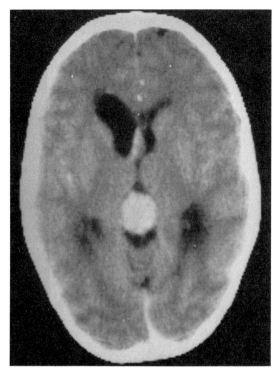 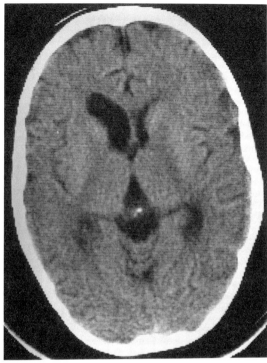

Fig. 13.4 Transaxial, enhanced CT scans of a 13-year-old boy with a pineal germ cell tumour. Left panel: before chemotherapy; right panel: after chemotherapy.

Bloom (1983) calculated the incidence of the various types of pineal tumours to be: germinoma 45%; glioma 17%; mature and anaplastic teratoma 16%; pineal parenchymal tumours 15%, and other 7%. In fact, in Japan and the Far East, the incidence of germinoma is even commoner, the tumour having a particular predisposition for young men.

The germinoma is therefore the commonest pineal tumour type, has its highest incidence in adolescent to young adult males, is relatively fast growing, and has a tendency for CSF dissemination. The pineal teratoma lineage tumours may secrete either AFP or βHCG, depending upon the presence of yolk sac or trophoblastic elements; they are therefore useful CSF markers. Except for the slower growing, non-secreting mature or differentiated teratomas, these tumours also have a tendency for CSF dissemination. (Our group also have experience of ventriculo-peritoneal shunt metastases of pineal choriocarcinoma to the peritoneum, in contrast to the above remarks on the rarity of this phenomenon in medulloblastoma.)

Pineoblastomas are fast growing tumours with a definite predisposition to spread to the whole neuraxis – particularly those arising in association with familial retinoblastoma. Pineocytomas are slower growing and have a lesser tendency to CSF dissemination.

Clinical presenting features are often due to hydrocephalus secondary to aqueduct obstruction. Pressure of a pineal tumour on the pretectal plate gives rise to Parinaud's syndrome – classic in pineal tumours. Germ cell tumours arising anteriorly in the IIIrd ventricle may present with visual difficulties and precocious puberty. Diagnosis is by CT scanning and stereotactic biopsy although a pineal mass and a high serum/CSF marker level might be accepted by many without recourse to biopsy.

Definitive microsurgical resection is indicated as primary therapy for mature teratomas, well differentiated pineocytomas and gliomas. On the other hand, no more than a diagnostic biopsy is indicated for germinomas, immature teratomas/choriocarcinoma and pineoblastoma, although immediate shunting may be necessary. All these latter tumour types are radiosensitive and, following neuraxis staging (as per medulloblastoma), neuraxis radiotherapy and a primary site boost leads to complete remission in a high percentage of cases. Overall, there is a 50–60% five-year survival rate for pineal tumours as a whole (Bloom, 1983; Berman *et al.*, 1986), but this rises to 80% for germinoma patients (Sung *et al.*, 1978; Jenkin *et al.*, 1978; Rich *et al.*, 1985).

Recently, the successes of chemotherapy for systemic germ cell tumours has led to its application as initial, pre-radiation therapy (on the same rationale as primary chemotherapy in medulloblastoma/PNET – see above) for pineal germ cell tumours. *Cis*-platin based chemotherapy is employed and this group have observed three out of four excellent responders (one IVth ventricular immature teratoma responding only transiently), Figure 13.4. This has encouraged us to employ pre-radiation chemotherapy routinely, and reduce standard neuraxis dose to staging negative cases.

Our group had very poor survival results in the series of 11 pineoblastomas/'trilateral' retinoblastoma children, reported by Kingston *et al.* (1985), with particular failure to control spinal metastases despite neuraxis radiotherapy. This, together with our encouraging recent chemotherapy data as palliative systemic therapy for advanced retinoblastoma patients has led us to pilot initial (platin based) chemotherapy prior to neuraxis radiotherapy in these children.

13.2.10 CHOROID PLEXUS TUMOURS

These usually occur in infants, the classic choroid plexus papilloma being a frond-like mass arising within the ventricles and secreting CSF. The infant usually presents with hydrocephalus and, following diagnosis, complete excision is curative. Approximately 10% of these tumours are more aggressive tumours and usually lead to death; following surgery for these so called 'carcinomas', radiotherapy is usually recommended although the evidence for its use is limited (Carpenter *et al.*, 1982).

13.2.11 PITUITARY ADENOMAS

Pituitary adenomas are less common in children than in adults and their clinical presentation is usually due to excessive hormone secretion by a functioning adenoma. These tumours have been of particular interest to our group.

Prolactinomas present with primary amenorrhoea or delayed/arrested puberty. We studied fourteen patients, ten girls/four boys (aged 14–25 years) who presented for the above reasons (Howlett *et al.*, 1989). The serum prolactin levels ranged from 920–104,300 mU/1 at presentation. CT scan showed macroadenomas in nine patients (the skull x-ray being grossly abnormal in eight), but only two patients had visual field defects. All patients were treated with bromocriptine which lowered the serum prolactin in all 14 and into the normal range in 11. Puberty thereafter progressed spontaneously in 13/14. In seven patients with macroadenomas, tumour shrinkage into the pituitary fossa was complete and in two others incomplete shrinkage was followed by transsphenoidal hypophysectomy. Seven patients (with macroadenomas) received pituitary radiotherapy (following bromocriptine shrinkage or surgery).

All patients remain well with tumour control (Howlett *et al.*, 1989).

Several important lessons can be learned from our experience above, when coupled with adult experience in the management of prolactinomas. Macroprolactinomas are managed with primary dopamine agonist medical therapy (with recourse to immediate transsphenoidal neurosurgery if any visual defects do not rapidly resolve). Dopamine agonist therapy is not definitive therapy (and cessation of this therapy may lead to severe tumour rebound expansion) and, following three months of such medical therapy, those tumours which have shrunk back into the fossa are treated with radiotherapy (Grossman and Plowman 1989; Plowman and Grossman, 1990). We have clearly demonstrated the effectiveness and safety of a three-field fixed, megavoltage x-ray dose prescription of 45 Gy in 25 fractions for this condition (Grossman *et al.*, 1984; Plowman, 1991). For tumours that have not shrunk back into the fossa after three months of dopamine agonist therapy, transsphenoidal surgery precedes radiotherapy. Microprolactinomas are treated by dopamine agonist therapy and a careful 'watch' policy in childhood. Tumour expansion or a girl's notification of the desire to conceive are indications for a more active management and we have reviewed elsewhere the arguments for surgery versus radiotherapy (Grossman and Plowman, 1989). There is a late incidence of anterior pituitary hormone dysfunction after radiotherapy (Tsagarakis *et al.*, 1990). It should be noted that hypothalamo-hypophyseal stalk disruption may lead to minor rises in serum prolactin levels in patients with non-functioning pituitary adenomas – so-called pseudoprolactinomas.

Growth hormone secreting adenomas usually present with the clinical stigmata of gigantism in the late teens and these patients usually have macroadenomas on investigation. Except for the fraction of patients with true mixed lactotroph/somatotroph tumours (Plowman and Grossman, 1990), the degree of shrinkage with primary dopamine agonist therapy is usually minor or absent in these patients. (It should be noted that a diagnosis of such mixed tumours cannot be made with certainty if there is a slightly raised prolactin level because of stalk disruption – see above.)

Management of gigantism patients with extrasellar extension is by transsphenoidal resection followed by post-operative radiotherapy; patients with tumours confined within the fossa may be successfully managed by radiotherapy alone. There is no longer any doubt but that radiotherapy achieves long-term cure of these patients (Ciccarelli *et al.*, 1988). Without radiotherapy, the relapse rate is high (Sheline, 1981; Plowman, 1991), but in post-operative patients who have undetectable random GH levels and on dynamic testing, we now have under careful observation a cohort of such patients, followed up without radiotherapy.

The principles of transsphenoidal surgery and post-operative radiotherapy also apply to childhood Cushing's disease (and Nelson's syndrome), although the documented radio-responsiveness of this disease in childhood (Jennings *et al.*, 1977) and the durability of control by radiotherapy (Howlett *et al.*, 1989), make many physicians believe that small tumours may be managed by radiotherapy alone.

13.3 THERAPEUTIC PRINCIPLES OF RADIOTHERAPY

There is no doubt that radiotherapy retains the major role as the non-surgical treatment of brain tumours but with recently acquired knowledge of radiation tolerance of the central nervous system, the concerns of mixed drug-radiation effects, and the late sequelae of radiotherapy to the young child's brain, more care and sophistication in radiotherapy is now required.

Of great clinical relevance to the subject of CNS tumours are the observations that with conventional external beam radiotherapy, the daily fraction size, the total dose delivered, the age of the child, and the volume of brain irradiated, are all relevant with regard to the degree of late CNS morbidity. Sheline (1980) quantified the importance of fraction size into a new isoeffect equation for CNS damage and, from this quantification of what earlier therapists had clinically discerned, it is usual to treat childhood brain tumours at daily fractional rates of 150–175 cGy. With regard to late tissue damage, the major CNS morbidity of radiotherapy, it is unlikely that the interfraction recovery interval is short. It is, for example, unlikely that it is the same few hours that are needed for 'Elkind' repair of radiation damage (Elkind *et al.*, 1965; Hall, 1978), and this augurs badly for trials of multiple daily fractionated radiotherapy for paediatric brain tumours – see below. Conversely, the time exponent (for longer than 24-hour interfraction intervals) is of much lesser consequence according to the new CNS isoeffect equation – so split course techniques are unlikely to reduce morbidity.

It is now standard practice to deliver radiotherapy to childhood gliomas by external beam megavoltage equipment, mapping the tumour from CT scan and allowing for target volume two centimetres around the CT perimeter. Usually, parallel opposed portals are used but small and lateralized gliomas may be best treated by wedged portals and multiple field plans. In infants and toddlers, total doses of up to 40 Gy in 150–160 cGy fractions are employed, whereas for older children with supratentorial astrocytomas a total dose of 50–55 Gy would be delivered. Respecting a longstanding clinical observation that the spinal cord and brainstem are more radiosensitive structures, the total doses to these structures should not exceed 40 Gy in young children, 45 Gy in under 10-year-olds. Only adolescents receive 50 Gy in 160 cGy

fractions. Although there was interest in multiple fractions per day radiotherapy for brainstem gliomas particularly, the results have not been promising and morbidity risks are considerable.

Neuraxis radiotherapy is employed for medulloblastoma/PNET, infratentorial and high grade ependymomas, pineal germ cell and pineoblastoma tumours and, incidentally, CNS leukaemia. In a prone 'shelled' child, a careful linear accelerator technique is employed to treat the entire cranial meninges (using shaped portals to exclude the orbits and structures below the meninges) through opposed lateral portals. A posterior spinal portal (which is perpendicular to the cranial portals) must be matched to the cranial portals and it is this 'matched junction' occurring at spinal cord depth (at our centre at C5), that is the most difficult part of neuraxis radiotherapy. The inferior border of the cranial portals is angled to match the angle of divergence of the superior border of the spinal portal, and a gap calculated and marked on the cervical portion of the head shell to allow match at depth (with several millimetres for safety). In young children and those who are staging negative (myelography and CSF cytology negative), the neuraxis receives 25–30 Gy in 160 cGy fractions. In older children or where staging is positive, 30 Gy (or 35 Gy in young high risk adults) is delivered; 'drop metastases' may be boosted further. Blood count monitoring twice weekly is mandatory for this myelosuppressive technique, particularly after induction chemotherapy. The platelets are at particular risk (Plowman, 1983).

Following neuraxis radiotherapy, the posterior fossa is boosted for medulloblastoma (by reduced portals – again parallel opposed). The fields should encompass the tumour bed but not the whole brainstem if the desired target dose of 55 Gy is to be delivered. For ependymomas and pineal tumours, a boost to 50–55 Gy is also directed at the primary –

in the case of pineal tumours by a three-field technique.

Arguing that the tumours requiring whole neuraxis radiotherapy are sensitive to low fraction size radiotherapy and, from recent radiobiological research, that low daily fractions of radiotherapy will cause less morbidity to the central nervous system, Plowman and Doughty (1991) have described a partial transmission block method for neuraxis radiotherapy which they anticipate will be less neuropsychometrically morbid to the developing child's brain. In this partial transmission block technique, a dose rate differential between the whole cranium (prophylactic area) and the primary site (high dose volume) is produced throughout the neuraxis radiotherapy prescription. Thereby, the daily dose (fraction size) to the whole neuraxis is kept low (circa 100–120 cGy/fraction) whilst the primary site (e.g. posterior fossa for medulloblastoma) is treated with orthodox daily dose (fraction size) prescriptions (around 165–180 cGy). The total dose to the whole brain and primary site (boost volume) are unchanged and the overall treatment time is not prolonged. It is predicted that serial neuropsychometric studies will show reduced late sequelae (Plowman and Janoun, in preparation). It is also predicted that this technique will prove advantageous for medulloblastoma/PNET/intracranial germ cell tumours/pineoblastoma/high risk ependymoma – i.e. all tumours where neuraxis radiotherapy has a standard use in therapy.

The historically useful test of delivering 20 Gy to the 'boost volume' first to identify radiosensitive pineal tumours is now outmoded owing to modern stereotactic biopsy techniques and should not be considered reliable (Murray *et al.*, 1989).

Where chemotherapy has been used, the interaction of methotrexate and neuraxis radiotherapy must be remembered (Bleyer and Griffin, 1980), and *cis*-platinum sensitization of the inner ear to radiotherapy can lead to profound deafness (Kirkbride and Plowman, 1989).

Newer focal radiotherapy techniques have a limited application in the management of childhood brain tumours. In the first method, stereotactically implanted sealed sources of [198]Au or ^{192}Ir are placed in a preplanned pattern to deliver a brachytherapy dose to the

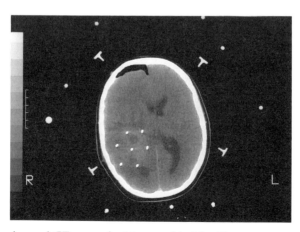

Fig. 13.5 Transaxial, enhanced CT scan of a 16-year-old girl with recurrence of low grade glioma one year after radical radiotherapy. A stereotactically implanted, seven iridium source implant is demonstrated. Eight months later the child is leading a normal life with a CT scan no longer showing any midline shift. (Thomson *et al.*, 1989, with permission of the editor of the *British Journal of Radiology*).

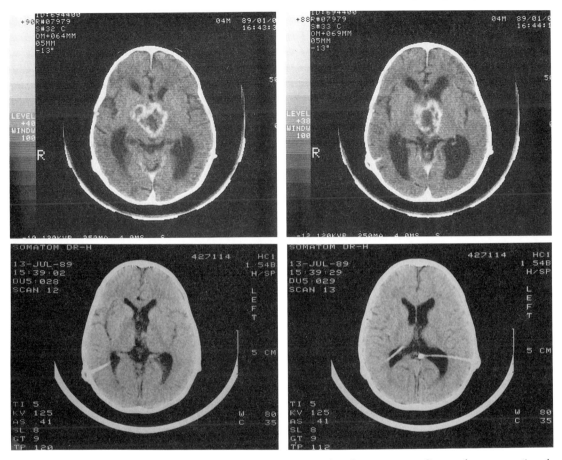

Fig. 13.6 Transaxial, enhanced CT scans of a 3-year-old child with a recurrent glioma after conventional external beam radiotherapy. Top: before converging arc, stereotactic, external beam radiotherapy (SMART); bottom: 6 months after SMART.

entire tumour and, by using the fast falling dose gradients at the periphery of the volume (due to the inverse square law), the surrounding brain does not receive a high dose. The Great Ormond Street/St. Bartholomew's Brain Tumour Group employs such brachytherapy for discrete recurrences of low grade gliomas after conventional therapy (surgery and external beam radiotherapy) has failed. Tumour recurrences up to 5 cm diameter and in sites technically safe to implant are considered in good performance status patients (Thomson *et al.*, 1989). Children have been returned to normal life and CT scans normalized after such brachytherapy (Fig. 13.5), although it is difficult to quantify the overall impact on the disease from the highly selected group chosen to receive this therapy. Nevertheless, there is now an established place for implant brachytherapy for low grade astrocytomas, (Thomson *et al.*, 1989), and we have implanted one small, low grade astrocytoma as definitive primary therapy (currently this child is 18 months post-radical implant, is disease free and by CT scan in complete remission).

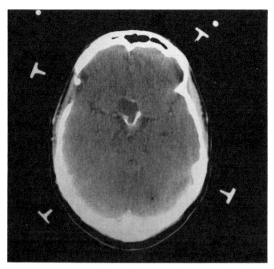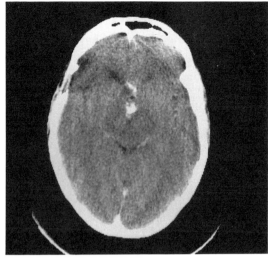

Fig. 13.7 Transaxial, enhanced CT scans of a 34-year-old woman: following conventional neurosurgical resection and external beam radiotherapy, she developed a cystic recurrence of her craniopharyngioma. In the one year leading up to ^{90}Y therapy, she required 3-monthly 'tappings' of 10–12 ml on each occasion. Left panel: before ^{90}Y instillation; right panel: 3 months after ^{90}Y instillation. One year after instillation she has required no further aspirations.

A second focal radiotherapy technique is now available. This external beam method was developed to treat arteriovenous malformations in the brain. In the St. Bartholomew's method, a stereotactic multiple arc rotational technique utilizing an isocentrically mounted linear accelerator is used. The lesion, having been stereotactically pin-pointed, is placed at the isocentre of the linear accelerator, and the accelerator treats the lesion whilst arcing around the lesion – i.e. only the lesion is being continuously irradiated during rotation. This external beam method is successful at sclerosing AVMs in the brain, but recently we have embarked on a programme of delivering a boost to the centre of discrete and small (up to 4.5 cm diameter) low grade astrocytomas that still show enhancement three months after conventional surgery and external beam radiotherapy (Fig. 13.6). This study is too early to report at this time. The advantage of this technique for focal radiotherapy is that it does not carry the risks of implant brachytherapy; conversely it can only treat a spherical volume (whereas the implant programme can treat any shaped volume). Both techniques risk focal/central radionecrosis.

The stereotactic multiple arc external beam radiotherapy (SMART) also has other applications (e.g. chordoma of clivus) and has become an important new radiotherapy capability that we now have routinely available. The proton beam in Boston has also been used for focal brain radiotherapy and chordoma of clivus in particular is well treated by this technique (Austin Seymour *et al.*, 1985).

For cystic recurrences of craniopharyngiomas, intracystic ^{90}Y installation is useful – utilizing the low penetrating beta emission to deliver a high (200 Gy) dose to the secretory epithelium without significantly dosing the sensitive adjacent neural structures (Fig. 13.7). Like Baklund, we have treated semi-cystic, semi-solid recurrences of craniopharyngioma with ^{90}Y installation to the cystic and SMART to the solid component. We do not consider that ^{90}Y (or any other radioisotope) instillation has a role in the management of cystic recurrences of astrocytomas as the underlying problem is not a thin secreting cyst wall.

For tumours that tend to relapse in the leptomeninges – often growing as monolayers of proliferating cells – there is current interest in the delivery of intrathecal/intraventricular radioisotope linked to monoclonal antibodies directed to specific tumour cell antigens. This technique has greatest potential in CNS relapse of acute lymphoblastic leukaemia and non-Hodgkin's lymphoma in children, but is also being applied for CNS relapse of medulloblastoma and PNET There are ongoing studies using panels of monoclonal antibodies or single monoclonal antibodies, linked to ^{131}I, and, in the Institute of Child Health, London, protocols, 11–60 mCi are delivered intrathecally, depending on the CSF volume/age of child and other dosimetric variables. The technique is less likely to be useful where there are macroscopic solid masses of tumour recurrence. Nevertheless, this is yet another area of research radiotherapy that may impact upon recommended paediatric neuro-oncology practice.

13.3.1 RETREATMENT RADIOTHERAPY

Focal radiotherapy salvage programmes aside, is retreatment external beam radiotherapy a fruitful and low risk procedure at relapse after radical external beam therapy previously? The answer to this question is complicated, particularly since the appreciation of the lower weighting to the time exponent in the Sheline isoeffect equation for CNS tolerance – implying that recovery with time from radiation effects is very small (Sheline, 1980). However, it has been the anecdotal

experience of many clinicians, including myself, that when a medulloblastoma patient relapses in the primary site some years after definitive radiation, that retreatment radiotherapy (with or without prior reoperation), to a dose of 30 Gy in 15–17 fractions (and not encompassing the whole brain stem), may offer good palliation without evidence of radionecrosis within the patient's lifetime. These observations have been extended to the retreatment of adults with late recurrences of gliomas preferably using different approach portals but nevertheless retreating the primary volume with good palliative effect and less than 10% evidence of radionecrosis within the patient's lifetime (Dritschilo *et al.*, 1981). Whether it is safe to employ this philosophy to supratentorial astrocytoma relapses in children must be more controversial and our present policy is to employ the brachytherapy programme outlined above.

13.4 THERAPEUTIC PRINCIPLES OF CHEMOTHERAPY

Despite despondence that an intact blood-brain barrier would prevent (particularly hydrophilic) drug molecules penetrating to CNS tumours, early drug trials in adult glioma patients examining adjuvant single agent nitrosourea chemotherapy demonstrated unequivocal prolongation of the median survival of patients receiving such chemotherapy (Shapiro, 1986). Nitrosoureas are small, hydrophobic drug molecules and despite some evidence that the blood-brain barrier is deficient within tumours, there remains considerable doubt that combination drug regimens will improve survival. Single agent CCNU delivered as 100–120 mg/m^2 orally every six weeks has a 17–35% response rate in astrocytomas (Fig. 13.8) and it is difficult to show that the San Francisco regime of CCNU/vincristine/procarbazine (Levin *et al.*, 1980), gives better results.

At a mid-eighties swimming pool party, a

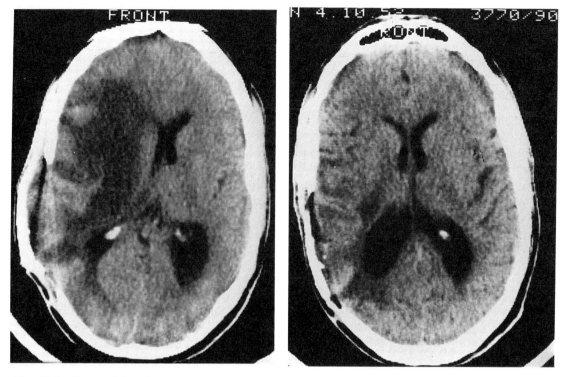

Fig. 13.8 Transaxial, enhanced CT scans of a young man with a high grade astrocytoma, recurrent after neurosurgery and conventionally fractionated external beam radiotherapy to radical dosage. Left panel: at recurrence; right panel: after 3 courses of CCNU (120 mg/m^2).

group of American workers decided to 'throw' every one of eight drugs thought to have activity against paediatric gliomas into a drug combination which achieved the notorious name of '8 drugs in one day'. All eight drugs (methylprednisolone, vincristine, CCNU, procarbazine, hydroxyurea, *cis*-platinum, cytosine arabinoside, DTIC) are given over 24 hours and out of 29 patients treated 36% had a partial or complete response (Pendergrass *et al.*, 1987). Some responses were indeed impressive but toxicity was considerable (Geyer *et al.*, 1988). A study comparing such aggressive combination chemotherapy versus standard dosage CCNU or even PCV should be performed before wide scale acceptance of toxic multi-agent chemotherapy in the palliative setting

of relapsed paediatric gliomas. Similar critical appraisal is required for the high dose BCNU and autologous BMT approach championed by some (Hochberg *et al.*, 1981).

Two excellent large, randomized two-armed studies have looked at the effect of adjuvant CCNU and vincristine following standard neurosurgical resection and neur-axis radiotherapy for medulloblastoma. It had been known for some time that when medul-loblastoma metastasized outside the CNS, the systemic metastases (usually in bone) were sensitive to alkylating agents (e.g. cyclophosphamide, CCNU), and vincristine – indeed they showed similar response to neuroblastoma. It therefore seemed logical to add CCNU plus vincristine (with or without steroid) to standard therapy. In the Chil-

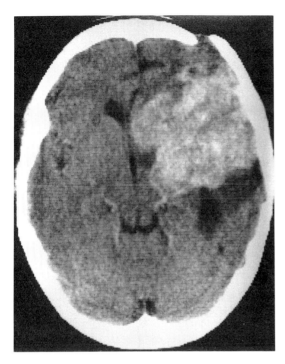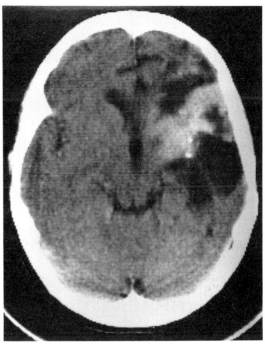

Fig. 13.9 Transaxial, enhanced CT scans of a 19-year-old girl with recurrent peripheral neurectodermal tumour (PNET) – after five neurosurgical resections, two courses of radiotherapy, and OPEC chemotherapy two years earlier. Left panel: before single agent carboplatin; right panel: after 6 courses of carboplatin.

dren's Cancer Study Group (CCSG) trial, 232 patients were entered and in the International Society of Pediatric Oncology (SIOP) Study, 276 children were entered. The results of both studies have been re-viewed by Allen *et al.* (1986): in summary, both trials showed a 10–15% relapse-free survival advantage (most clearly in higher risk patients) to the chemotherapy group at 4½ years, although subsequently the survival curves closed together. There are problems with higher dose CCNU/ nitrosourea chemotherapy after neuraxis radiotherapy due to myelosuppression.

In recent years, it has been appreciated that platinum analogues have activity in paediatric brain tumours, most notably medulloblastoma/PNET. At first *cis*-platin was demonstrated to be effective (Sexauer *et al.*,

1985) but prehydration (with the risk of worsening cerebral oedema, emesis and high tone hearing loss) detracted from the value of this drug. Later, Allen *et al.* (1987b), reported high single agent response rates with carboplatin in medulloblastoma, with lower toxicity to inner ear, and lesser emetic properties (now more easily controllable with $5HT_3$ antagonists).

In our own experience, 25 selected brain tumour relapse children (median age 14 years) were treated with platinum based combination chemotherapy – usually combined with vincristine and etoposide (Douek *et al.*, 1991). Eighteen of 25 evaluable patients had objective responses with a median duration of response of 12 months. Disease-specific response rates were: medulloblastoma/

PNET 9/11, with two complete responses (CR) and seven partial responses (PR) (Fig. 13.9), ependymoma 1/5, pineoblastoma 4/4 (2 CR, 2 PR), and primary brain germ cell tumours 4/4 (3 CR, 1 PR). Our experience in gliomas (only partially reflected in the ependymoma data just cited) is considerably less encouraging and in particular brain-stem gliomas have not responded well or durably.

With the extremely high response rates achievable in advanced/relapsed medullo-blastoma/PNET with this 'new' chemother-apy, there has been an obvious interest in moving it up into a neoadjuvant setting (Allen *et al.*, 1987a). Thus, our current com-bination regimen (carboplatin 175 mg/m² i.v. D1–3, etoposide 100 mg/m² i.v. D1–3, vincris-tine 1.5 mg/m² i.v. D1 q 3–4/52) is now being given as two full courses prior to neuraxis radiotherapy for all medulloblastoma/PNET children. The tolerance of the regimen is good and no difficulty has been experienced in achieving the desired neuraxis radiotherapy dose prescription after this induction chemo-therapy.

As our germ cell and pineoblastoma data on the same regimen has been equally encouraging, our current policy is to employ an identical induction strategy in the man-agement of these two tumour types prior to neuraxis radiotherapy. It will be noted that bleomycin and high dose methotrexate do not form part of the chemotherapy in our intracranial germ cell chemo-radiotherapy programme, for reasons to do with radiosen-sitization – a practice that should be com-pared with that of some other groups.

Furthermore, following the lead of others (Kretschmar *et al.*, 1988) it is our policy to treat infants with continuing chemotherapy until after their second or preferably third birthday – although long-delayed radiother-apy is not recommended in older children. Unfortunately, in the only paper with ade-quate follow-up of young children treated

with primary chemotherapy and delayed radiation, marked mental developmental retardation has still been observed (Mulhern *et al.*, 1989).

13.5 CNS TREATMENT MORBIDITY

The neuropsychological sequelae of paedi-atric radiotherapy in children with acute lymphoblastic leukaemia (ALL) receiving whole brain radiotherapy and in children surviving primary brain tumours treated by radiotherapy have been studied exhaus-tively.

Utilizing the Wechsler Intelligence Scales (WISC) (Wechsler, 1974) and Wide Range Achievement Test (WRAT) Jastak and Jastak (1978) – the latter concentrating on level of academic achievement in reading, spelling and arithmetic, or similar testing – there are now accumulating data that long-term sur-vivors of ALL have a significantly higher inci-dence of deficits than classmates, siblings or children with malignancy not receiving prophylactic cranial radiotherapy (Eiser and Lansdown, 1977; Meadows *et al.*, 1981; Moss *et al.*, 1981).

Different studies have looked at the age at time of cranial radiotherapy, the dose of radiation prescribed, and the influence of coadministered chemotherapy either by the systemic or intrathecal route.

Eiser and Lansdown (1977) first described that children under the age of five years and receiving cranial radiotherapy suffered most marked neuropsychological sequelae, and later work from Great Ormond Street demon-strated that children under three years were more affected than a 3–6 year old group (Jannoun, 1983). Other groups have pub-lished similar findings and it is now clear that children under 3–4 years are most vulnerable to late neuropsychological sequelae.

Throughout the 1970s the dose employed in cranial radiotherapy was 2400 cGy, but in the 1980s a dose of 1800 cGy has been shown to be equally effective at preventing CNS leukaemic relapse, at least in lower risk children. This has allowed study of neuro-psychological deficits in children after 2400 cGy and 1800 cGy of prophylactic whole brain radiation. To date, such studies have not demonstrated a significant difference although there is a trend to worse deficits after 2400 cGy (Trautman *et al.*, 1988; Harten *et al.*, 1984). However, where children have received more than 2400 cGy there are undoubtedly worse deficits. Thus in one study where 29 children had received two courses of cranial irradiation for isolated CNS relapse (i.e. a total of 4800 cGy to whole brain), 20% were functioning in the mentally retarded range with 8 having IQs below 70. Furthermore, with increasing time after the end of radiotherapy, the IQ scores appeared lower; they were also lower in children irradiated at younger ages (Mulhern *et al.*, 1987).

Co-administration of drugs may worsen late neuropsychological sequelae of whole brain radiotherapy, and may have contributed to some of the deficits mentioned above. Thus, Fallovollita *et al.*, (1987) studied 70 patients who had received whole brain irradiation to 2400 cGy either alone or with intrathecal methotrexate. Significantly lower scores were encountered in patients receiving methotrexate. In children less than five years old at diagnosis, the addition of methotrexate decreased the scores by an average of 10–11 points. From animal work and from drug:CNS penetration studies, it may well be that the sequence cranial radiotherapy followed by methotrexate is more damaging than methotrexate followed by brain radiotherapy.

Following whole brain prophylactic radiotherapy, several studies have attempted to correlate the neuropsychological sequelae with CT scan changes. Three CT scan changes: subacute leukoencephalopathy (CT areas of white matter hypodensity); (2) mineralizing microangiopathy (intracerebral calcifications on CT), and (3) cerebral atrophy/gyral thin-ning and ventricular and subarachnoid space dilatation on CT have been studied. In general, it may be said that a correlation exists between CT changes and neuropsychological deficits (Bronwers *et al.*, 1984; Mulhern *et al.*, 1987).

Studies on long-term survivors of primary brain tumours provide a number of interesting data that complement and augment the foregoing work. For example, local radiotherapy portals (i.e. less than whole brain) are commonly employed, and it now seems clear that whole brain radiotherapy (when compared with local field) is a significant contributor to neuropsychological dysfunction and that treatment volume is important.

Bloom *et al.* (1969) reported on work with 22 children surviving 5–17 years after treatment for medulloblastoma and found 18 (82%) were leading active lives, whilst only two were severely disabled. However, Silverman *et al.* (1984) made a case-controlled study of nine medulloblastoma survivors none of whom had had chemotherapy nor any supratentorial surgery. All had received cranio-spinal radiotherapy (3500–4080 cGy) at a median of seven years and posterior fossa boosts (4500–5460 cGy). Neuropsychological testing occurred 3–7.5 years after therapy and the patient group scored within the low–average to average range while the sibling control group scored average to high–average. Deficits were most pronounced in the younger patients.

In a review of the literature, Cohen and Duffner (1984) concluded that between 17% and 46% of children had IQs of less than 70 (a figure that applies to 2% of the normal population). It is interesting to contrast this overview result with the recently updated large personal experience of the late Dr Julian Bloom – a long-term champion of carefully executed and low daily dose fraction size radiotherapy. Jannoun and Bloom (1990) found overall that 15% of children so treated had IQs of less than 70. They found that children with supratentorial tumours or receiving whole neuraxis radiotherapy fared worst in terms of intellectual development and particularly affected were reduced powers of concentration and emotional and behavioural disturbances. Children who received treatment under the age of five were more adversely affected (average IQ 72) than those aged 6–10 (average IQ 93) and those aged 11–15 years (average IQ 107) (Jannoun and Bloom, 1990). These workers also noted that radiotherapy to the hypothalamic region seemed to have surprisingly marked late neuropsychological retardation. Lastly, in an optimistic conclusion to their paper, Jannoun and Bloom state that 3 to 20 years after receiving treatment for brain tumours, approximately 60% of surviving patients were functioning at an average level of intelligence or higher. From the Silverman *et al.* (1984) data it can be noted that the craniospinal dose of 3500–4080 cGy in children is now higher than is recommended (particularly for low risk young children) and that the absence of chemotherapy might have allowed some of the patients to retain average IQ as compared to the acute lymphoblastic leukaemia children who received retreatment drugs and radiation for CNS relapse.

13.5.1 NEUROENDOCRINE SEQUELAE OF BRAIN RADIOTHERAPY

Following radiotherapy to the pituitary and hypothalamus for either brain tumours or skull base tumours, in which this region receives above 40 Gy conventionally fractionated, late defects in anterior pituitary function, often manifesting some years later, have been observed and the cumulative incidence rises with time.

Defective growth hormone due largely to hypothalamic damage (Blacklay *et al.*, 1986) and impaired gonadotrophin secretion are commonest, but ACTH and TSH reserve may also suffer later – particularly where tumour

originally involved the anterior pituitary. Prolactin levels may also rise due to minor hypothalamic damage (Ciccarelli *et al.*, 1988).

Importantly, albeit rarely, precocious puberty may follow hypothalamic/pituitary irradiation in young children (Brauner *et al.*, 1984).

13.6 CONCLUSION AND CURRENT CONTROVERSIES

During the 1980s, much has been learnt concerning the potential for improving treatment results in children with brain tumours. Although high grade gliomas remain an insurmountable problem at present, this chapter has attempted to outline new and promising treatment developments in every other commonly encountered paediatric brain tumour.

13.6.1 TREATMENT IN INFANTS

Many groups, worried by the late morbidity of wide (or even limited) volume radiotherapy to infants, are currently evaluating combination chemotherapy for all infant brain tumours – hoping to postpone radiotherapy until 'the brain' is 2½ to 3 years old. Regimens varying from MOPP to platinum/etoposide have been used for glioma and non-glioma lineage tumours. There are an ever-accumulating number of, albeit anecdotal, successes to date but the practice must certainly remain controversial.

13.6.2 THE PLACE OF PRIMARY (POSTOPERATIVE) CHEMOTHERAPY IN THE MANAGEMENT OF MEDULLOBLASTOMA/PNET

With improved (platinum-based) chemotherapy, the early SIOP/CCSG/POG studies on CCNU/vincristine or methotrexate are now outmoded and the most important (and exciting) question relates to the role of modern neoadjuvant chemotherapy.

13.6.3 OPTIMAL MANAGEMENT OF PRIMARY INTRACRANIAL GERM CELL TUMOURS

There is now a large body of data that supports the use of chemotherapy as primary treatment of intracranial germ cell tumours. Platinum-based regimes (BEP and JOE [carboblatin, vincristine, etoposide]) are current best alternatives, the latter being preferred. There are few centres that would not add craniospinal radiotherapy after 2–3 courses of chemotherapy at present, certainly for teratomas/marker secreting tumours, but is it still needed for pure germinomas? This author believes that it is, but the subject remains controversial.

13.6.4 WHAT IS OPTIMAL CHEMOTHERAPY FOR GLIOMAS?

Here the controversy is to whether there is any chemotherapy better than nitrosoureas either alone or in combination (e.g. procarbazine, CCNU, vincristine). Some groups still use the eight in one day regimen mentioned above and other groups use platinum-based therapy; our own group is not impressed that the results are better than the less toxic nitrosourea-based therapy.

13.6.5 VERY HIGH DOSE CHEMOTHERAPY PLUS ABMT FOR GLIOMAS

This is an interesting concept but the lack of curative success with high dose/marrow ablative chemotherapy regimens has led to a large question mark as to whether such a labour intensive and potentially problematic procedure can be a justifiable procedure. It is not disputed that lengthy remissions in anecdotal cases have been achieved.

13.6.6 NEW RADIOTHERAPY TECHNIQUES

Accelerated fractionation schemes for brain-stem glioma is the subject of a current UK study, having failed to show promise in two North American schemes and despite data suggestive of increased CNS morbidity (Wong *et al.*, 1991; Dische, 1991).

Partial transmission block techniques for all craniospinal radiotherapy work are methods of reducing the daily dose to the neuraxis and thereby it is predicted to reduce late neuro-psychometric sequelae while not protracting the overall treatment courses (Plowman and Doughty, 1991).

Focal radiotherapy by both implants and stereotactic external beam methods has been discussed above. These techniques offer great potential advantages but the exact indications remain controversial.

REFERENCES

Allen, J.C., Bloom, J., Ertel, I. *et al.* (1986). Brain tumours in children: current co-operative and institutional chemotherapy trials in newly diagnosed and recurrent disease. *Sem. Oncol.*, **13**, 110–22.

Allen, J.C., Kim, J.H. and Packer, R.J. (1987a) Neoadjuvant chemotherapy for newly diagnosed germ cell tumours of the central nervous system. *J. Neurosurg.*, **67**, 65–70.

Allen, J.C., Walker, R., Luks, E. *et al.* (1987b) Carboplatin and recurrent childhood brain tumours. *J. Clin. Oncol.*, **5**, 459–63.

Amacher, A.L. (1980) Craniopharyngioma: the controversy regarding radiotherapy. *Child's Brain*, **6**, 57–64.

Austin Seymour, M., Munzenrider, J.E., Goitein, M. and Suit, H. (1985) Progress in low LET particle therapy: intracranial and paracranial tumours and uveal melanomas. *Radiat. Res.*, **104**, 5219–26.

Backlund, E.O. (1972) Studies on craniopharyngiomas. *Acta. Chir. Scand.*, **138**, 743–7.

Baskin, D.S. and Wilson, C.B. (1986) Surgical management of craniopharyngiomas. *J. Neurosurg.*, **65**, 22–7.

Berman, R., Plowman, P.N. and Jones, A.E. (1986) Third ventricular tumours, in *Tumours of the*

Brain, (ed. N.M. Bleehen), Springer, Berlin pp. 161–82.

Blacklay, A., Grossman, A., Savage, M. *et al.* (1986) Cranial irradiation in children with cerebral tumours – evidence for a hypothalamic defect in growth hormone release. *J. Endocrinol.*, **108**, 25–9.

Bleyer, A.W. and Griffin, T.W. (1980) White matter necrosis, mineralising microangiopathy, and intellectual abilities in survivors of childhood leukaemia: associations with central nervous system irradiation and methotrexate therapy, in *Radiation Damage to the Nervous System* (eds H.A. Gilbert and A.R. Kagan), Raven Press, New York, pp. 155–74.

Bloom, H.J.G. (1982) Medulloblastoma in children: increasing survival rates and further prospects. *Int. J. Radiat. Oncol. Biol. Phys.*, **8**, 2023–7.

Bloom, H.J.G. (1983) Primary intracranial germ cell tumours, in *Clinics in Oncology: Germ Cell Tumours* (eds K.D. Bagshaw, E.S. Newlands and R.H.J. Begent) W.B. Saunders, London pp. 233–57.

Bloom, H.J.G. (1986) Treatment of brain gliomas in children, in *Tumours of the Brain*, (ed. N.M. Bleehen), Springer, Berlin, pp. 121–40.

Bloom, H.J., Wallace, E.N. and Henk, J.M. (1969) The treatment and prognosis of medulloblastoma in children. *Am. J. Roentgenol.*, **105**, 43–62.

Bonnin, J.H. and Rubinstein, J.L. (1984) Immunohistochemistry of central nervous system tumours. *J. Neurosurg.*, **60**, 1121–33.

Brauner, R., Czernichow, P. and Rappaport, R. (1984) Precocious puberty after hypothalamic and pituitary irradiation in young children. *N. Engl. J. Med.*, **311**, 920–1.

Bronwers, P., Riccardi, R., Poplack, D. and Fediro, P. (1984) Attentional deficits in long-term survivors of childhood acute lymphoblastic leukaemia. *J. Clin. Neuropsych.*, **6**, 325–36.

Carpenter, D.B., Michelsen, W.G. and Hays, A.P. (1982) Carcinoma of the choroid plexus. *J. Neurosurg.*, **56**, 722–7.

Ciccarelli, E., Corsello, S.M., Plowman, P.N. *et al.* (1988). Prolonged lowering of growth hormone after radiotherapy in acromegalic patients followed for over 15 years. *Advances in the Biosciences*, **69**, 269–72.

Cohen, M.E. and Duffner, P.K. (1984) Ependymomas, in *Brain Tumours in Childhood: Principles of Diagnosis and Treatment*, (eds M.E. Cohen and P.K. Duffner) Raven Press, New York, pp. 136–55.

Cohen, M.E., Duffner, P.K., Heffner, R. *et al.* (1986) Prognostic factors in brain stem gliomas. *Neurology*, **36**, 602–5.

Danoff, B.F., Kramer, S. and Thompson, N. (1980) The radiotherapeutic management of optic gliomas in childhood. *Int. J. Radiat. Oncol. Biol. Phys.*, **6**, 45–50.

Deutsch, M. (1982) Radiotherapy for primary brain tumours in very young children. *Cancer*, **50**, 2785–9.

Deutsch, M. (1984) The impact of myelography on the treatment results for medulloblastoma. *Int. J. Radiat. Oncol. Biol. Phys.*, **10**, 999–1003.

Dische, S. (1991) Accelerated treatment and radiation myelitis. *Radiother. and Oncol.*, **20**, 1–2.

Douek, E., Plowman, P.N. and Kingston, J.E. (1991) Platinum based chemotherapy for recurrent non-gliomatous brain tumours in young patients. *J. Neurol. Neurosurg. Psych.*, **54**, 722–5.

Dritschilo, A., Bruckman, J.E. and Cassady, J.R. (1981) Tolerance of brain to multiple courses of radiation therapy I Clinical experience. *Brit. J. Radiol.*, **54**, 782–6.

Eifel, P.J., Cassady, J.R. and Belli, J.A. (1987). Radiation therapy of tumours of the brainstem and midbrain in children: experience of the joint center for radiation therapy and children's hospital medical centre (1971–1981). *Int. J. Radiat. Oncol. Biol. Phys.*, **13**, 847–52.

Eiser, C. and Lansdown, R. (1977) Retrospective study of intellectual development in children treated for acute lymphoblastic leukaemia. *Arch. Dis. Children*, **52**, 525–9.

Elkind, M.M., Sutton-Gilbert, H., Moses, W.B. *et al.* (1965) Radiation response of mammalian cells in culture. V. Temperature dependence of repair of x-ray damage in surviving cells. *Radiat. Res.*, **25**, 359–76.

Fallovollita, J., Bleyer, A., Robison, L. *et al.* (1987) Intellectual dysfunction after cranial irradiation in young children with acute lymphoblastic leukaemia: concurrent intrathecal methotrexate is a contributory factor. *Proc. Am. Soc. Clin. Oncol.*, **6**, 257.

Garret, P.G. and Simpson, W.J. (1983) Results of radiation treatment. *Int. J. Radiat. Oncol. Biol. Phys.*, **9**, 1121–4.

Geissinger, J. and Bucy, P. (1971). Astrocytomas of

the cerebellum of childhood: long term study. *Arch. Neurol.*, **29**, 125–35.

Geyer, J.R., Pendergrass, T.W., Milstein, J.M. and Bleyer, W.A. (1988) Eight drugs in one day chemotherapy in children with brain tumours: a critical toxicity appraised. *J. Clin. Oncol.*, **6**, 996–1000.

Grossman, A., Cohen, B.L., Charlesworth, M. *et al.* (1984) Treatment of prolactinomas with megavoltage radiotherapy. *Br. Med. J.*, **288**, 1105–9.

Grossman, A. and Plowman, P.N. (1989) Endocrine system, in *Cancer*, (eds K. Sikora and K. Halnan), Chapman and Hall, pp. 349–68.

Hall, E.J. (1978) Radiobiology for the radiologist, 2nd edn, Harper and Row, New York.

Harten, G., Stephani, U., Henze, G. *et al.* (1984) Slight impairment of psychomotor skills in children after treatment of acute lymphoblastic leukaemia. *Europ. J. Pediatr.*, **146**, 189–97.

Hochberg, F.H., Packer, L.M., Takvarian, T. *et al.* (1981) High dose BCNU with autologous bone marrow rescue for recurrent glioblastoma multiforme. *J. Neurosurg.*, **54**, 455–60.

Horwich, A. and Bloom, H.J.G. (1985) Optic gliomas: radiation therapy and prognosis. *Int. J. Radiat. Oncol. Biol. Phys.*, **11**, 1067–79.

Howlett, T.A., Plowman, P.N., Wass, J.A.H. *et al.* (1989) Megavoltage pituitary irradiation in the management of Cushing's disease and Nelson's syndrome: long-term follow-up. *Clin. Endocrinol.*, **31**, 309–23.

Howlett, T.A., Wass, J.A.H., Grossman, A. *et al.* (1989) Prolactinomas presenting as primary amenorrhoea and delayed or arrested puberty: response to medical therapy. *Clin. Endocrinol.*, **30**, 131–40.

Jannoun, L. (1983) Are cognitive and educational development affected by age at which prophylactic therapy is given in acute lymphoblastic leukaemia. *Arch. Dis. Children*, **58**, 953–8.

Jannoun, L. and Bloom, H.J.G. (1990) Long term psychological effects in children treated for intracranial tumours. *Int. J. Radiat. Oncol. Biol. Phys.*, **18**, 747–53.

Jastak, J.F. and Jastak, S. (1978) Wide range achievement test, revised edition. Jastak Associates, Wilmington, DE.

Jenkin, R.D.T., Simpson, W.J.K. and Keen, C.W. (1978) Pineal and suprasellar germinomas:

results of radiation treatment. *J. Neurosurg.*, **48**, 99–107.

Jennings, A.S., Liddle, G.W. and Orth, D.N. (1977) Results of treating childhood Cushing's disease with pituitary irradiation. *N. Engl. J. Med.*, **297**, 957–62.

Katz, E.L. (1975) Late results of radical excision of craniopharyngiomas in childhood. *J. Neurosurg.*, **42**, 86–90.

Kingston, J.E., Plowman, P.N. and Hungerford, J.L. (1985) Ectopic intracranial retinoblastoma in childhood. *Brit. J. Ophthalmol.*, **69**, 742–8.

Kirkbride, P. and Plowman, P.N. (1989) Platinum chemotherapy, radiotherapy and the inner ear: implications for 'standard' radiation portals. *Br. J. Radiol.*, **62**, 457–62.

Kramer, S. (1974) Radiation therapy in the management of craniopharyngiomas, in *Modern Radiotherapy and Oncology: Central Nervous System Tumours*, (ed. T.J. Deeley) Butterworths, London pp. 204–23.

Kretschmar, C., Loeffler, J., Lavally, B. *et al.* (1988) Response to chemotherapy before radiation in children with medulloblastoma. *Proc. Am. Soc. Clin. Oncol.*, **7**, Abstr 311.

Levin, V.A., Edwards, M.S., Wright, D.C. *et al.* (1980) Modified procarbazine, CCNU and vincristine combination chemotherapy in the treatment of malignant brain tumours. *Cancer. Treat. Rep.*, **64**, 237–41.

Mananka, S., Teramoto, A. and Takakura, K. (1985) The efficacy of radiotherapy for craniopharyngioma. *J. Neurosurg.*, **62**, 648–56.

Matson, D. (1956) Cerebellar astrocytoma in childhood. *Pediatrics*, **18**, 150–8.

Meadows, A.T., Gordon, J., Massari, D.J. *et al.* (1981) Declines in IQ score and cognitive dysfunctions in children with acute lymphoblastic leukaemia treated with cranial irradiation. *Lancet*, **ii**, 1015–18.

Moss, H.A., Nannis, E.D. and Poplack, D.G. (1981) The effects of prophylactic treatment of the central nervous system on the intellectual functioning of children with acute lymphoblastic leukaemia. *Am. J. Med.*, (Newton, MA) **71**, 47–52.

Mulhern, P.K., Ochs, J., Fairclough, D. *et al.* (1987) Intellectual and academic achievement status after CNS relapse: a retrospective analysis of 40 children treated for acute lymphoblastic leukaemia. *J. Clin. Oncol.*, **5**, 933–40.

Mulhern, R.K., Horowitz, M.E., Kovnar, E.H. *et al.* (1989) Neurodevelopmental status of infants and young children treated for brain tumors with preirradiation chemotherapy. *J. Clin. Oncol.*, **7**, 1660–6.

Murray, P.A., Harnett, A.N., Thompson, P.I. *et al.* (1989) Periventricular enhancement: a non-pathognomonic sign of intracerebral tumours. *Brit. J. Radiol.*, **62**, 1075–8.

Pendergrass, T.W., Milstein, J.M., Geyer, J.R. *et al.* (1987) Eight drugs in one day chemotherapy for brain tumours: experience in 107 children and rationale for pre-radiotherapy chemotherapy. *J. Clin. Oncol.*, **5**, 1221–31.

Peschel, R.E., Kapp, D.S. and Cardinale, F. (1983) Ependymomas of the spinal cord. *Int. J. Radiat. Oncol. Biol. Phys.*, **9**, 1093–6.

Plowman, P.N. (1983) The effects of conventionally fractionated, extended portal radiotherapy on the human peripheral blood count. *Int. J. Radiat. Oncol. Biol. Phys.*, **9**, 829–39.

Plowman, P.N. (1990) Neurone specific enolase as a marker for medulloblastoma. *Lancet*, **ii**, 1388 (letter).

Plowman, P.N. (1991) Pituitary radiotherapy in *Clinical Endocrinology*, (ed. A. Grossman), Blackwells, Oxford. In press.

Plowman, P.N. and Doughty, D. (1991) An innovative method for neuraxis radiotherapy using partial transmission block technique – a recently adopted treatment regime for medulloblastoma/primitive neurectodermal CNS tumour/intracranial germ cell tumours/pineoblastoma/high risk ependymoma. *Brit. J. Radiol.*, **64**, 603–7.

Plowman, P.N. and Grossman, A. (1990). Treatment of pituitary tumours. *Int. J. Radiat. Oncol. Biol. Phys.*, **19**, 229–30.

Reimer, R., Onofrio, B.M. (1985) Astrocytomas of the spinal cord in children and adolescents. *J. Neurosurg.*, **63**, 669–75.

Rich, T.A., Cassady, J.R., Straud, R. and Winston, K.R. (1985) Radiation therapy for pineal and suprasellar germ cell tumours. *Cancer*, **55**, 932–40.

Rorke, L.B. (1983) The cerebellar medulloblastoma and its relationship to primitive neuroectodermal tumours. *J. Neuropath. Exp. Neurol.*, **42**, 1–15.

Russell, D.R. and Rubinstein, L.J. (1977). *Pathology of Tumours of the Nervous System*, 4th edn, Williams and Wilkins, Baltimore.

Salazar, O.M., Casto-Vita, M., Van Houtte, D.

et al. (1983) Improved survival in cases of intracranial ependymoma after radiation therapy: late report and recommendations. *J. Neurosurg.*, **59**, 652–9.

Sexauer, C.L., Khan, A. and Burger, P.C. (1985) Cisplatinum in recurrent pediatric brain tumours. *Cancer*, **56**, 1497–501.

Shapiro, W. (1986) Therapy of adult malignant brain tumours: what have the clinical trials taught us? *Sem. Oncol.*, **13**, 38–45.

Sheline, G. (1980) Irradiation injury of the human brain: a review of clinical experience, in *Radiation Damage to the Nervous System*, (eds H.A. Gilbert and A.R. Kagan), Raven Press, New York, pp. 39–58.

Sheline, G. (1981) Pituitary tumours: radiation therapy, in *Clinical Endocrinology 1. The Pituitary*, (eds C. Beardwell and G.L. Robertson) Butterworths, London, pp. 106–39.

Shibamoto, Y., Takahashi, M., Dokoh, S. *et al.* (1989). Radiation therapy for brainstem tumour with special reference to CT features and prognosis correlations. *Int. J. Radiat. Oncol. Biol. Phys.*, **17**, 71–6.

Silverman, C.L. Palkes, H., Talent, B. *et al.* (1984) Late effects of radiotherapy on patients with cerebellar medulloblastoma. *Cancer*, **54**, 825–9.

Silverman, C.L. and Simpson, J.R. (1982) Cerebellar medulloblastoma: the importance of posterior fossa dose to survival and patterns of failure. *Int. J. Radiat. Oncol. Biol. Phys.*, **8**, 1869–76.

Sung, D., Harisiadis, L. and Chang, C.H. (1978) Midline pineal tumours and suprasellar germinomas: highly curable by irradiation. *Radiology*, **128**, 745–51.

Sung, D.I., Chang, C.H., Harisiadis, L. and Carmel, P.W. (1980) Treatment results of craniopharyngiomas. *Cancer*, **47**, 847–52.

Thomson, E.S., Afshar, F. and Plowman, P.N. (1989) Paediatric brachytherapy II Brain implantation. *Br. J. Radiol.*, **62**, 223–9.

Touzel, R., Rees, L.H., Besser, G.M. and Wass, J.A.H. (1989) Long term effects of radiotherapy for acromegaly on circulating prolactin. *Acta. Endocrinol.*, **121**, 827–32.

Trautman, P.D., Erickson, C., Shaffer, D. *et al.* (1988) Prediction of intellectual deficits in children with acute lymphoblastic leukaemia. *Dev. Behav. Pediatr.*, **9**, 122–8.

Tsagarakis, S., Plowman, P.N., Jones, A.E. *et al.*

(1991) Megavoltage pituitary irradiation in the management of prolactinomas: long term follow-up. *Clin Endocrinol.*, **34**, 399–406.

Wechsler, D. (1974) Manual for the Wechsler intelligence scale for children – revised. Psychological Corporation, New York.

Wong, C.S., Van Dyk, J. and Simpson, W.J. (1991) Myelopathy following hyperfractionated accelerated radiotherapy for anaplastic thyroid carcinoma. *Radiother. and Oncol.*, **20**, 3–9.

Chapter 14

Retinoblastoma

J. E. KINGSTON and J. L. HUNGERFORD

14.1 INTRODUCTION

Retinoblastoma (Rb), the most common intraocular tumour of childhood, can occur in two forms: a genetic or hereditary variant which is usually multifocal, and a non-genetic, non-hereditary variant which is unifocal. Patients with the genetic form of the disease have an increased susceptibility to the subsequent development of other malignant tumours (Meadows *et al.*, 1985; Draper *et al.*, 1986). Retinoblastoma confined to the eye has one of the best survival rates of all childhood cancers, but once spread outside the globe occurs, the prognosis for survival is dismal. Early diagnosis is, therefore, of paramount importance. In view of the fact that retinoblastoma is a rare neoplasm, optimal management is best achieved by concentrating expertize in a limited number of centres where there can be close collaboration between the ophthalmic surgeon, radiotherapist and paediatric oncologist working alongside experienced pathologists, radiologists and nursing staff.

14.2 EPIDEMIOLOGY

Retinoblastoma occurs in approximately one in every 20 000 live-births and, in the white caucasian population, accounts for between 2.5% to 4% of all cancers in children under the age of 15 years (Parkin *et al.*, 1988). The higher incidence reported in some African countries and in the Indian subcontinent, appears to reflect an increased incidence of the unilateral (non-genetic) form of retinoblastoma suggesting that there may be an environmental factor leading to the increased prevalence in these areas. There is no significant variation in incidence between the sexes. Seventy-five percent of cases are diagnosed before the age of three years, less than 5% after the age of five years. The peak incidence of age at diagnosis for children with unilateral disease is between 24 and 29 months and during the first 12 months for children with bilateral disease (Sanders *et al.*, 1988). In the UK, there are between 40 to 50 new cases of retinoblastoma per year, of which two-thirds have unilateral disease. There is no definite evidence that the incidence of retinoblastoma is increasing and the slight increase that has been reported in some countries, for example, in Holland (Schappert-Kimmijser *et al.*, 1966), is probably explained by more complete ascertainment and by the offspring of an increasing number of long-term survivors with the genetic form of the disease, rather than by an increased mutation rate.

14.3 AETIOLOGY AND GENETICS

The aetiology of retinoblastoma is still

unknown. Reported risk factors for sporadic hereditary retinoblastoma include high maternal and paternal age (DerKinderen *et al.*, 1990), and paternal employment in the metal industry (Bunin *et al.*, 1990). Knudson (1971) proposed a two-mutation hypothesis to explain the observed clinical differences between the genetic and non-genetic forms of retinoblastoma. He suggested that two independent events are required for a cell to acquire the potential to develop into a retinoblastoma. His hypothesis was based primarily on epidemiological data which indicated that children with the multifocal, genetic form of retinoblastoma developed tumours at an earlier age than those with the unifocal, non-genetic form. He proposed that, in children with the genetic form of retinoblastoma, loss or mutation of one allele of the retinoblastoma predisposition gene occurs prezygotically in the germ cell line and is present in every retinal cell, while the second event affects a somatic retinal cell. In children with the non-genetic form of the disease, both events occur sequentially in a somatic retinal cell and, therefore, tumours tend to appear at a later age. Knudson also proposed that the number of tumours acquired by a gene carrier seems to be a matter of chance since it follows a Poisson distribution, with a mean number of three tumours per person. The number of gene carriers who do not develop a tumour is unknown, but has been estimated to be of the order of 5%. Knudson noted that most of the genetic cases result from a new germ cell mutation probably arising as a result of spontaneous mutations at a 'background' mutation rate. Two recent studies, (Zhu *et al.*, 1989; Dryja *et al.*, 1989) have suggested that new germ-line mutations are more frequently derived from the paternal allele suggesting that germ-line mutations may occur more frequently during spermatogenesis rather than oogenesis.

Knudson (1976) suggested that the mutations leading to retinoblastoma involved chromosome 13 sub-band q14 and that the defect in the gene could be caused by either microscopic or submicroscopic change. In 1983, Cavenee and colleagues proposed that the mutated retinoblastoma gene is recessive at the cellular level, since inactivation or loss of the normal allele of the homologue appears to be necessary for tumorigenesis. Murphree and Benedict (1984) considered various possible mechanisms by which homozygosity or hemizygosity for the 'mutant' or inactive allele might arise at the cellular level. They proposed that the first event, which could occur at the germinal level or independently at the somatic level within the retinoblast, would either be a point or frameshift mutation that could not be detected microscopically, or a deletion that could be detected microscopically, resulting in a mutant, inactivated allele of the retinoblastoma gene (rb−). A second event involving the other normal allele (rb+) might then lead to homozygosity or hemizygosity at the retinoblastoma locus in which only the inactivated or deleted allele remained. This second event could be a nondisjunctional loss of the remaining allele, a mitotic recombination which included the rb− allele, a microscopic deletion, a point or frameshift mutation, or inactivation of the normal rb+ allele following a translocation of 13q14 to an inactive X chromosome. Homozygosity at the retinoblastoma locus could also occur if a nondisjunctional loss of the normal allele was followed by reduplication of the remaining rb− allele. Studies using restriction-fragment-length polymorphisms have confirmed that homozygosity of the mutant rb− allele in retinoblastoma is a not infrequent occurrence in both *in vitro* cultures of retinoblastoma cell lines (Cavenee *et al.*, 1983) and *in vivo* studies of retinoblastoma tumour tissue (Dryja *et al.*, 1984). These findings at the molecular level have recently been demonstrated at the cytogenetic level using high resolution banding techniques on retinoblastoma tumour cells in primary culture (Lemieux *et al.*, 1989).

The human retinoblastoma susceptibility gene (Rb1) is situated on the long arm of chromosome 13 at band q14 and is closely linked to the locus for esterase-D, a gene dose-dependent human polymorphic enzyme also assigned to 13q14 (Sparkes *et al.*, 1983). The Rb1 gene was first identified by Friend *et al.* in 1986 and subsequently cloned by Lee *et al.* (1987a). Fung *et al.* (1987) also found structural evidence for the authenticity of the human retinoblastoma gene. The Rb1 gene transcript is encoded in 27 exons dispersed over about 200 kilobases of genomic DNA (Hong *et al.*, 1989; McGee *et al.*, 1989). The gene product has been characterized as a 105 kilo-dalton nuclear phosphoprotein with DNA binding activity (Lee *et al.*, 1987b; Mihara *et al.*, 1989). Studies by Mihara *et al.* (1989) have shown that, when newly synthesized, the protein encoded by the Rb1 gene is not extensively phosphorylated, implying that it is 'underphosphorylated', in cells in the G0 and G1 phases but that it is phosphorylated at multiple sites in cells at the G1/S boundary and in the S phase. They suggest that the underphosphorylated protein may restrict cell proliferation and that phosphorylation may initiate tumorigenesis. It has been shown that the retinoblastoma protein can bind to the oncoproteins of certain transforming DNA viruses such as the E1A protein of adenovirus (Whyte *et al.*, 1988), the large-T antigen of SV40 (DeCaprio *et al.*, 1988) and the E7 protein of the human papilloma virus (Dyson *et al.*, 1989). It is suggested that binding of these viral oncoproteins to the retinoblastoma gene product, may inactivate its tumour-suppressing activity, thereby allowing tumour development.

The retinoblastoma susceptibility gene has been implicated in the development of other cancers including osteosarcoma (Benedict *et al.*, 1988), small cell carcinoma of the lung (Harbour *et al.*, 1988), bladder (Horowitz, *et al.*, 1989) breast (Lee *et al.*, 1988) and various soft tissue sarcomas (Weichselbaum, 1988;

Reissman *et al.*, 1989). It has recently been shown that abnormalities of the p53 gene frequently occur concurrently with inactivation of the retinoblastoma susceptibility gene (Stratton *et al.*, 1990).

14.3.1 CYTOGENETIC STUDIES

Approximately 5% of patients with retinoblastoma carry a constitutional deletion on the long arm of chromosome 13 (Cowell *et al.*, 1986). The association of retinoblastoma with deletion of part of a D-group chromosome in a child with bilateral retinoblastoma and developmental delay, was first described by Lele *et al.* in 1963. Subsequently, Yunis and Ramsay (1978), using sophisticated G-banding techniques with metaphase and prophase chromosome preparations, localized the deletion to band q14 of chromosome 13. Characteristic clinical features of the so-called D-deletion syndrome, which include mental retardation, developmental delay, facial dysmorphism and retinoblastoma, were described by Allerdice *et al.* in 1969. These features, particularly the degree of mental retardation, are variable in expression. Routine karyotypic analysis and identification of a D-deletion in babies presenting with congenital dysmorphism or failure to thrive, can lead to the diagnosis of retinoblastoma at an early stage (Seidmann *et al.*, 1987; Kingston *et al.*, 1990).

14.3.2 GENETIC COUNSELLING

An essential part of the initial assessment of a child with retinoblastoma should include a careful examination of both parents' eyes for the presence of spontaneously regressed retinoblastoma. Approximately 40% of children with retinoblastoma have the genetic form of the disease. In 10% to 15% of patients, there is a known family history of retinoblastoma whilst the remainder have either bilateral or unilateral, multifocal disease and therefore have the genetic form of the disease as a result of a new mutation.

The retinoblastoma gene has a high degree of penetrance, of the order of 80% to 100% (Vogel, 1979), so that the risk of retinoblastoma in the offspring of patients with the genetic form of the disease is 40% to 50%. Children born to such individuals should be regularly screened for retinoblastoma from birth to about the age of five years. Approximately one in ten patients with unilateral retinoblastoma are carriers of the retinoblastoma susceptibility gene and so the risk of retinoblastoma developing in the offspring of a unilateral case is approximately one in twenty.

The use of recombinant DNA probes to study DNA sequence polymorphism for discrimination of the parental origin of chromosome homologues was first described by Cavenee and colleagues in 1986 and now provides the basis for prenatal diagnosis and postnatal prediction of susceptibility to retinoblastoma. More recently, Yandell and colleagues (1989), described a method, using a sensitive technique of primer-directed enzymatic amplification, followed by DNA sequence analysis, to identify mutations as small as a single nucleotide in patients with retinoblastoma who had no family history of the disease. By applying this technique to both tumour and normal somatic cells from the same patient, they were able to identify which patients carried new germ line mutations and thus, were able to distinguish between the hereditary and the non-hereditary form of retinoblastoma.

All patients with the genetic form of retinoblastoma have an increased risk of developing second primary malignancies. There also appears to be an increased risk of osteosarcoma in unaffected gene carriers (Francois, 1977) and a generally increased risk of cancer in relatives of patients with retinoblastoma (Fedrick and Baldwin, 1978; Strong *et al.*, 1984; Sanders *et al.*, 1989).

14.4 HISTOLOGY AND CLINICAL PRESENTATION

14.4.1 HISTOPATHOLOGY

Although controversy still surrounds the histogenesis of retinoblastoma (Hungerford, 1990), recent work has shown that retinoblastoma is a tumour of neuroepithelial origin which may be classified as one of the primitive neuroectodermal tumours (PNETs) of childhood. It appears to arise from retinal precursor cells and the tumour cells bear certain structural similarities to retinal photoreceptor and amacrine cells. Retinoblastoma is characterized by a rapid growth pattern and as a consequence may outgrow its blood supply with resulting necrosis. Calcification occurs in the necrotic areas and is a common feature of large retinoblastomas.

Classically, two patterns of macroscopic growth have been described: (1) endophytic, in which the tumour grows towards the centre of the eye, breaking through the inner layers of the retina into the vitreous cavity, and (2) exophytic in which the tumour grows predominantly from the outer layers of the retina, away from the centre of the eye and towards the subretinal space. Large tumours with an exophytic growth pattern may cause detachment of the retina from the choroid with subsequent accumulation of fluid in the subretinal space. Both endophytic and exophytic growth patterns may be present in the same eye and neither pattern is significant in terms of prognosis. A third type of growth pattern, diffuse infiltrating retinoblastoma, is also recognized and is found in 1% to 2% of enucleated eyes, usually in older patients (Morgan, 1971).

The Flexner-Wintersteiner rosette is the characteristic morphological form of differentiation found in retinoblastoma and appears to represent an attempt to differentiate into photoreceptor cells (Fig. 14.1). Fleurettes which consist of 'bouquet-like' arrangements

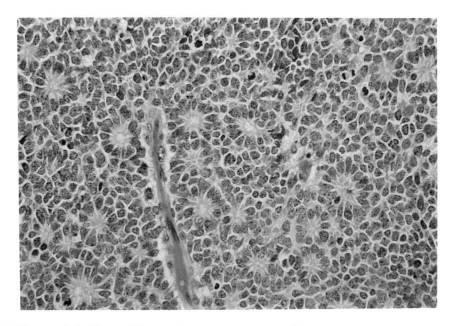

Fig. 14.1   Characteristic Flexner-Wintersteiner rosettes in retinoblastoma.

of cells with abundant pale cytoplasm, small nuclei and long cytoplasmic processes traversing a fenestrated membrane (Tso *et al.*, 1970) are less commonly seen in retinoblastoma. The undifferentiated cells in retinoblastoma are similar to those seen in other PNETs and are small cells with large basophilic nuclei of variable morphology, scant cytoplasm and containing few organelles (Sang and Albert, 1982). Immunohistochemical studies using an antibody to neurone-specific enolase (NSE) have demonstrated that many retinoblastomas stain positively for this glycolytic enzyme (Molnar *et al.*, 1984; Kyritsis *et al.*, 1984). Positivity to antibodies against glial fibrillary acidic protein has also been reported in retinoblastoma but may possibly be due to reactive astrocytes and it is thought that glial differentiation is a rare event in retinoblastoma (Hermann *et al.*, 1989). The product of the N-*myc* oncogene has been described in both retinoblastoma cell lines (Seshadri *et al.*, 1988) and in primary retinoblastomas (Yokoyama *et al.*, 1989) and these authors suggest that the level of the N-*myc* gene product may be inversely correlated with the differentiation of retinoblastoma cells and may relate to prognosis.

Very occasionally, an untreated retinoblastoma does not progress and remains undetected into adult life. Some workers consider that the lesion represents a spontaneous regression of a previously malignant retinoblastoma, (Steward *et al.*, 1956). The clinical appearance of such lesions is often very similar to that of active tumours successfully treated by radiotherapy, with clinical and histological evidence of necrosis (Smith, 1974). The phenomenon of late onset of retinoblastoma may be explained by reactivation of a previously spontaneously arrested growth, as a similar phenomenon has been observed in some patients with late recurrence of neuroblastoma following regression of stage 4S disease during infancy. An alternative hypothesis, proposed by Gallie *et al.*, (1982), is that the lesions are benign hyperplastic nodules or 'retinomas' which have developed from a mutation in relatively mature retinoblasts.

14.4.2 MODE OF PRESENTATION

This depends on the size of the tumour, on its site of origin, and on its growth pattern. The most common presentation is an abnormal or white reflex from the pupil, termed leucocoria (Fig. 14.2). This indicates a large tumour which has usually grown from the periphery before disturbing vision. Smaller tumours situated at or near the macula disturb central vision at an earlier stage causing strabismus before leucocoria is apparent. Occasionally, children with bilateral disease can present with deteriorating vision and if the tumour is very large and bleeding occurs, the child can present with painful, rubeotic glaucoma. Very occasionally, retinoblastoma can present with a pseudohypopyon with tumour cells in the anterior chamber or with a secondary cataract. A very small proportion of children, presenting to their general paediatrician with failure to thrive and abnormal facies, are found to have retinoblastoma on ophthalmological examination undertaken after cytogenetic analysis has revealed a deletion of chromosome 13q14.

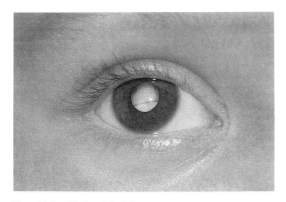

Fig. 14.2 Right-sided leucocoria as the presenting sign in a two-year-old boy with retinoblastoma.

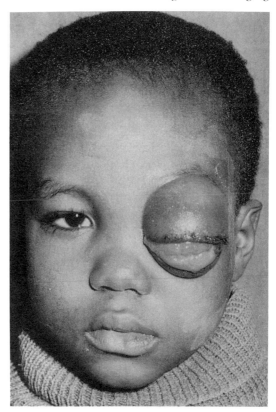

Fig. 14.3 Child with extra ocular extension.

Extra-ocular extension (Fig. 14.3) occurs late in the course of the disease and, although not an uncommon finding at presentation in developing countries, is rare in Western and developed countries.

14.5 DIAGNOSIS AND STAGING

The diagnosis of retinoblastoma is made on clinical grounds by ophthalmoscopic examination. To establish the full extent of the intraocular disease it is advisable to conduct the examination under general anaesthesia with the pupils fully dilated and with indirect ophthalmoscopy, including scleral indentation, to examine the pre-equatorial retina. The location and size of all the tumours

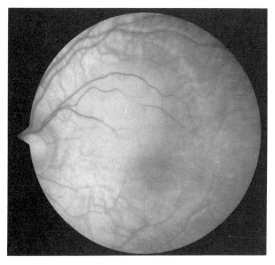

Fig. 14.4 Ocular fundus photograph of an early retinoblastoma confined to the retina.

should be recorded in a drawing or photograph. The characteristic appearance of retinoblastoma is of an elevated white mass sometimes with a large feeder vessel (Fig. 14.4). The tumour may be unifocal or multifocal and in tumours with an exophytic growth pattern, detachment of part or all of the retina may be observed. When retinoblastoma cells break off from the main tumour mass, they grow independently as spheroidal aggregates, a process known as seeding. Seeding may occur into either the subretinal space or the vitreous (Fig. 14.5). The intraocular pressure should be measured and the presence or absence of rubeosis noted. The differential diagnosis includes Coats' disease, toxocariasis, persistent hyperplastic primary vitreous, retrolental fibroplasia, endo-

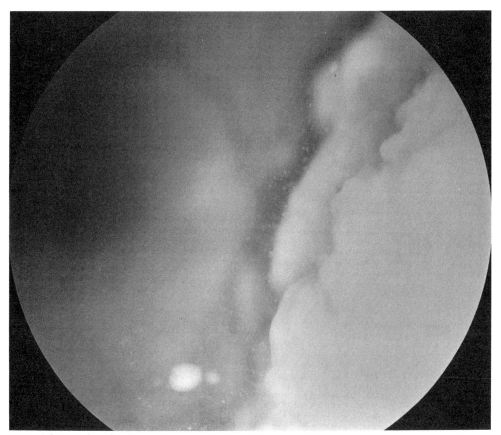

Fig. 14.5 Advanced endophytic retinoblastoma with vitreous seeding.

274

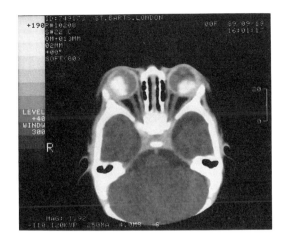

Fig. 14.6 Computed tomographic (CT) scan of orbits showing calcification in a child with bilateral retinoblastoma.

phthalmitis and astrocytic hamartomata. Coats' disease can usually be distinguished from retinoblastoma by the presence of telangiectatic vessels within the detached retina and by the absence of a mass lesion on two-dimensional B-scan ultrasonography. Calcification within retinoblastoma can be demonstrated by computerized tomographic (CT) scanning (Fig. 14.6) and in a study by Arrigg *et al.* (1983), 83% of tumours had evidence of calcification on CT scan. CT scanning is also useful in demonstrating extraocular extension of the tumour and as a baseline to exclude ectopic intracranial retinoblastoma. Magnetic resonance imaging (MRI) has also been used to try and identify extraocular disease (Schulman *et al.*, 1986) and may facilitate identification of intracranial extension of tumour. Intraocular biopsy to obtain tissue and aspiration of aqueous humour for enzyme studies are contraindicated because of the risk of spreading tumour cells outside the eye.

Systemic staging investigations are probably unnecessary in children with small intraocular tumours, (Pratt *et al.*, 1989). However, for children with large retinal tumours requir-

ing enucleation in whom adverse histological factors, such as extensive choroidal or optic nerve involvement are detected, cytological examination of the cerebrospinal fluid, in addition to ultrasonography of the eye and CT scanning of the head and orbits, should be undertaken. All children should have blood taken for cytogenetic analysis and estimation of esterase-D to exclude the possibility of a deletion of chromosome 13 (Cowell *et al.*, 1987).

14.5.1 STAGING CLASSIFICATION

There is no satisfactory staging system for the overall management of retinoblastoma. The classification in general use over the past three decades has been that defined by Reese and Ellsworth (1963) (Table 14.1). This was intended as a classification relating to the prognosis for retaining an eye with retinoblastoma and was not designed as a staging system with regard to prognosis for survival. Subsequently, Stannard *et al.* (1979), proposed a staging system based on histology and clinical features which could be used as a guide to prognosis and treatment (Table 14.2). Recently, an international committee has been set up to establish an internationally acceptable staging system which can form the basis for therapeutic trials.

14.5.2 TREATMENT

The aim of the clinician looking after a child with retinoblastoma is to preserve vision without compromising survival. The choice of treatment is determined by the number, location and size of the tumours and in bilateral disease, each eye is treated on its own merit. In severe bilateral disease, conservative management may be advised for both eyes, even when the visual outlook is poor, providing there is no risk to the life of the child from metastatic spread.

275

Retinoblastoma

Table 14.1 Reese-Ellsworth Classification of retinoblastoma

Group I: Very favourable
(a) Solitary tumour, less than 4 disk diameters* in size, at or behind the equator
(b) Multiple tumours, none over 4 disk diameters in size, all at or behind the equator.

Group II: Favourable
(a) Solitary tumour, 4 to 10 disk diameters in size, at or behind the equator
(b) Multiple tumours, 4 to 10 disk diameters in size, behind the equator

Group III: Doubtful
(a) Any lesion anterior to the equator
(b) Solitary tumours larger than 10 disk diameters in size, behind the equator

Group IV: Unfavourable
(a) Multiple tumours, some larger than 10 disk diameters
(b) Any lesion extending anteriorly to the ora serrata

Group V: Very unfavourable
(a) Massive tumours involving over half the retina
(b) Vitreous seeding

* 1 disk diameter = 1.5 mm

Table 14.2 Staging classification of retinoblastoma (Stannard *et al.*, 1979 with the permission of the editor of the *Br. J. Ophthalmol*).

Stage I: Lesions amenable to local, conservative therapy

Stage II: Lesions unsuitable for conservative local therapy and requiring enucleation but still confined to the eye and orbit. Subdivisions based on the histological assessment of the enucleated eye:
N0 = No invasion of the optic nerve
N1 = Invasion up to or into the *lamina cribrosa*
N2 = Invasion beyond the *lamina cribrosa* but resection line free
N3 = Resection line involved microscopically
C0 = No choroidal invasion
C1 = Superficial invasion of the choroid or ciliary body up to half thickness
C2 = Full thickness of choroid
C3 = Scleral invasion
C4 = Extrascleral invasion

Stage III: Lesions which have spread beyond the orbit but not yet undergone haematogenous metastasis
G1 = Preauricular nodes   G2 = Other nodes
B1 = Positive brain scan or malignant cells in CSF; B2 = Clinical malignant meningitis; B3 = Relapsing intracranial disease

Stage IV: Lesions which have undergone haematogenous metastases
M1 = bone marrow;   M2 = Clinical or radiological bone involvement;   M3 = Liver;   M4 = Multiple organs involved

276

(a) Focal therapy

Focal therapy may be used as the primary treatment of small and medium-sized retinoblastomas or as salvage treatment for small, new lesions or foci of residual disease following external beam irradiation. Photocoagulation and cryotherapy are available in most ophthalmology departments while radioactive plaques are only available in specialist centres.

(i) Indirect photocoagulation

Tumours up to 4 mm in diameter and located behind the equator may be treated by indirect xenon arc photocoagulation. A powerful beam of light is focused accurately on the retina around the base of the tumour and the tumour is encircled by one or two rows of burns in healthy retina. Regression depends on interruption of the blood supply to the tumour. Several treatments may be necessary and should be continued until a flat white scar remains. This method of therapy is not suitable for tumours very close to the optic disc on the temporal side or near to the macula because of possible damage to the macula or to the papillomacular bundle. Direct xenon arc photocoagulation of retinoblastoma should be avoided because viable tumour cells may be released into the vitreous by small explosions and lead to late vitreous recurrence.

(ii) Triple-freeze cryotherapy

Small lesions anterior to the equator are difficult to visualize using the direct ophthalmoscope supplied with most photocoagulators and are best treated with a cryoprobe. Tumours up to 7 mm in diameter can be treated by triple-freeze cryotherapy. The correct positioning of the cryoprobe over the external surface of the tumour is ascertained by indirect ophthalmoscopy and the tumour is

then treated by a triple 'freeze-thaw' method. It is important to allow complete thawing to take place before refreezing. The treatment may be applied through the conjunctiva for anterior lesions. When radiation-induced lens opacities are present, making photocoagulation difficult by direct ophthalmoscopy, the conjunctival sac may be opened and cryotherapy applied to posterior lesions. If the tumour is not inactive after three treatments a radioactive plaque or external beam radiotherapy should be considered.

(b) Radiotherapy

Retinoblastoma is a highly radiosensitive tumour and, fortunately, the retina itself is relatively radioresistant. The successful treatment of retinoblastoma with x-rays was first reported in 1903. Brachytherapy, in the form of radon seeds, for the treatment of retinoblastoma was first developed at St. Bartholomew's Hospital in London (Foster Moore, 1931). Subsequently, radioactive surface applicators were designed and have remained the primary treatment for certain localized tumours.

(i) Scleral plaque therapy

One or two tumours up to 10 mm in diameter may be treated simultaneously or sequentially using a radioactive scleral surface applicator such as an iodine, ruthenium or cobalt plaque. The original surface applicators used gamma emission from the decay of cobalt-60. These have the disadvantage that they cannot be shielded on their external surface and therefore deliver a significant dose of radiation to the orbital bones. Their advantage is that they can be used repeatedly because of their long half-life of 5.2 years. The use of shielded applicators, with either iodine-125 which has a lower emission energy, or ruthenium-106 which produces β rays, reduces the scatter dose to the surrounding tissues, but has the disadvantage that these isotopes have a shorter

277

half-life and therefore require regular reactivation.

Each form of applicator is available in a range of sizes and each has an inner radius of curvature corresponding to that of the eye. Under general anaesthetic, an applicator of appropriate size is sutured directly over the base of the tumour and removed once a dose of 40 Gy has been delivered to the apex of the tumour. The base of the tumour receives a much higher dose which may result in vascular occlusion and for this reason surface applicators should not be used for treating tumours near the optic disc or macula. However, single lesions that are situated away from the disc and macula are eminently suitable for treatment with a surface applicator and, where the fields do not overlap, two applicators can be applied simultaneously. Residual or recurrent disease following external beam radiotherapy can be treated by a surface applicator. However, radiation retinopathy may develop in areas of retina which have been irradiated twice and late vitreous haemorrhage may occur.

(ii) External beam radiotherapy

External beam radiotherapy is indicated in the following instances: when any single tumour is larger than 10 mm in diameter, when more than two scleral plaques would be required to treat multiple tumours less than 10 mm in diameter, when retinal detachment or vitreous seeding is present, and in cases where the tumour is within 3 mm of the optic disc or macula. Depending on the location of the tumour and on the presence or absence of vitreous seeding or retinal detachment, either a whole eye or a 'lens sparing' approach is used. For patients with anterior lesions, vitreous seedlings, or a retinal detachment extending to the ora serrata, a whole-eye approach is necessary.

At St. Bartholomew's Hospital, when a whole-eye approach is deemed necessary, treatment is given via an anterior field when the other eye is *in situ*. However, when the contralateral eye has been enucleated, a lateral beam is preferred as the exit dose will then traverse less critical tissues. When both eyes require whole eye external beam irradiation, parallel opposed portals are chosen. The tumour dose of 40 Gy, usually prescribed at a depth of 2 cm calculated to be the back of the eye, is given in 20 fractions over 28 days, treatment being administered every week-day. When there are multiple vitreous seedlings, the dose is increased to 44 Gy in 22 fractions. All radiotherapy is carried out with megavoltage photon apparatus using either a linear accelerator or telecobalt machine. Late morbidity from whole eye irradiation includes the development of cataract approximately 18 months after treatment, shrinkage of eyelids and ocular dryness which limits the tolerance of contact lenses after cataract surgery.

For children with posteriorly situated tumours, a lens sparing technique, first developed at Utrecht University (Schipper, 1983), and subsequently modified (Harnett *et al.*, 1987), is preferred. This technique allows screening of the lens and anterior chamber. A contact lens fitted to the cornea of the infant provides a fixed reference point from which all measurements can be made (Fig. 14.7). This point is connected accurately to a linear accelerator, the beam of which is split to minimize beam divergence; using an extended collimator, an anterior beam edge almost free of penumbra and divergence is produced. The distance from the front of the cornea to the back of the lens is ascertained by ultrasound. A head shell is made for each child to aid immobilization and facilitate a repeated, highly accurate set up each day. Planning marks on the shell also help to check the child's position. A lateral beam encompasses the retina up to the back of the lens and where the other eye is still *in situ*, is appropriately angled at 40 degrees to avoid an exit dose to the contralateral eye (Harnett *et al.*, 1987). This approach is recommended for posteriorly situated

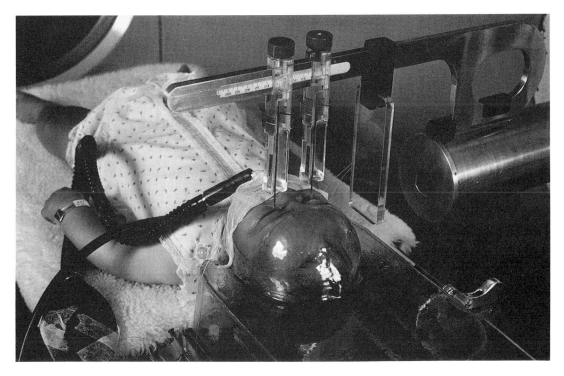

Fig. 14.7 Anaesthetized child receiving bilateral lens-sparing external beam radiotherapy.

tumours without vitreous seeding, particularly for lesions situated critically on the temporal side of the optic disc.

Response to scleral plaque or external beam irradiation, is assessed at about four weeks following completion of therapy. Various patterns of tumour regression may be observed. The two common ones are type I or 'cottage cheese' due to calcium deposition and type II or 'fish flesh', in which a homogeneous, avascular mass with an annulus of atrophic pigment around the base is observed. The expertise of an ophthalmologist familiar with the different regression patterns is essential to assess response.

(c) Enucleation

Enucleation is mandatory when there is involvement of the optic nerve, extrascleral extension, or conservative treatment has failed and it is recommended when the tumour involves more than half the retina, when there is evidence of glaucoma and when no useful vision is likely to be retained with conservative therapies. In a series of 516 children with retinoblastoma seen in the ocular oncology units at St. Bartholomew's and Moorfields Eye Hospitals during the period 1970–89, of the children with unilateral retinoblastoma, 80% had the affected eye enucleated whilst 72% of the bilateral cases had one eye removed and 12% had both eyes removed.

Enucleation is not an easy procedure, particularly in very young infants, and the most important aspect of the operation is to excise as much as possible of the orbital portion of the optic nerve along with the eye. Following enucleation of an eye containing retinoblastoma, it is important for the pathologist to

279

establish whether or not the optic nerve is invaded by tumour cells and to determine the extent of optic nerve invasion, that is, whether the involvement is pre-laminar, retrolaminar or to the resection margin itself, as this will influence further management. It is also necessary to ascertain whether the tumour cells are in the subarachnoid space or within the nerve parenchyma itself. Similarly, it is essential to assess the degree of choroidal invasion, that is, whether the tumour involves just the superficial layers or is more extensive, involving greater than half the thickness of the choroid. This latter finding is likely to indicate an increased risk of metastatic spread. The degree of choroidal invasion is frequently related to the extent of optic nerve invasion (Rootman *et al.*, 1978).

(d) Chemotherapy

The role of adjuvant chemotherapy in the management of retinoblastoma remains controversial. A multi-institutional study carried out by the Children's Cancer Study Group and the Pediatric Oncology Group in America (Wolff *et al.*, 1981), failed to show a benefit for adjuvant chemotherapy in children with unilateral, Reese Ellsworth group V retinoblastoma undergoing enucleation as primary treatment. Nevertheless, as a small proportion of children with tumours apparently confined to the eye develop metastatic disease following enucleation, it is important to identify the children at risk of this complication. It is in this group of patients that the use of adjuvant chemotherapy is likely to have a beneficial effect. Clinical and histological factors which have been reported to be associated with an increased risk of metastatic disease include optic nerve length <5 mm removed at enucleation (Rubin *et al.*, 1985), extensive choroidal invasion in the presence of retrolaminar optic nerve invasion (McCartney *et al.*, 1988) and extension of tumour to the cut end of the optic

nerve (Stannard *et al.*, 1979; Kopelman *et al.*, 1987). Prospective multi-institutional trials with patients staged by a common staging classification according to potentially predictive prognostic factors may provide a rationale for the role of chemotherapy in an adjuvant situation.

The role of chemotherapy in extra-ocular disease is not disputed but in view of the rarity of the problem there is a dearth of single agent data. In one of the few reported studies which attempted to look at the response of metastatic disease to single-agent therapy, Lonsdale *et al.* (1968), showed that cyclosphosphamide produced the best therapeutic effect (with a response rate of 47%). Ragab *et al.* in 1975 reported the outcome of six children with retinoblastoma treated with doxorubicin (adriamycin) as a single agent. One child showed a complete response but four had no response to the drug. Pratt *et al.* (1985) at St. Jude's Children's Research Hospital found the best responses in children treated with the alkylating agents cyclophosphamide and ifosfamide. Pratt's studies showed superior results for the combination of cyclophosphamide and vincristine. In view of the similarity of retinoblastoma to other neuroectodermal tumours such as neuroblastoma, multi-drug combinations containing platinum have been used and have been

Table 14.3 Indications for chemotherapy (data from St. Bartholomew's Hospital)

1 Extra ocular disease
  (a) orbital relapse
  (b) metastatic spread
  (c) ectopic intracranial retinoblastoma

2 Patients with extensive choroidal invasion and retrolaminar or cut end of optic nerve invasion

3 As part of salvage therapy of an only eye following failure of RT

4 Initial therapy, prior to radiotherapy in child with very extensive disease in both eyes

shown to be successful in achieving remissions in children with extraocular disease (Kingston *et al.*, 1987).

Chemotherapy plays an essential role in the treatment of orbital relapse (Goble *et al.*, 1990) and is also important in the management of ectopic intracranial retinoblastoma. It may have a role in the management in the primary treatment of extensive bilateral disease but this remains to be proven. The indications that are currently used for chemotherapy at St. Bartholomew's Hospital are shown in Table 14.3.

Laboratory and clinical research projects are essential in order to develop and test new chemotherapeutic agents. The human tumour clonogenic assay established by Hamburger and Salmon in 1977 has been used to test the chemosensitivity profiles of primary and cultured human retinoblastoma cells (Inomata and Kaneko 1987; Chan *et al.*, 1989). A xenograft model with heterotransplantation of human retinoblastoma cells into the anterior chamber of the nude mouse eye has been developed by White *et al.* (1989) and, using this model, the authors have shown that a new agent, diaziquone, is more effective than cyclophosphamide and other conventional agents against a retinoblastoma xenograft cell line.

14.6 PROGNOSIS AND RECURRENCE

The three-year survival rate for children with retinoblastoma in the UK is nearly 90% (Sanders *et al.*, 1988). These results have been achieved by the judicious use of surgery, radiotherapy and focal methods of treatment such as cryotherapy and photocoagulation. During the period 1960–88, 731 children with retinoblastoma were seen in the ocular oncology units in St. Bartholomew's and Moorfields Eye Hospitals. The actuarial overall five-year survival rate for all patients was 87% (Fig. 14.8). The corresponding survival for these patients by laterality of the tumour is shown

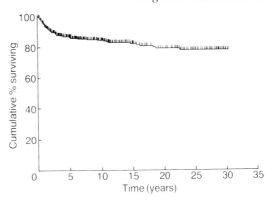

Fig. 14.8 Overall survival in retinoblastoma (data from St. Bartholomew's and Moorfields Eye Hospitals 1960–88).

in Fig. 14.9. This shows that children with unilateral retinoblastoma surviving for five years from diagnosis can be considered cured. This is not the case for patients with bilateral disease in whom the continuing attrition is due to deaths from ectopic intracranial retinoblastoma and second tumours.

In our series of 731 children, the commonest cause of death in children with both unilateral and bilateral retinoblastoma, was from metastatic disease, accounting for 97% of the deaths in children with unilateral dis-

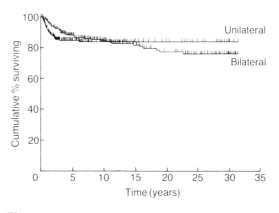

Fig. 14.9 Effect of laterality on survival in retinoblastoma (data from St. Bartholomew's and Moorfields Eye Hospitals 1960–88).

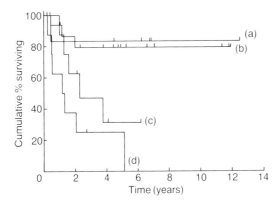

Fig. 14.10 Overall survival for patients with (a) invasion of cut end of optic nerve and either superficial or no choroidal invasion; (b) extensive choroidal invasion and either pre-laminar or no optic nerve invasion; (c) extensive choroidal invasion and retrolaminar optic nerve invasion; (d) extensive choroidal invasion and cut end of optic nerve involvement.

ease and for 50% of the deaths in children with bilateral disease. In children with bilateral retinoblastoma, there was a significant mortality from ectopic intracranial retinoblastoma (24%) and also from second malignant tumours (22%).

Poor survival rates have been reported for patients with invasion of the cut end of the optic nerve and heavy choroidal involvement (Stannard *et al.*, 1979; Rubin *et al.*, 1985) although the effect of choroidal invasion remains controversial (Redler and Ellsworth 1973; Kopelman *et al.*, 1987). Multivariate analysis of our data from 330 children undergoing enucleation showed that the deleterious effect of extensive choroidal invasion was lost in the absence of either retrolaminar or cut end of optic nerve invasion. The analysis revealed two groups with a particularly poor prognosis; children with retrolaminar extension and heavy choroidal invasion for whom the five-year survival was only 31% and children with both extensive choroidal and

cut end of optic nerve invasion, for whom the five-year survival rate was 25% (Fig. 14.10).

The prognosis for vision depends on the size and location of the tumours within the eye. Tumours involving the macula always lead to poor central visual acuity and in a series reported from Stanford by Egbert *et al.* (1978), this was the most common cause of reduced visual acuity.

14.6.1 ORBITAL RECURRENCE

Clinically, orbital recurrence is commonly manifested by poor fitting of the ocular prosthesis or the development of an obvious lump in the socket (Fig. 14.11) and usually presents within a year of enucleation. Orbital relapse has been associated with a poor prognosis for survival because in many cases extraorbital spread is detected at the time of the orbital recurrence or develops shortly afterwards.

In a series of 16 children with an orbital recurrence reported by Hungerford *et al.* (1987), 15 of the children died with a median survival of only 14 months from diagnosis of recurrence. Death resulted either from intracranial spread or from the development of distant metastatic disease. The one long-term survivor had been treated with adjuvant chemotherapy in addition to orbital radiotherapy and surgery. In a subsequent report

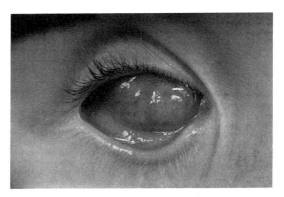

Fig. 14.11 Orbital recurrence of retinoblastoma.

from the same institution (Goble *et al.*, 1990), five children with an isolated orbital recurrence were successfully salvaged with combined modality treatment including lumpectomy, multi-agent systemic chemotherapy and orbital radiotherapy. Adjuvant chemotherapy would appear to play an essential role in the management of a child with an orbital relapse.

Factors predisposing to the development of an orbital recurrence include invasion of the cut end of the optic nerve, extrascleral extension, and an intraocular biopsy undertaken for diagnostic purposes (Stevenson *et al.*, 1989). To reduce the risk of an orbital recurrence, radiotherapy to the orbit should always be advised when there is evidence of invasion of the cut end of the optic nerve and in the presence of extra scleral extension.

14.6.2 ECTOPIC INTRACRANIAL RETINOBLASTOMA

In 1980, Bader and colleagues used the term 'trilateral' retinoblastoma to describe the clinical syndrome of bilateral retinoblastoma with an ectopic midline intracranial tumour. In a subsequent paper (Bader *et al.*, 1982), it was suggested that the development of an ectopic midline neuroblastic tumour in a patient with bilateral retinoblastoma, represented an additional focus of multicentric retinoblastoma rather than a second primary tumour.

The child with ectopic intracranial retinoblastoma presents either with symptoms and signs of raised intracranial pressure due to secondary hydrocephalus or, when the lesion arises in the suprasellar region, with symptoms of diabetes insipidus. The finding of a discrete, calcified, midline mass in the pineal or suprasellar region, on CT head scanning (Fig. 14.12) in a child with the genetic form of retinoblastoma, is sufficient for diagnosis.

In a series of 12 children with ectopic intracranial retinoblastoma reported by Kingston *et al.* (1985), the median interval from the initial diagnosis of intraocular retinoblastoma to the development of an isolated intracranial lesion was 34 months (range four to 70 months). All 12 children died, with a median survival of eight months. The four children who received no further treatment all died within four months (median survival two months). Treatment with radiation alone or in combination with chemotherapy appeared to prolong survival in the other eight children but did not achieve any durable remissions. The major cause of death in these patients was the development of spinal metastases. The poor prognosis for survival of children with ectopic intracranial retinoblastoma has been observed in other series (Bader *et al.*, 1982; Holladay *et al.*, 1991).

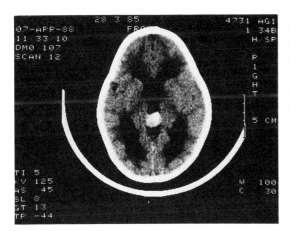

Fig. 14.12 Characteristic CT head scan appearances of child with ectopic intracranial retinoblastoma showing a calcified mass in the pineal region and secondary hydrocephalus.

14.6.3 METASTATIC DISEASE

Metastatic disease, like orbital relapse, usually manifests within a year of diagnosis. Retinoblastoma can spread by direct extension along the optic nerve into the central nervous system, through the blood vessels of the choroid, and via the lymphatics of the conjunctiva and lid. Haematogenous spread most frequently leads to metastases in bones, bone marrow and brain. Lymphatic spread commonly involves the pre-auricular and submandibular nodes and may be the cause of the subcutaneous deposits seen around the orbit and on the scalp. The patterns of metastatic spread have been reviewed by McKay *et al.* (1984).

The child with metastatic retinoblastoma usually shows a good initial response to chemotherapy but, unfortunately, these responses are often not sustained and there is subsequent early relapse and death (White, 1983; Kingston *et al.*, 1987a). However, there are an increasing number of reports now appearing in the literature, of long-term survival following metastatic retinoblastoma (Judisch *et al.*, 1980; Petersen, 1987; Saleh *et al.*, 1988).

14.6.4 COMPLICATIONS OF TREATMENT

The risk of cataract development is related both to the dose of radiation administered and to the technique of radiotherapy. In children given 40 Gy by a whole eye approach, significant lens opacities usually develop at 18 to 24 months post irradiation. Radiation damage to the lacrimal gland may result in decreased or absent lacrimal secretion with consequent drying of the surface of the eye; when this happens the surface of the cornea becomes rough and filaments can be seen in the epithelium of the cornea and conjunctiva leading to the 'dry eye' syndrome which is accompanied by considerable ocular discomfort. New radiotherapy techniques to spare the lens and anterior chamber, as outlined above, have been successful in preventing both cataract formation and the 'dry eye' syndrome.

Retinal vascular injury is a more serious complication and is likely to occur in eyes that need further radiation treatment for recurrent disease. There is some evidence that the administration of chemotherapy in addition to radiotherapy may increase the risk of radiation complications in the eye (Chan and Shukovsky, 1976).

Abnormalities of orbital bone growth may occur after both enucleation and radiotherapy. There is a significant reduction in growth of the orbit after enucleation (Osborne *et al.*, 1974) and both bone and soft tissue growth is retarded by radiotherapy; this may lead to asymmetry of the orbits when only one orbit is irradiated.

14.6.5 SECOND TUMOURS

It is now well recognized that patients with the genetic form of retinoblastoma have a significant risk of developing a second, histologically distinct, primary neoplasm (Abramson *et al.*, 1976; Meadows *et al.*, 1985; Draper *et al.*, 1986). Estimates of this risk have varied between 8.4% at 18 years (Draper *et al.*, 1986) to 90% at 30 years (Abramson *et al.*, 1984). In the series of 882 retinoblastoma patients reported by Draper *et al.* (1986) 30 developed second neoplasms. The cumulative incidence rate of second tumours was 4.2% at 18 years for the whole group and 8.4% for those with the genetic form of retinoblastoma. The incidence of second tumours in patients with the genetic form of retinoblastoma who had been irradiated was much greater than the incidence in patients with the non-genetic form who received radiation. In a series of 215 patients with bilateral retinoblastoma reported by Roarty *et al.* (1988), the cumulative incidence of second tumours at 30 years was 35.1% for the 137 patients who received radiation therapy compared with 5.8% for the 78 patients who were not irradiated. There is some evidence from these data of Draper *et al.* (1986) and Roarty *et al.* (1988) that patients with the genetic form of retinoblastoma may be particularly sensitive to the carcinogenic effect of radiation. However, although many sarcomas in patients with retinoblastoma develop within the radiation field and are therefore attributed to radiotherapy, similar numbers occur outside the radiation field and occur also in patients not treated with radiation (Abramson *et al.*, 1979).

Osteosarcoma is the commonest second malignancy occurring after retinoblastoma (Meadows *et al.*, 1980). Other common second malignancies reported include soft tissue sarcomas – mainly fibrosarcoma and leiomyosarcoma – central nervous system tumours, malignant melanoma, and acute leukaemia (Kingston *et al.*, 1987b). Tucker *et al.* (1987) suggested that the risk of bone tumours following retinoblastoma was approximately 1000 times the rate in the normal population. Hawkins *et al.* (1987) reported a relative risk of 415 for the development of a malignant bone tumour after genetic retinoblastoma and a relative risk of 130 for the development of a soft tissue sarcoma.

Aggressive management of the second primary tumour with combined modality therapy can achieve long-term remissions (Smith *et al.*, 1989).

14.7 CONCLUSION AND CURRENT CONTROVERSIES

Recognition of the retinoblastoma gene and the technology to identify point mutations within it will make it possible to offer antenatal diagnosis to an increasing number of patients. These advances at the molecular level will help to determine whether a new mutation is of somatic or germinal origin and thereby identify gene carriers. In future, it should be possible to screen offspring of retinoblastoma patients for the retinoblastoma susceptibility gene by a simple blood test. It will not then be necessary to subject these children to repeated ophthalmic examinations under anaesthetic as is current practice.

In addition, the growing understanding of the role of phosphorylation and binding of viral oncoproteins to the Rb1 gene product in the initiation of tumorigenesis is likely to facilitate the future development of techniques to return a deficient cell to normal and, possibly, to reverse the oncogenic process.

14.7.1 STAGING CLASSIFICATION

The Reese-Ellsworth grading system, based on size and location of tumours within the eye, was designed to predict visual outcome rather than survival. There is no universally accepted, comprehensive staging system which can be used as a guide for treatment and prognosis for survival. However, an international committee has been established and a new system is in the process of being drawn up. This takes into account the histological features of enucleated globes. Two of the major controversies are whether extensive choroidal invasion is an independent prognostic factor in the absence of retrolaminar nerve invasion, and whether laminar invasion should be classified as extra-ocular extension.

14.7.2 LENS-SPARING RADIOTHERAPY

There is a theoretical risk that lens-sparing radiotherapy could result in an increased number of anterior recurrences. This problem can be reduced to a minimum by (a) the use of cryotherapy to small tumours located anteriorly, prior to radiotherapy; (b) by ensuring that there is regular and careful follow-up post radiotherapy, so that any new tumours arising anteriorly can be treated at an early stage with cryotherapy, and (c) by careful selection of cases, avoiding lens sparing radiotherapy in patients with vitreous seedlings and in those with retinal detachments extending to the *ora serrata*.

14.7.3 ROLE OF CHEMOTHERAPY IN THE MANAGEMENT OF INTRAOCULAR RETINOBLASTOMA

Retinoblastoma is a chemosensitive tumour and chemotherapy is effective in intra-ocular tumours. Although there would seem to be little justification for using chemotherapy in children with unilateral tumours where there is normal vision in the remaining eye, in situations where there is extensive bilateral disease, chemotherapy can be used to shrink the tumours and may improve the local control rate subsequently achieved by radiotherapy. However, visual outcome in patients managed in this way has yet to be documented. In addition, children with bilateral retinoblastoma carry the Rb gene and are therefore prone to second tumour formation. It is possible that the addition of chemotherapy to radiotherapy may enhance this risk. Long-term survival may therefore be compromised at the expense of an attempt to preserve vision.

14.7.4 THE USE OF PHOTOCOAGULATION

The use of photocoagulation may predispose paediatric patients to the development of vitreous seedlings if there is injudicious use of the photocoagulator directed on to the tumour itself. Cryotherapy is therefore the focal treatment of choice wherever possible.

14.7.5 SPONTANEOUS REGRESSION

Do apparently inert tumours represent a benign variant of retinoblastoma sometimes called retinoma or are they malignant tumours which have undergone spontaneous regression as is seen in neuroblastoma, another childhood neuroectodermal tumour? Clinically, they are sometimes indistinguishable from lesions that have calcified following external beam radiotherapy. Whatever their histogenesis, they require regular observation as reactivation of an apparently spontaneously regressed lesion can occur after a period of several years.

14.7.6 GENETIC COUNSELLING

Retinoblastoma has a 90% cure rate. What,

therefore, is the justification for offering termination to parents of offspring carrying the Rb gene?

14.7.7 SECOND TUMOURS

Should the issue of second malignancies be discussed at the time of diagnosis or later when the parents have had time to come to terms with the primary problem? Views differ. Patients carrying the Rb gene should certainly be followed up and they themselves are probably best counselled during late adolescence.

REFERENCES

Abramson, D.H., Ellsworth, R.M. and Zimmerman, L.E. (1976) Nonocular cancer in retinoblastoma survivors *Trans. Am. Acad. Ophthalmol. Otolaryngol.*, **81**, 454–7.

Abramson, D.H., Ronner, H.J. and Ellsworth, R.M. (1979) Second tumours in nonirradiated bilateral retinoblastoma *Am. J. Ophthalmol.*, **87**, 624–7.

Abramson, D.H., Ellsworth, R.M., Kitchin, D. and Tung, G. (1984) Second nonocular tumors in retinoblastoma survivors. Are they radiation induced? *Ophthalmology*, **91**, 1351–5.

Allerdice, P.W., Davis, J.G., Miller, O.J. *et al.* (1969) The 13q- deletion syndrome. *Am. J. Hum. Genet.*, **21**, 499–512.

Arrigg, P.G., Hedges, T.R. and Char, D.H. (1983) Computed tomography in the diagnosis of retinoblastoma *Br. J. Ophthalmol.*, **67**, 588–91.

Bader, J.L., Miller, R.W., Meadows, A.T. *et al.* (1980) Trilateral retinoblastoma, *Lancet*, **ii**, 582–3.

Bader, J.L., Meadows, A.T., Zimmerman, L.E. *et al.* (1982) Bilateral retinoblastoma with ectopic intracranial retinoblastoma: trilateral retinoblastoma. *Cancer Genet. Cytogenet.*, **5**, 203–13.

Benedict, W.F., Fung, Y-KT. and Murphree, A.L. (1988) The gene responsible for the development of retinoblastoma and osteosarcoma. *Cancer*, **62**, 1691–4.

Bunin, G.R., Petrakova, A., Meadows, A.T. *et al.* (1990) Occupations of parents of children with retinoblastoma: a report from the Children's Cancer Study Group *Cancer Res.*, **50**, 7129–33.

Cavenee, W.K., Dryja, T.P., Phillips, R.A. *et al.* (1983) Expression of recessive alleles by chromosomal mechanisms in retinoblastoma. *Nature*, **305**, 779–84.

Cavenee, W.K., Murphree, A.L., Shull, M.M. *et al.* (1986) Prediction of familial predisposition to retinoblastoma *N. Engl. J. Med.*, **314**, 1201–7.

Chan, H.S., Canton, M.D. and Gallie, B.L. (1989) Chemosensitivity and multidrug resistance to antineoplastic drugs in retinoblastoma cell lines. *Anticancer Res.*, **9**, 469–74.

Chan, R.C. and Shukovsky, L.J. (1976) Effects of irradiation on the eye. *Radiology*, **120**, 673–5.

Cowell, J.K., Rutland, P., Jay, M. and Hungerford, J.L. (1986) Deletions of the esterase-D locus from a survey of 200 retinoblastoma patients *Hum. Genet.*, **72**, 164–7.

Cowell, J.C., Thompson, E. and Rutland, P. (1987) The need to screen all retinoblastoma patients for esterase D activity: detection of submicroscopic chromosome deletions. *Arch. Dis. Child.*, **62**, 8–11.

DeCaprio, J.A., Ludlow, J.W., Figge, J. *et al.* (1988) SV40 large tumor antigen forms a specific complex with the product of the retinoblastoma susceptibility gene. *Cell*, **54**, 275–83.

DerKinderen, D.J., Koten, J.W., Tan, K.E. *et al.* (1990) Parental age in sporadic hereditary retinoblastoma. *Am. J. Ophthalmol.*, **110**, 605–9.

Draper, G.J., Sanders, B.M. and Kingston, J.E. (1986) Second primary neoplasms in patients with retinoblastoma. *Br. J. Cancer*, **53**, 661–71.

Dryja, T.P., Cavenee, W., White, R. *et al.* (1984) Homozygosity of chromosome 13 in retinoblastoma. *N. Engl. J. Med.*, **310**, 550–3.

Dryja, T.P., Mukai, S., Petersen, R. *et al.* (1989) Parental origin of mutations of the retinoblastoma gene. *Nature*, **339**, 556–8.

Dyson, N., Howley, P.M., Munger, K. and Harlow, E. (1989) The human papilloma virus-16 E7 oncoprotein is able to bind to the retinoblastoma gene product. *Science*, **243**, 934–7.

Egbert, P.R., Donaldson, S.S., Moazed, K. *et al.* (1978) Visual results and ocular complications following radiotherapy for retinoblastoma. *Arch. Ophthalmol.*, **97**, 1826–30.

Fedrick, J. and Baldwin, J.A. (1978) Incidence of cancer in relatives of children with retinoblastoma. *Br. Med. J.*, **1**, 83–4.

Foster Moore, R. (1931) Retinal gliomata treated by radon seeds. *Br. J. Ophthalmol.*, **15**, 673–96.

Francois, J. (1977) Retinoblastoma and osteogenic sarcoma. *Ophthalmologica*, **175**, 185–91.

Friend, S.H., Bernards, R., Rogelj, S. *et al.* (1986) A human DNA segment with properties of the gene that predisposes to retinoblastoma and osteosarcoma. *Nature*, **323**, 643–6.

Fung, Y.K., Murphree, A.L., T'Ang, A. *et al.* (1987) Structural evidence for the authenticity of the human retinoblastoma gene. *Science*, **236**, 1657–61.

Gallie, B.L., Ellsworth, R.M., Abramson, D.H. and Phillips, R.A. (1982) Retinoma: spontaneous regression of retinoblastoma or benign manifestation of the mutation? *Br. J. Cancer*, **45**, 513–21.

Goble, R.R., McKenzie, J., Kingston, J.E. *et al.* (1990) Orbital recurrence of retinoblastoma successfully treated by combined therapy. *Br. J. Ophthalmol.*, **74**, 97–8.

Hamburger, A.W. and Salmon, S.E. (1977) Primary bioassay of human tumor stem cells. *Science*, **197**, 461–3.

Harbour, J.W., Lai, S-L., Whang-Peng, J. *et al.* (1988) Abnormalities in structure and expression of the human retinoblastoma gene in SCLC. *Science*, **241**, 353–7.

Harnett, A.N., Hungerford, J.L., Lambert, G. *et al.* (1987) Modern lateral external beam (lens sparing) radiotherapy for retinoblastoma. *Ophthalmic Paediatr. Genet.*, **8**, 53–61.

Hawkins, M.M., Draper, G.J. and Kingston, J.E. (1987) Incidence of second primary tumours among childhood cancer survivors. *Br. J. Cancer*, **56**, 339–47.

Hermann, M.M., Perentes, E., Katsetos, C.D. *et al.* (1989) Neuroblastic differentiation potential of the human retinoblastoma cell lines Y-79 and WERI-Rb1 maintained in organ culture system: an immunohistochemical electron microscopic, and biochemical study. *Am. J. Pathol.*, **134**, 115–32.

Holladay, D.A., Holladay, A., Montobello, J.F. and Redmond, K.P. (1991) Clinical presentation, treatment and outcome of trilateral retinoblastoma. *Cancer*, **67**, 710–15.

Hong, F.D., Huang, H.J., To, H. *et al.* (1989) Structure of the human retinoblastoma gene. *Proc. Natl. Acad. Sci. USA*, **86**, 5502–6.

Horowitz, J.M., Yandell, D.W., Park, S.H. *et al.*

287

(1989) Point mutational inactivation of the retinoblastoma antioncogene. *Science,* **243**, 937–40.

Hungerford, J.L., Kingston, J.E. and Plowman, P.N. (1987) Orbital recurrence of retinoblastoma. *Ophthal. Paediatr. Genet.,* **8**, 63–8.

Hungerford, J. (1990) Histogenesis of retinoblastoma. *Br. J. Ophthalmol.,* **74**, 131–2.

Inomata, M. and Kaneko, A. (1987) Chemosensitivity profiles of primary and cultured human retinoblastoma cells in a human tumor clonogenic assay. *Jpn. J. Cancer Res.,* **78**, 858–68.

Judisch, G.F., Apple, D.J. and Fratkin, J.D. (1980) A survivor 12 years after treatment for metastatic disease. *Arch. Ophthalmol.,* **98**, 711–13.

Kingston, J.E., Hungerford, J.L. and Plowman, P.N. (1985) Ectopic intracranial retinoblastoma in childhood. *Br. J. Ophthalmol.,* **69**, 742–8.

Kingston, J.E., Hungerford, J.L. and Plowman, P.N. (1987a) Chemotherapy in metastatic retinoblastoma. *Ophthal. Paediatr. Genet.,* **8**, 69–72.

Kingston, J.E., Hawkins, M.M., Draper, G.J. *et al.* (1987b) Patterns of multiple primary tumours in patients treated for cancer during childhood. *Br. J. Cancer,* **56**, 331–8.

Kingston, J.E., Clark, J., Santos, H. *et al.* (1990) Failure to thrive leading to early detection of retinoblastoma. *Pediatr. Hematol. Oncol.,* **208**, 191–5.

Knudson, A.G. (1971) Mutation and cancer: statistical study of retinoblastoma. *Proc. Natl. Acad. Sci. USA,* **68**, 820–3.

Knudson, A.G., Meadows, A.T., Nichols, W.W. and Hill, R. (1976) Chromosomal deletion and retinoblastoma. *N. Engl. J. Med.,* **295**, 1120–3.

Kopelman, J.E., McLean, I.W. and Rosenberg, S.H. (1987) Multivariate analysis of risk factors for metastasis in retinoblastoma treated by enucleation. *Ophthalmology,* **94**, 371–7.

Kyritisis, A.P., Tsokos, M., Triche, T.J. and Chader, G.J. (1984) Retinoblastoma – origin from a primitive neuroectodermal cell? *Nature,* **307**, 471–3.

Lee, EY-HP., To, H., Shew, J-Y. *et al.* (1988) Inactivation of the retinoblastoma susceptibility gene in human breast cancers. *Science,* **241**, 218–21.

Lee, W-H., Bookstein, R., Hong, F.D. *et al.* (1987a) Human retinoblastoma susceptibility gene: cloning, identification and sequence. *Science,* **235**, 1394–9.

Lee, W-H., Shew, J-Y., Hong, F.D. *et al.* (1987b) The retinoblastoma susceptibility gene encodes a nuclear phosphoprotein associated with DNA binding activity. *Nature,* **329**, 642–5.

Lele, K.P., Penrose, L.S. and Stallard, H.B. (1963) Chromosome deletion in a case of retinoblastoma. *Ann. Hum. Genet.,* **27**, 171–4.

Lemieux, N., Milot, J., Barsoum-Homsy, M. *et al.* (1989) First cytogenetic evidence of homozygosity for the retinoblastoma deletion in chromosome 13. *Cancer Genet. Cytogenet.,* **43**, 73–8.

Lonsdale, P., Berry, D.H., Holcomb, T.M. *et al.* (1968) Chemotherapeutic trials in patients with metastatic retinoblastoma. *Cancer Chemother. Reports,* **52**, 631–4.

MacFaul, P.A. and Bedford, M.A. (1970) Ocular complications after therapeutic irradiation. *Br. J. Ophthalmol.* **54**, 237–47.

MacKay, C.J., Abramson, D.H. and Ellsworth, R.M. (1984) Metastatic patterns of retinoblastoma. *Arch. Ophthalmol.,* **102**, 391–6.

McCartney, A.C.E., Olver, J.M., Kingston, J.E. and Hungerford, J.L. (1988) Forty years of retinoblastoma; into the fifth age. *Eye,* Suppl 2, S13–S18.

McGee, T.L., Yandell, D.W. and Dryja, T.P. (1989) Structure and partial genomic sequence of the human retinoblastoma susceptibility gene. *Gene,* **80**, 119–28.

Meadows, A.T., Strong, L.C., Li, F.P. *et al.* (1980) for the Late Effects Study Group. Bone sarcoma as a second malignant neoplasm in children. *Cancer,* **46**, 2603–6.

Meadows, A.T., Baum, E., Fossati-Bellain, F. *et al.* (1985) Second malignant neoplasms in children: An update from the Late Effects Study Group. *J. Clin. Oncol.,* **3**, 532–8.

Mihahara, K., Cao, X.R., Yen, A. *et al.* (1989) Cell cycle-dependent regulation of phosphorylation of the human retinoblastoma gene product. *Science,* **246**, 1300–3.

Molnar, M.L., Stefansson, K., Marton, L.S. *et al.* (1984) Immunohistochemistry of retinoblastoma in humans. *Am. J. Ophthalmol.,* **97**, 301–7.

Morgan, G. (1971) Diffuse infiltrating retinoblastoma. *Br. J. Ophthalmol.,* **55**, 600–6.

Murphree, A.L. and Benedict, W.F. (1984) Retinoblastoma: clues to human oncogenesis. *Science,* **223**, 1028–33.

Osborne, D., Hadden, O.B. and Deeming, L.W.

(1974) Orbital growth after childhood enucleation. *Am. J. Opthalmol.*, **77**, 756–9.

Parkin, D.M., Stiller, C.A., Draper, G.J. and Bieber, C.A. (1988) The international incidence of childhood cancer. *Int. J. Cancer*, **42**, 511–20.

Petersen, R.A., Friend, S.H. and Albert, D.M. (1987) Prolonged survival of a child with metastatic retinoblastoma. *J. Pediatr. Ophthalmol. Strabismus*, **24**, 247–8.

Pratt, C.B., Crom, D.B. and Howarth, C. (1985) The use of chemotherapy for extraocular retinoblastoma. *Med. Pediatr. Oncol.*, **13**, 330 3.

Pratt, C.B., Meyer, D., Chenaille, P. and Crom, D.B. (1989) The use of bone marrow aspirations and lumbar punctures at the time of diagnosis of retinoblastoma. *J. Clin. Oncol.*, **7**, 140–3.

Ragab, A.H., Sutow, W.W., Komp, D.M. *et al.* (1975) Adriamycin in the treatment of childhood solid tumors. Cancer, **36**, 1572–6.

Redler, L.D. and Ellsworth, R.M. (1973) Prognostic importance of choroidal invasion in retinoblastoma. *Arch. Ophthalmol.*, **11**, 106–14.

Reese, A.B. and Ellsworth, R.M. (1963) The evaluation and current concept of retinoblastoma therapy. *Trans. Am. Acad. Ophthalmol. Otolaryngol.*, **67**, 164–72.

Reissmann, P.T., Simon, M.A., Lee, W.H. and Slamon, D.J. (1989) Studies of the retinoblastoma gene in human sarcomas. *Oncogene*, **4**, 839–43.

Roarty, J.D., McLean, I.W. and Zimmerman, L.E. (1988) Incidence of second neoplasms in patients with bilateral retinoblastoma. *Ophthalmology*, **95**, 1583–7.

Rootman, J., Ellsworth, R.M., Hofbauer, J. and Kitchen, D. (1978) Orbital extension of retinoblastoma: a clinicopathological study. *Can. J. Ophthalmol.*, **13**, 72–80.

Rubin, C.M., Robison, L.L., Cameron, J.D. *et al.* (1985) Intraocular retinoblastoma group V: an analysis of prognostic factors. *J. Clin. Oncol.*, **3**, 680–5.

Saleh, R.A., Gross, S., Cassano, W. and Gee, A. (1988) Metastatic retinoblastoma successfully treated with immunomagnetic purged autologous bone marrow transplantation. *Cancer*, **62**, 2301–3.

Sanders, B., Draper, G.J. and Kingston, J.E. (1988) Retinoblastoma in Great Britain 1969–80: incidence, treatment and survival. *Br. J. Ophthalmol.*, **72**, 576–83.

Sanders, B.M., Jay, M., Draper, G.J. and Roberts, E.M. (1989) Non-ocular cancer in relatives of retinoblastoma patients. *Br. J. Cancer*, **60**, 358–65.

Sang, D.N. and Albert, D.M. (1982) Retinoblastoma: clinical and histopathologic features. *Hum. Pathol.*, **13**, 133–47.

Schappert-Kimmijser, J., Hemmes, G.D. and Nijland, R. (1966) The heredity of retinoblastoma. *Ophthalmologica*, **152**, 197–213.

Schipper, J. (1983) An accurate and simple method for megavoltage radiation therapy of retinoblastoma. *Radiother. Oncol.*, **1**, 31–41.

Schulman, J.A., Peyman, G.A., Mafee, M.F. *et al.* (1986) The use of magnetic resonance imaging in the evaluation of retinoblastoma. *J. Pediatr. Ophthalmol. Strabismus*, **23**, 144–7.

Seidman, D.J., Shields, J.A., Augsburger, J.J. *et al.* (1987) Early diagnosis of retinoblastoma based on dysmorphic features and karyotype analysis. *Ophthalmology*, **94**, 663–6.

Seshadri, R., Matthews, C., Norris, M.D. and Brian, M.J. (1988) N-*myc* amplified in retinoblastoma cell line FMC-RB1. *Cancer Genet. Cytogenet.* **33**, 25–7.

Smith, J.L.S. (1974) Histology and spontaneous regression of retinoblastoma. *Trans. Ophthalmol. Soc. UK*, **94**, 953–67.

Smith, L.M., Donaldson, S.S., Egbert, P.R. *et al.* (1989) Aggressive management of second primary tumors in survivors of hereditary retinoblastoma. *Int. J. Radiat. Oncol. Biol. Phys.*, **17**, 499–505.

Sparkes, R.S., Murphree, A.L., Lingua, R.W. *et al.* (1983) Gene for hereditary retinoblastoma assigned to human chromosome 13 by linkage to esterase-D. *Science*, **219**, 971–3.

Stannard, C., Lipper, S., Sealy, R. and Sevel, D. (1979) Retinoblastoma: correlation of invasion of the optic nerve and choroid with prognosis and metastases. *Br. J. Ophthalmol.*, **63**, 560–70.

Stevenson, K.E., Hungerford, J.L. and Garner, A. (1989) Local extraocular extension of retinoblastoma following intraocular surgery. *Br. J. Ophthalmol.*, **73**, 739–42.

Steward, J.K., Smith, J.L.S and Arnold, E.L. (1956) Spontaneous regression of retinoblastoma. *Br. J. Ophthalmol.*, **40**, 449–61.

Stratton, M.R., Moss, S., Warren, W. *et al.* (1990) Mutation of the p53 gene in soft tissue sarcomas: association with abnormalities of the RB1 gene. *Oncogene*, **5**, 1297–301.

Strong, L.C., Herson, J., Haas, C. *et al.* (1984) Cancer mortality in relatives of retinoblastoma patients. *J. Natl. Cancer Inst.*, **73**, 303–11.

Tso, M.O.M., Zimmerman, L.E. and Fine, B.S. (1970) The nature of retinoblastoma. I Photoreceptor differentiation: a clinical and histopathologic study. *Am. J. Ophthalmol.*, **69**, 339–49.

Tucker, M.A., D'Anjio, G.J., Boice, J.D. *et al.* (1987) Bone sarcomas linked to radiotherapy and chemotherapy in children. *N. Engl. J. Med.*, **317**, 588–93.

Vogel, F. (1979) Genetics of retinoblastoma. *Hum. Genet.*, **52**, 1–54.

Weichselbaum, R.R., Beckett, M. and Diamond, A. (1988) Some retinoblastomas, osteosarcomas, and soft tissue sarcomas may share a common aetiology. *Proc. Natl. Acad. Sci. USA*, **85**, 2106–9.

White, L. (1983) The role of chemotherapy in the treatment of retinoblastoma. *Retina*, **3**, 194–9.

White, L., Szirth, B. and Benedict, W.F. (1989) Evaluation of response to chemotherapy in retinoblastoma heterotransplanted to the eyes of nude mice. *Cancer Chemother. Pharmacol.*, **23**, 63–7.

Whyte, P., Buchkovich, K.J., Horowitz, J.M. *et al.* (1988) Association between an oncogene and an antioncogene the adenovirus E1A proteins bind to the retinoblastoma gene product. *Nature*, **334**, 124–9.

Wolff, J.A., Boesel, C.P. and Dyment, P.G. (1981) Treatment of retinoblastoma: a preliminary report. *Int. Congress Series*, **570**, 364–8.

Yandell, D.W., Campbell, T.A., Dayton, S.H. *et al.* (1989) Oncogenic point mutations in the human retinoblastoma gene: their application to genetic counseling. *N. Engl. J. Med.*, **321**, 1689–95.

Yokoyama, T., Tsukahara, T., Nakagawa, C. *et al.* (1989) The N-*myc*, gene product in primary retinoblastomas. *Cancer*, **63**, 2134–8.

Yunis, J.J. and Ramsay, N. (1978) Retinoblastoma and subband deletion of chromosome 13. *Am. J. Dis. Child.*, **132**, 161–3.

Zhu, X.P., Dunn, J.M., Phillips, R.A. *et al.* (1989) Preferential germline mutation of the paternal allele in retinoblastoma. *Nature*, **340**, 312–13.

Chapter 15

Soft tissue sarcomas

M. CARLI, M. GUGLIELMI, G. SOTTI,
G. CECCHETTO and V. NINFO

15.1 INTRODUCTION

Soft tissue sarcomas are a heterogeneous group of neoplasms showing different lines of differentiation according to the putative tissues of origin. These mainly include contractile, connective and supportive tissues, vascular tissue, adipose tissue and arguably, some derived from the neural crest. Soft tissue sarcomas constitute approximately 6.5% of all the childhood cancers.

In the United States, their annual incidence has been estimated to be eight per million white children under 15 years of age (Young *et al.*, 1986). A similar figure exists in Europe where data obtained from several Cancer Registries indicate that the incidence of soft tissue sarcoma ranges from 5.4 to 9.6 per million children (IARC, 1988).

Rhabdomyosarcoma (RMS) is the most common soft tissue sarcoma in children and young adults under the age of 21, accounting for approximately half to two-thirds of all sarcomas in this age group. Fibrosarcoma, synovial sarcoma, neurogenic sarcoma, extraskeletal Ewing's sarcoma, haemangiosarcoma, haemangiopericytoma, alveolar soft port sarcoma and peripheral neuroectodermal tumours (PNET) occur less frequently. For this reason, RMS has been the object of multi-institutional clinical trials, organized on a national or multinational basis both in Europe and the US, and the management of this tumour has become the model for practically all other paediatric soft tissue sarcomas.

15.2 RHABDOMYOSARCOMA

Rhabdomyosarcoma is a highly malignant tumour and is thought to arise from primitive mesenchymal cells committed to develop into striated muscles (Gaiger *et al.*, 1981). It can be found virtually anywhere in the body, including those sites where striated muscles are not normally found.

RMS accounts for 4% to 8% of all solid tumours in children with an annual incidence of 4.3 per million Caucasians under the age of 15. Of these 70% of cases occur before the age of ten. It shows two peaks of incidence, the first and most important in children two to five years of age, the second during adolescence. A slight male predominance (1.4–1.7:1) is generally reported.

15.3 AETIOLOGY AND GENETICS

The aetiology of childhood RMS is still unknown. Data derived from epidemiological studies, however, seem to indicate that genetic factors might play an important role in the aetiology of at least some childhood sarcomas.

An increased incidence of congenital anomalies, mostly involving the genitourinary and central nervous system have been associated with RMS. In particular, the incidence of genitourinary anomalies is comparable to that found in patients with Wilms' tumour (Ruymann *et al.*, 1988). RMS has also been associated with several congenital disorders including neurofibromatosis (Mckeen *et al.*, 1978), Gorlin's nevoid basal cell carcinoma syndrome (Beddis *et al.*, 1983) and fetal alcohol syndrome (Becker *et al.*, 1982). In addition, soft tissue sarcomas in children and young adults have been associated with an excess incidence of breast cancer in the mothers and other close relatives as well as with an excess of cancers (breast carcinoma, gliomas) in the siblings (Li and Fraumeni, 1969; Pastore *et al.*, 1987; Birch *et al.*, 1990).

According to Birch *et al.* (1990) this pattern of cancers is consistent with the well known Li-Fraumeni Cancer Family Syndrome.

Among the 24 families studied by Li *et al* (1988), bone and soft tissue sarcomas and breast cancer were the most frequent cancers, but brain tumours, leukaemias, and adrenocortical carcinomas had also occurred to excess in those below the age of 45. These findings have important implications in identifying a group of patients at high cancer risk who may benefit from genetic counselling and screening.

Birch *et al.* (1990) analysed 754 first-degree relatives of a population-based series of 177 children with soft tissue sarcoma. They were able to identify in the index child the following factors associated with high cancer risk in relatives: age younger than 24 months of age at diagnosis, histologic type such as embryonal RMS or other and unspecified soft tissue sarcoma, and male sex.

The improvement in molecular genetic and biological studies which has occurred in the past few years has made possible the identification of chromosomal abnormalities in several varieties of malignant soft-tissue tumours. In RMS, the translocation (2;13)(q35;q14) is consistently found in the alveolar subtype (Scrable *et al.*, 1989).

No karyotype abnormalities have been identified so far in the more common embryonal histologic subtype. However, the loss of constitutional heterozygosity at loci on the short arm of chromosome 11 has been detected in embryonal rhabdomyosarcoma (Scrable *et al.* 1989). This genotype change, which seems to distinguish between the embryonal and alveolar subtypes, suggests that a gene or genes on 11p are involved in malignant transformation.

Other specific cytogenetic abnormalities include the translocation (11;22)(q24;q12) in Ewing's Sarcoma and peripheral primitive neuroectodermal tumour (Whang-Peng *et al.*, 1985; Turc-Carel *et al.*, 1988) and the translocation (x;18)(p11.2;q11.2) in synovial sarcoma (Turc-Carel *et al.*, 1987).

15.4 CLASSIFICATION AND HISTOLOGICAL SUBTYPES

After the first report (Horn and Enterline, 1958), four types of rhabdomyosarcoma (RMS) have since been described on the basis of their cytoarchitectural features: embryonal, botryoid, alveolar and pleomorphic. Initially, no prognostic distinctions were made between these different histotypes, but with the introduction of multimodality therapy, it was found that some RMS responded better to treatment than others (Hays *et al.*, 1983). Several classifications have been proposed for RMS in an attempt to correlate the morphological appearance of the tumour with the prognosis. All these schemes claim to demonstrate good prognostic significance; an International Study Committee has recently been formed to ascertain any correspondence between the different classifications with a view to working out a standardized scheme (Newton *et al.*, 1991). A new prognostically significant classification has been created whereby RMS can be divided into two main classes, low grade and high grade RMS. This classification system excludes a pleomorphic category, very rarely observed in infancy.

15.4.1 LOW GRADE RMS

This category consists of embryonal RMS (ERMS) and its botryoid and spindle cell variants. ERMS is characterized by a loose myxoid stroma and a proliferation of spindle cells. The cells have round or oval eccentric hyperchromatic nuclei with uniformly distributed chromatin and small or absent nucleoli; the eosinophilic cytoplasm at times shows typical cross-striations (strap cell), or

has the characteristic angular irregular shape. Intermediate sized cells with eccentric nuclei and elongated eosinophilic 'comma' shaped cytoplasm (tadpole cells), as well as occasional large polygonal cells are usually scattered in the stroma. Pleomorphic cells are occasionally observed in classical ERMS. These cells show the same nuclear characteristics described above for ERMS and their presence does not affect the final prognosis.

A special variant of ERMS, botryoid RMS, is observed in hollow organs such as vagina, nasal sinuses, and bladder. Histologically this variant is defined by the presence of a discrete mucosal hypercellular zone called the 'cambium layer', and an abundant oedematous myxoid stroma, occasionally mimicking a myxoma.

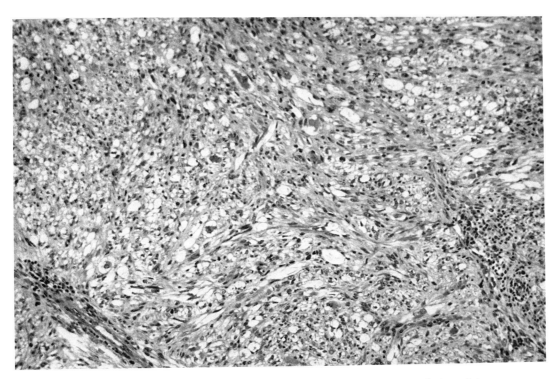

Fig. 15.1 Spindle cell RMS: fusiform cells arranged in fasciculated pattern simulating a leiomyosarcoma (H & E × 160).

myxoid stroma, occasionally mimicking a myxoma.

Short fascicles of eosinophilic spindle cells are frequently observed in ERMS; more rarely the tumour consists almost exclusively of long fascicles of spindle cells intersecting at right angles, simulating a leiomyosarcoma. This variant has therefore been tentatively called spindle-cell or leiomyomatous RMS (Cavazzana *et al.*, 1989) (Fig. 15.1). From an analysis of twenty-one cases studied by the German-Italian Soft Tissue Study, it was seen that this variant occurred chiefly in the para-testicular areas (12 cases) and the head and neck region (five cases). A clear male pre-dominance was documented (18M/3F). Micro-scopically, it may be confused with a leiomyo-sarcoma; scattered cytoplasmic cross-striations,

however, can be detected in the majority of cases. In this study, sufficient follow-up information was available in 17 cases, and fifteen patients were alive and well 24 to 89 months after diagnosis. Based on our find-ings, therefore, we believe this tumour to represent a very well differentiated variant of RMS, characterized by a low malignant potential.

15.4.2 HIGH GRADE RMS

This category consists of alveolar RMS (ARMS) and its variants. Microscopically, this tumour is characterized by the presence of alveolar spaces; these are usually lined with a single row of small or intermediate size cells with dark hyperchromatic nuclei,

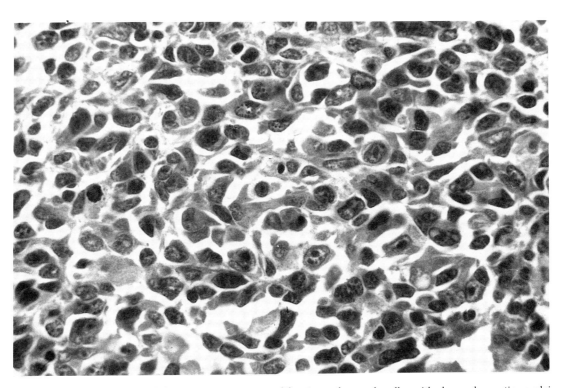

Fig. 15.2 Alveolar RMS, solid variant: compact proliferation of round cells with hyperchromatic nuclei and evident nucleolus and the same cellular pleomorphism as classical ARMS, with no evidence of alveolar pattern (H & E × 250).

evident nucleolus, and eosinophilic cytoplasm. Multinucleated giant cells are commonly observed. The term mixed type RMS has been advanced for cases in which areas of an embryonal or pleomorphic type of RMS are present within the alveolar tumour (Jaffe *et al.*, 1973; Gonzalez-Crussi and Black-Shaffer, 1979). Consequently, it was proposed that only tumour consisting of 70% alveolar spaces should be classified as ARMS (Bale *et al.*, 1986). However, no differences have been found in survival between cases with 70% alveolar spaces and those with few alveoli; thus tumours showing even a single alveolar space should be classified as ARMS (Harms *et al.*, 1985). At the periphery of ARMS, solid areas of closely packed round cells may be present, as originally observed by Riopelle and Theriault (1956). Recently, Tsokos *et al.* (1985) proposed that tumours consisting almost entirely of these solid areas should be considered a solid variant of alveolar RMS (Fig. 15.2). Microscopically, this variant presents a compact proliferation of round cells with hyperchromatic nuclei, evident nucleolus and scarce cytoplasm; any factors indicating a rhabdomyoblastic differentiation are rare or absent. Cross-striations are invariably absent whereas atypical mitoses as well as single cell necrosis and nuclear piknosis are frequently observed. No stroma is interspersed between the tumour cells, and an alveolar pattern, however vague, is seldom present. Cytologically, these cells are identical to those lining the alveolar spaces and show the same degree of cellular pleomorphism present in classical ARMS. The solid areas occasionally consist of sheets of small round monomorphous cells with the above described typical nuclear features. This variety, named monomorphous RMS by Palmer and Foulkes (1983), must be considered within the spectrum of possible morphologic variations of the solid variant of RMS and shows a very aggressive clinical course.

15.4.3 PRIMARY SITES

RMS may arise anywhere in the body. In order to reduce the differences of categorization of primary sites among different institutional and cooperative cancer clinical trial groups, a common classification of primary sites was adopted by European and US clinical investigators. The international definition of anatomical sites, adopted since 1986 in the workshop organized by the International Society of Pediatric Oncology (SIOP), is as follows:

1. Orbit;
2. Parameningeal head-neck;
3. Head-neck non PM
4. Genito-urinary tract;
   (a) bladder and prostate;
   (b) vagina, vulva, uterus, paratesticular;
5. Extremities
6. Others

The latter group includes wall of the trunk, intrathoracic, intraabdominal, pelvic, perineal and paravertebral regions. However, due to the fact that in some cases the determination of origin is uncertain, it was decided to describe the tumour by its assumed origin

Table 15.1 Distribution of primary site

	N	*Relative frequency (%)*
Orbit	95	10.5
Parameningeal HN	190	21
Head-neck non PM	83	9.5
Genito-urinary	211	23
B-P	89	10
non B-P	122	13
Extremity	124	14
Others	204	22

Data based on 907 cases enrolled in the following studies: International Society of Pediatric Oncology (SIOP) MMT-84; German Soft Tissue Sarcoma Study CWS-81 and CWS-86; Italian Rhabdomyosarcoma Study RMS-79.

and its possible secondary extension according to the topographical coding system described by Donaldson *et al.* (1986).

The relative frequency of occurrence at primary sites (SIOP 1984–88; CWS 81 and 86; ICG RMS 79–86), based on 907 RMS cases enrolled in four European studies, is given in Table 15.1.

15.4.4 PATTERN OF SPREAD

RMS is a very aggressive tumour which tends to infiltrate along fascial planes and into surrounding tissue as well as to disseminate through both lymphatic or haematogenous routes. About 20% of patients present with distant metastatic disease at diagnosis; the most common sites of metastases are lung, lymph nodes, bone, and bone marrow. More rarely, metastases can occur in the liver, brain and breast.

The frequency of regional lymph node involvement is still not precisely defined due to the fact that lymph node sampling is not routinely performed. Among 592 children with localized RMS enrolled in the first two Intergroup Rhabdomyosarcoma Studies (IRS) who had regional lymph node sampling, 14% presented with lymphatic spread. The incidence by primary site was: in the first two Intergroup Rhabdomyosarcoma Studies (IRS), the incidence of positive lymph nodes at presentation was 0% for orbital, 8% for non orbital head and neck, 12% for extremity, 24% for genito-urinary tract, 3% for trunk, and 23% for pelvis-retroperitoneum (Lawrence *et al.*, 1987). In the first Italian Study (RMS–79), 62 out of 145 patients received regional lymph node biopsy at diagnosis: of these 20 cases were positive, in particular 5/7 pelvis/retroperitoneum; 1/5 abdomen-thorax; 4/12 extremity; 6/13 non orbit-head and neck; 0/3 trunk; 4/22 genito-urinary tract.

The high incidence of retroperitoneal lymph node involvement previously reported in the paratesticular RMS (Raney *et al.*, 1978), was not subsequently confirmed (Olive *et al.*, 1984; Lawrence *et al.*, 1987; Cecchetto *et al.*, 1988).

It should be noted that these data may reflect a bias since some sites are much more frequently sampled that others and pathological evaluation is, in most instances, limited to the confirmation of clinically suspected lymph nodes. Thus the figure reported here is indicative rather than giving a picture of real differences in the incidence of lymphatic spread within these broad anatomic categories.

15.5 CLINICAL MANIFESTATION AND STAGING SYSTEMS

The initial signs and symptoms depend on the site of origin and on the extension of the tumour to contiguous organs or tissues or the presence of metastases.

The most important signs and symptoms of presentation are summarized in Table 15.2. Several peculiarities should be noted: tumours arising in parameningeal sites (nasopharynx, nasal cavity, paranasal sinuses, pterygoid-infratemporal fossae and middle ear mastoid) present a high risk of spreading to the meninges by contiguous bony destruction. Thus they may manifest with isolated or multiple cranial nerve palsies, sometimes with meningeal or increased intracranial pressure symptoms. This subtle presentation is the reason behind these patients' far advanced stage at diagnosis.

Bladder tumours are most frequently observed in young boys; they originate from neck or trigone, tend to proliferate intraluminally and to remain localized. In contrast, prostatic lesions are more aggressive and infiltrate the bladder neck and urethra and tend to metastatize earlier, mostly to the lungs. However, it is often difficult to clinically define whether a tumour is arising primarily in the bladder or in the prostate, unless the lesion is very small. Extremity lesions have a high propensity for involving the regional lymph nodes as well as for early

Table 15.2 Presenting signs and symptoms by primary site

Head-neck	Asymptomatic mass
Orbit	Proptosis, chemosis, ocular paralysis, eyelid mass
Nasopharynx	Airway obstruction, nasal voice, epistaxis, Local pain, dysphagia, cranial nerve palsies
Paranasal sinuses	Swelling, pain, sinusitis, obstruction, epistaxis, cranial nerve curve palsies
Neck	Hoarseness, dysphagia
Middle ear	Polypoid mass, chronic otitis media, haemorragic discharge, cranial nerve palsies
Larynx	Hoarseness, irritating cough
Genitourinary tract	Haematuria, urinary retention, polypoid vaginal extrusion of mucosanguinous tissue, vulval nodule or painless scrotal mass
Trunk	Asymptomatic mass (usually)
Retroperitoneum	Painless mass, ascites, gastrointestinal or urinary tract obstruction
Extremity	Painless mass (may be associated with bruising)

dissemination to distant lymph nodes, lung, bone marrow, bone and CNS.

Tumours of the trunk generally present as asymptomatic masses, but dyspnoea and thoracic pain associated with pleural effusion may also be present depending on the extension of the disease. Particular attention should be paid to neurological signs due to the possibility of thoracolumbar spine involvement.

Rare primary sites for RMS include the biliary tract. These lesions may present a clinical picture of asymptomatic jaundice or even as symptoms of acute cholecystitis. Unusual forms of the disease are represented by clinical symptoms characteristic of leukaemic patients: fever, bone pain, anaemia and pancytopenia, for example. The primary

tumour is often so small that it may at first go unnoticed. The differential diagnosis often requires special immunocytochemistry stains to reveal the nature of the nonhaemopoietic bone marrow infiltrate. In these cases the cytogenetic studies showing the translocation t(2:13)(q37;q14) may substantiate the diagnosis of alveolar RMS (Engel *et al.*, 1988). Thus the initial picture is not always obvious. A high degree of clinical suspicion is necessary in order to make an early diagnosis. In practice, diagnosis can only be made on biopsy.

15.5.1 STAGING INVESTIGATION

A precise definition of loco-regional extension of disease and a detailed investigation of the potential metastatic sites is mandatory before planning therapy. For histological diagnosis, an incisional biopsy is necessary. This approach generally gives sufficient material to avoid any difficulty in histopathological interpretation and allows a large variety of ancillary techniques such as cytogenetic or molecular biological studies to be performed, which could be helpful in differential diagnosis.

Pretreatment evaluation may vary depending on anatomical sites and clinical presentation, but for all patients it should include:

1. Complete physical examination with a precise definition of tumour site and size, and a careful regional lymph nodes assessment.
2. Laboratory studies: complete blood count, liver and renal function tests, serum electrolytes plus calcium, phosphorus and magnesium, uric acid, coagulation parameters.
3. CT scan and/or magnetic resonance imaging (MRI) of the primary lesion with three-dimensional measurement, if possible. Ultrasonography is also important, particularly in the assessment of pelvic tumours.

It avoids the use of irradiation and may be easily repeated in evaluating tumour volume reduction.

4. Bone marrow aspiration plus two trephine biopsies for Stage IV patients.
5. Technetium bone scan, with plain x-rays of abnormal sites.
6. Chest x-ray and computed tomography (CT) scan.
7. Biopsy of any clinically suspicious regional lymph nodes.

Other complementary investigations appropriate to the primary site include the following:

(a) parameningeal head and neck: brain CT scan and/or MRI and cerebrospinal fluid (CSF) cytology;
(b) genito-urinary: CT scan or MRI ± ultrasound of retroperitoneum. Uretrocystoscopy with biopsy for bladder prostate lesions;
(c) extremity: CT scan ± ultrasound of retroperitoneum for lower extremity. Brain CT scan should be considered as brain metastases seem more commonly associated with extremity primaries. Regional lymph node biopsy is highly recommended;
(d) trunk: spinal MRI or myelography if neurological signs of medullary compression are present;
(e) intra-abdominal: CT scan ± ultrasound of the liver.

CT scan is at present more often utilized than MRI, depending mostly on the local facilities available. However, in defining soft tissue tumours and intracranial extension, MRI appears to be superior to the CT scan. In addition, MRI has the ability to define vascular involvement without contrast enhancement as well as the ability to perform sagittal and coronal scans. Bone destruction, however, is more accurately defined on CT scan. Ultrasonography is also a useful, easily-repeated diagnostic technique for measuring therapy response. In summary, it can be said that these examinations are often complementary.

15.5.2 STAGING SYSTEMS

Two major systems have been utilized so far for the staging of childhood RMS: a post surgical and a pre surgical one. The most widely employed scheme of the post surgical systems has been the clinical pathological grouping system adopted by the IRS (Maurer, 1975). (Table 15.3). A major problem with these systems, based on whether or not excision is carried out and on its extent, is that patients with the equivalent extent of disease at diagnosis may be assigned different stages

Table 15.3 Surgical pathological IRS grouping system

Group I:	Localized disease, completely resected A. Confined to organ or muscle of origin B. Infiltration outside organ or muscle of origin; regional nodes not involved
Group II:	Regional disease, grossly resected A. Grossly resected tumours with microscopic residual B. Regional disease, completely resected, in which nodes may be involved and/or extension of tumour into an adjacent organ present C. Regional disease with involved nodes, grossly resected, but with evidence of microscopic residual
Group III:	Incomplete resection or biopsy with gross residual disease
Group IV:	Distant metastases present at onset

Table 15.4 Categories in pretreatment clinical staging system for childhood rhabdomyosarcoma (UICC)

T-1	Tumour confined to organ or tissue of origin
1a	5 cm or less in size
1b	more than 5 cm in size
T-2	Tumour involves contiguous organs or structures
2a	5 cm or less in size
2b	more than 5 cm in size
N-0	No clinical or radiographic evidence of involvement of regional lymph nodes (no histologic determination)
N-1	Clinical or radiographic evidence of regional lymph node involvement
M-0	No distant metastases on clinical, radiographic, or bone marrow assessment
M-1	Evidence of distant metastasis

on the basis of the prevailing institutional policies regarding resectability of primary tumours at different sites. This aspect has become more complex with the adoption of treatment policies which include pre-operative chemotherapy in the attempt to reduce the need for aggressive surgery or even to avoid it.

The pre surgical staging system such as the tumour node metastases (TNM) staging system proposed by the International Union Against Cancer (UICC) (Harmer, 1982) and adopted by the SIOP, allows patient categor-

Table 15.5 TNM staging system for childhood soft-tissue sarcomas reported by UICC (Harmer, 1982)

Clinic stage	Invasive-ness	Size	Nodal status	Metastasis status
I	T1	a or b	N0	M0
II	T2	a or b	N0	M0
III	T1 or T2	a or b	N1	M0
IV	T1 or T2	a or b	N0 or N1	M1

ization in advance of any therapeutic intervention. It is based on the description of local invasiveness and size of primary tumour, clinical status of regional lymph nodes, and the presence or absence of distant metastases as assessed by clinical examination and pretreatment radiological work-up (Tables 15.4 and 15.5).

The advantage of this staging system is that it allows a comparison of results between different Institutions or Cooperative Group Studies. This pre surgical staging system was recently chosen by both European and American investigators – together with other prognostic factors (for example, primary site) – as a basis for defining different groups of treatment in future childhood RMS studies (Rodary *et al.*, 1989).

15.6 PROGNOSTIC FACTORS

Several prognostic factors have so far been identified through different cooperative studies conducted in Europe and the US. Recently, an international workshop was held with the objective of identifying the most important pretreatment tumour characteristics for predicting survival (Rodary *et al.*, 1991).

The analysis was performed on 951 children with non metastatic RMS, enrolled in four European and US cooperative studies. Using univariate analysis, the following variables were identified as favourable prognostic factors: tumour invasiveness T1, tumour size ≤ 5 cm, negative regional lymph nodes, and primary site in orbit and genito-urinary non bladder prostate. The multivariate Cox regression analysis of the pooled data recognized tumour invasiveness, primary site, and the interaction between tumour invasiveness and primary site as significant predictive factors for survival, while lymph node involvement was no longer predictive. In particular the prognosis of orbital tumours was consistently favourable whereas the prognosis of 'other sites' was consistently unfavourable regardless of T status.

In addition, T status appeared to determine the relative risk of treatment failure for primary sites in the genito-urinary, head and neck, parameningeal and extremity sites. The risk was low for patients with tumour invasiveness T1 and primary sites in GU-non-BP, head and neck, and GU-BP, and high for patients with tumour invasiveness T2 and primary sites in extremity and parameningeal. In this study, tumour size was not considered for the multivariate Cox regression analysis, since it was not available for all centres. However, the multivariate analysis conducted on the Italian series of 145 children identified tumour size as a strong factor in predicting survival, whereas tumour invasiveness failed to be of prognostic significance (Rodary *et al.*, 1988; Treuner *et al.*, 1989b; Crist *et al.*, 1990; Carli *et al.*, 1991a).

All studies to date have also demonstrated the crucial role of disease extent, as defined by the post surgical clinical groups or the pre surgical TNM system, in predicting survival: survival in fact decreases from approximately 80% in Stage I patients to approximately 20% in Stage IV patients. The histopathological type of particular tumours is also an important variable. Although at present there is no general agreement that histology is an independent factor, many reports (Crist *et al.*, 1990; Carli *et al.*, 1991a) indicated that patients with alveolar RMS have a poorer survival than those with the embryonal subtype. No relationship with survival was found for age at presentation and, except in the SIOP series (Rodary *et al.*, 1988), for sex.

The response to treatment is another important variable and this must be taken into account in relationship to survival. In addition, the German Cooperative Soft Tissue Sarcoma Study has found a strong correlation between the degree of tumour reduction in response to induction chemotherapy,

and the relapse-free survival in Clinical Group III patients (Treuner *et al.*, 1989b).

15.7 TREATMENT MODALITIES

Multimodality therapy involving surgery, chemotherapy and radiotherapy is necessary in childhood RMS. The optimal time as well as the aggressiveness of these three treatment modalities must be planned, with regard to primary tumour, site, extent of disease, histology, and late effects of treatment.

15.7.1 SURGERY

Surgical management of RMS is less aggressive in children than in adults. *Primary* excision of tumours should be attempted only where the surgeon thinks it constitutes a complete but non mutilating procedure; primary surgery should otherwise be limited to biopsy alone and the child should undergo a *secondary* excision, if this becomes feasible, after chemotherapy ± radiotherapy. Not only does the surgical choice depend on the location, size and extent of the tumour and on the study design, but it is also influenced by the surgeon's own judgment and experience.

15.7.2 DIAGNOSTIC BIOPSY

The surgeon must carry out at least one initial diagnostic biopsy to identify the histological nature of the tumour. Needle cores or aspirates can establish malignancy, but rarely are they able to identify the subtypes of sarcoma and in many cases they are not able to supply the tissue required for biological research. Surgical biopsies are usually incisional. If the surgeon has carried out an excisional biopsy which indicates a sarcoma, this biopsy cannot be considered a radical excision: it should instead be considered as an excision where there is likely to be at least microscopic residual tumour.

Frozen sections prepared in the operating room can be sufficient for a generic diagnosis of sarcoma, making possible in some cases immediate definitive surgical excision if this is feasible.

15.7.3 PRIMARY EXCISION

The goal here is the complete removal of the tumour by a non mutilating procedure. Mutilating procedures are those which result in major functional or cosmetic impairment such as: orbital exenteration, head and neck dissection, total cystectomy or vaginectomy, pneumonectomy, permanent urinary or intestinal diversion, extremity amputation or local excision with great extremity impairment. Non mutilating operations are pulmonary lobectomy, partial intestinal or liver resection, nephrectomy, partial cystectomy, unilateral orchidectomy or ovariectomy or finger amputation. Excision is complete (radical) when no residue of the tumour remains. It is generally felt that an initial excision that leaves macroscopic residue does not offer any advantages over a biopsy and should therefore be discouraged. There are different opinions as far as initial excision with microscopic residue is concerned. If the tumour can be grossly resected, many surgeons prefer to undertake primary excision even when it is unlikely that a specimen with free microscopic margins can be obtained. However, microscopic residual disease receives local irradiation while the alternative choice of initial chemotherapy and secondary surgery would perhaps allow complete excision, making it possible to avoid radiotherapy (RT). Furthermore, in these patients the efficacy of chemotherapy cannot be monitored as microscopic residue is not a measurable target. For these reasons, the Italian group, for example, recommends primary excision only if there is reasonable probability that not even microscopic residue will be left; otherwise biopsy should be preferred.

The local microscopic spread of many sarcomas goes far beyond the macroscopic limits of the tumour. To obtain a specimen with free microscopic margins it is obviously necessary to resect the tumour together with some surrounding normal tissue. There are, however, no rules on how much apparently normal tissue should be resected to guarantee the absence of microscopic residual tumour. An adequate histological study is therefore necessary to decide whether or not the excision has been radical. Apart from the microscopic examination of the specimen margins, it is important that the surgeon performs further biopsies around the margins of the excision, especially in doubtful areas. In this way the risk of an incorrect evaluation of adequate surgery are minimized. When, after an initial excision specimen, margins or biopsies are found to be positive for microscopic disease, or when there are insufficient data on completeness, a wider local reexcision should be undertaken prior to any future therapy if complete surgical excision is possible by a non mutilating procedure (Hays *et al.*, 1989). This primary reexcision has the aim of avoiding local irradiation and is usually most useful in extremity and trunk sarcomas.

Adopting these criteria, initial surgery should be limited to biopsy for all parameningeal sarcomas and for the majority of orbital and other head and neck sarcomas. In order to preserve the urinary bladder, the endoscopic biopsy alone is also the initial procedure of choice for bladder and prostate sarcomas. Primary excision is nearly always indicated in paratesticular sarcomas and consists of inguinal orchidofunicolectomy without transscrotal biopsy to avoid scrotal contamination. Complete non mutilating excision should also be feasible in most extremity and trunk sarcomas. Surgical choice between excision or biopsy for pelvic, retroperitoneal and intrathoracic tumours requires great experience on the part of the surgeon: often these tumours cannot be completely resected and the operation is limited to biopsy.

An important aspect of all initial surgery regards the indications and techniques of regional lymph node exploration. In extremity sarcomas, regional lymph nodes should be explored both in the case of excision of primary tumour and in the case of biopsy. In other sites, it is common practice to explore lymph nodes immediately only if one has opted for the excision of the primary tumour; if the initial surgery is limited to biopsy, the regional lymph nodes should be eventually explored during a later operation following CT. However, in paratesticular sarcomas, a laparatomy in order to explore retroperitoneal (regional) lymph nodes is currently required by American protocols, while in European protocols the evaluation is based on clinical (imaging) data.

Lymph node exploration is essentially a diagnostic non therapeutic procedure. Radical lymph node dissections are discouraged. However, when nodes are clearly metastatic and the primary tumour has been radically removed, the surgeon should also remove all enlarged nodes if possible.

15.7.4 SECONDARY SURGERY

When the initial surgical approach has been a biopsy or an excision with macroscopic residue, the tumour mass may become surgically resectable after CT ± RT. Feasibility of secondary surgery depends on the tumour location and on the clinical response to therapy. However, the response evaluated by physical and imaging data often differs from the pathological findings during surgical exploration. In IRS III (Wiener *et al.*, 1991), 12% of Group III patients achieving a clinical CR after non operative therapy still had residual tumour at secondary surgical exploration; 46% of Group III patients achieving a clinical PR were without evidence of tumour

(that is, CR) at surgical exploration, and another 28% were converted to CR by excision of tumour residue. The most surprising fact was that 30% of Group III patients with no clinical response (NR) were CR at surgical exploration and another 43% could be converted to CR (i.e. completely resected) by the surgeon. In the Italian Study (Guglielmi and Cecchetto, 1990), secondary surgical exploration in 3/10 clinical CR patients confirmed CR in all three cases; in 13/21 clinical PR patients, surgical exploration showed no disease in two cases, and in eight cases residual disease could be completely removed: the surgeon explored 4/11 clinical NR patients and achieved complete excision of tumour in three cases. These data underline the importance of not excluding children from secondary surgery simply because of poor clinical response to chemotherapy.

Timing of secondary surgery depends on the study design. Generally at least two feasibility evaluations of the secondary exploration are suggested, the first after a period of chemotherapy alone, and the second after further chemotherapy associated with radiotherapy. The goal of surgical exploration after chemotherapy alone is that of avoiding RT. Local irradiation can be avoided when no further trace of tumour is found or when all residual tumour has been removed. Mutilating excisions at this time are discouraged. Lymph node sampling is highly recommended especially if it has not been previously performed. In clinical CR patients, surgical exploration after chemotherapy alone is undertaken only when it is easy to perform, otherwise it is omitted and the patient undergoes RT.

Sarcomas which are unresectable or non resected after initial chemotherapy, can be removed after further CT plus RT. At this point the aim is complete excision and any surgical procedure, mutilating or non mutilating, is acceptable if technically feasible.

15.7.5 RADIOTHERAPY

The role of radiotherapy in the management of childhood RMS is well known. High doses (60–65 Gy) and wide fields of irradiation have demonstrated that local control can be achieved in 90% of cases (Tefft *et al.*, 1981) but severe long-term morbidity results. Thereafter, several studies conducted in the USA and in Europe answered important clinical and biological questions about the behaviour of RMS; radiotherapy too underwent some changes. In IRS-I, patients in group I were randomized to receive or not receive post operative radiation. No significant advantage was apparent in the addition of radiotherapy to chemotherapy after surgery and it was concluded that group I patients do not require irradiation. Later patients in group I with unfavourable histology and/or extremity primary tumour treated without irradiation on IRS-II, Italian RMS-79 and German CWS-81 studies, showed an unexpectedly high local regional relapse rate. In the German study CWS-81, patients with RMS of the extremities (Stage I–III) who received radiotherapy, had a significantly better disease-free survival than patients that were not irradiated (60% versus 12%) (Treuner *et al.*, 1989b). For this reason, at present, nearly all protocols use radiation therapy for patients with unfavourable histology or extremity primary lesions even if they are in IRS group I.

Patients with parameningeal tumours who were enrolled on the IRS-I protocol had a lower relapse-free survival (46%) than those with other head and neck primaries. The reason for treatment failure in 35% of these patients was due to tumour invasion into the CNS and almost all patients died of this complication. The introduction of CNS directed therapy with whole brain irradiation in IRS-II increased the five-year survival to 65% compared to 45% in IRS-I. However, in IRS-I, 42% of relapsed patients received a radiation dose below 4000 cGy and in 58% of

cases the tumour volume irradiated was too small. These findings suggest that the dose delivered, the volume irradiated, or both might have influenced the clinical course (Raney *et al.*, 1987b).

Currently, it is recommended that the target volume is limited to the site of tumour plus a margin that includes the local meninges, reserving whole brain irradiation for patients who have evidence of intracranial meningeal extension. The IRS-I study was unable to show a dose-response curve but reported that doses below 40 Gy were associated with a higher local relapse rate in children aged six or older or with tumour diameters of 5 cm or above (Tefft *et al.*, 1981). For some years after this study almost all protocols utilized doses of 40–50 Gy with local control failure and local relapse rates ranging from 30% to 45%. In fact, despite a much better knowledge of risk factors and the improvement of multiagent chemotherapy, the lack of local control still represents the greatest problem in the treatment of RMS. An agreement has been reached that doses of about 40 Gy may be sufficient to sterilize microscopical residue after surgery, but doses of 50 Gy commonly used in macroscopical disease, are often inadequate for patients with large tumours or parameningeal primary with extensive bone erosion. However, higher radiation doses were found to be associated with unacceptable late effects. In an attempt to improve therapeutic effectiveness, maintaining a safety margin for late effects, the division of the daily dose into two or more small fractions (hyperfractionation) has been a subject of intense interest.

Several clinical studies in head and neck adult tumours, have confirmed that a daily dose of 200–250 cGy can be fractionated into two smaller fractions of 100–125 cGy, increasing the tolerance dose for late responding tissues and allowing an increase in total dose. Through a greater capacity for repair of sublethal injury, slow responding tissues are spared more by reducing dose per fraction than are tumours. In addition, studies conducted in weanling rats indicate that significant sparing of radiation-induced epiphysial growth arrest may be achieved using hyperfractionation, demonstrating that a portion of the epiphysial damage caused by ionizing radiation is recoverable during the six-hour interval between the two fractions (Eifel, 1988). These data are very important because the damaging of growing bone is a major dose-limiting factor in radiotherapeutic management of child cancer.

A pilot study of the IRS-IV is now testing a hyperfractionated programme of 5940 cGy in 54 fractions of 110 cGy each, given twice daily. Using the linear quadratic formula (Fowler, 1989), this would provide a 10% increased tumour response and similar late effects as compared to a standard schedule of 5040 cGy in 28 fractions of 180 cGy. A disadvantage of this strategy is the very high number of fractions and its overall length that may decrease the treatment compliance. It is possible to look for an improvement in radiotherapeutic regimens, by combining both a decrease in dose per fraction and a shortening overall treatment duration (hyperfractionated accelerated radiotherapy). An example of accelerated hyperfractionation would be to give a fraction size greater than 125 cGy and less than 180 cGy twice daily. In this way one might expect a decrease in late effects and an improvement in tumour control by hindering cell proliferation during treatment (Saunders *et al.*, 1989).

The limitation of accelerated hyperfractionation is acute toxicity that may require a rest period during the treatment. In order to maintain the advantage of acceleration, these pauses must be as short as possible. A hyperfractionated radiotherapy was adopted in a pilot study conducted at Memorial Sloan-Kettering Cancer Center from 1984 to 1986 on 12 children with gross residual disease. Radiotherapy was delivered at two daily frac-

tions of 150 cGy to a total dose of 5400 cGy in two courses respectively of 3000 cGy and 2400 cGy, alternating with intensive chemotherapy (Mandell *et al.*, 1988). Despite a rest period of four weeks between the two courses, so losing some of the benefits expected from hyperfractionation, the study proved to be both beneficial on local control (83% at two years) and well tolerated.

In 1986, the German CWS-86 study was the first to introduce a hyperfractionated accelerated radiotherapy given simultaneously with chemotherapy. Two daily fractions of 160 cGy were delivered to a total dose of 3200 cGy in patients who were good responders to chemotherapy (PR > 2/3). Poor responders received 5400 cGy in two courses of hyperfractionated radiotherapy, with a rest period of nine days. At the moment no definitive data are published although use of the reduced dose of 3200 cGy for good responders seems to be justified (Treuner *et al.*, 1991). The same hyperfractionated accelerated schedule is utilized in the Italian cooperative study RMS-88. Here, 160 cGy are given twice daily concomitantly with chemotherapy beginning at week 11. Patients with microscopic residuals after surgery or good responders to chemotherapy, received a total dose of 4000 cGy in 2.5 weeks. Gross residues are boosted with 1440 cGy (total dose 5440 cGy) after 10 days of rest in concomitance with the following cycle of chemotherapy. Up to now, the radiotherapeutic regimen has been well tolerated and no interruptions due to acute toxicity of irradiation have been recorded. The mucositis and the related symptoms decreased rapidly in 2–3 weeks.

At present a hyperfractionated accelerated radiotherapy is being tested in all Stage IV patients enrolled in the SIOP study MMT-89. Apart from dose and fractionation, another important radiotherapeutic issue in the management of RMS is the treatment volume. Local regional invasiveness is a salient feature in soft tissue sarcomas. Even if a pseudocapsule gives an impression that it confines the tumour, it is by no means an effective barrier, and tumour extensions can be typically identified far beyond it. In the IRS-I no significant difference was found in terms of local control between patients who received irradiation of the entire muscle or limited to the tumour bed or residual tumour with at least a 5 cm margin in all directions (Tefft *et al.*, 1981). In most current protocols the volume of irradiation suggested is based on the tumour's dimension before chemotherapy including a margin of 2–5 cm. The possibility of targeting irradiation to the residual tumour volume after completion of chemotherapy has been explored by SIOP studies and no excess of local relapse in field margins has been reported.

As a rule, 'prophylactic' irradiation of adjacent lymph nodes is not recommended. Regional nodes are only irradiated when they are clinically, radiologically or histologically involved. Usually the treatment volume should be gauged to encompass the level of the affected lymph node plus the adjacent one. In certain instances, when the tumour is clinically accessible and limited in volume, and in centres with special expertise, brachytherapy should be favoured. This approach is specially recommended in the SIOP Study in

patients with tumour, incompletely resected, of the perineum, bladder, prostate and genital tract. Late complications of brachytherapy appear lower than that caused by external radiotherapy. This is due to the small size of the target volume and probably also to a better tolerance by normal tissues over a continuous low-dose rate of irradiation in comparison with standard fractionated high-dose rate radiotherapy (Gerbaulet *et al.*, 1985).

15.7.6 CHEMOTHERAPY

Childhood RMS is a chemosensitive tumour. In the sixties and seventies, phase II single agent studies were used to identify the most effective agents. High tumour responses were reported mainly with vincristine (VCR) (59%), cyclophosphamide (CYC) (54%), adriamycin (ADR) (31%) actinomycin D (AMD) (24%) and DTIC (11%). (Green and Jaffe, 1978). More recently, other drugs such as cisplatin (CDDP) (Baum *et al.*, 1981), etoposide (VP-16) (Schniall, 1982), ifosfamide (IFO) (Stuart-Harris et al., 1982), high dose methotrexate (Bode, 1986) and melphalan – an alkylating agent similar to CYC – in conventional (Horowitz *et al.*, 1988) or (associated with bone marrow rescue) high dose (Bagnulo *et*

Table 15.6 Combination chemotherapy for RMS

VA	Pulse VAC
VCR 1.5 mg/m^2 (max 2 mg)	VCR 1.5 mg/m^2 (max 2 mg)
AMD 1.5 mg/m^2 (max 2 mg)	AMD 0.015 mg/kg/d × 5 d
or	or
VCR 1.5 mg/m^2/wk × 6 wks	AMD 1.5 mg/m^2 (max 2 mg)
AMD 0.015 mg/kg/d × 5 d	CYC 250 mg/m^2/d × 5–7 d
VADRC	VACA
VCR 2 mg/m^2 (max 2 mg)	VCR, 1.5 mg/m^2/wk
ADR 30 mg/m^2/d × 2 d	ADR 30 mg/m^2 × 2
CYC 10 mg/kg/d × 3 d	CYC 1200 mg/m^2/d
	AMD 0.5 mg/m^2/d × 3

Table 15.7 Ifosfamide-containing regimens

IVA (SIOP MMT-84)	VAIA (ICS RMS-88)
IFO 3 g/m²/d × 2d VCR 1.5 mg/m² max 2 mg AMD 0.9 mg/m² × 2 d	IFO 2 g/m²/d × 5 d AMD 1.5 mg/m² (max 2 mg) VCR 1.5 mg/m² (max 2 mg)
IVA (SIOP MMT-89)	VAIA (CWS-86)
IFO 3 g/m²/d × 3 d VCR 1.5 mg/m² (max 2 mg) AMD 1.5 mg/m² (max 2 mg)	IFO 3 g/m²/d × 2 d AMD 0.5 mg/m²/d (max 0.5 mg) × 3 d VCR 1.5 mg/m² (max 2 mg)

al., 1985), have been included in the list of the effective agents. Until recent years, the combinations most commonly utilized were the association of VCR, AMD, CYC, ADR in two-, three- and four-drug combinations. (Table 15.6).

In the early seventies, large cooperative national and international study groups on childhood RMS were begun. The IRS played a pivotal role in designing these clinical trials in which a variety of clinical questions were asked.

Patients were usually stratified according to the extent of the initial surgery. The first two studies (Maurer *et al.*, 1988; Maurer *et al.*, 1991), showed that a two-drug regimen with VCR and ACT-D (without local RT) is effective in achieving local tumour control in the majority of children with a group I (microscopically complete resection) non-alveolar RMS. The same regimen, in association with local RT, was as effective in maintaining local tumour control in group II RMS as a three-drug regimen including CYC (VAC). The addition of ADR to pulse VAC (VADRC–VAC regimen) did not significantly improve survival for patients with group III or IV disease.

The rate of complete clinical remission (CCR) after 6–8 weeks of chemotherapy of VAC ± ADR in patients with measurable tumour, is approximately 30% (Flamant *et al.*, 1985; Carli *et al.*, 1988; Maurer *et al.*, 1988,

1991. The need to improve the tumour response fostered research for new active agents and for more effective drug combinations.

Encouraging results with IFO-containing regimens (Table 15.7) were reported mainly in Europe in the late 1980s. The German Cooperative Soft Tissue Sarcoma Study Group obtained a higher response rate in their CWS-86 protocol (CR + tumour reduction $\geq 2/3 = 71\%$) in comparison with the previous one (CWS-81, 55%). This result was attributed to substitution of IFO for CYC (Treuner *et al.*, 1989a). Otten *et al.* (1989) reported the highest CR rate so far documented (59% within one year) with IVA regimen as sole treatment in RMS patients treated in SIOP-84 study.

The dose of IFO seems also to correlate with tumour reduction as indicated by the higher response rate observed with VAIA regimen incorporating IFO 10 g/m² in comparison to VAIA incorporating IFO 6 g (83% versus 68% of good responses) utilized by the German and Italian studies (Carli *et al.*, 1991) as pre-operative chemotherapy. IFO in combination with VP-16 was employed by Miser *et al.* (1987a) in patients with recurrent sarcoma of soft tissue and bone. A very favourable response rate of 69% has been obtained for 9 out of 13 patients with RMS.

CDDP-based combination regimens (such

as CDDP/VP-16 (Carli *et al.*, 1987) and CDDP/ADR Schimitt *et al.*, 1989) have also been shown to be effective, with response rates of 33% and 40% respectively in children with advanced RMS. Newer agents such as carboplatin (CBDCA) and epirubicin, analogues of CDDP and ADR, but with less documented neuro- and cardiotoxicity respectively, are presently under investigation.

A combination of CBDCA and high dose epirubicin has been utilized in newly diagnosed children with metastatic soft tissue sarcomas as front line therapy in the SIOP Study. Preliminary results of the ongoing trial indicate the effectiveness of this combination as demonstrated by the 56% response rate (CR + PR) achieved after a single course of such regimen (unpublished data).

Intrathecal (IT) chemotherapy including methotrexate (MTX) or the combination of MTX + cytosine arabinoside (ARA-C) + hydrocortisone has been utilized in association with whole-brain irradiation, to prevent the development of occult meningeal deposits in patients with parameningeal primary tumour and signs of extension to meningeal space such as erosion of the bones at the skull base, presence of cranial nerve palsy, and intracranial extension of the tumour (Maurer *et al.*, 1991). However, the role of ITCT in the marked improvement in survival observed in this group of patients is not clear.

Although great advances have been made in the treatment of RMS, progress is still needed, particularly for patients with locally advanced and metastatic disease. With this objective, more aggressive treatment must be utilized, with the goal of rapidly eliminating as many tumour cells as possible and preventing the development of drug resistance. An increased toxicity is likely to be expected, but the achievement of CR is of critical importance.

A recent observation pointed to the importance of dose intensity to achieve a maximal therapeutic effect (De Vita, 1986). This concept could potentially have an impact on the treatment of RMS. Summing up, the strategies to adopt for improving chemotherapy effectiveness in RMS must include:

1. the incorporation of as many active agents as possible to try and overcome drug resistance (Goldie and Coldman, 1984);
2. the use of chemotherapeutic regimens with higher dose intensity which may result in a higher CR rate.

Based on these chemotherapeutic concepts, chemotherapy as initial therapy is being utilized more and more, with the aim of using less aggressive methods of local treatment. In all European studies, primary intensive chemotherapy (IVA or VAIA) is given, unless complete non mutilating excision of primary tumour is feasible.

In the SIOP study MMT-89, primary chemotherapy alone is continued as long as tumour response is present before considering local treatment. Surgery or radiotherapy is reserved only for patients who do not respond well to chemotherapy, except for parameningeal tumour patients for whom radiotherapy is performed at day 40 in all children older than three years of age.

An example of the treatment guideline proposed in the SIOP MMT-89 study is shown in Fig. 15.3. The intensity and duration of chemotherapy is stratified according to site and the degree of tumour extent (and according to the TNM staging system). The major difference of the German (CWS-86) and the Italian (RMS-88) studies in comparison to SIOP, is the timing of local therapy. The objective of both these studies is to obtain better local tumour control as early as possible.

In the German study, irradiation (given in hyperfractionated doses, simultaneously to chemotherapy), is considered for all patients not in CCR after six weeks of primary chemo-

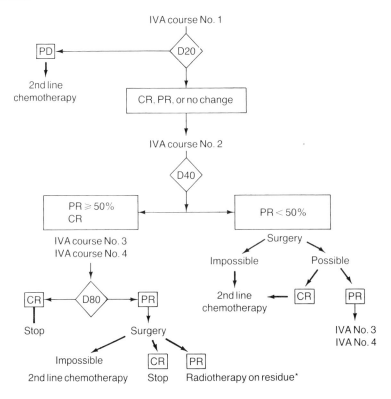

Fig. 15.3 Treatment scheme of Group B patients according to SIOP MMT-89 study guidelines.
◇ = assessment; □ = status; PD = progressive disease; CR = complete remission; PR = partial remission; ★ if impossible, 2nd line chemotherapy.

therapy. The irradiation starts at week seven, the dosage depending on the degree of tumour reduction. The Italian study plans secondary surgical exploration at week nine, attempting to remove the residual tumour or to histologically confirm the CCR. Local radiotherapy is not given in patients with histologically proven remission and with non alveolar histology: these patients will continue with chemotherapy alone. Hyperfractionated radiotherapy, in addition to chemotherapy, is considered for all other patients. Radiotherapy is delivered at week 11, the dosage given being in relation to the degree of tumour response achieved.

Aggressive chemotherapy has also been adopted in the IRS III study; combin-

ations of two to seven drugs (VCR, AMD, CYC, ADR, CDDP, VP-16 and DTIC) were utilized. Irradiation was delivered in all but group I favourable histology patients (Maurer *et al.*, 1989). Second- and third-look operations, to document tumour response and to excise residual tumour, were also included. Treatment duration (1–2 years) and intensity of chemotherapy were related to initial clinical group and histology.

In all studies, second line chemotherapeutic regimens together with radical surgery if feasible, and/or extensive radiotherapy, are considered for all patients who have tumour progression or only stable disease after first line chemotherapy. The duration of adjuvant chemotherapy required for patients who attain complete response is still unknown. The present tendency, with treatment programmes including high dose chemotherapeutic regimens, is to shorten treatment duration to 6–12 months.

High dose chemotherapy, followed by ABMT, may be an attractive strategy for selected patients. High dose melphalan + ABMT (Groot-Loonen *et al.*, 1988) or of an intensive regimen including TBI with VCR + ADR + CYC, with ABMT (Miser *et al.*, 1987c) were utilized after CR was achieved in patients considered of poor prognosis on standard therapy. The results so far reported in Gp IV patients are disappointing with a survival rate of approximately 25%. This approach, however, needs further investigation.

At present, the better quality of CR that can be achieved with the current most effective chemotherapeutic regimens, could be an optimal base for assessing high-dose CT followed by ABMT in improving survival in this group of patients.

The current SIOP-Intergroup European Study on metastatic RMS and other soft tissue sarcomas at diagnosis is evaluating whether a consolidation of CR with high dose melphalan and autologous bone marrow rescue will improve the cure rate of these patients for whom the relapse rate is still too high.

15.7.7 COMBINED MODALITY THERAPY FOR SPECIAL SITES

(a) Orbit

Chemotherapy in conjunction with radiation therapy is the preferred treatment in almost all cases. Surgical approach is usually limited to biopsy. No regional lymph node sampling is requested. Major efforts are now being made to limit the late effects of treatment by trying to reduce radiation therapy dose or even to avoid radiation altogether.

(b) Parameningeal head-neck

Primary excision is never indicated here and only in few cases does secondary excision becomes feasible. Radiation therapy starts after 6–10 weeks of primary chemotherapy. Whole brain irradiation is now limited to cases with intracranial tumour extension. In all other cases the radiotherapy field will include the skull base and the volume of the tumour with 2–3 cm margins. SIOP studies, MMT-84 and the current MMT-89 study do not consider irradiation for children less than three years of age, preferring local control with more intensive chemotherapeutic regimens.

(c) Bladder-prostate

All therapeutic efforts are directed towards avoiding cystectomy and limiting radiotherapy. The tumour response to primary chemotherapy (usually six weeks CT) indicates the following therapy. The patients who obtain a histologically proven complete response with chemotherapy ± conservative surgery, will continue with chemotherapy alone. Limited field radiotherapy or brachytherapy would be given only if micro or macroresidual disease can be demonstrated by endoscopy. The timing of delivering irradiation may vary depending on treatment policy. The SIOP study, for instance, suggested intensive chemotherapy be continued as long as the tumour showed response. Second line chemotherapy might be employed in poor response patients before proceeding to mutilating surgery.

(d) Paratesticular

The paratesticular type of tumour has a very favourable prognosis. Inguinal orchidofunicolectomy is the first therapeutic approach. In the European protocols, initial laparotomy for regional lymph node sampling is indicated only when imaging findings are doubtful. In patients with positive lymph node diagnosis, surgical retroperitoneal exploration should be performed after chemotherapy in order to decide whether radiotherapy is indicated.

15.8 TREATMENT RESULTS

The use of a multimodal approach to treatment has resulted in a dramatic improvement in the cure rate of childhood RMS; this has risen from less than 20% for the historical series (Sutow *et al.*, 1979) to 50–60% in the more recent ones (Maurer *et al.*, 1988; Treuner *et al.*, 1989b; Carli *et al.*, 1991a; Maurer *et al.*, 1991; Flamant *et al.*, 1991). The overall survival rate for non metastatic patients, according to the extent of disease, from four representative cooperative studies is given in Table 15.8.

The overall outcome for patients with metastatic disease at diagnosis, however, remains poor with survival rates ranging from 21% to 28%. (Maurer *et al.*, 1988; Treuner *et al.*, 1989b; Maurer *et al.*, 1991; Carli *et al.*, 1991a). Overall survival is also strongly influenced by primary sites as demonstrated by the analysis of 951 non metastatic patients evaluated in the International RMS Work-

shop (Rodary *et al.*, 1991) (Table 15.9). Moreover, alveolar RMS did not fare so well as embryonal RMS: the five-year survival rate in the IRS-II and the Italian RMS-79 studies was of 53% versus 67% and 41% versus 65% respectively (Heyn *et al.*, 1989; Carli *et al.*, 1990a). Patients who benefitted more from

Table 15.8 Five-year survival (%) by extent of disease

Studies	Clinical group*		
	I	II	III
IRS-I	83	70	52
IRS-II	82	78	64
ICS RMS-79	83	68	55
CWS-81 5-yr DFS	93	80	56
CWS-86 3-yr DFS	90	60	60
	TNM stage*		
SIOP-75 (3-yr survival)	76	40	47
SIOP-84	83	65	37

Note Group and Stage are incomparable (see text).
IRS = Intergroup RMS Study;
ICS = Italian Cooperative Study;
CWS = German Cooperative Study;
SIOP = International Society of Pediatric Oncology;
DFS = Disease-free survival

Table 15.9 Four-year survival by primary sites

Primary site	IRS II N	(% alive)	SIOP-75 N	(% alive)	SIOP-84 N	(% alive)	CWS-81 N	(% alive)	ICS-79 N	(% alive)
Orbit	36	(91)	32	(81)	25	(95)	16	(91)	20	(100)
H and N	44	(88)	48	(49)	37	(63)	10	(75)	10	(63)
PM	61	(65)	54	(33)	33	(58)	30	(56)	22	(47)
GU-BP	45	(67)	35	(54)	23	(81)	19	(70)	10	(75)
GU non BP	54	(94)	40	(88)	43	(85)	22	(95)	17	(100)
Extremity	63	(68)	28	(46)	32	(69)	22	(37)	20	(67)
Other	96	(57)	44	(36)	57	(45)	22	(77)	31	(28)

IRS-II = Intergroup RMS Study II;
SIOP-75 = International Society of Pediatric Oncology RMS-75 Study;
SIOP-84 = International Society of Pediatric Oncology RMS-84 Study;
CWS-81 = German Cooperative Soft Tissue Sarcoma Study 81;
ICS-79 = Italian Cooperative Study RMS-79.

an intensified treatment programme were those with extremity and parameningeal RMS (Maurer *et al.*, 1991).

A conservative approach in relation to organ preservation is feasible. This aspect, already achieved in orbit and extremity tumours, has also been reaffirmed for bladder-prostate tumours as shown by the 65% bladder salvage rate achieved in living patients, treated with intensive chemotherapeutic regimens with or without radiation therapy (Rodery *et al.*, 1990). No statistical difference in the overall survival rate was observed between older children and infants (< 1 year of age), despite the dosage reduction that is necessary in infants because of their greater susceptibility to chemotherapy-related toxicity (Carli *et al.*, 1990b). Local relapse is the main cause of treatment failure.

A review of relapse patterns in RMS patients (Carli and Periolongo, 1991) demonstrated that the first recurrence took the form of an isolated local or regional relapse in 50–60% of cases. Distant metastases occurred in 30% of cases while a combined distant and local relapse effected the remaining 10–20%. Specific patterns of tumour progression were also associated either with certain histological subtypes or with primary tumour location. The disease-free survival curve for childhood RMS seems to plateau at six years (Maurer *et al.*, 1988). Thus, if later recurrences can be ruled out, the recurrence time risk of this tumour is probably six years.

15.9 NON RHABDO SOFT TISSUE SARCOMAS

Non rhabdo soft tissue sarcomas (NRSTS) are a heterogeneous group of tumours of different origins and distinctive histological characteristics which are much more common in adults than in children. In the paediatric age group, NRSTS have two peaks of incidence, the first under the age of five years, the second in early adolescence. Peripheral neuroectodermal tumour (PNET) and extraosseous Ewing's sarcoma (EOE), fibrosarcoma, synovial sarcoma, malignant peripheral nerve sheath tumour (MPNST) are the prevalent entities (Dehner, 1987). Less common types include haemangiosarcoma, haemangiopericitoma, epithelioid sarcoma and alveolar soft part sarcoma. However, any histological entity of STS can be found in children and adolescents: even sporadic cases of liposarcoma, malignant fibrous histiocytoma and leiomyosarcoma are described in the literature.

NRSTS can be found anywhere in the body, but the most common sites are the extremities, the wall of the trunk and the retroperitoneum. The most important symptom is a painless mass that usually grows rapidly; indirect signs of vascular or peripheral nerve compression may be present; when the mass is retroperitoneal, intestinal obstruction is possible. Since these tumours are rare, and include different histological types, the diagnostic programme, staging systems, and general therapeutic strategies are the same as adopted for RMS. The definitive diagnosis is obtained by an incisional biopsy: at present, fine needle biopsy does not provide sufficient accuracy (Hays, 1990). Chemotherapy responsiveness is one of the main therapeutic problems and our knowledge in this field is incomplete particularly for the less common entities. Responsiveness depends on the histological type, but generally it is lower than that observed in RMS. Furthermore, not all authors agree on the indications and use of chemotherapy. According to Horowitz *et al.* (1986), for example, chemotherapy is unnecessary in completely removed tumours and not very effective in advanced forms of the disease. Olive *et al.* (1988) instead obtained good results by associating chemotherapy (ifosfamide, vincristine and actinomycin D) with surgical radical excision. Among 32 Stage III NRSTS patients registered in the Italian Studies, PNET and EOE have demonstrated a good response to primary chemotherapy (6/8 and 2/3 complete or very good partial remissions respectively); fibrosarcoma, MPNST and synovial sarcoma were less sensitive to chemotherapy regimens (1/2, 2/4, 1/3 partial responses respectively) (Carli *et al.*, 1986).

Generally, NRSTS show a higher tendency than RMS to local relapse. For this reason it is a common notion that local treatment should be more aggressive. A wide, non mutilating surgical resection, performed at diagnosis and completed by exploration of regional lymph-nodes, is of great importance. Radiotherapy can help in achieving the local control of the disease in patients with minimal residual disease; in some studies radiotherapy is utilized also when a radical excision is carried out. The results of combined conservative excision plus radiotherapy were compared to those obtained adopting mutilating surgery in both adults and children: survival at 5 years were of 69% and 72% respectively (Tepper and Smith, 1985). In tumours with minimal residue, the use of radiotherapy at doses of at least 40–50 Gy on the tumour bed can help to improve the prognosis. At present, however, all studies underline that NRSTS (excluding PNET and EOE) do not appear curable with

Table 15.10 Clinical features in paediatric NRSTS

	Age	*Site*	*Treatment-prognosis*
PNET and EOE	Adolescence	Chest-wall, head, extremities	Aggressive multimodal therapy. Stage related prognosis.
Fibrosarcoma infantile	< 5 y	Extremities (distal)	Excellent prognosis with surgery alone.
Adolescent	10–15 y	Extremities (proximal)	Aggressive excision. Poor response to CT, RT.
MPNST	Child, adolescent (20% associated with V. Recklinghausen disease)	Extremities, retroperitoneum	Surgical aggressive treatment. Poor response to CT, RT. Unfavourable prognosis.
Synovial sarcoma	Young adults	Legs (knee, foot)	Resection. Doubtful response to CT. Stage-related prognosis.
Haemangiosarcoma	Rare in children	Liver, head-neck	Multimodal treatment. High malignancy. Unfavourable prognosis.
Haemangiopericytoma child	< 1 y	Chest-wall, head, neck	Excellent prognosis with complete excision.
Young adult	15–20 y	Retroperitoneum, legs	Multimodal treatment. Stage-related prognosis.
Epithelioid sarcoma	Rare in children	Extremities (distal)	Radical excision and RT. Good prognosis if complete excision.
Alveolar soft tissue sarcoma	Adolescence (rare in children)	Head/neck (orbit and tongue)	Aggressive surgical exeresis. Stage-related prognosis.

Table 15.11 Differential diagnosis

Tumour	Morphology		Immunocytochemistry						
	Pattern of growth	Nuclear shape	S-100	NSE	Keratin	EMA	Desmin	Vimentin	Factor VIII
PNET	Lobular or diffuse	Oval-round	+	++	−	−	−	+	−
Fibrosarcoma	Herringbone	Sharp-pointed	−	−	−	−	−	+	−
Synovial sarcoma	Nodular and/ or biphasic	Spindle and/ or roundish	−	−	++	+	−	+	−
MPNST	Whorls	Comma	++	+	+−	−	−	+	−
Haemangiosarcoma	Lobular	Roundish and/ or spindle	−	−	+*	−	−	+	+
Epithelioid-sarcoma	Multinodular	Polygonal	−†	−	+	+	−	+	−
Alveolar soft tissue sarcoma	Alveolar	Large round	+−	−	−	−	+−	+	−

PNET Peripheral Neuroectodermal Tumour
MPNST Malignant Peripheral Nerve Sheath Tumour
NSE Neuron Specific Enolase
EMA Epithelial Membrane Antigen

* In epithelioid variant
† Occasionally positive

combinations of chemotherapy and RT alone; for this reason the local control of the disease must be surgically achieved. Furthermore, some histological types such as fibrosarcomas and MPNST show a very bad response to chemotherapy and radiotherapy; an aggressive surgical excision of the primary mass is the mainstay of the treatment for these entities.

Prognostic factors are: (1) extension of the disease at diagnosis: survival varies from 85% in patients with localized tumours to 7–10% in children with disseminated forms (Horowitz *et al.*, 1986); (2) histological type and consequent different responsiveness to combined treatments; (3) the primitive site of tumour: local control of the disease can be obtained only with greater difficulty in patients with thoracic or abdominal tumours: (4) age: children under five years of age seem to have a better prognosis. The clinical features and treatment of the most common NRSTS will be described. The clinical characteristics of these tumours and those of other less common histological types are illustrated in Table 15.10. The principal diagnostic morphological features of NRSTS are described in Table 15.11.

15.9.1 PERIPHERAL NEUROECTODERMAL TUMOURS (PNET) AND EXTRA-OSSEOUS EWING'S SARCOMA (EOE)

Since the clinical behaviour (and probably the histogenesis) of these tumours are similar, they have been put together in this chapter. PNET make up a controversial and poorly defined class of extracranial and extraspinal small round cell malignant tumours with 'neural' characteristics supposed of neuroectodermal origin (Dehner, 1986). Neuroblastoma and PNET are the two most representative members of this family. Recently, other entities have been added to this group (malignant small cell tumours of the thoracopulmonary region or Askin's tumours, PNET of bone, ectomesenchymoma, etc). Microscopically, PNET is composed of a uniform population of round cells arranged in lobular or diffused patterns, with small nucleoli and numerous mitoses; Homer-Wright or Flexner rosettes are frequently seen. Undifferentiated areas with Ewing-like appearance are occasionally observed, and PAS positive, diastase-sensitive material (glycogen) has been found in 40% of cases (Cavazzana, in press). The identification of neural characteristics (neuro-secretory granules) sometimes requires the use of electron microscopy and immuno-cytochemical analyses (presence of NSE, S-100 protein, and synaptophysin). PNET occurs in children and young adults with median age around 15–20 years; it is a very aggressive tumour most commonly found on the chest wall and extremities and has the tendency to metastasize to regional lymph-nodes, lung and bones. The overall prognosis is unfavourable with a survival rate below 50% even when a multimodal approach is adopted.

Extra-osseous Ewing's sarcoma (EOE) appears to be a very primitive member of the same neuroectodermal family on the basis of several common features (Cavazzana *et al.*, 1987). A specific cytogenetic abnormality involving chromosome 11 and 22 originally observed in Ewing's sarcoma on bone and PNET, was recently also reported in EOE (Casorso, 1989). This finding suggests a close histogenetic relationship between EOE and PNET. Therefore it seems convenient to use the term Ewing's sarcoma for undifferentiated blastematous soft tissue small round cell tumours that lack any morphologic or immunohistochemical evidence of neural differentiation. Generally, the best results for PNET and EOE seem to be linked to more aggressive treatments which include chemotherapy, radiotherapy and radical surgery. Because of the high incidence of local relapse, a wide surgical excision and accurate control of radicality are mandatory. Jurgens reports that in a study of 42 patients, ten of the 12

who developed a local relapse had had residual disease after the first excision (Jurgens *et al.*, 1988). Radiotherapy can be used effectively only in cases with minimal residuals; as far as chemotherapy is concerned, the best results are obtained with a combination of high doses of anthracycline and alkylating agents. Miser *et al.* (1987b) report that 16/17 patients obtained a complete response using chemotherapy and radiotherapy after surgical excision.

15.9.2 FIBROSARCOMA

Fibrosarcomas make up about 10–12% of paediatric STS. There are two peaks of incidence according to age: the first in children under four years of age (congenital and infantile fibrosarcoma) and the second in patients between 10 and 15 years (adult fibrosarcoma); furthermore, 50% of infantile fibrosarcoma are found during the first months of life (Chung and Enzinger, 1976). Microscopically, the tumour consists of small round or spindle-shaped fibroblasts, exhibiting variable collagen production and showing no evidence of other differentiation.

In adolescence, fibrosarcoma has clinical features similar to those found in adults. The most frequent sites are the proximal region of extremities, where the tumour is most aggressive. This form has an unfavourable prognosis and survival rate is less than 60%. The most effective treatment seems to be a radical surgery. Perhaps beneficial results can be obtained with radiotherapy on minimal residue. The role of chemotherapy remains uncertain both in unresectable or disseminated forms.

The infantile (or congenital) fibrosarcomas are usually located in the distal region of extremities. Even though these masses are fast growing and show a high cellularity, they are the most easily treatable forms of fibrosarcoma: surgery alone is able to cure the disease. Even if local relapses are around 30–40%, metastases are extremely rare and the overall survival is about 85–90% following second look operations (Soule and Pritchard, 1977). Nevertheless, recent reports have demonstrated a good response to primary chemotherapy (VAC combination) in patients with inoperable infantile fibrosarcoma (Ninane, 1991).

Other fibrous proliferations of infancy and childhood are the so-called fibromatoses. Because of their unusual histological features, they pose special diagnostic problems. Exuberant cellular proliferation, high mitotic index and infiltrative growth pattern do not necessarily indicate aggressive clinical behaviour. On the other hand innocent-appearing fibrous proliferation may relapse repeatedly. After the original series published by Stout (1954) on 'juvenile fibromatosis', many other entities have been recognized and categorized (Chung, 1985); of all the forms, infantile fibromatosis, desmoid-type, is the most controversial and difficult to delineate with precision (Ayala, 1986). In fact, it displays a considerable histological variability, from immature mesenchymal lesions to mature fibroblastic proliferations with abundant collagen production, which closely resemble adult musculoaponeurotic fibromatosis. Sometimes, in the more cellular variant of infantile fibromatosis, differential diagnosis from fibrosarcoma is a very difficult problem. Such difficulty in diagnosis is emphasized by the great variety of terms used in the past (aggressive fibromatosis, differentiated fibrosarcoma, fibrosarcoma Grade I desmoid type, etc). In general, in our experience, high mitotic rate, minor collagen production and destructive growth favour a diagnosis of infantile fibrosarcoma over fibromatosis. Fibromatosis does not usually metastatize but has high local aggressiveness; it requires complete surgical excision and must be distinguished from other NRSTS through a precise histological examination. Again, low

dose VA or VAC chemotherapy may be effective if the tumour is unresectable.

15.9.3 SYNOVIAL SARCOMA

Synovial sarcoma is common in young adults but rare in the paediatric age group. It is characterized by four histological subtypes: biphasic, monophasic-fibrous, monophasic-epithelial and poorly differentiated. The lower extremities, and in particular the knee, are the most common sites (80%). Many prognostic factors have been defined. The favourable factors seem to be: the earlier age (Buck *et al.*, 1981), the female sex (Wright *et al.*, 1982), the distal site (Treuner, *et al.*, 1987b) and the size of the tumour <5 cm (Hajdu *et al.*, 1977). The histological prognostic factors are more questionable. The best outcome seems to be linked to biphasic subtype (Cagle *et al.*, 1987; Flamant, 1989) particularly in those tumours in which a high percentage of glandular tissue and a low mytotic activity are evident. The presence of calcifications is also considered a favourable prognostic sign: in these cases the survival at five years is over 80% (Verela-Duran and Enzinger, 1982).

Because synovial sarcoma is rare, it has not been possible to establish precise therapeutic guidelines. A wide excision of the primitive mass offers the best chance of a favourable outcome in localized forms; about 60% of patients who undergo a simple excision relapse within one year. Radiotherapy is useful only in the treatment of microscopical residual disease. The effectiveness of chemotherapy is uncertain; however, in the German CWS-81 study, a cytostatic response rate of 77% (VACA combination) was registered for Stage III and IV patients (Treuner *et al.*, 1987a).

15.9.4 MALIGNANT PERIPHERAL NERVE SHEATH TUMOUR (MPNST) (MALIGNANT SCHWANNOMA)

MPNST represents about 5–10% of paediatric

315

STS. These tumours originate from the peripheral nerve sheaths. From 15% to 20% of patients with Von Recklinghausen disease develop a MPNST. The most common sites are the extremities and the trunk. This tumour has a poor response to chemotherapy and radiotherapy; as in the case of fibrosarcoma, surgical excision is the chosen treatment and is the most important prognostic factor. In a recent review of 24 patients, Raney *et al.* (1987a) found that 9/12 MPNST who had undergone a complete excision are alive without disease; none of the 12 who had residual disease had a favourable outcome. It is possible that chemotherapy may improve prognosis of the disease when a complete macroscopic resection has been performed but this has not been demonstrated to date.

15.9.5 LATE SEQUELAE

Late complications related to specific drugs may occur. Peripheral neuropathy and paralytic ileus may result from repeated doses of VCR as well as high frequency hearing loss and renal damage to high cumulative dose of CDDP. Infertility and haemorragic cystitis are the major complications following CYC administration; haemorragic cystitis is particularly severe if associated with bladder irradiation. Cardiac damage, including cardiac failure and dysrhythmias, have been described in patients receiving a high total dose of adriamycin (Steinhertz *et al.*, 1989). Nephrotoxicity after high-dose IFO has recently been reported. Proximal tubular impairment indicated by phosphaturia and hypophosphataemia, glycosuria, increased beta 2-microglobulin excretion, and generalized aminoaciduria, resulting in some cases in a clinical and radiological feature of rickets, is the most common damage. However, any part of the nephron may also be damaged and different combinations of clinical features may be seen (Skinner *et al.*, 1990).

Several ocular, dental and maxillofacial abnormalities have been described in long-term survivors of soft tissue sarcomas of the head and neck (Fromm *et al.*, 1986). Problems deriving from radio-chemotherapy for orbital RMS may be cataracts, xerophthalmia, keratitis, corneal ulcers, retinal injuries and orbital hypoplasia. Decreased vision in the treated eye was the most common functional problem and, in most patients, related to cataract formation which occurred in 90% of eyes (Heyn *et al.*, 1986).

Radiation to developing teeth may cause maldevelopment of roots and crowns; salivary gland irradiation, causing transient or permanent changes in salivation, may produce caries. Growth hormone deficiencies and growth failure after irradiation, including the hypophyseal region, have also been reported. Appropriate prophylactic and/or symptomatic management may often minimize the late effects of treatment.

The severity of these abnormalities is dependent on the stage of development of the specified irradiated organ and the radiation dose. Most severe damage developed in those patients who received a tumour dose of more than 50 Gy. Rare cases of leucoencephalopathy have been reported in patients with parameningeal tumour, intensively treated with whole brain irradiation and intrathecal chemotherapy (Fusner *et al.*, 1977). A satisfactory bladder function is present in most of the patients treated with chemotherapy ± radiotherapy ± partial cystectomy.

Mutilating surgery is, at present, very rarely performed; it may be considered for patients with progressive disease despite intensive chemo-radiotherapy programmes or for selected patients with recurrent disease. Bilateral retroperitoneal lymph node dissection is associated with a high incidence of ejaculatory impotence, and should be discouraged.

Second malignant neoplasms have been observed in children surviving from RMS who received multimodality therapy. Several cases of acute myeloid leukaemia and bone tumours, mostly in the field of radiation therapy, have been reported (Heyn *et al.*, 1991).

15.10 CURRENT CONTROVERSIES

15.10.1 WHICH PROGNOSTIC FACTORS ARE OF PROVEN CLINICAL VALUE?

For many years differences in clinical staging and histopathological definitions have be-devilled analyses of IRS and SIOP studies. The importance of alveolar pathology as an adverse factor has been questioned by the SIOP group, although a recent consensus has demonstrated that it is of value (Newton *et al.*, 1988; Rodary *et al.*, 1989; Caillaud *et al.*, 1989). The role of ploidy is also equivocal. American studies suggest that this is a clear prognostic indicator (Shapiro *et al.*, 1991), whereas data from the Kiel group has questioned this conclusion (K. Koscielniak, pers. comm.).

The emphasis by the SIOP group on regional extent of disease at presentation rather than clinical resectability as with the IRS, has led to two distinct staging systems making clinical outcome comparisons difficult. It has become increasingly accepted by the American groups, however, that the SIOP TNM staging is a more effective way of predicting outcome (Donaldson and Belli, 1984).

The German CWS group has suggested that speed of response is an important factor (Treuner *et al.*, 1989b) but differences in the timing of first reassessment between national groups makes this difficult to confirm. It seems likely, however, that this is an important factor and it is hoped that the current SIOP study will shed light on this by including guidelines regarding the timing of early reassessment of response.

15.10.2 HAS THERE REALLY BEEN ANY IMPROVEMENT OVER THE BASIC VAC CHEMOTHERAPY REGIMEN?

The inclusion of ifosfamide by the MMT group was based on the lack of cross-resistance between ifosfamide and cyclophosphamide in some relapsed patients. Apart from a small but significant difference in response rates in adults with soft tissue sarcomas (Bramwell *et al.*, 1986), no other randomized study has demonstrated an advantage to the inclusion of ifosfamide. More rapid cytoreduction has been described after ifosfamide (Treuner *et al.*, 1989a) but it seems likely that any benefit is simply due to a higher dose of alkylating agent. If the dose of cyclophosphamide was increased, possibly with bone marrow growth factors as support, equal efficacy could, perhaps, be achieved.

The addition of etoposide and cisplatin (IRS III) or the inclusion of doxorubicin (VACA) or high dose melphalan with autologous bone marrow rescue while probably reducing duration of chemotherapy has not produced any significant advance in disease-free survival (Pinkerton *et al.*, 1991).

15.10.3 THE ROLE OF LOCAL IRRADIATION

This remains the major area of contention between the IRS group and European centres. The continuing American conviction that extensive radiotherapy is necessary for adequate local control and cure has lead to an acceptance of many late sequelae, such as bone and soft tissue deformation and the possibility of second tumours. In the SIOP MMT-89 study, primary chemotherapy alone is continued as long as the tumour is responding and no local treatment is given if CCR is achieved. However, it remains for the SIOP group to demonstrate that overall survival is not compromised because of a significant salvage rate in patients who have a local relapse after radiotherapy has been omitted. Up to 35% local relapse rate was observed in patients in CR after chemotherapy alone, but 45% of them were alive two years after second line therapy (Flamant *et al.*, 1987, 1991).

The timing of local radiotherapy has also been an issue and it has been argued that if this modality is to be used it should be given early in treatment, i.e. within the first couple of months. In this situation extended fields are likely to be used whereas the SIOP strategy focuses on reduced fields given only to areas of residual disease following chemotherapy and conservative surgery; a strategy is designed to avoid late sequelae. The CWS and Italian groups introduce earlier local therapy (7–9 weeks) accepting that few patients will achieve CCR by this time. The high local relapse rate in RMS emphasizes the difficulty in detecting minimal residual disease. Histological confirmation of CR must be encouraged. It is possible that radiation dose can be modified with regard to the site and to the age of the child. Novel techniques such as interstitial radiation or the use of implantation moulds may be suitable for certain sites, such as head and neck or urogenital tract and may deliver effective doses without irradiating adjacent regions (Flamant *et al.*, 1990).

The role of radiotherapy in patients with metastatic disease differs between groups. Some argue that it is logical to irradiate all sites of distant disease where feasible, i.e. excluding bone marrow. Others feel that as there is almost certainly undetectable micrometastatic disease elsewhere, this type of 'spot welding' is a futile approach.

15.10.4 WHAT IS THE ROLE OF MULTIDRUG RESISTANCE IN RHABDOMYOSARCOMA?

The dramatic survival curves published by Chan *et al.* (1990), suggesting that MDR1

expression is an overriding prognostic factor irrespective of stage, need to be confirmed on a prospective multicentre basis. Because of problems reproducing the technique with formalin fixed tissue, this study may prove difficult as it would require fresh frozen tissue for immunohistochemistry or Northern blot assessment of MDR1 expression. It may be that the use of PCR to detect low levels of MDR1 expression may in the future be applicable to fixed tissue. Ideally, treatment strategies could be based on the presence of MDR, avoiding drugs such as vincristine, actinomycin or doxorubicin, known to be mediated by this resistance mechanism or possibly the elective use of an MDR reversing agent such as verapamil.

15.10.5 DOES CHEMOTHERAPY HAVE A ROLE IN NON-RMS SOFT TISSUE SARCOMAS?

Our knowledge regarding childhood non-RMS soft tissue sarcoma treatment must be improved. In particular, more information is needed concerning chemotherapy response in relationship to histological types. The treatment applied in RMS patients may be appropriate in some other sarcomas for which chemo-sensitivity has been demonstrated. To date, as a rule, a more aggressive local therapy than that adopted in RMS has been employed.

Fibrosarcoma and malignant peripheral nerve sheath tumour (MPNST) are considered poorly chemosensitive tumours and an aggressive loco-regional approach similar to that adopted in adult soft tissue sarcomas has been recommended. However, some reports indicate the effectiveness of chemotherapeutic regimens in infantile fibrosarcoma and fibromatosis MPNST (Stein, 1977; Weiss and Lackman, 1989; Ninane, 1991). Up until now the prognostic factors discussed have been based on the clinical and histological characteristics.

In the near future molecular genetic studies such as cellular DNA content (ploidy) and the research of structural cytogenetic abnormalities may give us more insight into the biological behaviour of these tumours and will help us to identify more precisely the different risk groups in relation to prognosis.

C.R.P.

REFERENCES

Ayala, A.G., Ro, J.Y., Goepfert, H. *et al.* (1986) Desmoid fibromatosis: A clinicopathologic study of 25 children. *Sem. Diagn. Pathol.*, **3**, 138–50.

Bagnulo, S., Perez, D.J., Barrett, A. *et al.* (1985) High dose melphalan and autologous bone marrow transplantation for solid tumors of childhood. *Eur. Paed. Haem. Oncol.*, **1**, 129.

Bale, P.M., Parson, R.E. and Stevens, M.M. (1986) Pathology and behavior of juvenile rhabdomyosarcoma. In: *Pathology of Neoplasia in children and Adolescents* (ed. M. Finegold), W.B. Saunders, Philadelphia pp. 196–222.

Baum, E.S., Gaynon, P., Greenberg, L. *et al.* (1981) Phase II trial of cisplatin in refractory childhood cancer: Children's Cancer Study Group report. *Cancer Treat. Rep.*, **65**, 815–22.

Becker, H., Zaunschirm, A., Muntean, W. and Domej, W. (1982) Alkoholembryopathie und maligner tumor. *Wien klin. Wochenschr.*, **94**, 364–5.

Beddis, I.R., Mott, M.G. and Bullimore, J. (1983) Case report: Nasopharingeal rhabdomyosarcoma and Gorlin's naevoid basal cell carcinoma syndrome. *Med. Pediatr. Oncol.*, **11**, 178–9.

Birch, J.M., Hartely, A.L., Blair, V. *et al.* (1990) Cancer in the families of children with soft tissue sarcoma. *Cancer*, **66**, 2239–48.

Bode, V. (1986) Methotrexate as relapse therapy for rhabdomyosarcoma. *Am. J. Pediatr. Hematol. Oncol.*, **8**, 70–2.

Bramwell, V.H.C., Mouridsen, H.T. and Santoro, A. *et al.* (1986) Cyclophosphamide versus ifosfamide: preliminary report of a randomized phase II trial in adult soft tissue sarcomas. *Cancer Chemother. Pharmacol.* **18** (2), 1–9.

Buck, P., Mickelson, M.R., Bonfiglio, M. (1981) Synovial sarcoma: a review of 33 cases. *Clin. Ortho Rel. Res.*, **156**, 211–15.

Cagle, L.A., Mirra, J.M. and Storm, F.K. (1987) Histologic features relating to prognosis in synovial sarcoma. *Cancer*, **59**, 1810–14.

Caillaud, J.M., Gerard-Marchant, R., Marsden, H.B. *et al.* (1989) Histopathological classification of childhood rhabdomyosarcoma: A report from the International Society of Pediatric Oncology Pathology Panel. *Med. Ped. Oncol.*, **17**, 391–400.

Carli, M., Grotto, P., Cavazzana, A. *et al.* (1990a) Prognostic significance of histology in childhood rhabdomyosarcoma: improved survival with a new histologic 'Leiomyomatous' subtype. *Proc. Am. Soc. Clin. Oncol.*, **9**, 297.

Carli, M., Grotto, P., Perilongo, G. *et al.* (1990b) Soft tissue Sarcomas in infants less than 1 year old: Experience of the Italian Cooperative Study RMS-79. In 'Cancer in the First Year of life. Leukemias; Neuroblastomas; Soft Tissue Sarcomas' (eds F. Lampert, L. Cordero di Montezemolo, A. Pession). *Contributions to Oncology* Vol. 41 (eds J.H. Holzner, W. Queiber), Karger, Basle.

Carli, M., Guglielmi, M., Sotti, G. *et al.* (1991a) Prognostic factors in children with rhabdomyosarcoma. Results of the Italian Cooperative Study RMS-79. Proc of XXIII SIOP Meeting *Med. Pediatr. Oncol.*, **19** (5), 398.

Carli, M., Pastore, G., Perilongo, P. *et al.* (1988) Tumor response and toxicity after single high-dose versus standard five-day divided-dose dactinomycin in childhood rhabdomyosarcoma. *J. Clin. Oncol.*, **6**, 4, 654–8.

Carli, M. and Perilongo, G. (1991) Pattern of treatment failure and the meaning of complete response in rhabdomyosarcoma. In *Rhabdomyosarcoma and Related Tumors in Childhood and Adolescence.* (eds H.M. Murer, F. Ruymann, C. Pochedly) CRC Press, Boca Raton, FL. (In press).

Carli, M., Perilongo, G., Cordero di Montezemolo, L. *et al.* (1987) Phase II trial of cisplatin and etoposide in children with advanced soft tissue sarcoma: A report from the Italian Cooperative Rhabdomyosarcoma Group. *Cancer Treat. Rep.*, **71**, 525–7.

Carli, M., Perilongo, G., Paolucci, P. *et al.* (1986) Role of primary chemotherapy in childhood malignant mesenchymal tumors other than rhabdomyosarcoma. Preliminary results. *Proc. Am. Soc. Clin. Oncol.*, **5**, 208.

Carli, M., Treuner, J., Koscielniak, E. *et al.* (1991b) Ifosfamide more is better? 6 vs 10 gr/mg in VAIA may influence the tumour response rate in childhood rhabdomyosarcoma. The experience of the German (CWS-86) and the Italian (ICS-RMS 88) Cooperative Studies. *Proc. Am. Soc. Clin. Oncol.*, **10**, 319.

Casorso, L., Pessia, L., Satimo, A. *et al.* (1989) Extraskeletal Ewing's tumor with translocation t(11:22) in a patient with Down's Syndrome. *Cancer Genet. Cytogenet.*, **37**, 79–89.

Cavazzana, A.O., Miser, J.S., Jefferson, J. *et al.* (1987) Experimental evidence for a neural origin of Ewing's sarcoma of bone. *Am. J. Pathol.*, **127**, 507–18.

Cavazzana, A.O., Ninfo, V., Roberts, J. *et al.* Peripheral neuroepithelioma: a light microscopy, immunocytochemical and ultrastructural study. *Med. Pathol.* (In press).

Cavazzana, A.O., Schmidt, D., Ninfo, V. *et al.* (1989) Spindle cell (leiomyomaous) rhabdomyosarcoma: an unusual variant of embryonal rhabdomyosarcoma. An anatomo-clinical study of 21 cases. *Path. Res. Pract.*, **185**, 35.

Cecchetto, G., Grotto, P., De bernardi, B. *et al.* (1988) Paratesticular rhabdomyosarcoma in childhood: Experience of the Italian Cooperative Study. *Tumori*, **74**, 645–7.

Chan, H.S., Thorner, P.S., Haddad, G. and Ling, V. (1990) Immunohistochemical detection of P glycoprotein: Prognostic correlation in soft tissue sarcoma of childhood. *J. Clin. Oncol.*, **8**, 689–704.

Chung, E.B. (1985) Pitfalls in diagnosis of benign soft tissue tumors in infancy and childhood. *Pathol. Annu.*, **20**, 2, 323–86.

Chung, E.B. and Enzinger, F.M. (1976) Infantile fibrosarcoma. *Cancer*, **38**, 729–39.

Crist, W.M., Garnsey, L., Beltangady, M. *et al.* (1990) Prognosis in children with rhabdomyosarcoma: A report of the Intergroup Rhabdomyosarcoma Studies I and II. *J. Clin. Oncol.*, **8**, 443–52.

De Vita, V.T. (1986) Dose-response is alive and well. *J. Clin. Oncol.*, **4**, 1157–9.

Dehner, L.P. (1986) Peripheral and central primitive neuroectodermal tumors. A nosologic concept seeking a consensus. *Arch. Pathol. Lab. Med.*, **110**, 997–1005.

Dehner, L.P. (1987) Soft Tissues Sarcomas, in *Pediatric Surgical Pathology*, 2nd edn Williams and Wilkins. pp. 869.

Donaldson, S.S. and Belli, J.A. (1984) A rational clinical staging system for childhood rhabdomyosarcoma. *J. Clin. Oncol.*, **2**, 135–9.

Donaldson, S.S., Draper, G.J., Flamant, F. *et al.* (1986) Topography of childhood tumours: Pediatric Coding System *Pediatr. Hematol. Oncol.*, **3**, 249–58.

Eifel, P.J. (1988) Decreased bone growth arrest in weanling rats with multiple radiation fractions per day. *Int. J. Radiat. Oncol. Biol. Phys.*, **15**, 141–5.

Engel, R., Ritterbach, J., Shwabe, D. *et al.* (1988) Chromosome translocation (2;13)(q37;q1) in a disseminated alveolar sarcoma. *Eur. J. Pediatr.*, **18**, 69–71.

Flamant, F. (1989) Tumeurs mesenchymateuse malignes en dehors du rhabdomyosarcoma, in *Cancer de l'Enfant*. Encyclopedie des Cancers. (ed J. Lemerle) Flammarion, Paris. pp. 446–56.

Flamant, F., Gerbaulet, A., Nihoul-Fekete, C. *et al.* (1990) Long-term sequelae of conservative treatment by surgery, brachytherapy, and chemotherapy for vulval and vaginal rhabdomyosarcoma in children. *J. Clin. Oncol.*, **8**, 1847–53.

Flamant, F., Rodary, C., Brunat-Mentigny, M. *et al.* (1987) SIOP MMT 84 Protocol – Interim rhabdomyosarcoma (RMS) analysis. *Proc. SIOP* 126–7.

Flamant, F., Rodary, C., Rey, A. *et al.* (1991) Assessing the benefit of primary chemotherapy in the treatment of rhabdomyosarcoma in children. Report from the International Society of Pediatric Oncology: RMS-84 study. *Proc. Am. Soc. Clin. Oncol.*, **10**, 309.

Flamant, F., Rodary, F., Voûte, P.A. *et al.* (1985) Primary chemotherapy in the treatment of rhabdomyosarcoma in children: Trial of the International Society of Pediatric Oncology (SIOP). Preliminary results. *Radiat. Oncol.*, **3**, 227–36.

Fowler, J.F. (1989) The linear-quadratic formula and progress in fractionated radiotherapy. *Brit. J. Radiol.*, **62**, 679–94.

Fromm, M., Littman, P., Raney, B. *et al.* (1986) Late effects after treatment of twenty children with soft tissue sarcomas of head and neck. Experience at a single institution with a review of the literature. *Cancer*, **57**, 2070–6.

Fusner, J.E., Poplack, D.G., Pizzo, P.A. *et al.* (1977) Leukoencephlopathy following chemotherapy for rhabdomyosarcoma: reversibility of cerebral changes demonstrated by computed tomography. *J. Pediatr.*, **91**, 77–9.

Gaiger, A.M., Soule, E.H. and Newton, W.A. Jr. (1981) Pathology of rhabdomyosarcoma: experience of the Intergroup Rhabdomyosarcoma Study, 1972–78. NCI Monogr. 56, 19–27.

Gerbaulet, A., Panis, X., Flamant, F. *et al.* (1985) Iridium after loading curietherapy in the treatment of pediatric malignancies. The Institute Gustave Roussy Experience. *Cancer,* **56**, 1274–9.

Goldie, J.H. and Coldman, A.J. (1984) The genetic origin of drug resistance in neoplasms: implication for systemic therapy. *Cancer Res.,* **44**, 3643–53.

Gonzalez-Crussi, F. and Black-Shaffer, S. (1979) Rhabdomyosarcoma of infancy and childhood. Problems of morphologic classification. *Am. J. Surg. Pathol.,* **3**, 157–71.

Green, D.M. and Jaffe, N. (1978) Progress and controversy in the treatment of childhood rhabdomyosarcoma. *Cancer Treat. Rev.,* **5**, 7–27.

Groot-Loonen, J.T., Pinkerton, R., Meller, S. *et al.* (1988) Rapid high-dose intensity chemotherapy including high dose melphalan for rhabdomyosarcoma. Proc. SIOP XX Meeting, *Med. Pediatr. Oncol.,* **16**, 430.

Guglielmi, M. and Cecchetto, G. (1990) Role of second look operations for children in group III soft-tissue sarcomas: Experience of the Italian Cooperative Study RMS 88. SIOP XXII Meeting. *Med. Ped. Oncol.,* **18**, 413.

Hajdu, S.I., Shin, M.H. and Fortner, J.G. (1977) Tenosynovial sarcoma. A clinicopathological study of 136 cases. *Cancer,* **39**, 1201–17.

Harmer, M.H. (1982) (ed) *TNM classification of paediatric tumors.* International Union Against Cancer, Geneva, pp. 23–8.

Harms, D., Schmidt, D. and Treuner, J. (1985) Soft-tissue sarcomas in childhood. A study of 262 cases including 169 cases of rhabdomyosarcoma. *Z. Kinderchir.,* **40**, 140–5.

Hays, D. (1990) New approaches to the surgical management of rhabdomyosarcoma in childhood. *Chir. Pediatr.,* **31**, 197–201.

Hays, D.M., Lawrence, W., Jr. *et al.* (1989) Primary reexcision for patients with 'microscopic residual' tumor following initial excision of sarcomas of trunk and extremity sites. *J. Ped. Surg.,* **24**, 5–10.

Hays, D.M., Newton, W.A., Soule, E.H. *et al.* (1983) Mortality among children with rhab-

domyosarcoma of the alveolar histological subtype. *J. Pediatr. Surg.,* **18**, 412.

Heyn, R., Beltangady, M., Hays, D. *et al.* (1989) Results of intensive therapy in children with localized alveolar extremity rhabdomyosarcoma: A report from the Intergroup Rhabdomyosarcoma Study. *J. Clin. Oncol.,* **7**, 200–7.

Heyn, R., Haeberlen, V., Newton, W.A. *et al.* (1991) Second malignant neoplasms in patients treated on Intergroup Rhabdomyosarcoma Studies I-II. *Proc. Am. Soc. Clin. Oncol.,* **10**, 311.

Heyn, R., Ragab, A., Romey, B. *et al.* (1986) Late effects of therapy in orbital rhabdomyosarcoma in children. A report from the Intergroup Rhabdomyosarcoma Study. *Cancer,* **57**, 1738–43.

Horn, R.C. and Enterline, H. (1958) Rhabdomyosarcoma: a clinicopathological study and classification of 39 cases. *Cancer,* **11**, 181–99.

Horowitz, M.E., Etcubanas, E., Christensen, N.L. *et al.* (1988) Phase II testing of melphalan in children with newly diagnosed rhabdomyosarcoma: A model for anticancer drug development. *J. Clin. Oncol.,* **6**, 308–14.

Horowitz, M.E., Pratt, C.B., Webber, L. *et al.* (1986) Therapy for childhood soft-tissue sarcomas other than rhabdomyosarcoma: a review of 62 cases. *J. Clin. Oncol.,* **4**, 559–64.

IARC (1988) *International Incidence of Childhood Cancer* (eds D.M. Parkin, C.A. Stiller, G.J. Draper, C.A. Bieber, B. Terracini and J.L. Young), IARC No. 87, pp. 364–5.

Jaffe, N., Filler, R.M., Farber, S. *et al.* (1973) Rhabdomyosarcoma in children. Improved outlook with multidisciplinary approach. *Am. J. Surg.,* **125**, 482–7.

Jurgens, H., Bier, V., Harms, D. *et al.* (1988) Malignant peripheral neuroectodermal tumors. A retrospective analysis of 42 patients. *Cancer,* **61**, 349–57.

Lawrence, W., Jr., Hays, D.M., Heyn, R. *et al.* (1987) Lymphatic metastases with childhood rhabdomyosarcoma. A report from the Intergroup Rhabdomyosarcoma Study. *Cancer,* **60**, 910–15.

Li, F.P. and Fraumeni, J.R., Jr. (1969) Rhabdomyosarcoma in children: Epidemiologic study and identification of a family cancer syndrome. *J. Natl. Cancer Inst.,* **43**, 1365–73.

Li, F.P., Fraumeni, J.R., Jr., Mulvihill, J.T. *et al.*

(1988). A cancer family syndrome in twenty-four kindreds. *Cancer Res.*, **48**, 5358–62.

Mandell, L.R., Ghavimi, F., Exelby, P. *et al.* (1988) Preliminary results of alternating combination chemotherapy and hyperfractionated radiotherapy in advanced rhabdomyosarcoma. *Int. J. Radiat. Oncol. Biol. Phys.*, **15**, 197–203.

Maurer, H.M. (1975) The Intergroup Rhabdomyosarcoma Study (N.I.H.): Objectives and Clinical Staging Classification. *J. Pediatr. Surg.*, **10**, 977–8.

Maurer, H.M., Beltangdy, M., Gehan, E.A. *et al.* (1988) The Intergroup Rhabdomyosarcoma Study-I. A final report. *Cancer*, **61**, 209–20.

Maurer, H.M., Gehan, E.A., Beltangady, M. *et al.* (1991) The Intergroup Rhabdomyosarcoma Study-II, *Cancer*, (In press).

Maurer, H.M., Gehan, E., Crist, W. *et al.* (1989) Intergroup Rhabdomyosarcoma Study (IRS) III: A preliminary report of overall outcome. *Proc. Am. Soc. Clin. Oncol.*, **8**, 296.

Mckeen, E.A., Bodurtha, J., Meadows, A.T. *et al.* (1978) Rhabdomyosarcoma complication multiple neurofibromatosis. *J. Pediatr.*, **93**, 992–3.

Miser, J.S., Kinsella, T.J., Triche, T.J. *et al.* (1987a) Ifosfamide with mesna uroprotection and etoposide: An effective regimen in the treatment of recurrent sarcomas and other tumors of children and young adults. *J. Clin. Oncol.*, **5**, 191–8.

Miser, J., Kinsella, T.J., Triche, T.J. *et al.* (1987b) Treatment of peripheral neuroepithelioma in children and young adults. *J. Clin. Oncol.*, **5**, 1752–8.

Miser, J., Kinsella, T., Triche, T.J. *et al.* (1987c) Treatment of high-risk sarcomas with an intensive consolidation followed by autologous bone marrow transplantation. *Proc. Am. Soc. Clin. Oncol.*, **6**, 218.

Newton, W.A., Jr., Soule, E.H., Hamoudi, A.B. *et al.* (1988) Histopathology of childhood sarcomas, Intergroup rhabdomyosarcoma studies I and II: Clinicopathologic correlation. *J. Clin. Oncol.*, **6**, 67–75.

Newton, W.A., Triche, T.J., Marsden, H. *et al.* (1991) International Childhood Soft Tissue Sarcoma Pathology Classification Study: design and implementation utilizing Intergroup Rhabdomyosarcoma Study II clinical and pathology data. *Proc. Am. Soc. Clin. Oncol.*, **10**, 317.

Ninane, J. (1991) Chemotherapy for infantile fibrosarcoma. *Med. Pediatr. Oncol.*, **19**, 209.

Olive, D., Flamant, F., Rodary, C. *et al.* (1988) Responsiveness of non RMS malignant mesenchimal tumors to primary chemotherapy. *Proc. XIX SIOP Meeting*. Trondheim.

Olive, D., Flamant, F., Zucker, J.M. *et al.* (1984) Paraaortic lymphadenectomy is not necessary in the treatment of localized paratesticular rhabdomyosarcoma. *Cancer*, **54**, 1283–7.

Otten, J., Flamant, F., Rodary, C. *et al.* (1989) Treatment of rhabdomyosarcoma and other malignant mesenchymal tumors of childhood with ifosfamide + vincristine + dactinomycin (IVA) as front-line therapy. *Cancer Chemother. Pharmacol.*, **24** (suppl), 30.

Palmer, N.F. and Foulkes, M. (1983) Histopathology and prognosis in the second Intergroup Rhabdomyosarcoma Study (IRS II). *Proc. Am. Soc. Clin. Oncol.*, **3**, 229.

Pastan, I.H. and Gottesman, H.M. (1988) Molecular biology of multidrug resistance in human cells, in *Important Advances in Oncology* (eds V.T. De Vita, Jr., S. Hellman, S.A. Rosemberg) J.B. Lippincott, Philadelphia. PA.

Pastore, G., Mosso, M.L., Carli, M. *et al.* (1987) Cancer mortality among relatives of children with soft tissue sarcoma: A national survey in Italy. *Cancer Letters*, **37**, 17–24.

Pinkerton, C.R., Groot-Loonen, J., Barrett, A. *et al.* (1991) Rapid VAC, high dose melphalan regimen. A novel chemotherapy approach in childhood soft tissue sarcomas. *Br. J. Cancer*, **64**, 381–5.

Raney, R.B., Jr., Hays, D.M., Lawrence, W., Jr. *et al.* (1978) Paratesticular rhabdomyosarcomas in childhood. *Cancer*, **42**, 729–36.

Raney, B., Schnauffer, L., Ziegler, M. *et al.* (1987a) Treatment of children with neurogenic sarcoma. Experience at the Children's Hospital of Philadelphia 1958–1984. *Cancer*, **59**, 1–5.

Raney, B., Tefft, M., Newton, W.A. *et al.* (1987b) Improved prognosis with intensive treatment of children with cranial soft tissue sarcomas arising in nonorbital parameningeal sites. *Cancer*, **59**, 147–55.

Riopelle, J.L. and Theriault, J.P. (1956) Sur une forme meconnue de sarcome des parties molles: le rhabdomyosarcome alveolaire. *Ann. Pathol.*, **1**, 88–111.

Rodary, C., Flamant, F. and Donaldson, S.S. (for the SIOP-IRS Committee) (1989) An attempt to use a common staging system in rhabdomyosarcoma: A report of an International Workshop initiated by the International Society of Pediatric Oncology (SIOP). *Med. Pediatr. Oncol.*, **17**, 210–15.

Rodary, C., Flamant, F., Treuner, J. *et al.* (1990) Bladder salvage in 109 non metastatic bladder and/or prostate rhabdomyosarcoma. A report from the International SIOP RMS Workshop Proc SIOP XXII Meeting. *Med. Pediat. Oncol.*, **149**, 405.

Rodary, C., Gehan, E., Flamant, F. *et al.* (1991) Prognostic factors in 951 nonmetastatic rhabdomyosarcoma in children: A report from the International Rhabdomyosarcoma Workshop. *Med. Pediatr. Oncol.*, **19**, 89–95.

Rodary, C., Rey, A., Olive, D. *et al.* (1988) Prognostic factors in 281 children with non-metastatic rhabdomyosarcoma at diagnosis. *Med. Pediatr. Oncol.*, **16**, 71–7.

Ruymann, F.B., Maddux, H.R., Ragab, A. *et al.* (1988) Congenital anomalies associated with rhabdomyosarcoma: An autopsy study of 115 cases. A report from the Intergroup rhabdomyosarcoma Study Committee. *Med. Pediat. Oncol.*, **16**, 33–9.

Saunders, M.I., Dische, S., Hong, A. *et al.* (1989) Continuous hyperfractionated accelerated radiotherapy in locally advanced carcinoma of the head and neck region. *Int. J. Radiat. Oncol. Biol. Phys.*, **17**, 1287–93.

Schimitt, C., Flamant, F. and Rodary, C. (1989) Efficacy of Cisplatin-Adriamycin in combination in children with rhabdomyosarcoma. *Proc. Am. Soc. Clin. Oncol.*, **9**, 306.

Schniall, H. (1982) Review of etoposide single agent activity. *Cancer Treat. Rev.*, **9** (suppl A): 21–30.

Scrable, H., Witte, D., Shimada, H. *et al.* (1989) Molecular differential pathology of rhabdomyosarcoma. *Genes Chromosomes Cancer*, **1**, 23–35.

Shapiro, D.N., Parham, D.M., Douglass, E.C. *et al.* (1991) Relationship of tumor-cell ploidy to histologic subtype and treatment outcome in children and adolescents with unresectable rhabdomyosarcoma. *J. Clin. Oncol.*, **9** (1), 159–66.

Skinner, R., Pearson, A.D., Price, L. *et al.* (1990) Nephrotoxicity after ifosfamide. *Arch. Dis. Child.*, **65**, 732–8.

Soule, E.H. and Pritchard, D.J. (1977) Fibrosarcoma in infants and children. A review of 110 cases. *Cancer*, **40**, 1711–21.

Stein, R. (1977) Chemotherapeutic response in fibromatosis of the neck. *J. Pediatr.*, **90**, 482–3.

Steinherz, L., Steinherz, P., Tan, C. *et al.* (1989) Cardiac toxicity 4–20 years after completing anthracycline therapy. *Proc. Am. Soc. Clin. Oncol.*, **8**, 296.

Stout, A.P. (1954) Juvenile fibromatoses. *Cancer*, **7**, 953–78.

Stuart-Harris, P., Harpe, C., Parkins, J.A. *et al.* (1982) High dose infosfamide in the treatment of soft tissue sarcoma. Abstract 15–0337, UICC Conference in Clinical Oncology.

Sutow, W., Sullivan, M.P., Ried, H.L. *et al.* (1979) Prognosis in childhood rhabdomyosarcoma. *Cancer*, **25**, 1384–91.

Tefft, M., Lindberg, R.D. and Gehan, A. (1981) Radiation therapy combined with systemic chemotherapy of rhabdomyosarcoma in children: local control in patients enrolled in the Intergroup Rhabdomyosarcoma Study. *NCI Monogr.*, **56**, 75–81.

Tepper, J.E. and Smith, H.D. (1985) The role of radiation therapy in the treatment of sarcoma of soft tissue. *Cancer Invest.*, **3**, 587–92.

Treuner, J., Flamant, F. and Carli, M. (1991) Results of treatment of rhabdomyosarcoma in the European Studies, in *Rhabdomyosarcoma and Related Tumors in Children and Adolescents* (eds H.M. Maurer, F. Ruymann, C. Pochedly) CRC Press, Boca Raton, FL. (In press).

Treuner, J., Jurgens, H. and Winkler, K. (1987a) The treatment of 30 children and adolescents of synovial sarcoma in accordance with the protocol of the German Multicenter Study for soft tissue sarcoma. *Proc. Ann. Soc. Clin. Oncol.*, **6**, 215.

Treuner, J., Koscielniak, E. and Keim, M. (1989a) Comparison of the rates of response to ifosfamide and cyclophosphamide in primary unresectable rhabdomyosarcoma. *Cancer Chemother. Pharmacol.*, **24** (suppl 1) 5, 48–50.

Treuner, J., Kuhl, J., Beck, J. *et al.* (1989b) New aspects in the treatment of childhood rhabdomyosarcoma: Results of the German Cooperative Soft-Tissue Sarcoma Study (CWS-81), in *Progress in Pediatric Surgery* Vol. 22, (eds L. Spitz, *et al.*), Springer-Verlag, Berlin, pp. 162–75.

Treuner, J., Suder, J., Gerein, V. *et al.* (1987b)

Behandlungsergebnisse der nichtrhabdomyosarkomosen Weichteilmalignome in Rahmen der CWS-81-Studie. *Klin. Padiatr.*, **199**, 209–17.

Tsokos, M., Miser, A., Wesley, R. *et al.* (1985) Solid variant of alveolar rhabdomyosarcoma: a primitive rhabdomyosarcoma with poor prognosis and distinct histology. Proceedings of SIOP XVIIth Meeting Venice, Italy, p. 71–4.

Turc-Carel, C., Aurias, A., Mugneret, F. *et al.* (1988) Chromosomes in Ewing's Sarcoma. An evaluation of 85 cases and remarkable consistency of t(11;22)(q24;q12). *Cancer Genet. Cytogenet.*, **32**, 229–38.

Turc-Carel, C., Dal Cin, P., Limon, J. *et al.* (1987) Involvement of chromosome X in primary cytogenetic change in human neoplasia: non random translocation in synovial sarcoma. *Proc. Natl. Acad. Sci. USA*, **84**, 1981–5.

Varela-Duran, J. and Enzinger, F.M. (1982) Calcifying synovial sarcomas. *Cancer*, **50**, 345–52.

Weiss, A.J. and Lackman, R.D. (1989) Low-dose chemotherapy of desmoid tumours. *Cancer*, **64**, 1192–4.

Whang-Peng, J., Triche, T.J., Krusten, *et al.* (1985) Chromosomal translocation in peripheral neuroepithelioma. *N. Engl. J. Med.*, **311**, 584–5.

Wiener, E., Lawrence, W., Hays, D.M. *et al.* (1991) Complete response or not complete response? Second look operations are the answer in children with rhabdomyosarcoma *Proc. Am. Soc. Clin. Oncol.*, **10**, 316.

Wright, P.A., Sim, F.H., Soule, E.H. *et al.* (1982) Synovial sarcoma. *J. Bone Joint Surg.*, **64-a**, 112–22.

Young, J.L., Jr, Ries, L.G., Silverberg, E. *et al.* (1986) Cancer incidence survival and mortality for children younger than age 15 years. *Cancer*, **58**, Suppl. 2, 595–602.

Chapter 16

Bone tumours

H. JÜRGENS, K. WINKLER and U. GÖBEL

16.1 INTRODUCTION

Bone tumours constitute approximately 10% of all malignant neoplasms in children and adolescents (Souhami, 1987). In European countries such as France, Germany, Italy or the United Kingdom, with a population between 60 and 80 million each, approximately 200 new cases are seen every year. More than 95% of the malignant bone tumours in children and adolescents fall into two main categories: osteosarcoma and Ewing's sarcoma, osteosarcoma being twice as common as the latter, making it the most common primary malignant bone tumour in children and adolescents. For this reason the discussion in this chapter will concentrate on these two major entities.

16.2 OSTEOSARCOMA: AETIOLOGY AND MANAGEMENT

Osteosarcoma is defined as a malignant tumour originating in bone consisting of a spindle cell stroma which produces osteoid or immature bone (Campanacci, 1990; Huvos, 1991). The annual incidence is estimated to be between two and three cases per million population. Osteosarcoma can occur at any age, however, approximately 60% of all patients are affected in the second decade of life. Males are slightly more frequently

affected than females, with the male to female ratio usually reported as about 1.4:1 (Fig. 16.1) (Huvos, 1991).

The typical age at presentation, the younger age of females at presentation, and the slight predominance of boys, all suggest a relationship between rapid bone growth and the development of this neoplasm (Link and Eilber, 1989). In addition, there is evidence that patients with osteosarcoma are taller than their age peers (Fraumeni, 1967). Osteosarcoma also characteristically occurs at the metaphyseal portion of the most rapidly growing bones in adolescents: the distal femur, the proximal tibia and the proximal humerus. In summary, this tumour appears most frequently at sites with the greatest increase in length and size of bone (Fig. 16.2). Thus osteosarcoma seems to be a malignant transformation of the rapidly proliferating bone forming cell, either as a result of a random event or induced by viral, chemical or physical agents (Link and Eilber, 1989; Huvos, 1991).

Evidence for a genetic predisposition is found in patients with hereditary retinoblastoma where subsequent development of osteosarcomas as second malignancies is also reported and occurs independently of therapy (Schimke *et al.*, 1974). In addition, there is evidence that the specific locus on chromosome 13 which is involved in the generation

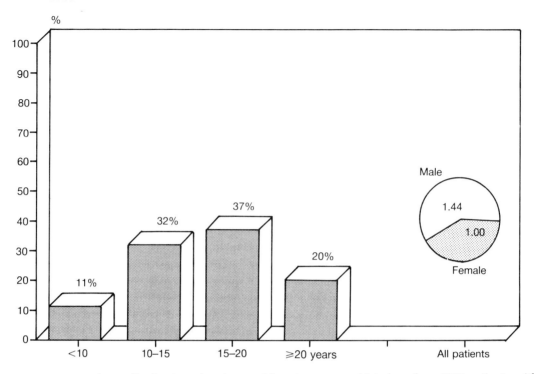

Fig. 16.1 Age and sex distribution of patients with osteosarcoma (data based on 1046 patients with osteosarcoma entered into the COSS trials).

of retinoblastoma is also implicated in the generation of osteosarcoma (Benedict *et al.*, 1988). It has also been shown recently that human osteosarcomas have rearrangements of the p53 gene, a fact that might have a crucial role in the oncogenesis (Miller *et al.*, 1990).

16.2.1 PATHOLOGY

Osteosarcomatous tissue is usually compact, whitish and, due to the presence of neoplastic osteoid, hard in consistency. The histological diagnosis of osteosarcoma depends on the presence of malignant sarcomatous spindle cell stroma with production of neoplastic osteoid. Great variability exists in the histological pattern of this tumour and the degree

of osteoid production (Campanacci, 1990; Huvos, 1991). Assuming that osteosarcoma originates from a primitive mesenchymal cell which is capable of differentiating, a number of histopathological variants of osteosarcoma have been defined. The largest subgroup is characterized by an abundant production of osteoid tissue and classified as osteoblastic osteosarcoma. Other histological subtypes are fibroblastic, (fibrosarcomatous, fibrohistiocytic), chondroblastic (chondrosarcomatous) and telengiectatic depending on the predominant stromal cell. The histopathological variety of osteosarcoma is complemented by a great variety in biological behaviour of this tumour, although most cases are malignant. Approximately 10% of osteosarcomas can be classified as a low or median grade malignant

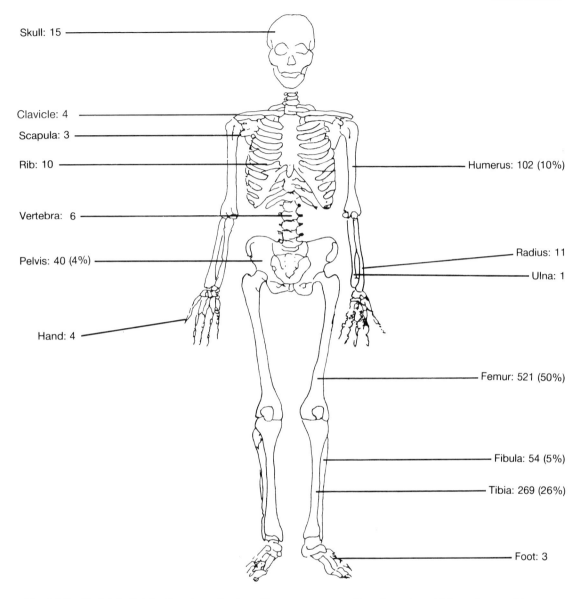

Skull: 15

Clavicle: 4

Scapula: 3

Rib: 10

Vertebra: 6

Pelvis: 40 (4%)

Hand: 4

Humerus: 102 (10%)

Radius: 11

Ulna: 1

Femur: 521 (50%)

Fibula: 54 (5%)

Tibia: 269 (26%)

Foot: 3

Fig. 16.2 Skeletal distribution in patients with osteosarcoma (data based on 1043 patients with osteosarcoma entered into the COSS studies).

process. Grading of osteosarcomas remains a controversial subject, primarily due to the tumour heterogeneity from area to area.

There is little doubt that tumours originating from the periosteum or paraosteal tissue at the surface of bone generally have a slower course. In contrast to classic high grade malignant osteosarcomas, paraosteal osteosarcomas have a favourable prognosis and recur locally rather than metastasize. Rarely, par-

327

aosteal osteosarcomas can be high grade; thus, the clinical course, the radiographic pattern and the histopathological appearance should be added together for exact classification and grading (Huvos, 1991).

In addition, primary osteosarcoma of the jaw, usually occurring in older patients, tends to be associated with a slower course with a tendency to local recurrences rather than distant metastases (Huvos, 1991). Finally, in a few instances, osteosarcoma presents as a multifocal tumour with multiple synchronous skeletal tumours suggesting a multicentric origin (Campanacci, 1990). Since osteosarcoma requires radical resection of all affected sites, the prognosis for those patients is extremely poor.

16.2.2 CLINICAL PRESENTATION AND DIAGNOSIS

As with other primary malignant bone tumours the earliest symptom is pain in the involved bone, initially transitory and gradually getting more severe. Swelling of the affected area becomes more prominent with time. Depending on the subtype of tumour, the swelling might be either hard and firm or soft. The skeletal distribution of osteosaroma is shown in Figure 16.2, above. Characteristically, the long tubular bones are affected, most frequently the distal femur, proximal tibia and proximal humeral metaphysis. In only approximately 10% of cases are the flat bones of the axial skeleton involved.

Due to the typical clinical presentation, with pain and swelling, a conventional x-ray is the first diagnostic step in most instances. Plain x-ray shows a destructive lesion with intense periosteal new bone formation and frequently breakage of the tumour through the cortex into the adjacent soft tissue (Fig. 16.3). Depending on the degree of ossification osteosarcomas may appear more osteosclerotic, more osteolytic or mixed. To estimate the true intramedullary and soft tissue exten-

sion of the tumour the conventional radiographic description must be complemented with additional CT-scanning and, if available, magnetic resonance imaging (MRI) (Fig. 16.4).

A radionuclide bone scan is required both for description of the primary tumour and also detection of metastatic deposits in intra- and extraosseous compartments. Both MRI and bone scan may be able to detect tumour deposits in other areas of the affected bone, so-called 'skip' lesions, which are known to occur in approximately 5% of osteosarcomas (Enneking and Kagan, 1975).

Arteriography may also be helpful, particularly when limb salvage procedures are planned; however, with the availability of MRI this option is now used less frequently.

Approximately 10 to 20% of patients present with visible metastases at diagnosis (Jürgens *et al.*, 1988a). The lungs are the first sites of metastases in 90% of patients. Hence conventional radiographs of the chest in two planes, complemented by CT-scanning of the chest, are mandatory for staging since the detection of mestastases at diagnosis is essential for treatment planning. The remaining 10% of patients with metastases at diagnosis present with metastases in other bones; here, the most sensitive method of detection is bone scanning with technetium diphosphonate.

Despite good evidence that tumour burden affects prognosis a generally accepted staging system for patients with osteosarcoma of bone does not exist. Most primary lesions fall into stage IIB of the Enneking staging system (Enneking, 1987), since although they originate within the bone there is also invasion of the soft tissue compartment. The only further categorization that is generally accepted is the distinction into patients with and without detectable metastases at diagnosis.

Given the correlation between osteoblastic activity within the tumour and serum levels of alkaline phosphatase, an elevation might serve as a tumour marker, both at diagnosis

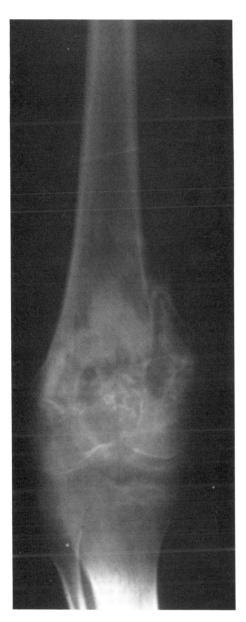

Fig. 16.3 X-ray appearance of distal femur osteosarcoma with pathological fracture in a 12-year-old girl.

mented in approximately 50% of patients. (Rosen, 1975).

(a) Differential Diagnosis

The more typical the radiographic picture, tumour site, and age of the patient, the less relevant are other diagnostic considerations. In non-typical areas, particularly the diaphysis of long bones or flat bones of the trunk, Ewing's sarcoma is the most common differential diagnosis (Huvos, 1991). Other considerations include bone metastases of other neoplasms, or in rare instances, bone lesions of Langerhans cell histiocytosis. Amongst non-malignant disorders, osteomyelitis must be considered as well as localized areas of *myositis ossificans* (Campanacci, 1990).

16.2.3 TREATMENT

Given its unresponsiveness to radiation, the approach to local treatment of primary osteosarcoma of bone is solely surgical. To minimize the risk of local recurrence radical removal of all gross and microscopic disease is mandatory. Hence ablative surgery has been considered the treatment of choice for a long period of time for most cases.

In view of the widely adopted use of systemic chemotherapy, given prior to definitive surgery, and better tumour definition with bone scanning, CT and MRI in order to define both the intramedullary extent of tumour and also to detect skip lesions within the affected bone, orthopaedic surgeons are increasingly able to select patients for limb salvage procedures. In a recent survey of the experience of the German Co-operative Osteosarcoma Studies (COSS) the proportion of ablative procedures decreased from 90% in the initial study COSS 77 to 34% in the latest study COSS 86 (Winkler *et al.*, 1991b).

The majority of limb salvage procedures are centered around the implantation of endoprosthetic devices, now readily available

and indicating relapse and/or metastases during follow-up (Huvos, 1991). An elevation of serum alkaline phosphatase can be docu-

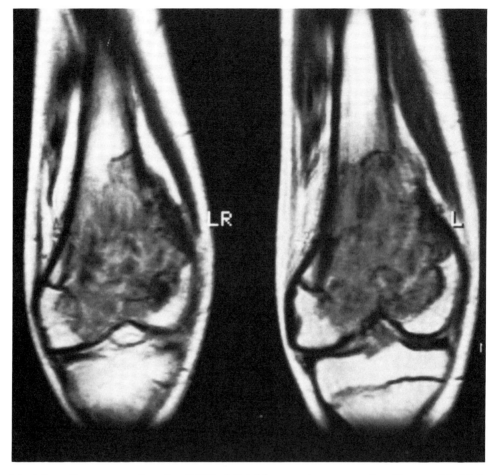

Fig. 16.4 Magnetic resonance imaging (MRI) of distal femur osteosarcoma in a 12-year-old girl showing outline of the medullary soft tissue tumour extension.

for tumours of the femur and tibia as well as of the humerus. Rotation plasties have been widely adopted, particularly in growing children with tumours of the femur, and have reached a proportion of 26% in the recent series (Winkler *et al.*, 1991). The rotation plasty involves excision of the turmour-bearing part of the femur with the adjacent muscle compartment and preservation of the lower leg maintaining an intact neuro- and often vascular bundle. The distal part of the

extremity is rotated 180 degrees and fixed to the proximal femur.

This procedure places the foot into an inverted position with the sole facing anteriorily and the ankle functioning as a knee joint. Fitting an external prosthesis, the patient is converted from an above the knee amputee to a functional below the knee amputee with considerable improvement in function (Salzer *et al.*, 1981; Winkelmann, 1986b).

The majority of limb salvage procedures

involve en-bloc-resections with different types of bone and joint reconstructions. The proportion of those procedures has increased from 10% in the initial Study COSS 77 to 41% in the latest series COSS 86 (Winkler *et al.*, 1991b).

While there is now wide experience in using endoprosthetic devices, the experience with biological approaches using autologous non-vascularized or vascularized grafts or allografts is limited (Link and Eilber, 1989).

Careful follow-up studies are needed to finally define valid guidelines for the safe local control of the tumour depending on the patient's age, tumour site and size. With the adoption of systemic chemotherapy to prevent disease dissemination, the disease-free survival rates reported now seem no different for ablative compared to limb salvage surgery (Winkler *et al.*, 1991b).

If, however, the results are analysed in detail for site of recurrence, patients with limb salvage procedures are found to have a higher rate of local recurrences. In the COSS trials the local control rate over four consecutive studies was 96%; 9.8% of patients with limb salvage surgery, however, developed local failures compared to 1.8% of patients who developed local recurrences following amputations (Winkler *et al.*, 1991b). The local recurrence rate following rotation plasties is as low as in patients with amputation (Winkler *et al.*, 1991b).

The increased recurrence rate in resections for osteosarcoma stresses the importance of en-bloc-resection of the whole affected area with a margin of normal uninvolved tissue. This principle also applies for patients with optimal tumour response to primary chemotherapy. Despite response to initial chemotherapy intralesional surgery will jeopardize disease-free survival (Winkler *et al.*, 1991b).

(a) Radiotherapy

Osteosarcoma is considered to be a highly radioresistant lesion (Spooner, 1987; Campanacci, 1990). Before the introduction of combination chemotherapy to the multidisciplinary approach to osteosarcoma, some investigators advocated the use of radiotherapy to the primary tumour and only aimed at ablative surgery in those patients who were free of metastatic disease approximately six months after diagnosis (Lee and Mackenzie, 1964). Currently, the only indication for radiotherapy lies in the attempt to control residual disease following debulking surgery in patients with unresectable lesions, e.g. primaries in the vertebrae. In addition, after debulking surgery and radiation, local recurrences are the rule and it is doubtful whether this will change with different schemes of fractionation and/or other techniques, e.g. hyperthermia (Spooner, 1987).

In the search for better ways of preventing metastases to the lungs, 20 Gy whole lung irradiation has been applied prophylactically. Results have shown a marginal benefit for radiated patients compared to a control group (Burgers *et al.*, 1988). Since the introduction of combination chemotherapy into systemic treatment of osteosarcoma the use of radiotherapy to the lungs has been abandoned (Link, 1986).

(b) Chemotherapy

Despite immediate surgery, even amputation, approximately 80% of all patients develop metastatic disease suggesting the presence of subclinical microscopic metastatic disease at the time of diagnosis (Campanacci, 1990; Huvos, 1991). Compared to other sarcomas in childhood, osteosarcoma has been considered a relatively drug-resistant tumour. Only with the availability of adriamycin and methotrexate in high doses followed by citrovorum factor rescue, cisplatin and, more recently, ifosfamide, has this changed (Link, 1986). Institutions and co-operative groups have been testing various schedules of combination chemotherapy in osteosarcoma starting a decade of controversy and dispute about the role of chemotherapy in the treatment of this disease (Carter, 1984; Holland, 1987). Following the introduction of high dose methotrexate with citrovorum factor rescue by Jaffé *et al.* (1974; 1977), and the incorporation of this treatment principle into a combination chemotherapy scheme mainly with adriamycin and alkylating agents by Rosen *et al.* (1975; 1979), co-operative groups such as the German Society of Paediatric Oncology (GPO) with a series of co-operative COSS trials, and the Paediatric Oncology Group (POG) have finally resolved this issue by demonstrating that long-term disease-free survival in the range of between 60% and 70% five to ten years after diagnosis can be obtained and maintained (Winkler *et al.*, 1984; Goorin *et al.*, 1985; Link *et al.*, 1986; Winkler *et al.*, 1990).

Initially aimed at bridging the time gap for fabricating custom-made endoprostheses to allow limb salvage surgery, primary chemotherapy after biopsy proven diagnosis has allowed the study of the 'in vivo' effect of chemotherapy on the primary tumour.

Depending on the intensity of presurgical initial chemotherapy, different grades of chemotherapy-induced tumour necrosis were seen on the surgical specimen and it could be shown that this histological response correlated strongly with prognosis (Rosen *et al.*, 1979; Jürgens *et al.*, 1981). Although different schemes of grading of histological response are being applied, most investigators agree that less than 10% viable tumour at the time of surgery indicates a favourable histological response and more than 10% viable tumour a poor histological response (Salzer-Kuntschik *et al.*, 1983; Huvos, 1991). The responsiveness of the primary tumour to preoperative chemotherapy was found to be the most powerful predictor of prognosis (Jürgens *et al.*, 1981).

It was shown in the German COSS trials

that by increasing the proportion of good responders with more intense preoperative chemotherapy the proportion of patients with favourable prognosis can be increased (Winkler *et al.*, 1991a). The intensity of initial therapy, therefore, seems to determine the treatment efficacy. Consequently, the current COSS regimen incorporates all known active agents in osteosarcoma in an intensive schedule in order to achieve a 'good response' in the range of 70 to 80%. Early hopes that patients with poor response could be salvaged with alternate chemotherapy regimens or late intensifications could not be confirmed by other groups and the evaluation of such regimens is the subject of currently ongoing trials (Rosen *et al.*, 1982; Winkler *et al.*, 1991a).

In order to increase the proportion of patients with favourable histological response, presurgical chemotherapy has also been administered intraarterially in order to maximize drug delivery to the tumour-bearing compartment. In particular *cis*-platin has been delivered by short-term or prolonged intraarterial infusion (Jaffé *et al.*, 1989).

The results being reported with the use of intraarterial chemotherapy are controversial; however, reports differ in the number of intraarterial treatment courses given, drug dose and time of exposure. The exact role of intraarterial chemotherapy in the treatment of osteosarcoma is yet to be determined (Jaffé *et al.*, 1989; Winkler *et al.*, 1990; Ruggierei *et al.*, 1990).

In view of the prognostic value of the histological response induced by preoperative chemotherapy, the value of postoperative chemotherapy or at least the optimal length of treatment are the subject of ongoing trials (Winkler *et al.*, 1991a). Until those trials are completed, it seems safe to continue chemotherapy following surgery for a total length of treatment between six to nine months following diagnosis, taking into consideration the long-term side effects of intensive combination chemotherapy. These are mainly related to the cumulative doses of individual agents or dose intensity, e.g. nephrotoxicity of cisplatin and ifosfamide, oto- and neurotoxicity of cisplatin and finally adriamycin-related cardiomyopathy.

(c) Immunotherapy

Immunological approaches to osteosarcoma have often been undertaken; however, convincing data supporting this approach are lacking (Link and Eilber, 1989). *In vitro* evidence of interferon activity against osteosarcoma cell lines have led to clinical trials which have demonstrated some benefit compared to historical groups, less, however, than that obtained with combination chemotherapy (Einhorn and Strander, 1978). In conjunction with chemotherapy, the European COSS 80 trial failed to show a benefit of additional β-interferon (Winkler *et al.*, 1984). Whether the definite 'in vitro' effect can be exploited with different interferons or scheduling is yet to be determined.

16.3 METASTATIC DISEASE

Most sarcoma patients who develop metastases on or off treatment have a poor prognosis. In osteosarcoma, however, most metastases are confined to the lungs and are in many cases less disseminated than those seen in other neoplasms (Jürgens *et al.*, 1988a). It has been shown over the last 15 years that complete surgical resection of all overt metastatic pulmonary disease can lead to salvage after relapse (Beattie *et al.*, 1975; Beron *et al.*, 1988). Patients not treated by thoracotomy, however, cannot be cured (Beron *et al.*, 1988). Removal of pulmonary lesions by wedge resections is considered the treatment of choice; removal of larger amounts of pulmonary tissue is rarely necessary (Martini *et al.*, 1974). If all lesions can be completely resected, disease-free survival following a single or

repeat thoracotomies is reported to be in the range of 40% to 50% (Jürgens *et al.*, 1988a; Beron *et al.*, 1988). The value of additional chemotherapy for patients with relapsed metastatic disease is being debated. Convincing data of controlled trials are lacking (Jürgens *et al.*, 1988a). Many investigators administer two to three courses of chemotherapy prior to thoracotomy and continue chemotherapy following surgery only in those patients who have had demonstrable effects of chemotherapy on resected metastatic nodules (Beattie *et al.*, 1975; Jürgens *et al.*, 1988a; Beron *et al.*, 1988).

16.4 PERSPECTIVES

The use of systemic combination chemotherapy has undoubtedly improved disease-free survival in patients with osteosarcoma. Tasks for the future include determination of the optimal length and schedule on chemotherapy and the tailoring of chemotherapy intensity and the number of active agents to the individual risk of relapse (Goorin *et al.*, 1985; Link, 1986; Winkler *et al.*, 1991b).

In conclusion, ablative surgery can be avoided in over 80% of patients. The question of function and duration of endoprosthetic devices remains unresolved; exact guidelines are also needed for situations where intracompartmental limb salvage surgery might jeopardize disease-free survival. The unresolved issues, including the as yet undetermined role of immunotherapy, should not detract from the exceptional advances made in the treatment of osteosarcoma during the last two decades (Kotz, 1978; Goorin, 1988).

16.5 EWING'S SARCOMA

Ewings's sarcoma is a malignant bone tumour histologically composed of small round cells (Campanacci, 1990; Huvos, 1991). In some instances, neuroepithelial markers are expressed, blurring the distinction from a malignant peripheral neuroectodermal tumour (Schmidt, *et al.*, 1987; Schmidt and Harms, 1990). Ewing's sarcoma is relatively common and accounts for 10 to 15% of all primary malignant bone tumours (Larsson and Lorentzon, 1974). The annual incidence is estimated at 0.6 per million population (Price and Jeffree, 1977).

Ewing's sarcoma rarely occurs in children below five years of age or in adults over the age of 30 years; the peak incidence is between ten and 15 years. The overall male to female ratio is approximately 1.5:1, is lower in younger children, and increases with age (Fig. 16.5). It is rare in Black and Chinese populations (Glass and Fraumeni, 1970; Huvos, 1991).

16.5.1 PATHOLOGY

Originating in the intramedullary cavity – which is often diffusely infiltrated – the tumour may break through the cortex, detach the periostium and extend into the soft tissue.

Macroscopically, the tumour tissue is soft, greyish white, and with areas of haemorrhage and necrosis. On histological examination, the tumour consists of a uniform pattern of small cells with round nuclei located close together. The cytoplasm is pale, the cellular borders ill defined (Campanacci, 1990; Huvos, 1991). In 90% of cases, the presence of glycogen can be demonstrated with periodic acid-Schiff (PAS) and diastase reactions (Schajowicz, 1959).

The presence of glycogen can no longer be considered pathognomonic for Ewing's sarcoma since it has also been demonstrated in other small cell sarcomas (Triche and Rosse, 1978). A large cell variant of Ewing's sarcoma, distinct from the common small cell type, has been described and according to some reports is associated with poorer survival (Nascimento, 1980).

Routine histological description has now

been supplemented by immunocytochemistry and cytogenetic studies to allow better distinction from other small round cell tumours (Schmidt *et al.*, 1987; Schmidt and Harms, 1990).

Clinically, the classical differential diagnosis is osteomyelitis, which may mimic Ewing's sarcoma in radiological appearance (Campanacci, 1990; Huvos 1991). On histological examination, Ewing's sarcoma must be differentiated from other small round cell tumours (Miser *et al.*, 1989). Myxoid changes and cross-striations are characteristic for rhabdomyosarcoma (Schmidt *et al.*, 1987; Schmidt and Harms, 1990). Immunocytochemical markers such as desmin, myoglobin and myosin are usually positive (Miser *et al.*, 1989). In children younger than five years of age, the classical differential diagnosis is neuroblastoma, characterized by its typical clinical presentation with disseminated osseous metastases (Berthold *et al.*, 1982). Immunocytochemistry is positive for neural markers such as NSE and S100 (Schmidt *et al.*, 1987; Schmidt and Harms, 1990). The presence of neural markers is also characteristic for the variant of Ewing's sarcoma usually referred to as peripheral neuroectodermal tumour (PNET) or malignant peripheral neuroectodermal tumour (MPNT) (Schmidt *et al.*, 1989; Israel *et al.*, 1989). Round cell tumours of the chest wall, occurring predominantly in adolescents, as first described by Askin and colleagues (1979), also fall into this category of primitive neuroectodermal tumours. Both tumours share the same characteristic chromosomal translocation t(11;22) (Aurias *et al.*, 1983; Whang-Peng, 1984).

This fact and the observation that some Ewing's sarcoma cell lines in culture develop neural characteristics (van Valen and Jürgens, 1991) support the hypothesis that both tumours are strongly related and may represent different stages of differentiation of the same malignancy (Schmidt *et al.*, 1985; Israel *et al.*, 1989). A recently described specific

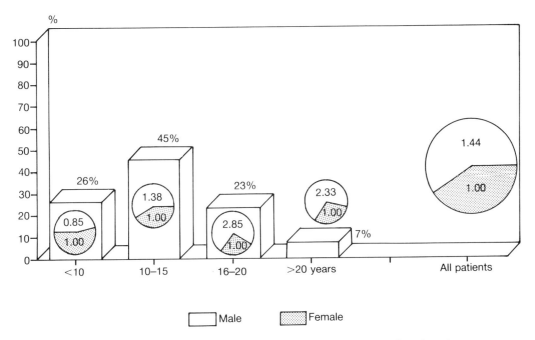

Fig. 16.5 Age and sex distribution of patients with Ewing's sarcoma (data based on 300 patients entered into the CESS trials).

marker, the expression of the *mic*2 gene was also demonstrated on both Ewing's sarcoma and neuroepithelioma (Ambros *et al.*, 1990). Hence there was difficulty in drawing a clear borderline between these tumours. Ambros *et al.* (1990) have recently proposed the presence of at least two neural markers for a neuroepithelioma.

The presence of extracellular matrix, particularly tumour osteoid, is characteristic for small cell osteosarcomas (Sim *et al.*, 1979). Malignant cartilage may lead to the diagnosis of mesenchymal chondrosarcoma (Huvos *et al.*, 1983). Another consideration in the differential diagnosis of Ewing's sarcoma is primary lymphoma of bone, although in children this only rarely presents without disseminated lymph node, visceral, meningeal or bone marrow involvement (Askin *et al.*, 1979). Again immunocytochemistry is helpful for distinction, showing positive reactivity with lymphoid markers.

Ewing's sarcoma in rare cases presents as extraskeletal tumour (EES) and in that case the predominant site of initial presentation is the trunk (Angervall and Enzinger, 1975). Distinct from Ewing's sarcoma of bone, here, there is no predominance in boys. The same rules as for Ewing's sarcoma of bone apply for diagnostic work-up, differential diagnosis, and also for treatment. However, as there appears to be a higher risk for lymphatic spread, local therapy particularly with radiation has to be planned according to the same principles as applied to embryonal rhabdomyosarcoma (Kinsella *et al.* 1983b).

16.5.2 CLINICAL PRESENTATION AND DIAGNOSIS

As in other primary malignant bone tumours, the predominant symptoms are persistent pain and swelling of the affected area; both symptoms may increase rapidly over a short

335

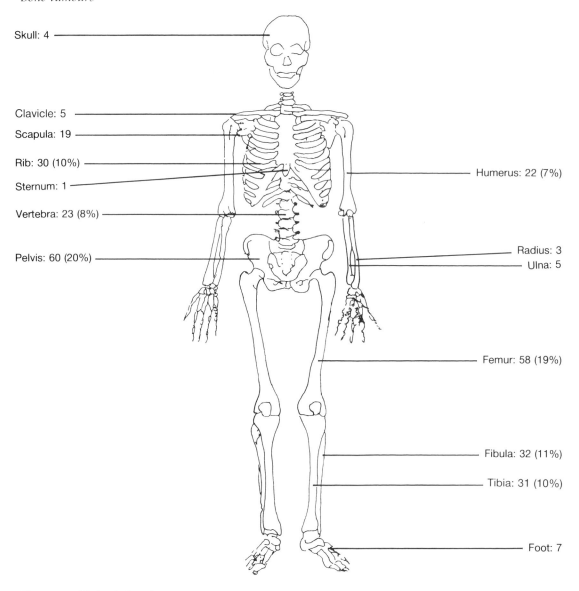

Skull: 4

Clavicle: 5

Scapula: 19

Rib: 30 (10%)

Sternum: 1

Vertebra: 23 (8%)

Pelvis: 60 (20%)

Humerus: 22 (7%)

Radius: 3

Ulna: 5

Femur: 58 (19%)

Fibula: 32 (11%)

Tibia: 31 (10%)

Foot: 7

Fig. 16.6 Skeletal distribution in patients with Ewing's sarcoma (data based on 300 patients entered into the CESS trials).

period of time or remain constant for months. Involvement of peripheral nerves may produce neurological symptoms (Rosen, 1976). Slight to moderate fever is common, more so in advanced disease (Huvos, 1991).

Most commonly affected sites are the pelvis, femur, tibia and fibula, making up about 60% of all primary sites (Fig. 16.6). Compared with osteosarcoma, the flat bones of the trunk are more often involved. In long bones the tumour usually originates from the diaphysis, either centrally or towards the

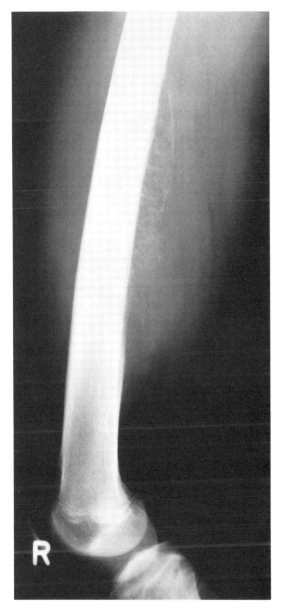

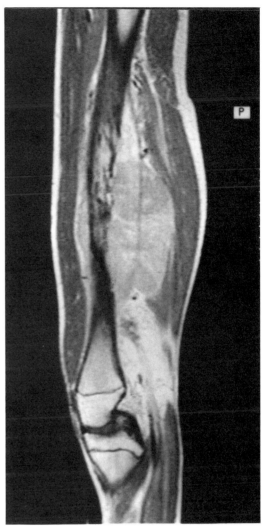

Fig. 16.8 Magnetic resonance imaging (MRI) of a femoral Ewing's sarcoma in a 17-year-old male patient showing outline of the intramedullary and soft tissue tumour extension.

Fig. 16.7 X-ray appearance of a femoral Ewing's sarcoma in a 17-year-old male patient.

end, but distinct from the typical metaphyseal presentation of osteosarcoma (Campanacci, 1990; Huvos, 1991).

Given the presenting symptoms of pain and swelling, the initial diagnostic step usually is a conventional x-ray of the affected area. Often a patchy 'moth-eaten' pattern of bone destruction with poorly defined margins and a parallel 'onion skin' periosteal lamellation is seen, with a varying degree of soft tissue extension of tumour (Fig. 16.7) (Campanacci, 1990). A pathological fracture is noted in about 5% of cases. Rib lesions are often associated with pleural effusion. The conventional x-ray evaluation should be complemented by CT-scans and/or magnetic resonance imaging (MRI). The latter is particularly helpful in outlining the exact intramedullary tumour extension (Fig. 16.8) (Dalinka *et al.*, 1990). A whole body radionuclide bone scan is required to determine the extent of the primary tumour within the affected bone and also to detect other sites of osseous involvement within the skeleton (Fig. 16.9).

To evaluate the lungs for metastases, PA and lateral x-rays are required, preferably complemented by full chest tomography and/or CT-scan of the chest. Bone marrow aspiration and/or biopsy (preferably obtained from several sites) are needed to search for bone marrow infiltration.

Ewing's sarcoma is a rapidly disseminating neoplasm. In the literature, the proportion of patients presenting with detectable metastases at diagnosis varies between 15 and 35% (Hayes *et al.*, 1987; Wessalowski *et al.*, 1988). Of these, about 50% present with pulmonary metastases and about 40% with multiple bone involvement and/or diffuse bone marrow contamination. Lymphatic spread is seen in less than 10% of cases. CNS involvement, either as meningeal spread or parenchymal metastases, is extremely rare at initial presentation but may occur in advanced disease (Mehta and Hendrickson, 1974).

Laboratory studies usually show a moderately elevated erythrocyte sedimentation rate and may show some degree of anaemia and leucocytosis. An elevated serum LDH is associated with less favourable outcome (Glaubiger *et al.*, 1981), probably due to its correlation with tumour burden. In some patients, the neuron-specific enolase (NSE) is elevated in serum, possibly more so in patients with small cell sarcomas with neural differentiation (Marangos and Polak, 1986). Its relationship to prognosis has yet to be determined.

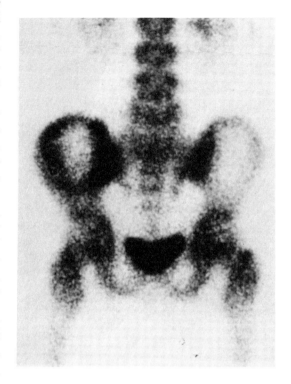

Fig. 16.9 Bone scan of a 12-year-old female patient with pelvic Ewing's sarcoma.

However typical the radiographic or CT/MRI image may be, histological confirmation is required in all cases, both to confirm the diagnosis of malignancy and also to distinguish between the various subcategories of small cell sarcomas.

16.5.3 TREATMENT

Prior to the era of effective systemic treatment, over 90% of patients died within two to five years following the initial diagnosis from systemic pulmonary and/or multiple bone metastases (Falk and Alpert, 1967). This was the case in spite of the fact that it had been noted by James Ewing that this sarcoma, as distinct from osteosarcoma, could be controlled with radiation. (Ewing, 1921; 1924; 1939).

(a) Radiotherapy

Given its radiosensitivity, radiotherapy conventionally plays a major role for local control in Ewing's sarcoma (Donaldson, 1981). With longer metastasis-free survival as a result of effective systemic treatment, the problem of local failures following radiation has become more evident (Rosen *et al.*, 1981a; Thomas *et al.*, 1984), advocating an increasing role for surgery (Pritchard, 1980; Kinsella *et al.*, 1984). Due to the variability of initial presentation of Ewing's sarcoma and also the variability in radiation technique, an exact assessment of the risk of local failures following radiation is difficult (Kotz *et al.*, 1977, 1978; Kinsella *et al.*, 1984). However, there is accumulating evidence that its radiocurability is related to tumour bulk and also correlates with chemosensitivity as assessed clinically by tumour regression during initial chemotherapy (Göbel *et al.*, 1987; Dunst *et al.*, 1988; 1991).

Whenever a partial resection of the tumour-bearing bone is considered to have removed all visible tumour, postoperative radiotherapy is often given to control microscopic or undetectable residual disease (Bacci *et al.*, 1982). In view of the effect of primary chemotherapy, this practice, however, may be adapted to the precise surgical margins and also the histological evaluation of response to chemotherapy (Dunst *et al.*, 1988; Hayes *et al.*, 1989; Dunst *et al.*, 1991).

It may well be that radiotherapy can be omitted in situations of clearly wide resections according to the Enneking criteria (1987), particularly in those cases with demonstrably good histological response to the initial chemotherapy, defined as less than 10% viable tumour present in the surgical specimen. The application of the Enneking criteria classifying tumour surgery into intralesional, marginal, wide and radical procedures (Enneking, 1987) and the exact determination of the proportion of viable tumour present in the surgical specimen are essential to define individual treatment guidelines (Hayes *et al.*, 1989; Dunst *et al.*, 1991).

Conventionally, radiotherapy portals must deliver treatment to the entire affected bone with an additional boost to the region of visualized bulky disease (Tefft *et al.*, 1977). Treatment planning is based upon the extent of initial tumour. It was shown in the first Intergroup Ewing's Sarcoma Study (IESS I) that radiotherapy volumes failing to include the entire bone or less than a 5 cm safety margin to gross disease, were associated with an increased local failure rate (Perez *et al.*, 1977; Razek *et al.*, 1980). In the German cooperative trial, it has become evident that limited portals following impressive tumour shrinkage under initial chemotherapy were associated with an increased risk of local recurrences, particularly in larger primaries (Sauer *et al.*, 1987; Jürgens *et al.*, 1988b). Other investigators, however, have reported excellent results with limited surgery and/or radio therapy following initial chemotherapy (Hayes *et al.*, 1989) and the question of the optimal scheduling and timing of local therapy is still under investigation.

In no case, however, is chemotherapy at present sufficient to control gross disease (Jürgens *et al.*, 1988b). Regarding the adequate dose of radiation, most investigators consider doses above 50 Gy in combination with chemotherapy as the treatment of choice to control initially gross disease (Tepper *et al.*, 1980; Thomas *et al.*, 1984).

Recent data suggest that the definitive dose of radiation should be related to tumour size, unless surgery is considered as the treatment of choice for larger tumours (Mendenhall *et al.*, 1983; Marcus and Million, 1984; Göbel *et al.*, 1987). To control microscopic disease, a compartment dose of 45 Gy is considered adequate by most investigators (Donaldson, 1981; Dunst *et al.*, 1991).

The standard therapeutic technique involves a fraction size of 1.5 to 2 Gy/day five days per week avoiding joints and epiphyses whenever justifiable. Conventional fractionation requires avoiding radiation sensitizers, e.g. adriamycin or actinomycin D, during the period of radiation. Alternate schedules of fractionation, e.g. hyperfractionation 1.6 Gy twice daily are currently under investigation for their impact on local control and acute or late side effects (Dunst *et al.*, 1991); results are pending. In growing children the inclusion of the epiphysis may result in an unacceptable functional deficit due to length discrepancies of the extremities. In many instances this justifies surgery as the primary choice of treatment (Gonzales-Gonzales and Breur, 1983; Kinsella *et al.*, 1983a).

(b) Surgery

Problems related to the effectiveness of radiotherapy in controlling the primary lesion and also those related to late side effects have made it necessary to reconsider the role of surgery in the treatment of the primary lesion (Kotz *et al.*, 1977; Pritchard, 1980; Rosen *et al.*, 1981a). Local recurrence rates vary as a function of primary site and tumour size, ranging from 5–50% (Göbel *et al.*, 1987; Jürgens *et al.*, 1988b). Local control following radiotherapy has been found to be best in patients with small primaries, particularly in the distal part of extremities compared to the high rate of local failures in lesions of the proximal parts of the extremity or the trunk, which are usually located in deeper areas and are of larger size. Tumour bulk appears to be of more influence than site on local control achieved by radiation (Göbel *et al.*, 1987; Jürgens *et al.*, 1988b).

Ewing's sarcoma of the pelvis requires particular attention since this site is associated with an unfavourable prognosis (Pritchard, 1980; Li *et al.*, 1983; Nesbit *et al.*, 1990). In only rare cases is a pelvic tumour small and primarily resectable. Most pelvic tumours are large, with an extensive soft tissue mass invading the pelvic cavity (Mendenhall, 1983). There is, however, good evidence that the prognosis of extensive pelvic lesion can be improved, when following tumour shrinkage induced by initial chemotherapy the residual intraosseous disease is resected (Jürgens *et al.*, 1991). Radiotherapy follows surgical resections in most instances.

(c) Chemotherapy

Single drug data have demonstrated the chemosensitivity of Ewing's sarcoma. Alkylating agents such as cyclophosphamide (Samuels and Howe, 1967), nitrogen mustard, chlorambucil and recently ifosfamide (Jürgens *et al.*, 1989a; 1989b) are effective. Other agents studied include vincristine, actinomycin D, 5-fluorouracil, mithramycin and in particular adriamycin (Oldham and Pomeroy, 1972).

The improved long-term disease-free survival rates above 50% now being reported are the result of intensive combination chemotherapy regimens (Rosen *et al.*, 1981a; Bacci *et al.*, 1982; Jürgens *et al.*, 1988b; Nesbit *et al.*, 1990). The first Intergroup Ewing's sarcoma study (IESS I) has convincingly shown the superiority of a four-drug regimen with vincristine, actinomycin D, cyclophosphamide and adriamycin (VACA) over a three-drug regimen with vincristine, actinomycin D and cyclophosphamide (VAC), both in terms of disease-free survival (74% versus 54%) and also the effectiveness of local control (96% versus 86%) (Nesbit *et al.*, 1981; 1990).

Results reported by Rosen from the Memorial Sloan Kettering Cancer Center (MSKCC) confirmed the effectiveness of the four-drug regimen and gave evidence that the use of these four effective agents in combination rather than sequentially has further improved the results (Rosen *et al.*, 1981a; 1981b).

Recently, the impact of treatment intensity

was shown by the analysis of IESS II, where high dose intermittent chemotherapy was compared to moderate dose continuous chemotherapy resulting in a significant benefit for the more intensive regimen of 68% versus 48% disease-free survival at five years (Burgert *et al.*, 1990). The first co-operative Ewing's sarcoma study of the German Society of Paediatric Oncology (GPO) (CESS 81) has shown the prognostic significance of tumour burden at diagnosis and histological response to initial chemotherapy and also stressed the impact of surgery on the safety of local control (Jürgens *et al.*, 1988b). Consequently, in a follow-up study CESS 86 patients with large primaries (more than 100 ml tumour volume) received a more intensive chemotherapy regimen, where conventional doses of cyclophosphamide (1200 mg/m²/course) were replaced by high doses of ifosfamide (6000 mg/m²/course) in combination with the other agents (Jürgens *et al.*, 1988c; Dunst *et al.*, 1991). The results show a significant benefit to high risk patients from the more intensive regimen, again stressing the impact of treatment intensity on disease-free survival.

The combination of ifosfamide and etoposide was recently shown to be highly effective in patients who had failed previous chemotherapy and has now been incorporated in first line chemotherapy (Miser *et al.*, 1987). Increasing evidence that high cumulative doses of ifosfamide are associated with considerable renal tubular dysfunction stresses the importance to tailor treatment according to the individual risk of relapse (Skinner *et al.*, 1989; Patterson and Khojasteh, 1989).

16.6 METASTATIC DISEASE

Of those patients with Ewing's sarcoma, between 10 and 35% present with detectable metastatic disease at diagnosis (Hayes *et al.*, 1987; Wessalowski *et al.*, 1988). The survival of these patients is poor compared to patients presenting with primary tumours only (Glaubiger, 1980), but seems better for patients with pulmonary metastases compared to those with multiple bone disease (Wessalowski *et al.*, 1988). Treatment involves combination chemotherapy as outlined for patients with primary Ewing's sarcoma and in addition, if pulmonary disease is present, radiation to both lungs with doses between 14–20 Gy depending on the patient's age administered in 1.5 Gy fractions per day on five days per week. For multiple bone lesions all involved areas require local treatment; however, it may not be possible to irradiate the entire bone at all sites affected since this may limit the tolerance of chemotherapy (Vietti *et al.*, 1981; Pilepich *et al.*, 1981; Wessalowski *et al.*, 1988).

The survival of patients with multiple bone disease has been extremely poor despite an initial response to intensive systemic and local treatment (Glaubiger *et al.*, 1980; Wessalowski *et al.*, 1988). The disease-free survival of these patients is less than 10% two years following diagnosis and is therefore comparable to the prognosis of patients with disseminated neuroblastoma. Recently encouraging results have been reported with autologous or allogeneic bone marrow transplantation, particularly when performed in first remission (Pinkerton *et al.*, 1986; Burdach *et al.*, 1991). Conditioning regimens containing total body irradiation in combination with high dose chemotherapy seem superior to solely chemotherapeutic conditioning regimens; however, the current experience is too sparse to allow definitive conclusions (Burdach *et al.*, 1991). Consolidation with a megatherapy regimen followed by bone marrow transplantation is solely aimed at controlling residual systemic disease. It is essential to obtain local control of bulky disease prior to such a procedure since the results of bone marrow transplantation performed in partial remissions were discouraging (Craft, 1987).

In patients who developed metastatic disease on or off therapy, survival is poor and with the exception of some late recurrences off therapy second remissions are usually shortlived (Craft, 1987). Attempts are being made to increase salvage with the use of bone marrow transplantation following intensive chemoradiotherapy regimens. In responsive relapses this might be of value; results in patients with resistant disease have so far been disappointing (Burdach *et al.*, 1991).

16.7 PROGNOSTIC FACTORS

Disease-free survival rates of 50% and more necessitate the search for prognostic factors to allow treatment stratification. The tumour site, serum LDH levels at diagnosis and sex are usually recognized as prognostic discriminators for patients with Ewing's sarcoma (Pomeroy and Johnson, 1975; Gehan *et al.*, 1981; Glaubiger *et al.*, 1981). It must, however, be pointed out, that prognostic factors are treatment-dependent and may also be interrelated. A Cox regression analysis of the CESS 81 trial has identified tumour volume and histological response to initial chemotherapy as the major determinators of prognosis (Jürgens *et al.*, 1988b). High serum LDH-levels are linked to large tumour burden and this may explain the prognostic significance of serum LDH (Glaubiger *et al.*, 1981). As has been said, morphological characteristics as in the large cell variant of Ewing's sarcoma are associated with a poor prognosis (Nascimento, 1980).

To what extent the expression of immunochemically detectable markers, e.g. the expression of neural characteristics, offer a possibility of prognostic discrimination is yet to be determined (Ambros *et al.*, 1990). Above all, the presence of visible metastases at the time of initial diagnosis remains the most significant prognostic factor (Glaubiger *et al.*, 1981). Hence the importance of initial staging cannot be overstressed since patients with detectable metastases may benefit from treatment intensification such as irradiation to both lungs in the case of pulmonary metastases or megatherapy in first remission in patients with disseminated skeletal disease (Burdach *et al.*, 1991).

16.8 PERSPECTIVES

Since Ewing's sarcoma is fundamentally a systemic disease, only the combination of both safe local control with surgery and/or radiation, and effective systemic combination chemotherapy has been able to improve the disease-free survival rates from approximately 10% with local therapy only to its present 50 to 70%. The impact of chemotherapy intensity on disease-free survival must be weighed against late side effects. The incidence of adriamycin cardiomyopathy seems to be less under the current policy of not exceeding cumulative doses of more than 500 mg/m² adriamycin and administering the dose per course on two to three consecutive days rather than administering the whole dose per course in one single day (Jürgens *et al.*, 1988c). Infertility is associated particularly with high cumulative doses of alkylating agents and also depends on the patient's age at diagnosis. Prepubertal children are known to tolerate higher doses (Chapman, 1982). Since alkylating agents play an essential role in the combination chemotherapy of Ewing's sarcoma, this cannot be avoided at present other than to stratify treatment intensity according to the individual risk of relapse. With increasing use of high doses of ifosfamide there is now evidence that this might lead to severe, if not irreversible, renal tubular damage (Skinner *et al.*, 1989; Patterson and Khojasteh, 1989). To what extent this risk can be minimized, by different schedules of administering ifosfamide and the protective agent mesna or by limiting the administration of ifosfamide to a particular cumulative dose, is to be investigated.

Secondary malignant neoplasms following treatment of Ewing's sarcoma, e.g. osteosarcomas in the radiation field or acute myeloid leukaemias, are considered a risk, the incidence varying between 5 and 20% after a period of observation of about 20 years (Smithon *et al.*, 1978; Meadows *et al.*, 1985). The principle risk seems to be the association between high doses of radiation and administration of high cumulative doses of alkylating agents. Both the preferred use of surgery for local control and limits to the cumulative doses of chemotherapeutic agents may help to minimize the risk of secondary malignant neoplasms.

The impact of treatment intensity on disease-free survival may justify the use of growth factors to ameliorate chemotherapy-induced myelosuppression allowing the safe administration of higher doses of chemotherapy during a shorter period of time (Andreeff and Welte, 1989; Burdach, 1991). In addition, Ewing's sarcoma cell lines respond *in vitro* to the combination of tumour necrosis factor α and gamma-interferon (van Valen *et al.*, 1990), suggesting a possible application for biological response modifiers in treatment.

Such new developments and the need for clearly defined guidelines for local control, weighing the risk and benefit of radiotherapy and surgery, emphasize the necessity of continuing large scale clinical trials in order to optimize treatment for patients with primary and metastatic Ewing's sarcoma.

16.9 CURRENT CONTROVERSIES

16.9.1 HOW INTENSIVE DOES CHEMOTHERAPY NEED TO BE?

(a) Osteosarcoma

In chemotherapy for osteosarcoma, the Medical Research Council has demonstrated that two drugs are as effective as five and is currently comparing the doxorubicin/cisplatin combination against the traditional Rosen T 10 protocol which has been regarded by many as the gold standard. Duration of treatment is limited by cumulative drug toxicity but there is little evidence that it need be longer than six months.

(b) Ewing's sarcoma

Although not proven by randomized studies, the outcome following regimens containing high doses of ifosfamide such as the German CESS or United Kingdom CCSG ET2 protocols for example, appear superior to those using cyclophosphamide at conventional doses, i.e. 1 g/m^2 or less. There is concern, however, regarding the late effects of ifosfamide and, in addition, about the complexities of its administration and the necessity for mesna uroprotection. It has been suggested as part of a planned joint CESS/UKCCSG study that good prognostic subgroups, such as those with small disease bulk or peripheral sites, may be cured by cyclophosphamide-based regimens, so reserving the more intensive ifosfamide protocols for those with bulky tumours or axial primaries.

The role of very high dose chemotherapy with bone marrow rescue is unclear and although high response rates have been reported with melphalan-containing regimens, the potential of this strategy for high risk patients in first remission remains to be demonstrated (Hartmann *et al.*, 1986; Bagnulo *et al.*, 1985; Miser, 1990).

With the advent of more sophisticated prostheses, aggressive surgery has become incorporated into some protocols, in particular those of the German group. Although this may improve local control, it necessitates extensive rehabilitation and functional outcome is not always ideal. It is possible that with more effective systemic chemotherapy the use of limited field radiotherapy may be as appropriate. It should be noted that there is concern about the incidence of secondary tumours where high dose, extended field radiation has been given (Bacci *et al.*, 1989).

16.9.2 HOW SHOULD SOFT TISSUE EWING'S/PRIMITIVE NEUROECTODERMAL TUMOURS (PNET) OF BONE BE TREATED?

It has become increasingly clear on the basis of immunohistochemical and cytogenetic studies that these tumours are part of a spectrum of the same disease (Dehner, 1990). The management of soft tissue Ewing's or PNET has varied between centres. It may be the same as for soft tissue sarcoma (Rud *et al.*, 1989), neuroblastoma (Marina *et al.*, 1989) or Ewing's sarcoma of bone (Kinsella *et al.*, 1983b). As local control is less of a problem than in Ewing's of bone, less emphasis can be put on aggressive surgery or radiotherapy. In contrast, PNET of bone should probably be regarded in the same light as Ewing's sarcoma and call for aggressive local treatment. Since soft tissue Ewing's/PNET share the typical translocation of boney Ewing's, and as Ewing's of bone is generally cisplatin-refractory, it is more appropriate to use IVA, IVAd or VAC regimens for the soft tissue variant.

16.9.3 CAN LOCAL CONTROL BE IMPROVED BY NOVEL RADIOTHERAPY STRATEGIES?

In Ewing's sarcoma the use of accelerated, hyperfractionated irradiation schedules is being assessed by the German CESS group and novel schedules such as those involving concomitant aggressive chemotherapy and breaks of two to three weeks between courses of irradiation have been suggested (Dunst *et al.*, 1991). This avoids reducing chemotherapy during the radiation period, something which may adversely affect control of micrometastatic disease; such joint therapy could also lead to beneficial synergism between irradiation and actinomycin D. In osteosar-

coma, radiotherapy is generally limited to palliative use. The question of whether irradiation to incomplete surgical margins after conservative surgery can avoid amputation is debatable.

16.9.4 ARE LOCALIZED LUNG METASTASES SURGICALLY CURABLE?

There is little role for surgery in Ewing's sarcoma since persisting detectable disease is a reflection of chemoresistance at other sites. In osteosarcoma, however, surgery may be curative. The need for and timing of chemotherapy with limited pulmonary metastatic disease at relapse has been debated. The cure rate in patients who have metastatectomy, often involving bilateral thoracotomies either as single or separate procedures, has discouraged the entry of such patients into phase II studies of second line chemotherapy (Rosenberg *et al.*, 1979). It seems appropriate, however, that a trial of chemotherapy is given prior to metastatectomy in order to provide a basis for second line adjuvant chemotherapy following surgery. In patients who have relapsed after a doxorubicin/cisplatin regimen, the use of high dose methotrexate and BCD is appropriate. Where these drugs have been included in the first line regimen, other agents such as carboplatin, ifosfamide or etoposide are worthy of study. There appears to be no role for radiotherapy other than for palliation of local pain.

16.9.5 CAN NEW PROGNOSTIC FACTORS BE USED TO DECIDE THE INTENSITY OF CHEMOTHERAPY?

Recent studies suggest that in osteosarcoma ploidy may separate good and bad risk patients with hyperploidy being an adverse factor (Look *et al.*, 1988). Expression of neural markers in Ewing's sarcoma may be a favourable factor (Pinto *et al.*, 1989).

16.9.6 ARE LOWER LIMB PROSTHESES JUSTIFIED IN THE YOUNG CHILD?

Children under eight years of age are generally not considered suitable for conservative prosthetic procedures of the lower limbs because of the amount of growth remaining. Replacement of a knee involving the epiphyseal ends of both tibia and femur will result in a short and often useless limb. The development of expandable prostheses may help but, even with this, multiple surgical procedures may be required with the necessity for intensive rehabilitation post-operatively. It may be that an amputation and rapid adaptation to an artificial leg is the most appropriate procedure for these young children. The pros and cons of rotation plasty with regard to function versus psychological effects have been the subject of debate (Craft, 1986).

C.R.P.

REFERENCES

Ambros, I.M., Ambros, P.F., Strehl, S. *et al.* (1990) MIC2 is a specific marker for Ewing's sarcoma and peripheral primitive neuroectodermal tumors. Evidence for a common histogenesis of Ewing's sarcoma and peripheral primitive neuroectodermal tumors from MIC2 expression and specific chromosome aberration. *Cancer*, **67**, 1886–93.

Andreeff, M. and Welt, K. (1989) Hematopoietic colony-stimulating factors. *Semin. Oncol.*, **16**, 211–29.

Angervall, L. and Enzinger, F.M. (1975) Extraskeletal neoplasm resembling Ewing's sarcoma. *Cancer*, **36**, 240–51.

Askin, F.B., Rosai, J., Sibley, R.K., Dehner, L.P. and McAlister, W.H. (1979) Malignant small cell tumor of the thoracopulmonary region in childhood. *Cancer*, **43**, 2438–51.

Aurias, A., Rimbaut, C. Buffe, D. *et al.* (1983) Chromosomal translocation in Ewing's sarcoma. *N. Engl. J. Med.*, **309**, 469–97.

Bacci, G., Picci, P., Gitelis, S. *et al.* (1982) The treatment of localized Ewing's sarcoma: experience at the Istituto Ortopedico Rizzoli in 163 cases treated with and without adjuvant chemotherapy. *Cancer*, **49**, 1561–70.

Bacci, G., Toni, A., Avella, M. *et al.* (1989) Long-term results in 144 localized Ewing's sarcoma patients treated with combined therapy. *Cancer*, **63**, 1477–86.

Bagnulo, S., Perez, D.J., Barrett, A. *et al.* (1985) High dose melphalan and autologous bone marrow transplantation for solid tumours in childhood. *Eur. J. Paed. Haem. Oncol.*, **1**, 129–33.

Beattie, E.J., Martini, N. and Rosen, G. (1975) The management of pulmonary metastases in children with osteogenic sarcoma with surgical resection combined with chemotherapy. *Cancer*, **35**, 618–21.

Benedict, W.F., Fung, Y.K.T. and Murphree, A.L. (1988) The gene responsible for the development of retinoblastoma and osteosarcoma. *Cancer*, **62**, 1691–4.

Beron, G., Winkler, K., Beck, J. *et al.* (1988) Prognosis after metastasis in osteosarcoma: Experience from the COSS studies. *Contr. Oncol.*, **30**, 143–9.

Berthold, F., Kracht, J., Lampert, F. *et al.* (1982) Ultrastructural, biochemical, and cell-culture studies of a presumed extraskeletal Ewing's sarcoma with special reference to differential diagnosis from neuroblastoma. *J. Cancer Res. Clin. Oncol.*, **103**, 293–304.

Burdach, S. (1991). The granulocyte/macrophage-colony stimulating factor (GM-GSF): Basic science and clinical application. *Klin. Pädiatr.*, **203**, 302–10.

Burdach, S., Peters, C., Paulussen, M., *et al.* (1991) Improved relapse free survival in patients with poor prognosis Ewing's sarcoma after consolidation with hyperfractionated total body irradiation and fractionated high-dose melphalan followed by high dose etoposide and hematopoietic rescue. *Bone Marrow Transplant.* In press.

Burgers, J.M.V., van Glabbeke, M., Busson, A. *et al.* (1988) Osteosarcoma of the limbs. Report of the EORTC-SIOP 03 trial 20781 investigating the value of adjuvant treatment with chemotherapy and/or prophylactic lung irradiation. *Cancer*, **61**, 1024–31.

Burgert, E.O., Nesbit, M.E., Garnsey, L.A. *et al.* (1990) Multimodal therapy for the management of nonpelvic localized Ewing's sarcoma of bone:

Intergroup Study IESS–II. *J. Clin. Oncol.*, **8**, 1514–24.

Campanacci, M. (1990) *Bone and Soft Tissue Tumors*, Springer, Berlin.

Carter, S.K. (1984) Adjuvant chemotherapy in osteogenic sarcoma: The triumph that isn't? *J. Clin. Oncol.*, **2**, 147–8.

Chapman, R.M. (1982) Effect of cytotoxic therapy on sexuality and gonadal function. *Semin. Oncol.*, **9**, 84–94.

Craft, A.W. (1986) Osteosarcoma and Chondrosarcoma, in *Cancer in Children Clinical Management*, (eds P.A. Voûte, A. Barrett, H.J.G. Bloom, J. Lemerle and M.K. Neidhardt), Springer-Verlag, Berlin.

Craft, A.W. (1987) *Chemotherapy of Ewing's Sarcoma*. Baillière Clinical Oncology 1, 205–21.

Dalinka, M.K., Zlatkin, M.B., Chao, P. *et al.* (1990) The use of magnetic resonance imaging in the evaluation of bone and soft-tissue tumors. *Radiol. Clin. North Am.*, **28**, 461–70.

Dehner, L.P. (1990) Whence the primitive neuroectodermal tumor? *Arch. Pathol. Lab. Med.*, **114**, 16–17.

Donaldson, S.S. (1981) A story of continuing success – radiotherapy for Ewing's sarcoma. *Int. J. Radiat. Oncol. Biol. Phys.*, **7**, 279–81.

Dunst., J., Sauer, R., Burgers, J.M.V., *et al.* (1991) Radiation therapy as local treatment in Ewing's sarcoma. Results of the cooperative Ewing's sarcoma studies CESS 81 and CESS 86. *Cancer*, **67**, 2818–25.

Dunst. J., Sauer, R., Burgers, J.M.V. *et al.* (1988) Radiotherapie beim Ewing-Sarkom: Aktuelle Ergebnisse der GPO Studien CESS 81 und CESS 86. *Klin. Pädiatr.*, **200**, 261–6.

Einhorn, S., and Strander, H. (1978) Interferon therapy for neoplastic diseases in man. *In vitro* and *in vivo* studies. *Adv. Exp. Med. Biol.*, **110**, 1159–74.

Enneking, W.F. (1987) *A System of Staging Musculoskeletal Neoplasms*. Baillière's Clinical Oncology, **1**, 97–110.

Enneking, W. and Kagan, A. (1975) 'Skip' metastases in osteosarcoma. *Cancer*, **36**, 2192–205.

Ewing, J. (1921) Diffuse endothelioma of bone. *Proc. N.Y. Pathol. Soc.*, **21**, 17–24.

Ewing, J. (1924) Further report of endothelial myeloma of bone. *Proc. N.Y. Pathol. Soc.* **24**, 93–100.

Ewing, J. (1939) A review of the classification of bone tumors. *Surg. Gynecol. Obstet.*, **68**, 971–6.

Falk, S. and Alpert, M. (1967) Five-year survival of patients with Ewing's sarcoma. *Surg. Gynecol. Obstet.*, **124**, 319–24.

Fraumeni, J. (1967) Stature and malignant tumors of bone in childhood and adolescence. *Cancer*, **20**, 967–73.

Gehan, E.A., Nesbit, M.E., Burgert, O.E. *et al.* (1981) Prognostic factors in children with Ewing's sarcoma. *Natl. Cancer Inst. Monogr.*, **56**, 273–8.

Glass, A.G. and Fraumeni, Jr. J.F. (1970) Epidemiology of bone cancer in children. *J. Natl. Cancer Inst.*, **44**, 187–99.

Glaubiger, D.L., Makuch, R., Schwarz, J. *et al.* (1980) Determination of prognostic factors and their influence on therapeutic results in patients with Ewing's sarcoma. *Cancer*, **45**, 2213–19.

Glaubiger, D.L., Makuch, R.W. and Schwarz, J. (1981) Influence of prognostic factors on survival in Ewing's sarcoma. *Natl. Cancer Inst. Monogr.*, **56**, 285–8.

Gonzales-Gonzales, D. and Breur, K. (1983) Clinical data from irradiated growing long bones in children. *Int. J. Radiat. Oncol. Biol. Phys.*, **9**, 841–6.

Goorin, A.M., (1988) Adjuvant chemotherapy for osteogenic sarcoma. *Int. J. Cancer Clin. Oncol.*, **24**, 113–15.

Goorin, A.M., Abelson, H.T., and Frei, E. (1985) Osteosarcoma, Fifteen years later. *N. Engl. J. Med.*, **313**, 1637–42.

Göbel, V., Jürgens, H., Etspüler, G. *et al.* (1987) Prognostic significance of tumor volume in localized Ewing's sarcoma of bone in children and adolescents. *J. Cancer Res. Clin. Oncol.*, **113**, 187–91.

Hartmann, O., Benhamou, E., Beaujean, F. *et al.* (1986) High-dose busulphan and cyclophosphamide with autologous bone marrow transplantation support in advanced malignancies in children: A Phase II study. *J. Clin. Oncol.*, **4**, 1804–10.

Hayes, F.A., Thompson, E.I., Meyer, W.H. *et al.* (1989) Therapy for localized Ewing's sarcoma of bone. *J. Clin. Oncol.*, **7**, 208–13.

Hayes, F.A., Thompson, E.I., Parvey, L. *et al.* (1987) Metastatic Ewing's sarcoma: Remission induction and survival. *J. Clin. Oncol.*, **5**, 1199–204.

Holland, J.F. (1987) Adjuvant chemotherapy of

346

osteosarcoma: No runs, no hits, two men left on base. *J. Clinic. Oncol.*, **5**, 4–6.

Huvos, A.G. (1991) *Bone Tumours. Diagnosis, Treatment and Prognosis*, W.H. Saunders, Philadelphia.

Huvos, A.G., Rosen, G., Dobska, M. and Marcove, R.C. (1983) Mesenchymal chondrosarcoma, *Cancer*, **51**, 1230–7.

Israel, M.A., Miser, J.S., Triche, T.J. and Kinsella, T. (1989) Neuroepithelial Tumors, in *Principles and Practice of Pediatric Oncology*, (eds P.A. Pizzo and D.G. Poplack) J.B. Lippincott, Philadelphia, pp. 623–34.

Jaffé, N. (1974) Progress report on high-dose methotrexate (NSC-740) with citrovorum rescue in the treatment of metastatic bone tumors. *Cancer Chemother. Rep.*, **58**, 275–80.

Jaffé, N., Frei, E., Traggis, D. *et al.* (1977) High-dose methotrexate with citrovorum factor in osteogenic sarcoma – Progress Report II. *Cancer Treat. Rep.*, **61**, 675–9.

Jaffé, N., Raymond, A.K., Ayala, A. *et al.* (1989) Effect of cumulative courses of intraarterial *cis*-diamminedichloroplatin-II on the primary tumor in osteosarcoma. *Cancer*, **63**, 63–7.

Jürgens, H., Bier, V., Dunst, J. *et al.* (1988c) Die GPO cooperativen Ewing-Sarkom Studien CESS 81/86: Bericht nach 6 1/2 Jahren. *Klin. Pädiatr.*, **200**, 243–52.

Jürgens, H., Dunst., J. Göbel, U. *et al.* (1991) Improved survival in Ewing's sarcoma with response based local therapy and intensive chemotherapy. Proc. ASCO **10**, 316, Abstract No. 1112.

Jürgens, H., Exner, U., Gadner, H. *et al.* (1988b) Multidisciplinary treatment of primary Ewing's sarcoma of bone. A 6-year experience of a European Cooperative Trial. *Cancer*, **61**, 23–32.

Jürgens, H., Exner, U., Kühl, J. *et al.* (1989b) High-dose ifosfamide with mesna uroprotection in Ewing's sarcoma. *Cancer Chemother. Pharmacol.*, **24** (Suppl.): S40–S44.

Jürgens, H., Kosloff, C., Nirenberg, A. *et al.* (1981) Prognostic factors in the response of primary osteogenic sarcoma of preoperative chemotherapy (high-dose methotrexate with citrovorum factor) *Natl. Cancer Inst. Monogr.*, **56**, 221–6.

Jürgens, H., Treuner, J., Winkler, K. and Göbel, U. (1989a) Ifosfamide in pediatric malignancies. *Semin. Oncol.*, **16**, 46–50.

Jürgens, H., Winkler, K., Winkelmann, W. and

Göbel, U. (1988a) Metastatic osteosarcoma. *Sem. Orthop.*, **3**, 13–20.

Kinsella, T.J., Lichter, A.S., Miser, J. *et al.* (1984) Local treatment of Ewing's sarcoma: radiation therapy versus surgery. *Cancer Treat. Rep.*, **68**, 695–701.

Kinsella, T.J., Loeffler, J.S., Fraass, B.A., and Tepper, J. (1983a) Extremity preservation by combined-modality therapy in sarcomas of the hand and foot: an analysis of local control, disease-free survival and functional results. *Int. J. Radiat. Oncol. Biol. Phys.*, **9**, 1115–19.

Kinsella, T.J., Triche, T.J., Dickman, P.S., *et al.* (1983b) Extraskeletal Ewing's sarcoma: results of combined-modality treatment. *Am. J. Clin. Oncol.*, **1**, 489–95.

Kinsella, T.J., Triche, T.J., Dickman, P.S. *et al.* (1983c) Extraskeletal Ewing's sarcoma: Results of combined modality treatment. *J. Clin. Oncol.*, **1** (8), 489–95.

Kotz R. (1978) Osteosarkom 1978. Die Wende der Prognose durch adäquate Chirurgie und adjuvante Chemotherapie. *Wien Klin. Wschr.*, **90**, Suppl. 93: 1–25.

Kotz, R., Kogelnik, H.D., Salzer-Kuntschik, M. *et al.* (1977) Problems of local recurrence in patients with Ewing's sarcoma. *Osterr. Z. Onkol.*, **4**, 7–12.

Larsson, S.E. and Lorentzon, R. (1974) The geographic variation of the incidence of malignant primary bone tumors in Sweden. *J. Bone Joint Surg. (Am).*, **56**, 592–600.

Lee, S. and MacKenzie, D. (1964) Osteosarcoma: A study of the value of preoperative megavoltage radiotherapy. *Br. J. Surg.*, **51**, 252–74.

Li, W.K., Lane, J.M., Rosen, G., Marcove, R.C. *et al.* (1983) Pelvic Ewing's sarcoma. Advances in treatment. *J. Bone Joint Surg.*, **65**, 738–47.

Link, M.P. (1986) Adjuvant therapy in the treatment of osteosarcoma, in *Important Advances in Oncology*, (eds V.T. Devita, S. Hellman and S.A. Rosenberg) J.B. Lippincott, Philadelphia, pp. 193–207.

Link, M.P. and Eilber, F. (1989) Osteosarcoma, in *Principles and Practice of Pediatric Oncology*, (eds P.A. Pizzo and D.G. Poplack) J.B. Lippincott, Philadelphia, pp. 689–711.

Link, M.P., Goorin, A.M., Miser, A.W. *et al.* (1986) The effect of adjuvant chemotherapy on relapse-free survival in patients with osteosarcoma of the extremity. *N. Engl. J. Med.*, **314**, 1600–606.

Look, A.T., Douglass, E.C. and Meyer, W.H. (1988). Clinical importance of near-diploid tumor stem lines in patients with osteosarcoma of an extremity. *N. Engl. J. Med.*, **318**, 1567–72.

Marangos, P.J. and Polak, J.M. (1986) Neurone-specific enolase (NSE) as a marker for neuroendocrine tumors, (eds G.E.J. Stahl and C.W.M. van Veelen) in *Markers of Human Neuroectodermal Tumours*. CRC Press, Boca Raton, pp. 109–17.

Marcus, R.B. and Million, R.R. (1984) The effect of primary tumor size on the prognosis of Ewing's sarcoma. *Int. J. Radiat. Oncol. Biol. Phys.*, **10**, 88.

Marina, N.M., Etcubanas, E., Parham, D.M. *et al.* (1989) Peripheral primitive neuroectodermal tumor (peripheral neuroepithelioma) in children. A review of the St. Jude experience and controversies in diagnosis and management. *Cancer*, **64**, 1952–60.

Martini, N., Bains, M.S., Huvos, A.G. and Beattie, E.J. (1974) Surgical treatment of metastatic sarcoma to the lung. *Surg. Clin. North Am.*, **54**, 841–8.

Meadows, A.T., Baum, E., Fossati-Bellani, F. *et al.* (1985) Second malignant neoplasms in children: An update from the late effects study group. *J. Clin. Oncol.*, **3**, 532–8.

Mehta, Y. and Hendrickson, R. (1974) CNS involvement in Ewing's sarcoma. *Cancer*, **33**, 859–62.

Mendenhall, C.M., Marcus, R.B., Enneking, W.F., *et al.* (1983) The prognostic significance of soft tissue extension in Ewing's sarcoma. *Cancer*, **51**, 913–17.

Miller, C.W., Aslo, A., Tsay, C. *et al.* (1990) Frequency and structure of p53 rearrangements in human osteosarcoma. *Cancer Res.*, **50**, 7050–954.

Miser, J.S. (1990) Autologous bone marrow transplantation for the treatment of sarcomas, in *Bone Marrow Transplantation in Children*, (eds F.L. Johnson and C. Pochedly), Raven Press, New York, pp. 289–99.

Miser, J.S., Kinsella, T.J., Triche, T.J. *et al.* (1987) Ifosfamide with mesna uroprotection and etoposide: An effective regimen in the treatment of recurrent sarcomas and other tumors of children and young adults. *J. Clin. Oncol.*, **5**, 1191–8.

Miser, J.S., Triche, T.J., Pritchard, D.J. and Kinsella, T. (1989) Ewing's sarcoma and the nonrhabdomyosarcoma soft tissue sarcomas of childhood,

in *Principles and Practice of Pediatric Oncology*, (eds P.A. Pizzo and D.G. Poplack) J.B. Lippincott, Philadelphia, pp. 659–88.

Nascimento, A.G. (1980) A clinicopathologic study of 20 cases of large-cell (atypical) Ewing's sarcoma of bone. *Am. J. Surg. Pathol.*, **4**, 29–36.

Nesbit, M.E., Gehan, E.A., Burgert, E.O. *et al.* (1990) Multimodal therapy for the management of primary nonmetastatic Ewing's sarcoma of bone: a long-term follow-up of the First Intergroup Study. *J. Clin. Oncol.*, **8**, 1664–74.

Nesbit, M.E., Perez, C.A., Tefft, M. *et al.* (1981) Multimodal therapy for the management of non-metastatic Ewing's sarcoma of bone: an intergroup study. *Natl. Cancer Inst. Monogr.*, **56**, 255–62.

Oldham, R.K. and Pomeroy, T.C. (1972) Treatment of Ewing's sarcoma with adriamycin (NSC-123,127). *Cancer Chemother. Rep.*, **56**, 635–9.

Patterson, W.P. and Khojasteh, A. (1989) Ifosfamide-induced renal tubular defects. *Cancer*, **63**, 649–51.

Perez, C.A., Razek, A., Tefft., M. *et al.* (1977) Analysis of local tumor control in Ewing's sarcoma. Preliminary results of a cooperative intergroup study. *Cancer*, **40**, 2864–73.

Pilepich, M.V., Vietti, T.J., Nesbit, M.E. *et al.* (1981) Radiotherapy and combination chemotherapy in advanced Ewing's sarcoma – Intergroup Study. *Cancer*, **47**, 1930–6.

Pinkerton, R., Philip, T., Bouffet, E. *et al.* (1986) Autologous bone marrow transplantation in paediatric solid tumours. *Clin. Hematol.*, **15**, 187–203.

Pinto, A., Grant, L.J., Hayes, F.A. *et al.* (1989) Immunohistochemical expression of neuron-specific enolase and Leu 7 in Ewing's sarcoma of bone. *Cancer*, **64**, 1266–73.

Pomeroy, T.C. and Johnson, R.E. (1975) Prognostic factors for survival in Ewing's sarcoma. *Am. J. Roentgenol. Radium Ther. Nucl. Med.*, **123**, 598–606.

Price, C.H.G. and Jeffree, G.M. (1977) Incidence of bone sarcomas in SW England, 1946–74, in relation to age, sex, tumor site and histology. *Br. J. Cancer*, **36**, 511–22.

Pritchard, D.J. (1980) Indications for surgical treatment of localized Ewing's sarcoma of bone. *Clin. Orthop.*, **153**, 39–43.

Razek, A., Perez., C.A., Tefft., M. *et al.* (1980)

Intergroup Ewing's Sarcoma study. Local control related to radiation dose, volume and site of primary lesion in Ewing's sarcoma. *Cancer*, **46**, 516–21.

Rosen, G. (1975) The development of an adjuvant chemotherapy program for the treatment of osteogenic sarcoma. *Front. Radiat. Ther. Onc.*, **10**, 115–33.

Rosen, G. (1976) Management of malignant bone tumors in children and adolescents. *Pediat. Clin. North Am.*, **23**, 183–213.

Rosen, G., Caparros, B., Huvos, A.G., et al. (1982) Preoperative chemotherapy for osteogenic sarcoma: Selection of postoperative adjuvant chemotherapy based on the response of the primary tumor to preoperative chemotherapy. *Cancer*, **49**, 1221–30.

Rosen, G., Caparros, B., Nirenberg, A. et al. (1981a) Ewing's sarcoma: ten year experience with adjuvant chemotherapy. *Cancer*, **47**, 2204–13.

Rosen, G., Jürgens, H., Caparros, B. et al. (1981b) Combination chemotherapy (T-6) in the multidisciplinary treatment of Ewing's sarcoma. *Natl. Cancer Inst. Monogr.*, **56**, 289–99.

Rosen, G., Marcove, R.C., Caparros, B. et al. (1979) Primary osteogenic sarcoma. The rationale for preoperative chemotherapy delayed surgery. *Cancer*, **43**, 2163–77.

Rosen, G., Tan, C., Sanmaneechai, A. et al. (1975) The rationale for multiple drug chemotherapy in the treatment of osteogenic sarcoma. *Cancer*, **35**, 936–45.

Rosenberg, S.A., Flye, M.W., Conkle, D. et al. (1979) Treatment of osteogenic sarcoma. II. Aggressive resection of pulmonary metastases. *Cancer Treat. Reports*, **63**, 753–6.

Rud, N.P., Reiman, H.M., Pritchard, D.J. et al. (1989) Extraosseous Ewing's sarcoma. A study of 42 cases. *Cancer*, **64**, 1548–53.

Ruggierei, P., Picci, P., Marangolo, M. et al. (1990) Neoadjuvant chemotherapy for osteosarcoma of the extremities (OE): preliminary results in 116 patients treated preoperatively with methotrexate (MTX) (IV), *cis*platinum (CDP) (IA) and adriamycin (ADM). Proc ASCO 9:310.

Salzer, M., Knahr, K., Kotz, R. and Kristen, H. (1981) Treatment of osteo-sarcomata of the distal femur by rotation-plasty. *Arch. Orthop. Traumat. Surg.*, **99**, 131–6.

Salzer-Kuntschik, M., Delling, G., Beron, G. and

Sigmund, R. (1983) Morphological grades of regression in osteosarcoma after polychemotherapy – Study COSS 80. *J. Cancer Res. Clin. Oncol.*, **106** (Suppl.), 21–4.

Samuels, M.L. and Howe, C.D. (1967) Cyclophosphamide in the management of Ewing's sarcoma. *Cancer*, **20**, 961–6.

Sauer, R. Jürgens, H., Burgers, J.M.V. et al. (1987) Prognostic factors in the treatment of Ewing's sarcoma. *Radiother. Oncol.*, **10**, 101–10.

Schajowicz, F. (1959) Ewing's sarcoma and reticulum cell sarcoma of bone. With special reference to the histochemical demonstration of glycogen as an aid to differential diagnosis. *J. Bone Joint Surg.* (Am)., **41**, 349–56.

Schimke, R., Lowman, J. and Cowan, G. (1974) Retinoblastoma and osteogenic sarcoma in siblings. *Cancer*, **34**, 2077–9.

Schmidt, D. and Harms, D. (1990) The applicability of immunohistochemistry in the diagnosis and differential diagnosis of malignant soft tissue tumors. a reevaluation based on the material of the Kiel Pediatric Tumor Registry. *Klin. Pädiatr.*, **202**, 224–9.

Schmidt, D., Harms, D. and Burdach, S. (1985) Malignant peripheral neuroectodermal tumors of childhood and adolescence. Virchows Arch. (Pathol. Anat.), **406**, 351–65.

Schmidt, D., Harms, D. and Jürgens, H. (1989) Maligne periphere neuro-ektodermale Tumoren. Histologische und immunhistochemische Befunde an 41 Fällen. *Zentralbl. Allg. Pathol. Anat.*, **135**, 257–67.

Schmidt, D., Harms, D. and Pilon, V.A. (1987) Small-cell pediatric tumors: histology, immunohistochemistry and electron microscopy. *Clin. Lab. Med.*, **7**, 63–89.

Sim, F.H., Unni, K.K., Beabout, J.W. and Dahlin, D.C. (1979) Osteosarcoma with small cells simulating Ewing's sarcoma. *J. Bone Joint Surg.*, (A), **61A**(2), 207–15.

Skinner, R., Pearson, A.D.J., Price, L. et al. (1989) Hypophosphataemic rickets after ifosfamide treatment in children. *Br. Med. J.*, **298**, 1560–1.

Smithon, W.A., Burgert, E.O., Jr., Childs, D.S. and Hoagland, C.H. (1978) Acute myelomonocytic leukemia after irradiation and chemotherapy for Ewing's sarcoma. *Mayo Clin. Proc.*, **53**, 757–9.

Souhami, R. (1987) *Incidence and Aetiology of Malig-*

nant Primary Bone Tumors. Baillière's Clinical Oncology, **1**, 1–20.

Soule, E.H., Newton, W. Jr., Moon, T.E. and Tefft, M. (1978) Extraskeletal Ewing's sarcoma: a preliminary review of 26 cases encountered in the Intergroup Rhabdomyosarcoma Study. *Cancer*, **42**, 259–64.

Spooner, D., (1987) *The Role of Radiotherapy in the Management of Primary Bone Tumours*. Baillière's Clinical Oncology **1**, 243–59.

Tefft, M., Chabora, B. and Rosen, G. (1977) Radiation in bone sarcomas. *Cancer*, **39**, 806–16.

Tepper, J., Blaubiger, D., Lichter, A. *et al.* (1980) Local control of Ewing's sarcoma of bone with radiotherapy and combination chemotherapy. *Cancer*, **46**, 1969–73.

Thomas, P.R., Perez, C.A., Neff, J.R. *et al.* (1984) The management of Ewing's sarcoma: role of radiotherapy in local tumor control. *Cancer Treat. Rep.*, **68**, 703–10.

Triche, T.J. and Rosse, W.E. (1978) Glycogen-containing neuroblastoma with clinical and histopathologic features of Ewing's sarcoma. *Cancer*, **41**, 1425–32.

Vietti, T.J., Gehan, E.A., Nesbit, M.E. *et al.* (1981) Multimodal therapy in metastatic Ewing's sarcoma: an Intergroup study. *Natl. Cancer Inst. Monogr.*, **56**, 279–84.

van Valen, F. and Jürgens, H. (1991) Expression of functional Y_2 receptors for neuropeptide in ten human Ewing's sarcoma cell lines in culture. *J. Cancer Res. Clin. Oncol.* In press.

van Valen, F., Piechot, G., Burdach, S. *et al.* (1990) Cytostatic and cytolytic synergism between tumor necrosis factor-α and interferon-α, -β and

-gamma in human peripheral neuroepithelioma cells in culture. SIOP XXII Meeting, Rome, Italy. *Med. Pediatr. Oncol.*, **18**, 367. Abstract No. 16.

Wessalowski, R., Jürgens, H., Bodenstein, H. *et al.* (1988) Behandlungsergebnisse beim primär metastasierten Ewing-Sarkom: Eine retrospektive Analyse von 48 Patienten. *Klin. Pädiatr.*, **200**, 253–60.

Whang-Peng, J., Triche, T.J., Knutsen, T., *et al.* (1984) Chromosome translocation in peripheral neuroepithelioma. *N. Engl. J. Med.*, **311**, 584–5.

Winkelmann, W. (1986) Hip rotationplasty for malignant tumors of the proximal part of the femur. *J. Bone Jt. Surg.*, **68A**, 362–70.

Winkler, K., Beron, G., Kotz., R., *et al.* (1984) Neoadjuvant chemotherapy for osteogenic sarcoma: Results of a cooperative German/Austrian study. *J. Clin. Oncol.*, **2**, 617–24.

Winkler, K., Bielack, S., Delling, G., *et al.* (1990) Effect of intraarterial versus intravenous cisplatin in addition to systemic doxorubicin, high-dose methotrexate, and ifosfamide on histologic tumor response in osteosarcoma (Study COSS-86) *Cancer*, **66**, 1703–10.

Winkler, K., Bielack, S.S., Delling, G., *et al.* (1991a) Treatment of osteosarcoma: experience of the Cooperative Osteosarcoma Study Group (COSS). *Pediatr. Oncol.* In press.

Winkler, K., Bieling, P., Bielack, S. *et al.* (1991b) Local control and survival from the cooperative osteosarcoma study group studies (COSS) of the German Society of Pediatric Oncology (GPO) and the Vienna Bone Tumour Registry (WKGR). *Clin. Orthop.* In press.

Chapter 17

Neuroblastoma

J. NINANE

17.1 INTRODUCTION

Neuroblastoma is a malignant tumour derived from the sympathetic nervous system. It is the most frequent extracranial solid tumour occurring in children. Until recently it remained fatal for children over one year of age who had reached the metastatic phase. A boom in clinical and basic research on this particularly aggressive tumour has made it possible to improve the short-term prognosis over the last decade. The combination of a better understanding of the natural history of the disease, more sophisticated investigative methods, and a resolutely new therapeutic approach has raised the two-year survival rate of children with advanced neuroblastoma to 50%. The aim of this chapter is to review some well understood and well accepted characteristics of neuroblastoma and to focus on some current controversies.

17.2 EPIDEMIOLOGY

Neuroblastoma accounts for roughly 10% of all the solid malignancies encountered in paediatric practice. Its annual incidence is between six and eight per million children under 15 years of age. The median age of onset is two years, making neuroblastoma the most frequent malignant tumour of early childhood. Moreover, age is an independent prognostic factor – the age of onset is usually inversely proportional to the survival rate. The existence of less advanced stages in

Table 17.1 Primary sites of neuroblastoma

References	Adrenal N	%	Abdomen N	%	Pelvis N	%	Thorax N	%	Neck N	%	Other N	%	Total N
Gross, 1959	89	41	28	13	12	6	25	12	4	2	59	27	217
Bodian, 1959	48	37	41	32	10	8	14	11	7	5	9	7	129
Fortner, 1968	67	50	25	19	5	4	11	8	3	2	22	17	133
Stella, 1970	42	29	62	43	5	3	24	17	4	3	6	4	143
Wilson, 1974	112	23	155	32	32	7	80	46	0	0	108	22	487
Total	358	32	311	28	64	6	154	14	18	2	204	18	1109

Neuroblastoma

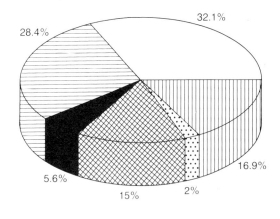

- ☐ Adrenal
- ☰ Abdomen
- ⠿ Neck
- ▨ Thorax
- ■ Pelvis
- ▥ Other

Fig. 17.1 Primary sites of neuroblastoma (n=1310).

younger patients only partly explains the correlation with the prognosis.

Table 17.1 and Fig. 17.1 present 1310 cases of neuroblastoma taken from seven studies of more than 100 cases each. The most frequent anatomical sites of the primary tumours are, in decreasing order of frequency, the adrenal gland, paravertebral retroperitoneum, posterior mediastinum, pelvis, and cervical area. The number of 'unknown' primary sites (17%) is rather high when compared with recent series. This is probably due to the fact that, before 1975, CT scan, ultrasound, MRI (magnetic resonance imaging) and *meta*-iodobenzylguanidine (*m*IBG) were not used in the staging of children with neuroblastoma.

As for other malignant tumours, neuroblastoma tends to metastasize to specific sites, i.e. bones, bone marrow and lymph nodes. Liver and skin are less frequent sites of metastases while lungs and brain are

only exceptionally affected (de la Monte *et al.*, 1983).

17.3 CLINICAL PRESENTATION

The initial symptoms of neuroblastoma are frequently non-specific and may mimic a wide variety of more common paediatric conditions. This is due to the numerous possible sites of both the primary tumour and metastases and to some symptoms that can be attributed to the associated metabolic disturbances. A growing infiltrative tumour in the neck, the thorax, the abdomen or pelvis may

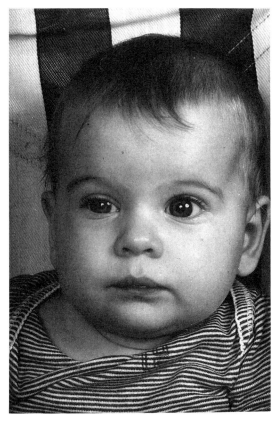

Fig. 17.2 Horner's syndrome: miosis, ptosis and enophthalmia in a 9-month-old girl with a neuroblastoma of the right cervical sympathetic side-chain.

invade and compress surrounding structures. In the head and neck region, a palpable mass and Horner's syndrome (Fig. 17.2) can be the first symptoms. In the chest, the tumour can cause respiratory distress, dysphagia and venous compression. A palpable mass, with or without abdominal pain, is usually the sign of an abdominal tumour, whereas pelvic tumours may be revealed by troubles in defaecation and voiding urine. Tumours growing through the intra-vertebral foramina and compressing the spinal cord ('dumb-bell' neuroblastoma) may present with neurological symptoms such as flaccid paralysis of the legs and/or urinary dysfunction with distension of the bladder.

The clinical symptoms due to metastases also vary widely. In infants, the first sign is usually a rapidly enlarging liver, sometimes accompanied by skin nodules with a bluish colour and bone marrow involvement. Older children show a different pattern of metastasic spread due to the change in circulation from the fetal type of blood circulation to the new-born type. Symptoms due to metastases in older children include bone pain and lymph node enlargement. Signs and symptoms can sometimes be confused with those of leukaemia, consisting of anaemia and mucosal or skin haemorrhage due to pancytopaenia caused by bone marrow infiltration by neuroblastoma cells (Fig. 17.3)

The metabolic effects of the tumour can also cause systemic symptoms. The high level of catecholamines and sometimes vasoactive intestinal peptides (VIP) produced by neuroblastoma cells can result in bouts of sweating and pallor associated with watery

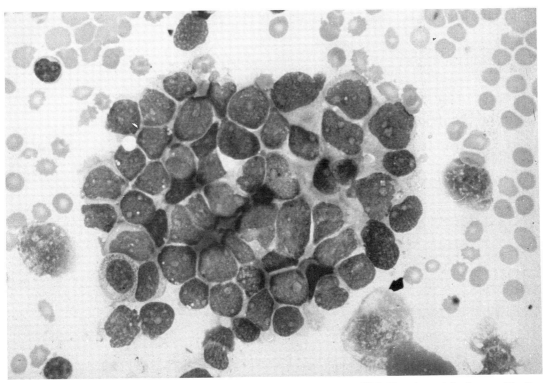

Fig. 17.3 Cluster of neuroblastoma cells in a bone marrow smear. H & E stain, original magnification × 600.

diarrhoea and hypertension. These symptoms are probably unrelated to the site and size of the tumour and regress following successful therapy. Finally, the tumour may be disclosed by a routine clinical examination.

17.4 STAGING SYSTEMS: TOWARDS A CONSENSUS?

Up to 1988, the following three major staging systems were used for neuroblastoma throughout the world, making communication between clinicians and researchers very difficult: (1) the system used by the Children's Cancer Study Group (CCSG) in the USA as well as many others (Evans *et al.*, 1971); (2) the system utilized by St Jude's Children's Research Hospital (SJCRH) and the Pediatric Oncology Group (POG) (Hayes

Table 17.2 Staging systems in neuroblastoma

1. *The CCSG staging system* (Evans *et al.*, 1971)

Stage I	Tumour confined to the organ or structure of origin.
Stage II	Tumour extending in continuity beyond the organ or structure of origin but not crossing the midline. Regional lymph nodes on the ipsilateral side may be involved.
Stage III	Tumour extending in continuity beyond the midline. Regional lymph nodes may be involved bilaterally.
Stage IV	Remote disease involving the skeleton, organs, soft tissue and distant lymph nodes groups.
Stage IV-S	(Special category). Patients who would be otherwise Stage I or II but who have remote disease confined to liver, skin, or bone marrow, and who have no radiographic evidence of bone metastases on complete skeletal survey.

2. *The TNM classification* (UICC-TNM, 1987)

Stage I	T1	Single tumour, <5 cm in diameter
	No	No evidence of lymph node involvement
	Mo	No evidence of distant metastases
Stage II	T2	Single tumour, >5 cm but <10 cm
	No	No evidence of lymph node involvement
	Mo	No evidence of distant metastases
Stage III	T1/T2	Single tumour, <5 cm in diameter/Single tumour, >5 cm but <10 cm
	N1	Regional lymph node involvement
	Mo	No evidence of distant metastases
	T3 any N Mo	Single tumour, >10 cm Regional lymph nodes involved/not involved/cannot be assessed No evidence of distant metastases
Stage IVA	T1/T2/T3	Single tumour, <5 cm in diameter/Single tumour, >5 cm but <10 cm/Single tumour, >10 cm
	any N	Regional lymph nodes involved/not involved/cannot be assessed
	M1	Evidence of distant metastases
Stage IVB	T4	Multiple simultaneous tumours
	any N	Regional lymph nodes involved/not involved/cannot be assessed
	any M	Distant metastases evident/not evident/cannot be assessed

T = Primary tumour; N = Regional lymph nodes; M = Distant metastases.

Table 17.2 *Continued*

3. *INSS – international staging system for neuroblastoma* (Brodeur *et al.*, 1988)

Stage 1	Localized tumour confined to the area of origin; complete gross excision, with or without microscopic residual disease; identifiable ipsilateral and contralateral lymph nodes negative macroscopically.
Stage 2a	Unilateral tumour with incomplete gross excision; identifiable ipsilateral and contralateral lymph nodes negative microscopically.
Stage 2b	Unilateral tumour with complete or incomplete gross excision; with positive ipsilateral regional lymph nodes; contralateral lymph nodes negative microscopically.
Stage 3	Tumour infiltrating across the midline with or without regional lymph node involvement; or, unilateral tumour with contralateral regional lymph node involvement; or, midline tumour with bilateral regional lymph node involvement.
Stage 4	Dissemination of tumour to distant lymph nodes, bone, bone marrow, liver and/or other organs (except as defined in Stage 4S).
Stage 4S	Localized primary tumour as defined for Stage 1 or 2 with dissemination limited to liver, skin and/or bone marrow.

4. *Incidence and survival by INSS stage*

Stage 1	Incidence	5%
	5-year survival	≥90%
Stage 2a + 2b	Incidence	10%
	5-year survival	70–80%
Stage 3	Incidence	20%
	5-year survival	40–70% (depends on surgical resection)
Stage 4	Incidence	60%
	5-year survival	60% if age <1 year
		20% if age >1 year and <2 year
		10% if age >2 year
Stage 4-S	Incidence	5%
	5-year survival	>80%

et al., 1983); and (3) the TNM system proposed by the International Union Against Cancer (UICC) (1987). Modifications of these staging systems were employed by the Italian Cooperative Working Group, the Malignant Tumour Committee of the Japanese Society of Pediatric Surgeons, and others. In general, the various staging systems gave comparable results in distinguishing low-stage, good-prognosis patients from high-stage, poor prognosis patients. However, some of the differences between these different staging systems are substantial, particularly when applied to individual patients. The results of clinical trials or studies performed by different groups thus cannot be readily compared. Points of disagreement include: (1) the prognostic importance of tumours crossing the mid-line; (2) the prognostic importance of ipsilateral and/or contralateral lymph nodes involvement. (Ninane *et al.*, 1982); and (3) the importance of resectability of the primary tumour.

Agreement on the definition of stage with regard to these and other issues has been achieved (Brodeur *et al.*, 1988). This will facilitate the comparison of different studies. It is to be hoped that this new staging system, known as INSS (International Neuroblastoma Staging System) will be used widely. For comparison, Table 17.2 shows the CCSG, TNM and INSS systems for staging neuroblastoma patients. Incidence and survival by stage, using the consensus staging system (INSS), are given at the end of the same table.

17.5 TUMOUR MARKERS: FACTS AND CONTROVERSIES

The 'ideal' tumour marker is a specific mole-cule produced by the malignant cells, measurable at the time of diagnosis, absent during remission periods, and again present in relapse. In this section, four 'circulating' markers, detectable either in patients' blood or in their urine will be discussed: catecholamines, neurone-specific enolase, ferritin and gangliosides.

17.5.1 CATECHOLAMINES

In 1959, excessive secretion of vanillylmandelic acid (VMA) was noticed in children with ganglioneuroma and ganglioneuroblastoma. Today, the fact that neuroblastoma cells secrete large amounts of one or more catechol-

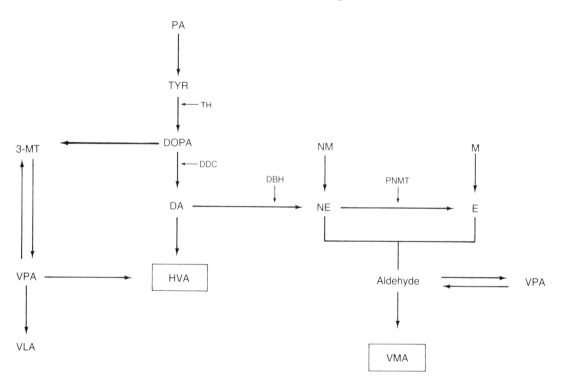

Fig. 17.4 Enzymes: TH (tyrosine hydroxylase), DDC (dopa-decarboxylase), PNMT (Phenylethanolamine-N-methyl transferase), DBH (dopamine-β-hydroxylase). Catecholamines, metabolites and precursors: PA (phenylalanine), TYR (tyrosine), DOPA (3,4-dihydroxylphenylalanine), DA (dopamine), NE (norepinephrine), E (epinephrine), VMA (vanillyl-mandelic acid), HVA (homovanillic acid), NM (normethanephrine), M (methanephrine), 3-MT (3-methoxytyramine), VLA (vanillactic acid), VPA (vanilpuric acid), VG (vanilglycol).

amines, in addition to their metabolites, is well documented. Despite the fact that VMA and homovanillic acid (HVA) are relatively easy to measure and are usually raised in neuroblastoma patients, there are 'non-secreting' tumours for which less frequently measured metabolites may be useful e.g. dopamine. A good understanding of the synthesis and metabolism of catecholamines is therefore useful, although for practical clinical reasons, HVA and VMA are the most widely used in diagnosis and follow-up (Fig. 17.4).

During the past 20 years, the measurement of urinary VMA and HVA has become a routine test for diagnosis and follow-up of patients with neuroblastoma. However, recent developments have questioned this procedure.

(a) Random samples versus 24-h collections

Recently Tuchman and co-workers challenged the statement that a 24-h collection was necessary: they showed that random urinary HVA and VMA levels were adequate not only for diagnosis but also for follow-up (Tuchman *et al.*, 1985). A three-year study performed by the same authors led them to conclude that prolonged urine collections for HVA and VMA determination in the diagnosis of neuroblastoma are no longer necessary (Tuchman *et al.*, 1987).

(b) Mass screening for neuroblastoma

Age and stage at diagnosis are the two most important prognostic variables in neuroblastoma. It thus seems logical to try to detect the disease in its early stage, especially during infancy. Since 1973, Sawada and his colleagues in Kyoto, Japan, have organized what they call a 'mass screening' and, on reading their results, one must admit that they have been successful. In their hands,

neuroblastoma screening at six to seven months of age was estimated to include around 70% of area births (Sawada *et al.*, 1984). They have demonstrated that this technique, aimed at the prevention of advanced disease, is effective since they have recorded a 92% disease-free survival among the first 25 children detected by screening almost half a million infants (Sawada and Tuchman, 1987). In the USA (Woods and Tuchman, 1987) and in Europe, there is a trend towards embarking on such a programme since the Japanese data is provocative. However, there are important methodological limitations to these programmes: (1) preliminary reports suggest that the incidence of neuroblastoma may be increased by screening, probably by detecting cases which would have spontaneously regressed and disappeared (Nishi *et al.*, 1987); and (2) the Japanese did not attempt to address the natural biases that screening introduces in the long-term outcome of any cancer (Prorok and Connor, 1986). Collaborators in North America have embarked on a large scale mass screening programme, which may be able to answer these important questions.

(c) Prognostic significance of HVA:VMA ratio

Conflicting results have been reported concerning the prognostic significance of HVA and VMA levels in pretreatment urines of children with neuroblastoma. In the study by Gitlow *et al.* (1973), high initial VMA levels were associated with a poorer prognosis whereas in more recent reports no significant correlation was found between the levels of HVA or VMA or the HVA:VMA ratio and prognosis (Siegel *et al.*, 1980; Ninane *et al.*, 1986).

(d) Plasma HVA and VMA

In one recent study, Gahr and Hunneman

357

(1987) determined the plasma levels of HVA and VMA in 84 newly diagnosed children with histologically confirmed neuroblastoma as well as in 15 patients in relapse. The urinary levels were measured at the same time. Their data showed that plasma levels of catecholamine metabolites could be used with reliability for monitoring neuroblastoma. Furthermore, in some children, elevated plasma levels were found whereas urine levels were normal. These data seem to confirm the findings of Krivit and co-workers (1980) who showed that serum HVA and VMA levels tended to parallel urinary levels in children with Stage IV neuroblastoma. The logical next step would be to compare plasma-serum levels and random urine determination of HVA and/or VMA.

17.5.2 NEURONE-SPECIFIC ENOLASE

Enolase is a glycolytic enzyme: brain and neuroendocrine tissues contain two forms of enolases, denoted $\alpha\alpha$ and $\gamma\gamma$ to indicate that they are dimers of biochemically immunologically distinct subunits. A hybrid form ($\alpha\gamma$) is also present in these tissues. The γ-enolase is found in neurones and therefore has been called neurone-specific enolase (NSE). In children, although high serum NSE levels are suggestive of neuroblastoma, increased levels have been reported in other malignancies like Wilms' tumour, Ewing's sarcoma, non-Hodgkin's lymphoma, soft tissue sarcoma, and acute leukaemias (Cooper *et al.*, 1987). Caution should thus be exercised in using NSE as a diagnostic test in children with a malignant disease. Furthermore, the test is not particularly sensitive since raised serum NSE levels have been described in all stages of neuroblastoma at diagnosis. In general, a low level predicts a good prognosis and a high level a poor outcome, this being mainly due to the fact that children with advanced disease present with higher serum NSE levels (Zeltzer *et al.*, 1986). It is interest-

ing to observe that patients with 4S neuroblastoma (see below), which generally present with a large tumour burden, but have a good prognosis, usually have lower NSE levels than children with Stage IV disease of equivalent tumour bulk. This is further evidence that the biological characteristics of 4S neuroblastoma are different to the other stages of the disease. In summary, NSE is a 'marker' of neuroblastoma but not a very good one since it lacks both good specificity and good sensitivity.

17.5.3 FERRITIN

Children with advanced neuroblastoma frequently present with an increased level of ferritin and the levels usually decrease during treatment and may reach normality when the patients are in clinical remission. Increased amounts of serum ferritin in patients with neuroblastoma can, in theory, be due to the following: tissue damage caused by tumour invasion, an increase of unused iron associated with anaemia, a leakage of neuroblastoma cell ferritin during tumour necrosis, or to an augmented synthesis of ferritin by neuroblastoma cells and subsequent secretion in plasma. There is now clear evidence that tumour cells are, at least in part, responsible for the increased amount of serum ferritin in some neuroblastoma patients (Hann *et al.*, 1986).

Prognostic significance of serum ferritin

Ferritin is not frequently elevated in sera from children with Stage I and II disease but is abnormally raised in some patients with Stage III and IV disease (Hann *et al.*, 1985). In one study on prognostic factors in neuroblastoma, it was possible to define three groups of children with different prognoses: good (normal ferritin; age less than two years: two-year survival 93%), intermediate (normal ferritin; age two years or older: two-year survival of 58%), and poor (raised ferritin; two-year survival of 19%) (Evans *et al.*, 1987). At the present time, we unfortunately lack prospective studies from other cooperative study groups to definitively ascertain the prognostic significance of serum ferritin as an independent variable in neuroblastoma even if the references cited above look convincing.

17.5.4 GANGLIOSIDES

Gangliosides, sialic-acid-containing glyco-sphingolipids, are mainly detected in the cell surface membrane. These membrane-bound glycolipids are shed or released *in vitro* by a variety of cells, particularly tumour cells. It now appears that these markers are present in both the tumours and the plasma of most children with neuroblastoma. Elevated con-centrations of disialoganglioside G_{D2} to more than 50 times the normal value have been demonstrated in the plasma of children with active neuroblastoma. Sequential determin-ation of circulating G_{D2} has revealed that plasma levels decreased in children respond-ing to treatment and reappeared in patients in relapse. In contrast, raised circulating G_{D2} has not been demonstrated in the plasma of children with ganglioneuroblastoma or gang-lioneuroma (Ladisch and Wu, 1985).

Ganglioside composition of neuroblastoma cells as a prognostic factor

Preliminary studies of the ganglioside com-position of neuroblastoma have suggested that the lack of G_{T1_b} might indicate a poorer diagnosis. This finding has now been con-firmed and is particularly striking for children with mediastinal neuroblastoma. Indeed, tumours of patients with thoracic primaries were found to contain more complex gang-liosides of the b series – $G_{D_{1b}}$ and G_{T1b} – and fewer monosialogangliosides, suggesting a

more differentiated cellular composition (Schochat *et al.*, 1987). Only one child of the 20 with a mediastinal primary lacked GT_{1b} in his tumour and died of disease. These interesting data, if confirmed, suggest that the better prognosis universally reported in children with thoracic neuroblastoma, as compared with other sites, is probably due to a biological difference within the membrane of tumour cells.

In summary, the ideal neuroblastoma mar-ker has yet to be found. It is a molecule of neuroblastoma cell origin, released in the circulation and/or in the urine in amounts easily detectable and proportional to the stage of the disease. This molecule should disappear when the child is in remission and reappear in advance of clinical evidence of relapse. Not all of the above criteria for an ideal neuroblastoma marker are met by catecholamines, NSE, ferritin and ganglio-sides when taken individually.

17.6 CLINICAL AND HISTOLOGICAL FEATURES

Virchow described for the first time a child presenting with an abdominal neuroblast-oma, to which he gave the name 'glioma' in 1864. In 1891, Marchand defined the relation-ship between the sympathetic nervous sys-tem and tumours of the adrenal medulla. It was not until 1910 that Wright showed con-vincingly that the tumour developed from embryonal neuroblasts of the sympathetic system (sympathogonia); he was also the first to propose the name 'neuroblastoma' for this malignant disease.

17.6.1 HISTOPATHOLOGY

The terminology of 'neuroblastoma' has been confused in the past but the current nomen-clature generally classifies three types of tumour: (1) undifferentiated neuroblastoma; (2) ganglioneuroblastoma, a tumour with

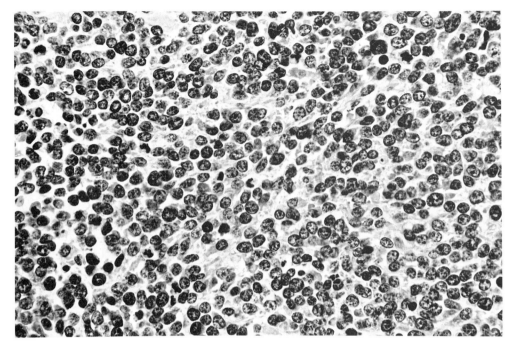

Fig. 17.5a   Undifferentiated neuroblastoma (H & E × 130).

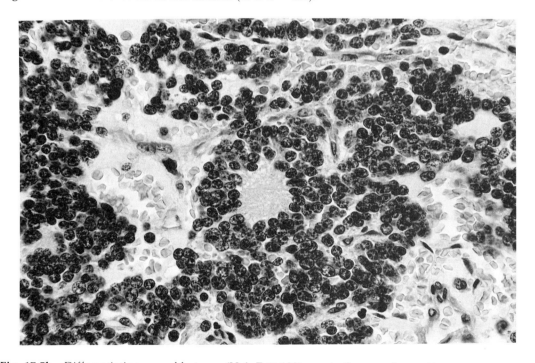

Fig. 17.5b   Differentiating neuroblastoma (H & E × 130) – note the pseudo-rosettes.

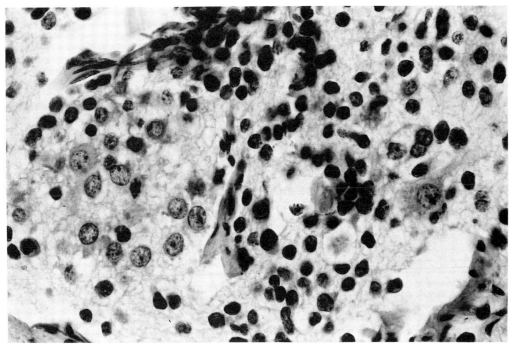

Fig. 17.5c Complex ganglioneuroblastoma with both mature and undifferentiated tumour cells (H & E × 130).

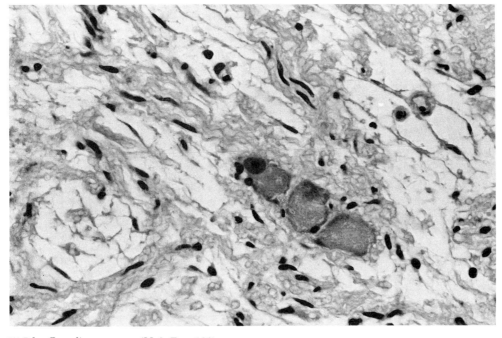

Fig. 17.5d Ganglioneuroma (H & E × 130).

both maturing or mature ganglion cells together with neuroblasts; and (3) ganglioneuroma, the most mature end of the spectrum.

The microscopic appearance of undifferentiated neuroblastoma (Fig. 17.5a) is that of diffusely arranged sheets of cells showing some focal evidence of aggregation. Differentiating neuroblastoma (Fig. 17.5b) show definite evidence of neurofibril formation: neurofibrils may be arranged at the centre of 'pseudorosettes'. Ganglioneuroblastoma contains both neuroblasts and ganglion cells in two histological patterns: (a) complex ganglioneuroblastoma (Fig. 17.5c) in which the tumour has a lobular arrangement and undifferentiated neuroblasts are intermixed with ganglion cells and intermediate forms, all within any lobule; and (b) composite ganglioneuroblastoma, in which undifferentiated neuroblasts and mature ganglion cells are located in different parts of the tumour.

Ganglioneuroma (Fig. 17.5d) consists of mature ganglion cells lying against a background of neurofibrils and fibrous tissue. Although it is clear that the prognosis for ganglioneuroma is extremely good and that for ganglioneuroblastoma considerably better than for neuroblastoma, it is not always easy to demonstrate prognostic correlations within the neuroblastoma subtypes. Systems for histological grading must take into account varying degrees of differentiation from field to field within a tumour since the potential for metastasis is probably determined, at least in part, by the most undifferentiated component. In general, there is a correlation between more neural differentiation and better prognosis (Beckwith and Martin, 1968; Hugues *et al.*, 1974). An age-related classification has been proposed by Shimada and co-workers (1984). This system is based on the amount of stroma, tumour cell differentiation, and an index of mitosis and karyorrhexis in the tumour. Using these criteria, Shimada *et al.* (1984) showed a correlation

between histology and survival, the better prognosis being achieved within the 'favourable stroma-poor group' with more than 80% survival at two years from diagnosis. However, this age-related classification seems difficult to apply world-wide due to its complexity and it remains to be demonstrated in prospective studies whether the correlation to prognosis is not mainly due to the introduction of the patients' age.

17.6.2 CYTOGENETICS

Chromosome 1 is the chromosome most frequently involved in structural and numerical abnormalities in neuroblastoma cells. These include deletions or rearrangements leading to the loss of material from the short arm (1p) and additional long arm segments (1q). Chromosome 17 has also been reported to be frequently involved. Besides chromosomes 1 and 17, there are individual case reports enumerating structural and numerical abnormalities that involve almost all the autosomes. Other cytogenetic findings include homogeneously staining regions (HSR) and double minutes (DM). The HSR is a chromosome segment that is usually longer than any single band in the standard karyotype, staining with intermediate density over its length and not showing the alternating pattern of dark and light bands that are characteristic of a normal karyotype. The HSR shows the staining properties of the DMs which are paired chromatin bodies lacking centromeres. It has been reported that DMs either form or are breakdown products of HSRs. Both HSRs and DMs have been shown to be the site of gene amplification.

17.6.3 MOLECULAR BIOLOGY

In neuroblastoma, a hyperdiploid DNA content has been reported to predict a better response to therapy than diploidy, particularly in children less than 18 months old at the time of diagnosis (Look *et al.*, 1984). N-*myc* is a member of the cellular growth control gene family, generally referred to as cellular oncogenes. N-*myc* has been located on chromosome 2 at 2p23–24. The association of N-*myc* amplification with advanced stages of neuroblastoma has been shown to be of prognostic significance since children with a high number of genomic N-*myc* copies have a poorer prognosis than those with a single copy of the gene (Seeger *et al.*, 1985).

17.6.4 IMMUNOCYTOLOGY

Neuroblastoma can be confused clinically and histologically with other so-called 'small round and blue cell tumours'. These include rhabdomyosarcoma, Ewing's sarcoma, lymphoma, neuroectodermal tumours and some forms of Wilms' tumour. The diagnosis is particularly difficult – especially between Ewing's, neuroblastoma and neuroectodermal tumours – when the metastatic site is the major clinical presentation. Recent developments in immunohistology and immuno-cytology techniques now provide new tools for the differential diagnosis of neuroblastoma from other small round and blue cell tumours. Many of the surface antigens on neuroblastoma cells have been identified and through the use of various monoclonal antibodies, neuroblastoma cells have been well characterized. However, most antibodies are not specific for neuroblastoma and cross-react with other tumours and normal tissues. Therefore, a panel of several monoclonal antibodies 'highly specific' for neuroblastoma cells is required for an accurate diagnosis. In addition to anti-neuroblastoma monoclonal antibodies, the panel should include antisera to neurone-specific enolase (NSE) and S-100 protein even if NSE and S-100 protein are not specific to neuroblastoma. Finally, in addition to neuroblastoma markers, the diagnostic panel should include leucocyte markers, intermediate filament markers for desmin (muscle cells), vimentin (mesenchymal cells) and cytokeratin (epithelial cells) to exclude other malignancies in case of doubt (Sugimoto *et al.*, 1984; Oppedal *et al.*, 1987).

Electron microscopy and tissue culture studies are also helpful in the diagnosis of neuroblastoma. However, since the recent development of immunohistochemistry, modern cytogenetics and molecular biology, these two expensive and time-consuming techniques appear less useful, at least for diagnostic purposes.

17.7 CLINICAL EVALUATION

The diagnostic methods are numerous, and include a growing number of 'imaging techniques', bone marrow biopsies and trephines, blood sampling and urine collection for the search of tumour markers, and open or closed biopsy of the primary tumour for histology grading and biological studies.

17.7.1 LOCOREGIONAL INVOLVEMENT

Ultrasound should always be the first investigation performed when an abdominal or pelvic mass is detected or suspected. Following echography, CT-scan is usually indicated, particularly when primary or delayed surgery is contemplated. Ultrasounds and CT-scan (Fig. 17.6) are capable of accurately localizing masses and providing anatomic information: in particular, they offer information regarding both intra- and extraperitoneal structures in the case of an abdominal mass. Both techniques also differentiate cystic from solid tumours and define the extent of a primary tumour as well as its relationship to other structures. These examinations also detect small calcifications in a neuroblastoma that cannot be demonstrated with standard x-ray studies.

Recently, MRI (magnetic resonance imaging) has proven to be a very powerful method of investigation (Fig. 17.7). It should be noted that CT-scan and MRI often necessitate sedation and sometimes general anaesthesia in small children.

17.7.2 EVALUATION OF METASTASES

Bone marrow metastases are best looked for by means of aspirations and trephine biopsies. It seems that many different sites of aspirates are necessary to exclude bone marrow involvement, either at diagnosis or following primary chemotherapy. Aspirates can be studied by cytology, immunocytochemistry or flow cytometry. Histology of bone marrow shows that 10% of marrow involvement by neuroblastoma can be missed when aspirates only are performed. The study of at least four different sites is therefore recommended with both aspirates and trephine biopsies (Bayle *et al.*, 1985; Franklin and Pritchard, 1983; Kemshead and Pritchard, 1984). Neuroblastoma has a predilection to metastasize widely to the skeletal system. Radiographic bone changes on skeletal x-ray survey can occur very rapidly. Skeletal metastases are generally more frequent in children aged two years or older. The frequency of detecting skeletal metastases with

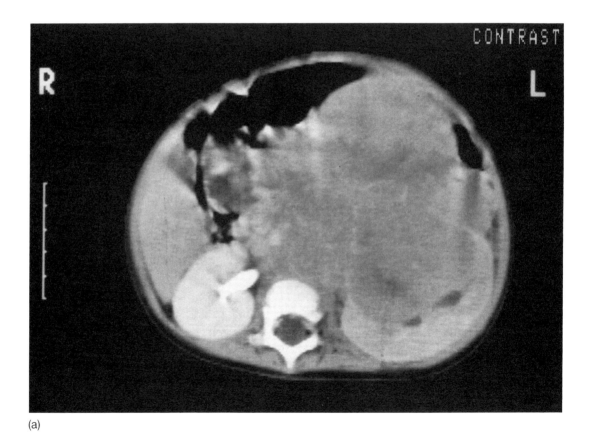

(a)

Fig. 17.6 An 18-month-old girl with Stage III neuroblastoma of the left adrenal gland (a) pre-treatment CT scan; (b) (overleaf) pre-operative CT scan following four courses of chemotherapy. Note that the entire tumour looks 'necrotic', showing good response to chemotherapy.

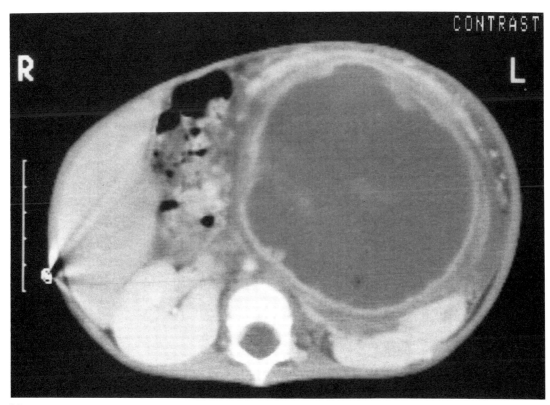

(b)

Fig. 17.6 *continued*

standard radiography at the time of the initial diagnosis is approximately 50–60%. With the introduction of the ^{99m}Tc methylene diphosphate for bone imaging, the accuracy in detecting metastatic bone disease in children has improved dramatically with 80% of metastases detected. More recently, *meta-iodobenzylguanidine* (*m*IBG), a guanethidine analogue, labelled with iodine-131 (^{131}I), has been successfully used for the diagnosis and follow-up of children with neuroblastoma. ^{131}I-*m*IBG scintigraphy correctly demonstrates primary, residual and recurrent tumour masses, as well as diffuse bone marrow infiltration and skeletal, lymph node and soft tissue metastases (Hoefenagel *et al.*, 1987). Cumulative reported findings in the literature concerning 550 patients with neuroblastoma, indicate that more than 90% of these tumours are able to concentrate ^{131}I-*m*IBG (Gelfand and Hoefenagel, 1988). Follow-up of marrow and skeletal metastases during and after therapy should include ^{131}I-*m*IBG scintigraphy coupled with bone marrow aspirates and trephines. It has recently been demonstrated that MRI could detect focal marrow and bone abnormalities in case of neuroblastoma (Cohen *et al.*, 1984). However, this technique is too expensive and necessitates general anaesthesia in small children: it can not therefore be recommended as a routine follow-up test for children with neuroblastoma.

In conclusion, during the past ten years, the development of computerized tomography, ultrasonography, MRI and radionuclide

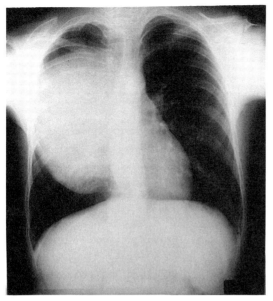
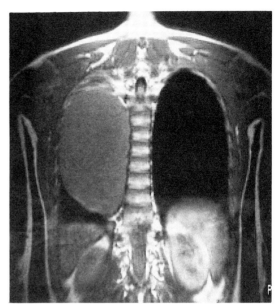

Fig. 17.7 An 8-year-old boy with Stage IIa mediastinal ganglioblastoma (A) chest x-ray; (B) magnetic resonance imaging.

imaging has improved accuracy in the diagnosis, staging and follow-up of children with neuroblastoma. These technical advances and the need for cost containment place new responsibilities on the paediatric oncologist to consult the surgeon and the radiologist in selecting the most appropriate diagnostic modalities: the temptation to test excessively must be resisted.

17.8 TREATMENT STRATEGIES

Neuroblastoma has been studied extensively for more than a century and has fascinated both clinicians and scientists. The treatment is still, however, one of the most important challenges in paediatric oncology. The treatment strategy depends on at least two factors: what are the criteria of response to therapy and what are the prognostic factors for a given child affected with the disease. Having answered these two questions, the oncologist, together with the surgeon and the radiotherapist, may offer the child the best

treatment – this should be 'aggressive' for an aggressive tumour and 'light' for a good prognosis neuroblastoma. Unfortunately, things are not that easy, and Dargeon's statement in 1962 that 'neuroblastoma is an unpredictable tumour' is still true in the 1990s (Dargeon, 1962).

17.8.1 DEFINITION OF RESPONSE TO TREATMENT

Criteria for determining the response to therapy vary from one institution or cooperative group to another, as well as the time following diagnosis at which the assessment of response should be made. The same tests that are used for staging the disease (see above) should be used to assess response of primary tumour and metastases to therapy. When a patient responds, the tests that were negative at diagnosis should of course not all be repeated but a relapsing child should, on the contrary, be reassessed as a newly diagnosed patient. Table 17.3 summarizes

366

Table 17.3 Definitions of response to treatment (Adapted from Brodeur *et al.*, 1988)

Response[1]	Primary	Metastases	Tumour markers
CR	No tumour	No tumour	HVA/VMA normal
VGPR	Reduction 90–99%	No tumour	HVA/VMA decreased 90–99%
PR	Reduction 50–90%	No tumour except bone; no new bone lesion, all previous lesions improved	HVA/VMA decreased 50–90%
MR	No new lesions; >50% reduction of any measurable lesion (primary or metastases) with <50% reduction in any other; >25% increase in any existing lesion[2]		
NR	No new lesions; <50% reduction but <25% increase in any existing lesion[2]		
PD	Any new lesions; increase of any measurable lesion by >25%; previous negative marrow positive for tumour		

[1] CR: complete response; VGPR: very good partial response; PR: partial response; MR: minimal response; NR: no response; PD: progressive disease
[2] Quantitative assessment does not apply to bone marrow.

the International Neuroblastoma Response Criteria (Brodeur *et al.*, 1988). Implementation of these criteria should facilitate communication between different clinical and laboratory study groups dealing with neuroblastoma.

17.8.2 PROGNOSTIC FACTORS

Prognostic factors in neuroblastoma patients result from a correlation between survival on the one hand and age, stage and biological parameters on the other (Oppedal *et al.*, 1988; Ninane *et al.*, 1986). Using a multivariate analysis, Evans and co-workers (1987) suggested that combinations of age, stage, serum ferritin and histology could define three populations according to prognosis: one favourable with more than 80% 2-year survival, one unfavourable with less than 20%, and one intermediate. Age at diagnosis is still the single most important prognostic factor, with children less than one year old at diagnosis having the best prognosis. Other prognostic factors include stage and primary site. The prognosis for INSS Stage 1 and 4S chil-

Table 17.4 Prognostic factors in neuroblastoma

Factors	Prognosis		
	Good	Intermediate	Poor
Age (years)	<1	1–2	>2
Stage (INSS)	1; 2a; 4S	2b; some 3	some 3; 4
Primary site	Mediastinal	Pelvic, cervical	Retroperitoneal
Histology	Ganglioneuroblastoma	Differentiated neuroblastoma	Undifferentiated neuroblastoma
Ferritin levels	Normal	–	Abnormal (raised)
NSE levels (ng/ml)	<20	20–100	>100
No. of N. *Myc* copies	2	3–10	>10
Ploidy	Hyperdiploid		Diploid
Chromosome 1	Normal		Abnormal

dren is better than for children with more advanced disease (Table 17.2). Retroperitoneal and in particular adrenal neuroblastoma are associated with the poorest prognosis while mediastinal neuroblastoma have the better prognosis. Signs of differentiation within the primary tumour is a favourable prognostic factor. Flow cytometry studies of tumour cell DNA content may help in distinguishing the group of tumours with hyperdiploid neuroblastoma that respond better to therapy. This is particularly true in small children. Finally, studies in molecular biology have shown that amplification of N-*myc* oncogene is an independent prognostic factor. The RNA levels (N-*myc* expression) do not show the same correlation to prognosis. Table 17.4 summarizes the most important prognostic factors in neuroblastoma children.

17.8.3 CHEMOTHERAPY

(a) Single-agent drugs

At conventional doses, six drugs have shown definite activity when used as monotherapy in children with neuroblastoma (Carli *et al.*, 1982) (Table 17.5). They include vincristine, cyclophosphamide, *cis*-platin, doxorubicin, epipodophyllotoxins (etoposide/VP-16; teniposide/VM-26) and melphalan. More recent studies have demonstrated that ifosfamide

(de Kraker *et al.*, 1987) and carboplatin (Pinkerton *et al.*, 1989) are also active as single agents in neuroblastoma.

(b) 'Conventional' chemotherapy regimen

Until 1980, most chemotherapy regimens included vincristine and cyclophosphamide with or without adriamycin (Ninane *et al.*, 1981). The long-term results were quite disappointing for children aged more than one year with advanced neuroblastoma since the two-year survival rate rarely exceeded 10%. The addition of *cis*-platin and epipodophyllotoxin had a significant influence on the initial response rate but long-term remissions are not the rule (Shafford *et al.*, 1984; Philip *et al.*, 1987a; Hartmann *et al.*, 1988; Bernard *et al.*, 1987).

(c) 'High-dose' chemotherapy

Due to the high relapse rate of children treated with 'conventional' chemotherapy, several 'megatherapy' regimens – also called 'consolidation' therapy – have been designed in the hope of increasing the number of long-term survivors. 'Megatherapy' usually refers to very high-dose chemotherapy (and sometimes total body irradiation) followed by bone marrow rescue. Optimistic preliminary results were published a few years ago that

Table 17.5 Chemotherapy for neuroblastoma

Single agents	Combination (conventional chemotherapy)					High dose regimen (with marrow rescue)			
Vincristine	X	X	X	X	X	X			
Cyclophosphamide	X		X	X	X				
Doxorubicin			X		X			X	
Cis-platin			X	X	X			X	
Melphalan						X	X	X	X
VM26/VP-16	X	X	X	X	X		X		X
Carboplatin	X								
BCNU							X		

are summarized in Table 17.6. The clinical status of the children at the time of consolidation treatment as well as the time of 'megatherapy' differs in the various studies. However, despite the patients' heterogeneity, and methodological differences in the treatment administered, three important points can be made: (1) the patients who received megatherapy after complete response or good partial response survived longer than those who were treated in relapse; (2) at two years, high-dose melphalan administered as single-drug therapy yielded comparable results to those of intensive multiple chemotherapy, even if the latter was combined with total body irradiation; (3)

mortality due to treatment was lower in the ENSG study. High-dose therapy given as consolidation treatment to children with advanced neuroblastomas in complete or good partial response increases the children's two-year survival rate significantly, although the toxicity of the treatment cannot be discounted. The value of purging the marrow of residual malignant cells when cytologically and histologically it appears normal remains to be demonstrated.

Where are we now with more than five years' follow-up for the first patients included in the intensive chemotherapy regimen? Data are available for two studies; in a French Cooperative Group (LMCE), the median

Table 17.6 Megatherapy and bone marrow (BM) rescue

Cooperative groups [1]	ENSG-1 (a)	LMCE group (b)	IGR (c)	CCSG (d)
No. children	30	37	26	47
Stage	III–IV	V	III–IV	IV
Status [2]	CR/GPR	CR/GPR	CR/GPR/PR	REL (28) CR/GPR/PR (19)
Randomization	Yes	No	No	No
Megatherapy[3]	HDM	TBI + VCR + HDM	HDM (15) HDM + BCNU + VM-26 (11)	TBI + HDM + other drugs
BM rescue[4]	ABMT	ABMT (35) BMT (2)	ABMT	ABMT (26) BMT (21)
Ex vivo treatment of BM[5]	No	MoAb	ASTA-Z (11)	No
2-year survival	54%	44%	?	25%
Toxic deaths	2 (7%)	7 (19%)	3 (12%)	15 (32%)

(a) Pritchard *et al.*, 1986
(b) Philip *et al.*, 1987b
(c) Hartmann *et al.*, 1985
(d) D'Angio *et al.*, 1985
(1) Cooperative groups
    ENSG: European Neuroblastoma Study Group
    LMCE: Lyon, Marseille, Paris, Curie, East of France
    IGR: Institut Gustave Roussy
    CCSG: Children's Cancer Study Group
(2) Status at the time of megatherapy
    CR: Complete response
    GPR: Good partial response
    PR: Partial response
    REL: Relapse

(3) Megatherapy
    HDM: High-dose melphalan
    TBI: Total body irradiation
    VCR: Vincristine
    BCNU: Carmustine
    VM-26: Teniposide
(4) BM rescue
    ABMT: Autologous bone marrow transplantation
    BMT: Allogeneic bone marrow transplantation
(5) *Ex-vivo* treatment of BM-cells
    ASTA-Z: Mafosfamide
    MoAb: Monoclonal antibodies

observation time is 55 months for the 62 unselected Stage 4 patients over one year old at diagnosis grafted between 1983 and 1987: 22 in CR/VGPR, and 40 in PR. Survival progression-free for the grafted children is 40% at two years, 25% at five years and 13% at seven years. However, in the group of children grafted with complete response at the metastatic sites – regardless of the primary tumour status – the progression-free survival is 37% at both two *and* seven years (Philip *et al.*, 1990). An Italian group has also updated its results on 34 children grafted for more than one year between 1984 and 1987. This group of patients is, however, less homogeneous since it includes children in relapse and selected and unselected Stage 4 patients. The progression-free survival at 45 months is 29% (Dini *et al.*, 1990). TBI is still in use in many pre-transplant regimens but its contribution has not yet been evaluated in prospective randomized studies.

In summary, high-dose chemotherapy – with or without TBI – is able to prolong survival in a small group of children with Stage 4 neuroblastoma who have their metastatic sites cleared by chemotherapy *before* embarking on megatherapy. Since short- and long-term side effects, including second malignancies, are already reported, megatherapy should still be considered as an area of clinical research.

17.8.4 SURGERY

Previously, only children with localized disease were subjected to surgery. At present, even children with advanced localized or metastatic diseases are treated surgically. Metastases may be cleared by chemotherapy, leaving only a small primary tumour to be excised. These operations are frequently very difficult, but complete or near-complete excision is now possible for the majority of patients. Furthermore, the role of the surgeon is essential in primarily unresectable Stage 3

neuroblastoma. All patients should undergo a second or even a third operation if the primary tumour continues to respond to chemotherapy and complete resection becomes feasible (Haase *et al.*, 1989).

17.8.5 RADIOTHERAPY

Theoretically, external beam radiotherapy may be used for residual tumour. Some tumours may, however, recur within the field of radiotherapy. Moreover, the long-term side effects of radiotherapy given to small children are now well recognized. Two kinds of radiotherapy treatments are particularly used in neuroblastoma patients. As part of the ablative regimen in poor prognosis patients total body irradiation is used prior to bone marrow transplantation. Secondly, radio-nuclide treatment using *m*IBG labelled with iodine-131 has been successful as targeted radiotherapy in the treatment of neuroblastoma. The immediate results are quite impressive: 50% of Stage 4 patients, heavily pretreated and resistant to chemotherapy, do respond to ^{131}I-*m*IBG (Rome Workshop, 1986). Additionally, Mastrangelo *et al.* (1989) have reported on a ten-month-old child with Stage 3 neuroblastoma who is alive, with no evidence of disease, 18 months from diagnosis: that particular child was treated only with ^{131}I-*m*IBG.

17.8.6 TREATMENT BY STAGE

(a) Stage 1:

These tumours are often discovered by chance: the homolateral Claude Bernard Horner's syndrome associated with a cervical tumour may be the only sign. Surgery alone is curative for Stage 1 tumours. Furthermore, surgery will permit a precise histological diagnosis and confirmation of the stage. Long-term follow-up of these children is nevertheless necessary to make sure that there is no local recurrence of the disease or distant metastases.

(b) Stage 2a:

These tumours are curable by surgery involving an approach identical in all respects to that for Stage 1. Microscopic residual tumour tissue following surgery is probably not an indication for adjuvant therapy in Stage 2a disease. Two studies have indeed shown that the disease-free survival of children with Stage 2a neuroblastoma is 100% whether they are given post-operative treatment or not (Ninane *et al.*, 1982; Hayes *et al.*, 1983). The only exception is the 'dumb-bell' form of paravertebral neuroblastoma, in which case adjuvant chemo- or radiotherapy may be given. There is, however, no evidence that this peculiar form of neuroblastoma needs a different therapeutic approach.

(c) Stage 2b:

In contrast, surgical treatment should be followed by chemotherapy in children with this stage, according to their ages. It is not clear whether chemotherapy is needed in children under six months as their young age is an independent favourable prognostic factor. The advantage of youth diminishes between six months and one year, warranting 'conventional' (vincristine and cyclosphosphamide) chemotherapy of short duration. The prognosis for children over one year of age with Stage 2b is intermediate to that of Stage 2a and advanced neuroblastoma. More intensive chemotherapy is thus necessary (Ninane *et al.*, 1982; Hayes *et al.*, 1983).

(d) Stage 3 (when unresectable) and Stage 4:

Metastatic tumours have to be treated with chemotherapy and surgery (and possibly radiotherapy). Children with Stage 4 disease who are more than one year old at diagnosis should be considered for investigational protocols, as effective treatment for all of them remains elusive, and thus specific recommendations regarding drug treatment cannot be made. Two principles are, however, of importance and should be taken into account: (1) aggressive surgery is essential in Stage 3; (2) Stage 4 disease patients less than one year old have a better prognosis than older children and probably do not need intensification chemotherapy with bone marrow rescue.

To date, no initial chemotherapy combination has been proven to be superior to the basic OPEC regimen (vincristine, *cis*platin, etoposide, cyclophosphamide) (Shafford *et al.*, 1984) despite recent variations (Pinkerton *et al.*, 1990; Hartmann *et al.*, 1988; Bernard *et al.*, 1987).

(e) Stage 4S:

Children – and much more often infants – with the classic Stage 4S disease, showing metastasis to the skin, bone marrow and liver, have usually a good prognosis (Table 18.2). Chemotherapy is indicated if significant liver involvement or bone marrow infiltration is present. This chemotherapy is usually 'à la carte': a few courses of vincristine and cyclophosphamide preceding or following surgery to the primary tumour is usually sufficient. However, rarely, some patients are resistant to this treatment and need a more aggressive chemotherapy approach.

17.9 CONCLUSIONS

Although the two-year disease-free survival of children with advanced neuroblastoma has increased over the past decades, thanks to intensive treatment, it is still far too low. The outcome for children older than one year of age with Stage 4 neuroblastoma remains poor. The long-term disease-free survival was about 5% in the early sixties (when only vincristine and cyclophosphamide were available) and around 10–20% in the seventies (after the introduction of multiagent chemotherapy, surgery and radiotherapy). The use of late intensification-megatherapy followed by bone marrow transplantation in good responders has had only a marginal effect on the cure rate: only 20% of Stage 4 children older than one year are likely to be long-term survivors. Besides chemotherapy, surgery and radiotherapy, other types of treatment therefore should be explored, preferably in children with no evidence of clinical disease after consolidation therapy: they include the following: 'targeting' with radiolabelled *m*IBG or monoclonal antibodies, adoptive immunotherapy with tumour necrosis factor (TNF), or lymphokine-activated killer cells (LAK) and different 'maturating agents' (retinoids). Their respective roles – together with the place of 'megatherapy' – are discussed in later chapters of this book.

17.10 CURRENT CONTROVERSIES

17.10.1 IS SCREENING FOR NEUROBLASTOMA IN INFANTS OF ANY VALUE?

This issue has been widely debated following suggestions by workers in Kyoto, and then nationally in Japan, that the incidence of Stage 4 disease had been dramatically reduced by screening of infants using urinary catecholamines (Sawada, 1984; Woods and Tuchman 1987). The main objection to this strategy is the undoubted overdiagnosis of 'disease' in infants. It is clear from the Japanese data that the incidence of neuroblastoma was increased by the introduction of screening, and that a number of children were subjected to what was almost certainly unnecessary laparotomies

and, in some cases, chemotherapy and radiotherapy. The likely spontaneous resolution of the majority of small primary tumours in this age group makes the development of management strategies difficult once raised catecholamines have been observed. The current conclusion by an international review group is that, while it is worth continuing prospective studies in view of the significance of their findings with regard to the biology and natural history of this disease, there is no clear supportive evidence for a more general acceptance of this strategy (Murphy, 1991).

17.10.2 ARE THERE ADVERSE RISK FACTORS WITHIN THE INSS STAGING SYSTEM?

Although the majority of Stage 4S patients will resolve spontaneously and remain free of disease, a small number will die due to complications associated with the initial disease. These complications are largely avoidable by intensive supportive care and perhaps also low dose chemotherapy or radiotherapy. It is possible that patients who subsequently recur and develop true Stage 4 disease show adverse biological features, such as n-*myc* amplification and diploid-tetraploid karyotype. It has been suggested that in the presence of n-*myc* amplification, a Stage 4S patient should be treated with aggressive systemic chemotherapy (Bourhis, 1989).

The relevance of node positivity in Stage II patients remains debatable. It has been suggested that node-positive patients do significantly worse and should therefore be given adjuvant chemotherapy (Ninane, 1982; Hayes, 1983). This view has been questioned and other data indicate that there is no significant difference between these two groups of patients (Rosen, 1984). However, the need for surgical node assessment still is debated (Castleberry, 1991).

The outcome of Stage 3 patients varies widely between the international groups, ranging from 20 to 60%. Only a minority of patients will have n-*myc* amplification, and completeness of surgery following chemotherapy appears to be an important prognostic factor (Haase, 1989). The need for intensification of chemotherapy with megatherapy and autograft remains debatable, and it seems likely that it is necessary where complete resection of tumour is not achieved.

Within the Stage 4 group, recent analyses have revealed that factors such as n-*myc* and ploidy may identify patients with up to a 50% chance of long-term survival. If this is borne out in larger studies there may be a subgroup where high morbidity therapy may not be necessary, and conversely a subgroup with a prognosis so bleak that it is appropriate to carry out innovative phase II studies at the onset of treatment.

17.10.3 DOES SURGERY HAVE ANY SIGNIFICANT ROLE IN STAGE 4 DISEASE?

Traditionally, prolonged aggressive surgery is undertaken following initial chemotherapy in patients with Stage 4 disease who have cleared their distant metastases with intensive chemotherapy. Because of the overall poor outcome, the role of prolonged surgical procedures has been questioned (Malone, 1990). It seems probable that complete resection of tumour is of value in patients who have truly achieved complete remission at metastatic sites, similar to its beneficial role in Stage 3 patients. This beneficial effect is, however, blurred by the inability of systemic chemotherapy to ablate all micrometastatic disease which remains despite an apparently complete clinical remission. It seems likely that chemosensitive patients will also have tumours which can be resected within three to four hours' operating time; the six to seven hour procedures simply reflect the lack of chemosensitivity and are almost certainly not worthwhile.

17.10.4 IS THERE A ROLE FOR RADIOTHERAPY IN STAGE 3 AND 4 DISEASE?

The contribution of radiation treatment to macroscopic or microscopic residual disease in Stage 2 patients has been shown to be insignificant (Matthay, 1989). Randomized studies in Stage 3 patients indicate that it may be beneficial (Castleberry, 1989). Targeted radiotherapy using radiolabelled *m*IBG or G_{D2} antibody is under evaluation and may have a useful role in both Stage 3 and 4 disease (Klingebiel, 1989; Cheung, 1989).

17.10.5 WHO BENEFITS FROM DOSE ESCALATION?

In one of the few prospective randomized studies evaluating the role of dose escalation, high dose melphalan significantly prolonged progression-free survival (Pritchard *et al.*, 1986; Pinkerton, 1987). Dose escalation is usually ineffective, following recurrent disease, although some long-term survivors who were transplanted in CR2 do exist. Specific subgroups may benefit (Philip *et al.*, 1991) but there is clearly a need for further randomized studies (Shuster *et al.*, 1991). It is possible that multiple procedures using bone marrow growth factors may be a therapeutic option in the future (Neidhart *et al.*, 1989) and high dose intensity regimens without marrow rescue appear promising (Cheung and Heller, 1991; Pearson *et al.*, 1990).

17.10.6 *m*IBG IMAGING: IS IT OF CLINICAL VALUE?

[131I]*m*IBG is a useful diagnostic tool in patients whose tumour diagnosis is equivocal. However, in the vast majority of patients there is little doubt about the diagnosis on the basis of histology and urinary catecholamines. [131I]*m*IBG scanning at presentation is unlikely to upstage a significant number of patients who have adequate bone marrow evaluation and technetium bone scan. It does, however, have a useful role for evaluation of minimal residual disease following chemotherapy. This may be of importance in deciding whether an autologous bone marrow procedure is appropriate, as it may detect minimal residual bone marrow involvement not detected on routine cytology and histology. Moreover, at this stage, [131]I*m*IBG therapy to [131]I*m*IBG positive disease is probably of benefit. Despite initial suggestions to the contrary, there is no doubt that false negative *m*IBG scans may occur, particularly in patients who have a more differentiated component to their tumour; conversely, false positive scans may result from a highly differentiated but inactive residual tumour.

17.10.7 IS THERE A ROLE FOR *CIS*RETINOIC ACID?

*Cis*retinoic acid has been shown to produce ganglionic differentiation in undifferentiated neuroblastoma cell lines (Hill, 1986). Although there are anecdotal reports of clinical responses in patients with measurable marrow disease, its efficacy in this context is unlikely to be dramatic. It may, however, have a role in patients with minimal residual disease, and this is being evaluated by the European Neuroblastoma Study Group (ENSG V) in a placebo controlled double blind study where children are given *cis*retinoic acid for a two-year period following attainment of CR or VGPR (Lie, 1990).

C.R.P.

ACKNOWLEDGEMENTS

Photographs of histopathology have been provided by Dr S. Gosseye and of imaging by Dr Ph. Clapuyt. Their contribution to the illustration of this chapter is greatly appreciated.

REFERENCES

Bayle, C., Allard, T., Roday, C. *et al.* (1985). Detection of bone marrow involvement by neuroblastoma: comparison of two cytological methods. *Eur. Paediatr. Haematol. Oncol.*, **2** 123–8.

Beckwith, J.B. and Martin, R.F. (1968) Observations on the histopathology of neuroblastomas. *J. Pediatr. Surg.*, **3**, 106–10.

Bernard, J.L., Philip, T., Zucker, J.M. *et al.* (1987) Sequential cisplatin/VM26 and vincristine/cyclophosphamide/doxorubicin in metastatic neuroblastoma: an effective alternating non-cross resistant regimen? *J. Clin. Oncol.*, **5**, 1952–9.

Bodian, M. (1959) Neuroblastoma. *Pediatr. Clin. North Am.*, **6**, 449.

Bourhis, J., Hartmann, O., Benard, J. *et al.* (1989) Relapse from a Stage IV-S neuroblastoma and N-*myc* amplification. *Eur. J. Cancer Clin. Oncol.*, **25**(11), 1653–5.

Brodeur, G.M. Seeger, R.C., Barrett, A. *et al.* (1988) International criteria for diagnosis, staging and response to treatment in patients with neuroblastoma. *J. Clin. Oncol.*, **6**, 1874–81.

Carli, M., Green, A.A., Hayes, F.A. *et al.* (1982) Therapeutic efficacy of single drugs for childhood neuroblastoma: a review, in *Pediatric Oncology*. (eds E. Raybaud, R. Clément, G. Lebreuil, J.L. Bernard) Excerpta Medica, Amsterdam, pp. 141–50.

Castleberry, L., Kun, J., Shuster, G., *et al.* (1991) Radiotherapy (RT) improves the outlook for children older than 1 year with POG stage C neuroblastoma (NB). *J. Clin. Oncol.*, **9**, 789–95.

Castleberry, R.P., Smith, E.I., Cantor, A. *et al.* (1991) Surgico-pathologic staging of neuroblastoma. *J. Clin. Oncol.* **9** (1), 189–93.

Cheung, N-K.V., Munn, D., Kushner, B.H. *et al.* (1989) Targeted radiotherapy and immunotherapy of human neuroblastoma with G_{D2} specific monoclonal antibodies. *Nucl. Med. Biol.*, **16** (2), 111–20.

Cheung, N-K.V. and Heller, G. (1991) Chemotherapy dose intensity correlates strongly with response, median survival and median progression-free survival in metastatic neuroblastoma. *J. Clin. Oncol.*, **9**, 1050–8.

Cohen, M.D., Klatte, E.C., Baehner, R. *et al.* (1984) Magnetic resonance imaging of bone marrow disease in children. *Radiology*, **151**, 715–18.

Cooper, E.H., Pritchard, J., Bailey, C. and Ninane, J. (1987) Serum neurone-specific enolase in children's cancer. *Br. J. Cancer*, **56**, 65–7.

D'Angio, G.J., August, C., Elkins, W. *et al.* (1985) Metastatic neuroblastoma managed by supralethal therapy and bone marrow reconstitution. Results of a four-institutions Children's Cancer Study Group pilot study, in *Advances in Neuroblastoma Research*, (eds A.E. Evans, G.J. D'Angio, R. Seeger) Liss, New York, pp. 557–63.

Dargeon, H.W. (1962) Neuroblastoma. *J. Pediatr.*, **61**, 456–71.

de Kraker, J., Pritchard, J., Hartmann, O. and Ninane, J. (1987) Single-agent Ifosfamide in patients with recurrent neuroblastoma. (ENSG Study 2). *Pediatr. Hematol. Oncol.*, **4**, 101–4.

de la Monte, S.M., Moore, G.W. and Hutchins, G.M. (1983) Non random distribution of metastases in neuroblastic tumours. *Cancer*, **52**, 915–20.

Dini, G., Garaventa, A., Lanino, E. *et al.* (1990) Marrow ablative therapy (MAT) and unpurged autologous bone marrow transplantation (ABMT) for neuroblastoma (NB): an update of 34 patients. SIOP XXII – Rome, Italy 2–5 October 1990. *Med. Pediatr. Oncol.*, **18**, 389–90 (abstract).

Evans, A.E., D'Angio, G.J. and Randolph, J. (1971) A proposed staging for children with neuroblastoma. Children's Cancer Study Group A. *Cancer*, **27**, 374–8.

Evans, A.E., D'Angio, G.J., Propert, K. *et al.* (1987) Prognostic factors in neuroblastoma. *Cancer*, **59**, 1853–9.

Franklin, I.M. and Pritchard, J. (1983) Detection of bone marrow invasion by neuroblastoma is improved by sampling two sites with both aspirates and trephine biopsies. *J. Clin. Pathol.*, **36**, 1215–18.

Gelfand, M.J. and Hoefnagel, C.A. (1988), in *Textbook of Pediatric Radiology*.

Gitlow, S.E., Dziedzig, L.G., Strauss, L. *et al.* (1973) Biochemical and histologic determinants in the prognosis of neuroblastoma. *Cancer*, **32**, 898–905.

Gahr, M. and Hunneman, D.H. (1987) The value of determination of homovanillic and vanillylmandelic acids in plasma for the diagnosis and follow-up of neuroblastoma in children. *Eur. J. Pediatr.*, **146**, 489–93.

Gross, R.E., Farber, S. and Martin, L.W. (1959) Neuroblastoma sympatheticum: a study and report of 217 cases. *Pediatrics*, **23**, 1179.

Haase, G.M., Wong K.Y., de Lorimier, A.A. *et al.* (1989) Improvement in survival after excision of primary tumor in stage III neuroblastoma. *J. Pediatr. Surg.*, **24**, 194–200.

Hann, H.L., Evans, A.E., Siegel, S.E. *et al.* (1985) Prognostic importance of serum ferritin in patients with stage III and IV neuroblastoma: the Children's Cancer Study Group experience. *Cancer Res.*, **45**, 2843–8.

Hann, H.L., Stahlut, M.W. and Evans, A.E. (1986) Source of increased ferritin in neuroblastoma: studies with cocanavillin A-sepharose binding. *J. Natl. Cancer Inst.*, **76**, 1031–3.

Hartmann, O., Kalifa, C. and Beaujean, F. (1985) Treatment of advanced neuroblastoma with two consecutive high-dose chemotherapy regimens and ABMT, in *Advances in Neuroblastoma Research* (eds A.E. Evans, G.J. D'Angio and R.D. Seeger) Liss, New York, pp. 565–8.

Hartmann, O., Pinkerton, C.R., Philip, T. *et al.* (for ENSG) (1988) Very high dose cisplatin and etoposide in children with untreated, advanced neuroblastoma. *J. Clin. Oncol.*, **2**, 742–6.

Hayes, F., Green, A., Hutsu, O. *et al.* (1983) Surgicopathologic staging of neuroblastoma: Prognostic significance of regional lymph node metastases. *J. Pediatr.*, **102**, 59–62.

Hill, B.T. (1986) Neuroblastoma – an overview of laboratory studies aimed at inducing tumor regression by initiation of differentiation or administration of antitumor drugs. *Pediatr. Hematol. Oncol.*, **3** 73–88.

Hoefnagel, C.A., Voûte, P.A., de Kraker, J. and Marcuse, H.R. (1987) Radionuclide diagnosis and treatment of neural crest tumours using iodine-131-meta-iodobenzylguanidine. *J. Nucl. Med.*, **28**, 308–14.

Hugues, M., Marsden, H.B. and Palmer, M.K. (1974). Histologic patterns of neuroblastoma related to prognosis and clinical staging. *Cancer*, **34**, 1706–11.

Kemshead, J.T. and Pritchard, J. (1984) Neuroblastoma: recent developments and current challenges. *Cancer Surv.*, **3**, 691–708.

Klingebiel, T., Treuner, J. Ehninger, G. *et al.* (1989) [131I]-Meta-iodobenzylguanidine in the treatment of metastatic neuroblastoma. Clinical, pharmacological and dosimetric aspects. *Cancer Chem. Pharmacol.*, **25**, 143–8.

Krivit, W., Mirkin, B.L., Freier, E. *et al.* (1980)

Serum catecholamine metabolites in stage IV neuroblastoma, in *Advances in Neuroblastoma Research*, (ed. A.E. Evans) Raven Press, New York, pp. 33–42.

Ladisch, S. and Wu, Z.L. (1985) Shedding of G_{D2} ganglioside by human neuroblastoma. *Int. J. Cancer.*, **39**, 73–6.

Lie, S.O. (1990) 13-*Cis* retinoic acid as continuation therapy in children with advanced neuroblastoma in complete or good partial remission. A toxicity study. *Med. Paed. Oncol.*, **18** (5), 384.

Look, A.T., Hayes, F.A., Nitschke, R. *et al.* (1984) Cellular DNA content as predictor of response to chemotherapy in infants with unresectable neuroblastoma. *N. Engl. J. Med.*, **311**, 231–5.

Malone, P.S., Marwaha, R.K., Kiely, E.M. *et al.* (1990) The role of radical surgery in the management of advanced abdominal neuroblastoma. *Med. Pediatr. Oncol.* **18** (5), 377.

Mastrangelo, R., Trocone, L., Lasorella, A. *et al.* (1989) ^{131}I-Meta-iodobenzylguanidine in the treatment of neuroblastoma at diagnosis. *Am. J. Pediatr. Hematol. Oncol.*, **11**, 28–31.

Matthay, K.K., Sather, H.N., Seeger, R.C. *et al.* (1989) Excellent outcome of Stage II neuroblastoma is independent of residual disease and radiation therapy. *J. Clin. Oncol.*, **7** (2), 236–44.

Murphy, S.B., Cohn, S.L., Craft, A.W. *et al.* (1991) Do children benefit from mass screening for neuroblastoma? Consensus statement from the American Cancer Society Workshop on Neuroblastoma Screening. *Lancet*, **337**, 344–6.

Neidhart, J., Mangalik, A., Kohler, W. *et al.* (1989) Granulocyte colony-stimulating factor stimulates recovery of granulocytes in patients receiving dose-intensive chemotherapy without bone marrow transplantation. *J. Clin. Oncol.*, **7** (11), 1685–92.

Ninane, J., Pritchard, J. and Malpas, J.S. (1981) Chemotherapy of advanced neuroblastoma: does adriamycin contribute? *Arch. Dis. Child.*, **56**, 544–8.

Ninane, J., Pritchard, J., Morris Jones, P.H. *et al.* (1982) Stage II neuroblastoma. Adverse prognostic significance of lymph node involvement. *Arch. Dis. Child.*, **57**(6), 438–42.

Ninane, J., Vangyseghem, S., Andre, F. *et al.* (1986) Long term survivors of advanced neuroblastoma: factors effecting prognosis. An ENSG study. (Abstract) International Society of Paediatric Oncology, XIII Meeting, Belgrade, Yugoslavia, September 15–20.

Nishi, M., Miyake, H., Takeda, T. *et al.* (1987) Effects of the mass screening of neuroblastoma in Sapparo City. *Cancer*, **60**, 433–6.

Oppedal, B.R., Brandtzaeg, P. and Kemshead, J.T. (1987) Immunohistochemical differentiation of neuroblastoma from other small round cell neoplasms of childhood using a panel of mono- and polyclonal antibodies. *Histopathol.*, **11**, 363–74.

Oppedal, B.R., Storm-Mathisen, I., Lie, S.O. *et al.* (1988) Prognostic factors in neuroblastoma. Clinical, histopathologic and immunohistochemical features and DNA ploidy in relation to prognosis. *Cancer*, **62**, 772–80.

Pearson, A.D.J., Pinkerton, C.R., Gerard, M. *et al.* (1990) High dose rapid schedule chemotherapy for disseminated neuroblastoma. *Med. Ped. Oncol.*, **18**, 384.

Philip, T., Ghalie, R., Pinkerton, R. *et al.*, (1987a) A phase II study of high dose *Cis*platinum and VP16 in neuroblastoma. *J. Clin. Oncol.*, **5**, 941–50.

Philip, T. Zucker, J.M. Bernard, J.C. *et al.* (1990) High-dose chemotherapy with BMT as consolidation treatment in neuroblastoma – The LMCE1 unselected group of patients revisited with a median follow-up of 55 months after BMT. SIOP XXII – Rome, Italy 2–5 October, 1990. *Med. Pediatri. Oncol.*, **18**, 385 (abstract).

Philip, T., Zucker, J.M., Bernard, J.L. *et al.* (1991) Improved survival at 2 and 5 years in the LMCE unselected group of 72 children with Stage IV neuroblastoma older than 1 year of age at diagnosis: Is cure possible in a small subgroup? *J. Clin. Oncol.*, **9**, 1037–44.

Philip, T., Bernard, J.L., Zucker, J.M. *et al.*, (1987b) High dose chemo-radiotherapy with bone marrow transplantation as consolidation treatment in neuroblastoma: an unselected group of stage IV patients over 1 year of age. *J. Clin. Oncol.*, **5**, 266–72.

Pinkerton, C.R., Zucker, J.M., Hartmann, O. *et al.* (1990) Short duration, high dose, alternating chemotherapy in metastatic neuroblastoma (ENSG 3C induction regimen). *Br. J. Cancer*, **62**, 319–23.

Pinkerton, C.R., Lewis, I.J., Pearson, A.D.J. *et al.* (1989) Carboplatin or Cisplatin *Lancet*, **ii**, 161 (letter).

Pinkerton, C.R., Pritchard, J. deKraker, J. *et al.* (1987) ENSG 1 – Randomised study of high dose melphalan in neuroblastoma, in *Autologous Bone Marrow Transplantation* (eds K.A. Dicke, G. Spitzer and S. Jagonnoth) University of Texas Press, pp. 401–5.

Pritchard, J., Germond, F.N. and Jones, D. (1986) High dose melphalan (HDM) of value in treatment of advanced neuroblastoma (AN): preliminary review results of a randomized trial by the European Neuroblastoma Study Group (ENSG). Proceedings ASCO, p. 205.

Prorok, P.C. and Connor, R.J. (1986) Screening for the early detection of cancer. *Cancer Invest.*, **4**, 225–38.

Rome Workshop 1986 (1987) ^{131}I-Meta-iodobenzyl-guanidine in therapy, diagnosis and monitoring of neuroblastoma. *Med. Pediatr. Oncol.*, **15**, 4.

Rosen E.M., Cassady, J.R., Kretschmar, C. *et al.* (1984) Influence of local-regional lymph node metastases on prognosis in neuroblastoma. *Med. Pediatr. Oncol.*, **12** 260–3.

Sawada, T., Nakata, T., Takasugi, N. *et al.* (1984) Mass screening for neuroblastoma in infants in Japan. Interim report of a Mass Screening Study Group. *Lancet*, 271–3.

Sawada, T. and Tuchman, M. (1987) Mass screening for neuroblastoma in infants in Japan: Interim report of a mass screening study group. *Lancet*, **ii**, 271–3.

Schochat, S., Corbelletta, N., Repman, M. and Schengrund, C.L. (1987) A biochemical analysis of thoracic neuroblastomas: a pediatric oncology group study. *J. Pediatr. Surg.*, **22**, 660–4.

Seeger, R.C., Brodeur, G.M., Sathe, H. *et al.* (1985) Association of multiple copies of the N-*myc* oncogene with rapid progression of neuroblastomas. *N. Engl. J. Med.*, **313**, 1111–16.

Shafford, E.A., Roger, D.W. and Pritchard, J. (1984) Advanced neuroblastoma: improved response-rate using a multiagent regimen (OPEC) including sequential *cis*platinum and VM26. *J. Clin. Oncol.*, **5**, 1952–9.

Shimada, H., Chatten, J., Newton, W.A. *et al.* (1984) Histopathologic prognostic factors in neuroblastic tumours. Definition of subtypes of ganglio-neuroblastoma and an age-linked classification of neuroblastomas. *J. Natl. Cancer Inst.*, **73**, 405–9.

Shuster, J.J., Cantor, A.B., McWilliams, N. *et al.* (1991) The prognostic significance of autologous bone marrow transplant in advanced neuroblastoma. *J. Clin. Oncol.*, **9**, 1045–9.

Siegel, S.E., Laug, W.E., Harlow, P.J. *et al.* (1980) Patterns of urinary catecholamine metabolite excretion in neuroblastoma, in *Advances in Neuroblastoma Research*, (ed. A.E. Evans) Raven Press, New York, pp. 25–32.

Stella, J.G., Schweisguth, O. and Schlienger, M. (1970) Neuroblastoma: a study of 144 cases treated in the Institute Gustave Roussy over a period of 7 years. *Am. J. Roetgenol.*, **108**, 324.

Sugimoto, T., Tatsumi, E., Kemshead, J.T. *et al.* (1984) Determination of cell surface membrane antigens, common to both human neuroblastoma and leukemia-lymphoma cells lines by a panel of 38 monoclonal antibodies. *J. Natl. Cancer Inst.*, **73**, 51–7.

Tuchman, M., Morris, L., Ramnaraine, M. *et al.* (1985) Value of random urinary homovanillic acid and vanillylmandelic acid levels in the diagnosis and management of patients with neuroblastoma: comparison with 24-hour urine collections. *Pediatrics*, **75**, 324–8.

Tuchman, M., Ramnaraine, M., Woods, W. and Krivit, W. (1987) Three years of experience with random urinary homovanillic and vanillylmandelic acid levels in the diagnosis of neuroblastoma. *Pediatrics*, **79**, 203–5.

UICC-TNM (1987) *Classification of malignant tumours*. 4th edn, Springer Verlag, Berlin.

Wilson, L.M.K. and Draper, G.J. (1974) Neuroblastoma: its natural history and prognosis – a study of 487 cases. *Br. Med. J.*, **3**, 301.

Woods, W.G. and Tuchman, M. (1987) Neuroblastoma: the case for screening infants in North America. *Pediatrics*, **79**, 869–73.

Zeltzer, P.M., Marangos, P.J., Evans, A.E. *et al.* (1986) Serum neurone-specific enolase in children with neuroblastoma. Relationship to stage and disease course. *Cancer*, **57**, 1230–4.

Chapter 18

Wilms' tumour and renal carcinoma

J. DE KRAKER

18.1 HISTORICAL INTRODUCTION

In his classical monograph of 1899, Wilms reviewed the literature of kidney tumours in children (Wilms, 1899). Since then these tumours have been known as Wilms' tumours. Over the years, this tumour has served as a model for progress in treatment results, as well as for significant advances in the knowledge of pathology, genetics and histogenetics. One of the main problems concerning this tumour is to determine the level of treatment needed to cure the patient at low risk and to ensure that patients survive as healthy young adults.

18.2 HISTOLOGY AND GENETICS

Wilms' tumour (WT), also called nephroblast-oma, originates in the developing renal tissue, the metanephrogenic blastema. At birth the blastema has vanished in most newborns; in many patients with WT, however, it can still be found. This persisting and proliferating blastema is considered to be a possible substrate for tumour development.

WT is often found in combination with congenital anomalies. A Japanese study showed congenital anomalies in 58% of patients with this tumour (Nakissa *et al.*, 1985). In a Dutch study, reporting 38.3% of congenital anomalies of the genito-urinary tract among 133 patients, a comparison was made between the incidence of each detected malformation in a group of patients and in the general population. Some anomalies appeared to be specifically associated with nephroblastoma. As a possible explanation

Table 18.1 Incidence of congenital anomalies in patients with WT

	Lemerle 1976a N=248	Pendergrass 1976 N=547	Pastore 1989 N=1040	Total N=2170	%
Aniridia	4	6	11	21	0.97
Hemihypertrophy	4	16	32	52	2.40
Genitourinary anomaly	19	24	59	102	4.70

for this relationship it has been suggested that these defects share the same basic embryological disorder (Smeets *et al.*, 1989). In support of this hypothesis, a disproportionately high incidence of sporadic aniridia, hemihypertrophy, and the renal anomalies mentioned above has been observed in WT (Table 18.1).

A number of examples of WT occurring in monozygous twins have been reported (Maurer *et al.*, 1979). Sometimes WT has been found in only one of the children, with none of the stated abnormalities. In another example, aniridia with psychomotor retardation was present in both children, but WT was found in only one of them. These findings are consistent with the two-mutation model first proposed by Knudson and Strong (1972) – assuming that both twins share an inherited gene predisposing to WT. The second mutational event, however, which is also necessary for tumour development, occurred in only one of them. The observation that certain abnormalities are associated with WT indicates that there are hereditary and sporadic forms of this tumour. The increasing rate of long-term survivors will consequently increase our insight into the genetic patterns of inheritance of WT and its related somatic abnormalities. In sporadic aniridia patients, 33% will go on to develop WT (Brodeur, 1984). Of these, 5% are bilateral. The combination of a higher frequency of bilaterality and occurrence of WT at an earlier age in patients with sporadic aniridia, supports the hypothesis that aniridia and Wilms' tumours are linked by the heritable form of mutation (Mesrobian, 1988).

The aniridia-Wilms' tumour association (AWTA) has become a known clinical syndrome with more than 50 patients reported until 1978, when a small interstitial deletion of band 11p13 was found to be the underlying defect (Riccardi *et al.*, 1978). The fact that not all children with constitutional del(11)p(13) develop a Wilms' tumour is evi-dence that either additional genetic changes are required for complete transformation to the malignant phenotype (Mannens *et al.*, 1988) or that small, as yet undetected differences exist in the size of the deletion (Slater, 1986).

18.3 EPIDEMIOLOGY

The incidence of WT is remarkably constant among the different countries on both sides of the Atlantic (Table 18.2). The frequency of WT among boys and girls is approximately equal. At the time of diagnosis 75% of the patients are less than five years of age. There is no significant difference in occurrence rate between children of diverse ethnic background and geographic location. This has made WT the index tumour of childhood cancer distribution. However, recent reports on an increase in risk of WT for the offspring of fathers exposed to certain chemicals, have cast doubt on this (Terracini, 1983).

Table 18.2 Incidence of Wilms' tumour

	Rate*
Finland	9.5
Sweden	8.3
USA	7.8
Australia (Queensland)	7.2
Italy (Turin)	6.5
The Netherlands	6.5
UK (Manchester)	5.1

* Cases/10^6 children less than 15 years of age/year

18.4 PATHOLOGY

Macroscopically, Wilms' tumour presents as an expansive, in most cases encapsulated, tumour causing deformation of the pyelocalyceal cavities. The tumour is often large and heterogeneous, with pseudocystic, necrotic and haemorrhagic parts. In rare cases the cut-surface shows many thin-

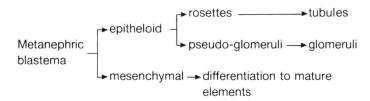

Fig. 18.1 Normal differentiation of metanephric blastema.

walled cysts: the so-called multicystic type of nephroblastoma. It is possible to have invasion of surrounding tissues: renal vein, the inferior vena cava, and with even atrial involvement, the renal pelvis, and the ureter (Ritchey *et al.* 1988). In 7–10% of cases it involves regional lymph nodes and distant metastases formed by haematogeneous spread.

Microscopically, three elements are nearly always present. These are undifferentiated blastema and, differentiating from this structure, epithelial and stromal elements (Fig. 18.1). Central reviewing is one of the important advantages of the national and international study groups. This has allowed pathologists to discriminate between prognostically favourable, normal, and poor risk groups.

The panel of pathologists of the International Society of Paediatric Oncology (SIOP) consider the multicystic, tubular, and fibroadenomatous types as having favourable histology. Tumours with foci of marked cytological atypism (anaplasia) and those with predominantly sarcomatous stroma – the bone metastasizing clear cell sarcoma of kidney (CCSK) – have an unfavourable prognosis.

The 'rhabdoid' variant is considered separately (see below).

18.5 CLINICAL PRESENTATION

A Wilms' tumour is discovered more often by the parents than by the physician. The firm, irregular abdominal mass is often the only clinical sign. Other presenting symptoms are non-specific and include: gastrointestinal

Table 18.3 Necessary investigations for the diagnosis of WT (in Amsterdam)

	Investigation	*Purpose*
Day one	1. Start to collect 24-hr. urine while on a standardized diet	To exclude neuroblastoma without interference by contrast medium; to establish kidney function and test for haematuria and tumour cells
	2. Ultrasound	To establish if this is an intrarenal process; is it cystic or solid? To look for the opposite kidney
	3. Plain x-ray of the chest	To exclude pulmonary metastases
Day two	Intravenous urogram + lateral view	Is it retroperitoneal, intrarenal with calyces displaced and deformed?

upset, fever, and abdominal pain. Haematuria occurs in one out of four patients. This is the case when the tumour penetrates the calyceal cavity. Such tumours originate close to the renal pelvis and are diagnosed in an early phase which explains the favourable outcome in most of the patients with this symptom.

After taking the history, paying special attention to the use of drugs in the prenatal period, symptoms suggestive of recent infections, and the family history of neoplasia, one should look for congenital aniridia, hemihypertrophy of the whole body or part of it and urogenital malformations. The kidneys are normally obscured for the palpating hand by muscles on the back with the liver and intestines covering them in the front. This helps to explain why WT is often discovered in a relatively late stage. It also explains why, when gently palpating this tumour, the intestines can be felt moving under one's hand. This is called by some people the 'Wilms' sign'. The diagnosis of WT can be made relatively quickly and unnecessary investigations can be avoided (Table 18.3). Only in cases in which there is still doubt in diagnosis after having followed this programme, should investigations such as computerized tomography (CT), renal-arteriography, or thin needle biopsy be considered. Finally, there are several diseases which can mimic WT, including neuroblastoma, cystic diseases of the kidney, and mesoblastic nephroma.

The definitive diagnosis can be made at laparotomy and after confirmation by the pathologist. At this point the stage of the tumour can be determined and the next therapeutical steps taken.

18.6 PROGNOSTIC FACTORS

A wide range of factors, including renal vein invasion, age of the patient, and histology have been studied to determine the likelihood of relapses among patients treated for WT.

Based on histology, three categories have been identified: unfavourable histology – with anaplastic elements and sarcomatous changes; favourable histology – the fibroadenomatous type and multicystic type and thirdly, the so-called standard histology. Other factors with poor prognostic implications are spread of the tumour and the presence of lymph node involvement. Survival rates decrease from Stage I through to Stage III. Patients with Stage IV or Stage V have survival rates of 83% and 70% respectively in the recent SIOP studies (de Kraker *et al.*, 1990; Coppes *et al.*, 1989).

18.7 RARE CLINICAL PRESENTATIONS

18.7.1 HYPERTENSION

Wilms' tumour is sometimes associated with arterial hypertension; a fall in blood pressure to the normal range can be observed after removal of the affected kidney. Reports of plasma renin activity in WT make it plausible that high plasma renin concentration contributes to this phenomenon (Voûte *et al.*, 1971). It has been shown that significant quantities of renin are found in the tumour tissue of pre operative hypertensive patients, despite the fact that no renin could be detected in the normal renal cortex of the affected kidney nor in the tumour tissue of two other normotensive patients with WT (Mitchell *et al.*, 1970).

18.7.2 NEPHROTIC SYNDROME

There are two different forms of nephrotic syndrome in combination with WT. Focal glomerulosclerosis as a late sequelae of WT is one of them (Welch and McAdams, 1986). Glomerular disease developed after ten to 20 years of disease-free survival. The causative factor is not known. The hypothesis is that progressive glomerular damage is the result of hyperfiltration, an adaptive part of compensatory hypertrophy after nephrectomy. Thus far, treatment has not been satisfactory; it may, however, be prudent to consider a low protein intake diet for children with multifocal nephroblastoma or who have had more than a unilateral nephrectomy.

The second form of nephrotic syndrome is the Drash-syndrome. This is a complex disorder characterized by diffuse mesangial sclerosis, abnormal sexual differentiation, and gonadal or renal neoplasms. Renal failure often progresses rapidly. The diagnosis of WT is seldom made after the age of 12 months and is bilateral in a large number of patients (Habib *et al.*, 1985; Manivel *et al.*, 1987).

18.7.3 THE BECKWITH-WIEDEMANN SYNDROME (BWS)

The criteria for the diagnosis of BWS are not precise. Children with a congenital assymmetry have the potential for development of neoplasia. It is important to recognize patients with incomplete forms of BWS because of this oncogenic potential.

18.8 CLASSIFICATION AND STAGING

At the beginning of this century, the survival

Table 18.4 Staging of Wilms' tumours

Stage	Definitions and comments
I	*Tumour limited to the kidney and completely excised* The renal capsule is intact. The tumour has not ruptured nor been punctured before its excision. No tumour is observed in the renal bed, and histological examination confirms that the capsule is intact.
II	*Tumour extends outside the kidney, but is completely excised* There is a local extension of the tumour, in particular: – penetration of the tumour into the perirenal tissues beyond the false capsule of the tumour and 'adhesions' that are confirmed histologically to be due to tumour – Invasion of the para-aortic nodes, confirmed histologically; the pathologist must make a careful search of all the excised nodes for foci of tumour cells. – Invasion of the renal vessel walls outside the kidney or thrombosis caused by tumour in these vessels. Thrombosis which is apparently non-neoplastic may contain islands of tumour cells; thrombi must be examined very carefully – Invasion of the renal pelvis and ureter
III	*Incomplete excision, without haematogenous metastases* This stage has been reached if one or several of the following conditions are present: – Tumour rupture before or during surgery – Peritoneal metastases, as distinguished from the simple tumour adhesions of Stage II – Invasion of lymph nodes beyond the abdominal periaortic nodes – Complete excision impossible (e.g. infiltration of the vena cava)
IV	*Haematogenous metastases* Involving lung, liver, bones, brain, etc.
V	*Bilateral renal tumours*

rate of WT when surgery only was performed was 8%. At that time the operative mortality rate was 23%. Those who were cured were probably the patients with what is now called Stage I disease. The stage of the disease remains one of the most important prognostic factors. In order to be able to make a comparison between several treatment modalities it is important for clinicians to agree the use of the same staging system.

Both the USA National Wilms' Tumour Study (NWTS) and the International Society of Paediatric Oncology (SIOP) use a classification as shown in Table 18.4 The TNM classification system is used by the International Union against Cancer (UICC). This system is based on the assessment of the following components:

T: the extent of the primary tumour;
N: the condition of the regional lymph nodes and in certain regions of the juxta-regional lymph nodes;
M: the absence or presence of distant metastases.

Table 18.5 TNM clinical stage-grouping

Stage I	T1	NO, NX	MO
Stage II	T2	NO, NX	MO
Stage III	T1,T2	N1	MO
	T3	Any N	MO
Stage IV	T1, T2, T3	Any N	M1
Stage V	T4	Any N	Any M

This system is used as a pre-treatment clinical classification and as a post-surgical histopathological (pTNM) classification. Moreover it is possible to use the TNM classification to group patients into the different stages (Table 18.5).

18.9 MANAGEMENT

Surgery, radiotherapy and chemotherapy are the three major modalities of treatment in children with Wilms' tumour. It is a continuing challenge to find out the best way of using and combining these treatment strategies.

The question of pre-operative treatment was investigated by the first clinical trial of

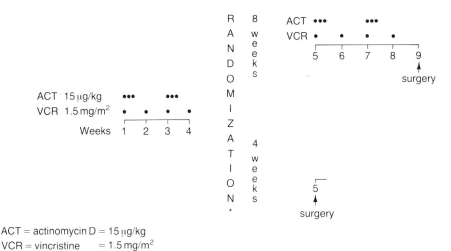

Fig. 18.2 The two pre-operative CT arms of SIOP-trial No. 9.

the International Society of Paediatric Oncology (SIOP). Pre-operative irradiation facilitated surgery and reduced the frequency of tumour spillage. Since whole abdominal irradiation is often given after tumour rupture, pre-operative therapy meant that fewer patients required large field irradiation. This observation was extended to pre-operative chemotherapy (CT) in SIOP study 5. Children with tumours confined to the kidney post chemotherapy were not irradiated. This means that abdominal irradiation can be avoided in half the number of patients. Encouraged by these results and the finding that only 1.5% of the registered patients were given CT for a benign lesion of the kidney,

Stage I: nephroblastoma > 6 months, standard histology and anaplasia

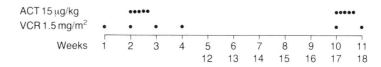

ACT = actinomycin D = 15 µg/kg
VCR = vincristine = 1.5 mg/m^2

Stage II N$^-$ (negative lymphnodes): nephroblastoma standard histology

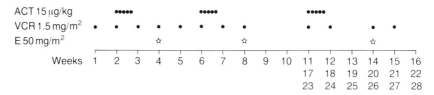

ACT = actinomycin D = 15 µg/kg
VCR = vincristine = 1.5 mg/m^2
E = epirubicin = 50 mg/m^2

Stage II N$^+$ (positive lymph nodes) and Stage III: nephroblastoma standard histology

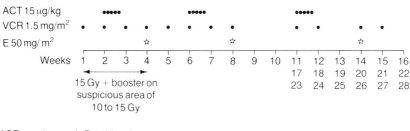

ACT = actinomycin D = 15 µg/kg
VCR = vincristine = 1.5 mg/m^2
E = epirubicin = 50 mg/m^2

Fig. 18.3 Post-operative treatment of Wilms' tumour (SIOP 9 protocol).

SIOP 9 study is looking at the effect of a prolonged pre-operative CT treatment (Fig. 18.2).

This policy is supported by the fact that in Stage IV patients with a prolonged and intensified pre-operative treatment, the number of Stage I abdominal tumours has increased. The approach of the National Wilms' Tumor Society (NWTS) is a different one. In this study pre-operative treatment is not employed. The reason for this lies in the fear of obscuring prognostic clues which govern management in individual patients. Both studies, however, showed very clearly the effectiveness of multiple courses of a combination of vincristine (VCR) and actinomycin D (ACT D) in that it lowered the proportion of cases with subsequent metastases from 50% to 20% (D'Angio *et al.*, 1976). The need to investigate which of the two drugs has an advantage over the other, as was done earlier, then became redundant.

The highest incidence of WT occurs in children aged between two and five years. In order to prevent unnecessary late sequelae, it is necessary to make as little use of aggressive treatment as possible. Both the NWTS and SIOP studies showed that Stage I normal risk patients need only a short post-operative treatment with two drugs (D'Angio *et al.*, 1989a,b).

The addition of adriamycin (ADR) in Stage II (with involved regional nodes) and in Stage III, decreased the incidence of relapse in these groups. As a consequence, WT is now pretreated in most parts of Europe with ACT D and VCR. What post-operative treatment is given, depends on the stage of the tumour and the histological report (Fig. 18.3). Management by stage is as follows:

Stage I: including anaplastic tumours will have a two-drug treatment of short duration;

Stage II: with negative lymph nodes will have a three-drug schedule of 28 weeks;

Stage II: with positive nodes and Stage III receive radiotherapy to the tumour bed as well as a three-drug regimen for 28 weeks.

18.9.1 TREATMENT OF PATIENTS WITH LUNG METASTASES AT DIAGNOSIS

A recent study by de Kraker *et al.* (1990) demonstrated that the majority of these children do not need lung irradiation routinely. After a six-week pre-operative three-drug regimen only those patients with persistent inoperable pulmonary metastases will be given radiotherapy and abdominal irradiation depending on the stage of the abdominal tumour.

18.9.2 BILATERAL CASES

In 5% of patients with WT, there is, at diagnosis, a tumour in both kidneys. Each case of synchronous bilateral WT needs individual therapy. It is highly recommended to treat these patients in centres experienced both in WT and the multi-modality approach to childhood malignancy.

To preserve renal function, chemotherapy plays a major role in shrinking the tumour, thereby opening the way to limited surgery and probably reducing the need for RT to what is left of both or one of the kidneys. Actinomycin D and vincristine will be the drugs of choice, but in case of minimal response, addition of other drugs is indicated.

18.9.3 TREATMENT OF RECURRENCES

In case of pulmonary metastases, surgery is indicated in patients with easily resectable tumours. If the excision is histologically complete, no RT is needed. Otherwise irradiation will be given to both lungs. Multiple or bulky disease needs a more intensive chemotherapy to start with. After the optimum response, local adjuvant surgery and radiotherapy are indicated in most of these patients.

18.9.4 NEW DRUGS IN WILMS' TUMOUR

In patients with recurrent disease, and in certain non-responding bilateral cases, the following new drugs have been used by some centres. Ifosfamide 3000 mg/m^2 for two consecutive days has been used, among others, by Tournade *et al.*, with six complete responses and five partial responses out of 21 patients (Tournade *et al.*, 1988). Carboplatin 400–600 mg/m^2 in one day or 800–1000 mg/m^2 in 4–5 days is now under study as is etoposide. So far small non-published results only exist, but it is worthwhile to continue studying these drugs as single agents or in combination.

It should be borne in mind that most of these patients have only one kidney at the time of the treatment. These drugs can be nephrotoxic and renal function should be monitored carefully during therapy.

18.10 COMPLICATIONS OF TREATMENT

New modes of multimodality treatment have increased the overall survival rate of patients with this disease. The long-term normal tissue toxicity of such therapy is well recognized. In WT, the tissues at risk are osseous, renal, pulmonary, hepatic and those of the reproductive organs. It should be added that the carcinogenic potential of chemotherapy and radiotherapy is now well recognized.

In a study by Dubousset among 59 consecutive Wilms' tumours treated between 1950 and 1963, 65% of the patients showed kyphosis of over 10%. Scoliosis was observed in 40% (Dubousset, 1980). In order to prevent these deformities, symmetric irradiation and early bracing are important. Evaluation is only possible after the growth spurt has occurred.

Late effects of renal origin, sometimes even ten years after ceasing treatment, include proteinuria as a consequence of a glomerulosclerosis, a rise in serum creatinine despite the compensatory hypertrophy of the contralateral kidney, and hypertension. Hypertension is nearly always observed in patients who have had abdominal irradiation.

After pulmonary irradiation, diffuse interstitial pneumonitis may sometimes have a prolonged course. The aetiology is unknown in the majority of these patients.

In a small number of patients, loss of renal function caused by the neoplasm, treatment, or both, necessitates haemodialysis or renal transplantation. There is no direct oncological reason not to put such a patient on haemodialysis or continuous ambulatory peritoneal dialysis. The time between dialysis and transplantation is important. Patients who received homografts less than a year after treatment of the tumours had a 47% incidence of recurrence or metastasis compared to a zero incidence of these problems in those whose transplants were delayed for a longer period (Penn, 1979). A disease-free period of two years after stopping therapy seems reasonable. Those who survive without evidence of disease can most probably be regarded as cured. However, judging from the results reported by DeMaria, and the increasingly successful hemi-nephrectomies, the best chance for a patient with extensive disease in both kidneys is conservative surgery which avoids the need for transplantation (DeMaria, 1979). In a retrospective cohort study of 47 WT survivors and their 77 sibling controls, female survivors had four times more risk for any adverse livebirth outcome, including birth defects, compared with their sibling controls (Byrne *et al.*, 1988).

Preliminary results from patients registered at the National Wilms' Tumour studies, demonstrate that the relative risk of a second malignant tumour is 10.8% among irradiated patients and 5% among nonirradiated patients (Breslow *et al.*, 1988).

18.11 OTHER MALIGNANT DISEASES OF THE KIDNEY

Renal carcinoma or Grawitz tumour is the only other malignant tumour that originates from the kidney. The incidence is very low in children. Among 1258 registered cases at the Wilms' tumour office of the SIOP, only 21 patients were diagnosed as having such a tumour. The age of these patients is normally higher than those with WT. An abdominal tumour is found after haematuria made the patient see the doctor. Without histology it is impossible to distinguish between this tumour and WT. The pre-operative treatment, therefore, will be the same as in WT. After the operation and the histopathological findings, RT (40–50 Gy) is advised for all patients with residual disease. In Stage I tumours, nephrectomy alone seems to be sufficient.

18.12 CONCLUSIONS AND CURRENT CONTROVERSIES

In the past (1930) only 10% of patients with a WT survived. Nowadays only around 10% of patients die. The aim now is to further increase survival and disease-free survival rates, and at the same time improve the quality of life of those who survive. This can be done both by looking carefully at prognostic markers and decreasing the amount of radiotherapy and chemotherapy in prognostically favourable cases. In high risk patients and relapsed patients, new effective drugs should be used. Attention should also be paid to new developments in the identification of children at risk of developing this disease. In this way the incidence rate may be reduced and in the future prevention of this disease may become a possibility.

18.12.3 PREOPERATIVE CHEMOTHERAPY IN NON-METASTATIC DISEASE

This is the most controversial subject in Wilms' tumour. As stated above, the SIOP group believes that there is every merit in treating the disease with systemic therapy first (and they are now studying prolonged primary chemotherapy) before proceeding to delayed nephrectomy on a much reduced and more easily operable primary tumour.

The NWTS workers hold that omission of an initial diagnosis based on tissue biopsy (diagnosis in SIOP studies can be made on clinical grounds alone) is open to error, both with regard to subtypes of Wilms' and even in terms of identifying the tumour in the first place. Without initial surgery, the SIOP patients are exposed to over-treatment (of those found to be Stage I cases with favourable histology at initial operation), or under-treatment (actinomycin/vincristine chemotherapy) in more advanced stage/unfavourable histology patients, and perhaps the omission of postoperative radiotherapy where it is needed (Zucker *et al.*, 1968). The incorrect diagnosis rate in SIOP studies is 4% and in Britain pretreatment needle biopsy avoids this problem. With needle aspiration focal adverse histological features may be missed, but initial chemotherapy does not alter histology and, if necessary, treatment may be intensified after delayed surgery.

The UKCCSG WT3 study addresses this issue in a randomized study of early versus delayed surgery in all potentially operable patients. Using initial needle biopsies, this study should clarify whether preoperative chemotherapy has any adverse effect on outcome for reasons of downstaging or altered histology.

18.12.4 LENGTH OF CHEMOTHERAPY IN STAGE II, III, IV CASES

This remains an unsolved subject. Chemo-therapy for six months seems adequate for Stage II disease, but could it be shorter in Stage II with favourable histology? In addition, in the context of aggressive three or four agent regimens do we really need chemotherapy for a minimum of one year for Stage IV?

18.12.5 FLANK RADIATION DOSAGE

In sequential NWTS trials, it was demonstrated that Stage I-II patients with normal histology did not have a higher local relapse rate if radiotherapy was omitted, provided two-drug chemotherapy was given (D'Angio *et al.*, 1981). With regard to Stage III normal histology patients, the NWTS 3 trial showed a slightly higher risk of flank recurrence in those receiving 1000 cGy versus 2000 cGy (in 180 cGy fractions) in addition to two-drug (actinomycin and vincristine) chemotherapy. This was not the case with triple drug chemotherapy (with the addition of adriamycin). It was concluded that the addition of adriamycin and only 1000 cGy flank dosage was preferable, particularly for late local effects and possibly with regard to metastatic relapse. There remains the question of adriamycin-related cardiotoxicity versus the sequelae of 2000 cGy of radiotherapy for these patients with good prognosis, which has made other groups more reticent about adopting this modification. The UKCCSG study still recommends 2000 cGy in 11 fractions.

A dosage of 2000 cGy with a boost to regions suspect for residual malignant cells of 4000 cGy is recommended for more locally advanced tumours, bulk residual disease after surgery and cases of unfavourable histology.

18.12.6 LUNG RADIOTHERAPY

Whole lung radiotherapy to the modest dose of 1200 cGy in eight fractions (150 cGy per fraction) is advocated by the NWTS in Stage IV patients with pulmonary metastases, having achieved remission in the lungs with primary chemotherapy. Although safe within the radiation tolerance of the lungs, there are late musculoskeletal growth sequelae and breast hypoplasia in girls. The survival results in the early British studies using identical chemotherapy to the NWTS studies but without lung irradiation for pulmonary metastases were unquestionably inferior to the NWTS results. As the only difference in therapy was lung irradiation, albeit this was a suboptimal comparative study by statisticians' standards, it seems logical to recommend lung radiotherapy in these patients. In the current UKCCSG study, there is a compromise recommending that those in whom chest x-ray is not clear after eight weeks of chemotherapy should receive radiotherapy. A recent study by SIOP (de Kraker *et al.*, 1990) indicated that only those patients with multiple, inoperable metastases after a three drug preoperative regimen require for lung irradiation.

18.12.7 CAN SALVAGE THERAPY BE SUCCESSFUL?

In a recent study by Groot-Loonen *et al.* (1990), 71 out of 381 children relapsed after modern treatment regimens, and of those only 17 survived, suggesting that 'first time' cure must still be the goal. In this study, as in one from the NWTS (Grundy *et al.*, 1989), early relapse, unfavourable histology and relapse after triple drug chemotherapy with or without radiotherapy were all bad prognosticators for ultimate survival. In patients who were non-aggressively treated initially, early relapse may well be salvageable; chemotherapy, irradiation and surgery may be important treatment methods either in isolation or in combination.

18.12.8 ALTERNATIVES TO NEPHRECTOMY

With increasing surgical expertise, partial nephrectomy is becoming technically possible and extracorporeal 'bench surgery' of the kidney may allow this practice to develop further. Achieving clear tumour margins is desirable if the flank is not to require subsequent irradiation (Bishop *et al.*, 1985), therefore the argument for conservative surgery balanced against a possible increase in local recurrence remains to be proven. The long-term impact, if any, of nephrectomy on renal function or blood pressure remains unclear (Welch and McAdams, 1986).

At the other extreme, controversy continues as to whether bilateral nephrectomy with a dialysis programme is indicated for bilateral synchronous Wilms' tumours, where partial nephrectomy has not been possible; in particular, the question is how long one should wait before transplantation (Coppes *et al.*, 1989).

18.12.9 POTENTIAL NEW DRUGS

Cyclophosphamide, although active in Wilms' tumour, adds little to the three-drug therapy. It has a role in relapsed tumours, and its analogue ifosfamide is probably even more effective but is avoided due to its associated renal toxicity. Etoposide has produced encouraging response rates in relapsed patients (Pein *et al.*, 1988), and there is an argument to try and replace adriamycin with this drug due to its lesser late effects. Cisplatin is relatively inactive, but its less nephrotoxic analogue carboplatin may have some promise.

P.N.P.

REFERENCES

Bishop, H.C., Betts, J. and Chatten, J. (1985) Partial nephrectomy for Wilms' tumor in a child with hemihypertrophy. Proceedings of the

Tumor Board of the Children's Hospital of Philadelphia. *Med. Pediatr. Oncol.*, **13**, 37–9.

Breslow, N.E., Norkool, P.A., Alsahn, A. *et al.* (1988) Second malignant neoplasms in survivors of Wilms' tumor: A report from the national Wilms' tumor study. *J. Natl. Cancer Inst.*, **80**, 592–5.

Brodeur, G.M. (1984) Genetic and cytogenetic aspects of Wilms' tumor, in *Wilms' Tumor: Clinical and Biological manifestations.* (eds C. Pochedly and E.S. Baum). Elsevier, New York, **9**, pp. 125–45.

Byrne, J., Mulvikill, J.J., Conelly, R.R. *et al.* (1988) Reproductive problems and birth defects in survivors of WT and their relatives. *Med. Pediatr. Oncol.*, **16**, 233–40.

Coppes, M.J., Kraker, J. de, Dijken, P.J. van *et al.* (1989) Bilateral Wilms' Tumour: Long-term survival and some epidemiological features. *J. Clin. Oncol.*, Vol. 7, No. 3. pp. 310–15.

D'Angio, G.J., Beckwith, J.B., Breslow, N. *et al.* (1989a) Wilms' tumor (nephroblastoma, renal embryoma, in *Principles and Practice of Pediatric Oncology*, (eds P.A. Pizzo, D.G. Poplack) J.B. Lippincott, Philadelphia. pp. 583–606.

D'Angio, G.J., Breslow, N., Beckwith, B. *et al.* (1989b) Treatment of Wilms' Tumor. Results of the third National Wilms' Tumor Study. *Cancer*, **64**, 349–60.

D'Angio, G.J., Evans, A.E., Breslow, N. *et al.* (1976) The treatment of Wilms' tumor: results of the National Wilms' Tumor Study. *Cancer*, **38**, 633–46.

D'Angio, G.J., Evans, A., Breslow, N. *et al.* (1981) The treatment of Wilms' tumor: Results of the Second National Wilms' Tumor Study. *Cancer*, **47**, 2302–11.

DeMaria, J.E., Hardy, B.E., Brezinski, A. and Churchill, B.M. (1979) Renal transplantation in patients with bilateral Wilms' Tumor. *J. Pediatr. Surg.*, Vol. 14, No. 5. 577–9.

Dubousset, J. (1980) Déformations rachidiennes post-radiothérapique après traitement du nephroblastome chez l'enfant. *Revue de chirurgie orthopédique*, **66**, pp. 441–51.

Groot-Loonen, J.J., Pinkerton, C.R., Morris-Jones, P.H. *et al.* (1990) How curable is relapsed Wilms' tumour? *Arch. Dis. Childh.*, **65**, 968–70.

Grundy, P., Breslow, N., Green, D.M. *et al.* (1989) Prognostic factors for children with recurrent Wilms' tumor: Results from the Second and Third National Wilms' Tumor Study. *J. Clin. Oncol.*, **7**, 638–47.

Habib, R., Loirat, C., Gubler, M.C. *et al.* (1985) The nephropathy associated with male pseudohermaphroditism and Wilms' tumor (Drash syndrome): a distinctive glomerular lesion – report of 10 cases. *Clin. Nephrol.*, Vol. 24, No. 6 pp. 269–78.

Knudson, A.G. and Strong, J.C. (1972) Mutation and Cancer: A model of Wilms' tumor of the kidney. *J. Natl. Cancer Inst.*, **48**, 313–24.

Kraker, J. de, Lemerle, J., Voûte, P.A. *et al.* (1990) Wilms' tumour with pulmonary metastases at diagnosis: the significance of primary chemotherapy (CT). *J. Clin. Oncol.*, **8**, (7), 1187–90.

Lemerle, J., Tournade, M., Gerard, Marchant, R. *et al.* (1976a) Wilms' tumour: natural history and prognostic factors. *Cancer*, **37**, 255.

Lemerle, J., Voûte, P.A., Tournade, M.F. *et al.* (1976b) Preoperative versus postoperative radiotherapy, single versus multiple courses of actinomycin D, in the treatment of Wilms' tumor. *Cancer*, **38**, 647–54.

Manivel, J.C., Sibley, R.K. and Dehmer, L.P. (January 1987) Complete and incomplete Drash syndrome: A clinicopathologic study of five cases of a dysontogenetic-neoplastic complex. *Hum. Pathol.*, Vol. 18, No. 1. pp. 80–9.

Mannens, M., Slater, R., Heyting, C. *et al.* (1988) Molecular nature of genetic changes resulting in loss of heterozygosity of chromosome 11 in Wilms' tumours. *Hum. Genet.*, **81**, 41–8.

Marsden, H.B., Lawler, W. and Kumar, P.M. (1978) Bone metastazing renal tumor of childhood. *Cancer*, **42**, 1922–8.

Maurer, H.S., Pendergrass, T.W., Borges, W. and Honig, G.R. (1979) The role of genetic factors in the etiology of Wilms' tumor. *Cancer*, **43**, 205–8.

Mesrobian, H.J. (1988) Wilms' tumor: Past, present, future. *J. of Urol.*, Vol. 140, pp. 231–8.

Mitchell, J.D., Baxter, T.J., Blair-West, J.R. and McCredie, D.A. (1970) Renin levels in nephroblastoma (Wilms' tumour). Report of a Renin Secreting Tumour. *Arch. Dis. Child.*, **45**, 376–84.

Nakissa, N., Constine, L.S., Rubin, P. and Strohl, R. (1985) Birth defects in three common paediatric malignancies: Wilms' tumour, neuroblastoma and Ewing's sarcoma. *Oncology*, **42**, 358–63.

Pastore, G., Carli, M., Lemerle, J. *et al.* (1988) Epidemiological features of Wilms' tumour:

results of studies by the International Society of Paediatric Oncology (SIOP). *Med. Ped. Oncol.*, **16**, 7–11.

Pein, F., Tournade, M-F., Brunat-Mentigny, M. *et al.* (1988) A phase II study of etoposide in the treatment of relapsed Wilms' tumors. Proc. ASCO, **259**, (Abst. 1003).

Pendergrass, T.W. (1976) Growth anomalies in children with Wilms' tumour *Cancer*, **37**, 402.

Penn, K. (1979) Renal transplantation for WT: report of 20 cases. *J. Urology*, Vol. 122. pp. 793–4.

Pritchard, J., Barnes, J.M., Gough, D. *et al.* (1988) Preliminary results of the first UKCCSG Wilms' Tumour Study. *Med. Ped. Oncol.*, **16**, 413.

Raine, J. Bowman, A., Wallendszus, K. and Pritchard, J. (1991) Hepatopathythrombocytopenia syndrome – a complication of dactinomycin therapy for Wilms' tumor: A report from the United Kingdom Children's Cancer Study Group. *J. Clin. Oncol.*, **2**, 268–73.

Riccardi, V.M., Sujansky, E., Smith, A.C. and Francke, U. (1978) Chromosomal inbalance in the aniridia-Wilms' tumor association: 11p interstitial deletion. *Pediatrics*, **61**, 604–10.

Ritchey, M.L., Kelalis, P.P., Breslow, N. *et al.* (November 1988) Intracaval and atrial involvement with nephroblastoma: review of national Wilms' tumor study-3. *J. Urol.*, Vol. 140.

Slater, M.R. (1986) The cytogenetics of Wilms' tumor. *Canc. Genet. Cytogenet.*, **19**, 37–41.

Smeets, R.M.M., Voûte, P.A., Vos, A. and Delemarre, J.F.M. (1989) Congenitale afwijkingen van de tractus urogenitalis bij patiënten met een Wilms tumor. *Ned. Tijdschr. Geneesk.*, **133**, No. 37.

Terracini, B., Pastore, G. and Segnan, N. (1983) Association of father's occupation and cancer in children. *Biol. Res. Preg. Perinatol.*, **4**, 40–5.

TNM Classification of Paediatric Tumours (1982) (ed. M.H. Harmer) International Union Against Cancer. Geneva.

Tournade, M.F., Lemerle, J., Brunat-Mentigny, M. *et al.* (1988) Ifosfamide is an active drug in Wilms' tumor: A phase II study conducted by the French society of pediatric oncology. *J. Clin. Oncol.*, **6**, 793–6.

Tournade, M.-F., Lemerle, J., Sarrazin, D. and Valayer, J. (1986) Tumours of the kidney. In *Cancer in children, Clinical Management* (eds P.A. Voûte, A. Barrett, H.J.G. Bloom, J. Lemerle and M.K. Heidhardt) 2nd edn. Springer-Verlag, Berlin. pp. 252–64.

Voûte, P.A., Meer, J. van de and Stangaard-Kloosterhiel, W. (1971) Plasma renin activity in Wilms' tumour. *Acta Endocrinol.* **67**, 197–202.

Weeks, D.A., Beckwith, J.B. and Luckey, D.W. (1987) Relapse-associated variables in stage I favorable histology Wilms' tumor. *Cancer*, **60**, 1204–12.

Weeks, D.A., Beckwith, J.B., Mierau, G.W. and Luckey, D.W. (1989) Rhabdoid tumor of kidney. A report of 111 cases from the National Wilms' Tumor Study Pathology Center. *Am. J. Surg. Path.*, **13**, 439–58.

Welch, T.R. and McAdams, J.A. (0000) Focal glomerulosclerosis as a late sequela of Wilms' tumor. Clinical and laboratory observations Vol. 108, No. 1 pp. 105–9.

Welch, T.R. and McAdams, A.J. (1986) Focal glomerulosclerosis as a late sequela of Wilms' tumor. *J. Pediatr.*, **108**, 105–9.

Wilimas, J.A., Douglass, E.C., Magill, H.L. *et al.* (1988) Significance of pulmonary computed tomography at diagnosis in Wilms' tumor. *J. Clin. Oncol.*, **6**, 1144–6.

Wilms, M., Die Mischgeschwülste der Niere (1899) von Arthur Georgi, Verlag, Leipzig, pp. 1–90.

Chapter 19

Malignant germ cell tumours

C.R. PINKERTON

19.1 PATHOGENESIS

Pathological definitions and classifications in germ cell tumours (GCT) lead to almost as much confusion as those in non-Hodgkin's lymphoma. The overlap and mix of histological subtypes which inevitably occurs in a tumour of germ cell origin has given rise to various descriptive subdivisions.

In the human embryo, the first germ cells can be identified in the extra-embryonal yolk sac at four weeks. From here the cells migrate through the middle and dorsal mesentery and are seen in the germinal epithelium of the gonadal ridge at six weeks. They then populate either the developing testis or ovary (Fig. 19.1)

The commonest sites of extra-gonadal germ cell tumours, namely, the sacrococcygeal area, retroperitoneum, mediastinum, neck and pineal area of the brain, can be explained by aberrant migration along the gonadal ridge which lies adjacent to the vertebral column from the cervical to lower lumbar region. It has been suggested that malignant transformation, occurring when gonadal tissue strays from the normal developmental pathway, may be due to a loss of growth regulation normally controlled by the notochord and contiguous structures. In children, 70% of germ cell tumours arise in extra gonadal sites.

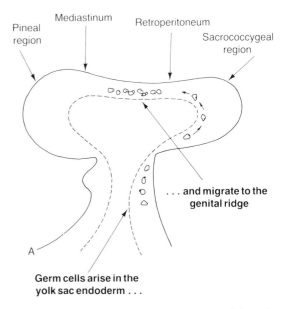

Fig. 19.1 Diagrammatic representation of the origin and migration of germ cell from yolk sac to gonadal ridge, showing possible aberrant sites of migration.

The morphological subtype reflects the pathway of differentiation to which the cell is committed prior to malignant transformation. The cell line may remain in the germinal state as a dysgerminoma or seminoma, or the transforming event may occur in a population which differentiates towards either embry-

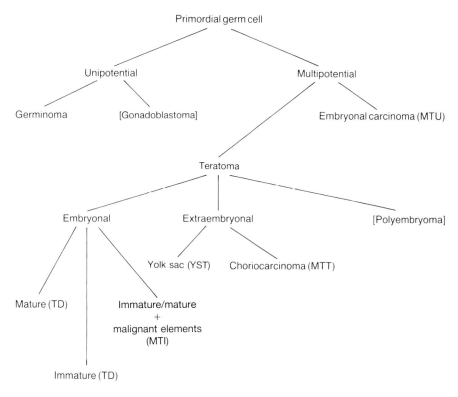

Fig. 19.2 Schema of differentiation pathway for germ cell tumours.

onal or extra-embryonal cell types (Fig. 19.2). The degree of differentiation will range from a completely undifferentiated embryonal carcinoma to the benign, fully differentiated teratoma leading to the definitions MTU, MTI & MTD (Tables 19.1 and 19.2). Mature or immature teratomas may include somatic tissues from the three basic embryonal layers – mesoderm, ectoderm and endoderm.

In the case of tumour developing in cells destined to form extra-embryonal tissues, differentiation is toward either yolk sac or placenta. This produces either malignant yolk sac tumour (endodermal sinus tumour) or choriocarcinoma.

Germ cell tumours (GCT) account for approximately 3% of childhood malignancies. The true incidence is difficult to ascer-

tain as many of the benign germ cell tumours will not be registered with central cancer registries. Two-thirds of GCTs occur in extragonadal sites and the incidence of the commonest GCT, the sacrococcygeal teratoma, is one in 35 000 live births. These are two to four times more common in girls than in boys. The incidence of malignant germ cell tumours (MGCT), per annum, in the Manchester Children's Tumour Registry, is three per million children under 15 years. Epidemiological studies have shown a bimodal age distribution with one peak in children under three years of age and a second peak after twelve years of age. The early peak reflects the incidence of sacrococcygeal tumours, the latter malignant germ neoplasms of the testis, accounting for the male preponderance at

Table 19.1 Classification of germ cell tumours in childhood (Dehner, 1986)

I.   Germinoma
          A. Intratubular germ cell neoplasia
          B. Invasive (dysgerminoma, germinoma)

II.   Teratoma
          A. Polydermal
              1. Mature
              2. Immature
                  a. Indeterminant biological behaviour
                  b. Malignant
          B. Monodermal

III.   Embryonal carcinoma (adult type)

IV.   Endodermal sinus tumour (infantile type of embryonal carcinoma, yolk sac carcinoma)

V.   Choriocarcinoma

VI.   Gonadoblastoma
          A. Pure
          B. With invasive component

VIII.   Malignant germ cell tumour of mixed histological pattern
          A. Germinoma and teratoma
          B. Endodermal sinus tumour and teratoma
          C. Endodermal sinus tumour, teratoma, and choriocarcinoma
          D. Germinoma, endodermal sinus tumour, teratoma and choriocarcinoma

Table 19.2 Classification of germ cell tumours in childhood (Ablin and Isaacs, 1989)

I.   Teratoma
          A. Mature
          B. Immature = MTD
          C. With malignant germ cell tumour component(s) = MTI

II.   Germinoma

III.   Embryonal carcinoma = MTU

IV.   Yolk sac tumour (endodermal sinus)

V.   Choriocarcinoma = MTT

VI.   Gonadoblastoma

VII.   Polyembryoma

          MTD = Malignant teratoma differentiated
          MTI = Malignant teratoma intermediate
          MTU = Malignant teratoma undifferentiated
          MTT = Malignant teratoma trophoblastic

this age (Mann *et al.*, 1989; La Vecchia *et al.*, 1983; Flamant *et al.*, 1984; Ablin, 1982). It is of interest that orbital teratomas are commonly found in females, whereas those in the gastric, mediastinal and central nervous systems tend to affect males.

Karyotypic studies of fresh tumour and cell lines have shown a number of characteristic features. There may be duplication or deletion of the short arm of chromosome 1, or an isochromosome 12. The latter is of particular

interest as it has been used as a diagnostic marker, both at presentation and also to evaluate the malignant potential of residual tumour following chemotherapy (Castedo *et al.*, 1989).

Congenital anomalies associated with sacrococcygeal teratomas may involve the genito-urinary tract, hind gut and lower vertebrae. The syndrome of ataxia-telangiectasia has also been associated with germ cell tumours, as have neuroblastoma and haematological malignancies.

19.2 TUMOUR MARKERS

Because the majority of malignant germ cell tumours in childhood involve extra-embryonal differentiation, i.e. have at least some component of yolk sac tumour or choriocarcinoma, serum markers are of great value both in diagnosis and management. Alpha 1 globulin alpha-fetoprotein (αFP), is produced in the fetal yolk sac and later in embryonal hepatocytes and the gastro-intestinal tract.

Concentrations of αFP are detectable in the fetus at around 15 weeks of gestation and full-term infants may have levels in excess of 50 000 ng/ml (Tsuchida *et al.*, 1978). This is of great importance in the evaluation of tumours in new-born and in young infants, where a raised αFP cannot be taken as indicative of malignancy, provided there is a normal decline over the following weeks.

The beta sub-unit of human chorionic gonadotrophin (β-HCG) is produced by placental cells. Any tumour with trophoblastic elements, i.e. choriocarcinoma, will produce β-HCG.

Details of serum markers and their role in patient management are described in Chapter 6 but in the case of a morphologically undifferentiated tumour, where diagnostic difficulty arises, an elevated αFP or β-HCG may be the only clue to the diagnosis and appropriate curative chemotherapy (Mann *et al.*, 1978; Vugrin *et al.*, 1984). The failure of a tumour marker to fall with treatment is suggestive of unresponsive disease and may be an indication for either early surgical intervention or a change of chemotherapy. Conversely, a rapid fall in a tumour marker, even in the absence of change in bulk disease, may reflect a good response in the malignant component of the tumour and only benign differentiated teratoma may remain. In this context changing chemotherapy would be appropriate. The wait-and-watch approach in localized, completely resected tumours using serum marker is considered below (Peckham *et al.*, 1982).

19.3 MORPHOLOGICAL CATEGORIES

The Dehner classification is shown in Table 19.1 (Dehner, 1986). Table 19.2 shows the paediatric application of this classification as suggested by Ablin and Isaacs (1989). The British Testicular Tumour Panel definitions are also added for clarity as these terms are in common usage (Einhorn *et al.*, 1989). The following discussion will describe pathological subtypes in order of the degree of differentiation as indicated in Figure 19.2. The clinical features and common anatomical sites of the different histological subtypes are listed in Table 19.3.

19.3.1 GERMINOMA

The germinoma is a tumour developing in the undifferentiated germ cell and does not, by definition, show features of differentiation towards embryonal or extra-embryonal tissue. When occurring in the testis, this tumour is called a seminoma and when occurring in the ovary, a dysgerminoma. When the tumour occurs at an extra-gonadal site the term germinoma is used. This histological subtype is often found combined with others rather than in the pure form. In children the pure form is confined to ovarian

Table 19.3 Sites of different histological subtypes

Germinoma	*Teratoma*	*Embryonal carcinoma*	*Yolk sac tumour*	*Choriocarcinoma*
Ovary	Sacrococcyx	Usually mixed with	Ovary	Pineal
Pineal	Ovary	yolk sac or	Sacrococcyx	Third ventricle
Mediastinum	Head and neck	choriocarcinoma	Testis	Mediastinum
Testis	Abdomen/pelvis		Pineal	Ovary
	– Retroperitoneum		Mediastinum	Testis
	– Stomach			
	– Liver			
	– Vagina			

tumours in adolescent females and the region of the pineal gland/third ventricle in the teenage male. It may also be occasionally found in the anterior mediastinum and testis. Germinoma is the commonest MGCT to occur in the dysgenetic gonad or undescended testis (Dehner 1986). Histologically, the tumour contains a monotonous infiltrate of large mononuclear cells which, when occurring as a mediastinal mass, must be distinguished from non-Hodgkin's lymphoma. The microscopic pattern may be of fibrous septae and lymphoid infiltrate, with necrosis and granulomatous reactions. The latter may be very prominent. Rarely intracranial dysgerminomas may contain syncytiotrophoblasts which produce β-HCG. This accounts for the raised levels of this marker in serum and cerebrospinal fluid in some patients with pineal tumours.

19.3.2 TERATOMA

It is within this subgroup that most terminological confusion arises. Three main subgroups should be considered, namely mature, immature and tumour with malignant components. The mature teratoma is a benign, highly differentiated tumour, composed of tissue derived from ectoderm, endoderm or mesoderm. The sacrococcygeal teratoma, for example, is a predominantly cystic tumour with mucoid or keratinous content. Histologically, there may be mature neuroglia, bone, hair or cartilage. Glandular structures resembling pancreas, cysts with retinal differentiation, hepatocytes and smooth muscle, may all be found. By definition the mature teratoma should not contain any evidence of extra-embryonal tumour or embryonal carcinoma.

The immature teratoma should probably not be regarded as a 'malignant' teratoma as in childhood its natural history is almost invariably benign. The term malignant should be restricted to tumours containing either embryonal carcinoma, yolk sac or choriocarcinoma. The immature teratoma will contain some fully mature tissue but also embryonal tissues at varying degrees of differentiation. Neuroectoderm is commonly seen with primitive medullary structures, neuroblasts and neuroblastoma-like rosettes. Again, epithelial structures may be seen. Immature teratomas have been further graded on the basis of the amount of embryonal tissue present but this is of little relevance in paediatric practice and is not predictive of which tumours will convert to an unfavourable malignant type. In general, immature teratomas in children have a good prognosis and chemotherapy is rarely required.

The third subgroup, teratoma with malignant components, is a tumour of mixed histology with a background of mature or immature teratoma containing either immature embryonal carcinoma or evidence of extra-embryonal differentiation. In some cases elevated serum markers may be the only clue to the presence of malignancy. In practical terms, evidence of the latter is an indication for clinical management identical to that of pure yolk sac or pure chorioncarcinoma, i.e. treatment should be directed to the most malignant element.

19.3.3 EMBRYONAL CARCINOMA

Embryonal carcinoma has been divided into adult and infantile type based on histological differences. The infantile type is essentially a yolk sac tumour and should be classified as such. Cellular anaplasia, mitotic activity, embryoid bodies, necrosis and haemorrhage are indicative of the 'adult' embryonal carcinoma. Pure embryonal carcinoma is one of the commoner types of germ cell neoplasm in the testis of young adults and occasionally is seen in the ovary. By definition pure carcinoma will not produce αFP or β-HCG (Kurman and Norris, 1976).

19.3.4 YOLK SAC TUMOUR

This is also known as endodermal sinus tumour because of its structural similarity to the mouse endodermal sinus. Like the term 'yolk sac carcinoma', this term is unhelpful. It is the commonest type of malignant germ cell tumour in children and is found in 10–20% of sacrococcygeal tumours. Other common sites are the ovary and testis. Less commonly, the pineal region, mediastinum, vagina and retro-peritoneum may be involved. Although four histological patterns have been described, namely pseudo-papillary, reticular, polyvesicular vitelline and solid, the pseudopapillary type is the commonest. Papillary projections associated with characteristic perivascular sheets of cells give rise to the term endodermal sinus and are also known as Schiller-Duval bodies. In most cases there are intracellular and extra-cellular hyaline droplets which are PAS and αFP positive. αFP is clearly demonstrable using immuno-histochemical techniques.

19.3.5 CHORIOCARCINOMA

Pure choriocarcinoma is rare in children and more commonly is a feature of mixed histological subtypes. Pure tumour may however be found in the pineal region, mediastinum, ovary and testis. In the neonate, multiple visceral metastasis from gestational placental neoplasms have been reported. Tumours in the posterior aspect of the third ventricle occur almost exclusively in young males. Anterior lesions may occur in females. Mediastinal choriocarcinoma is more common in young adults (Witzleben and Bruninga, 1968).

Microscopically, choriocarcinoma consists of two components: syncytiotrophoblasts and cytotrophoblasts. The former form syncytial knots and contain abundant vacuoles containing β-HCG. Considerable haemorrhage and necrosis may be seen.

19.3.6 POLYEMBRYOMA AND GONADOBLASTOMA

These very rare tumours are occasionally seen in children. The polyembryoma occurs in ovary and mediastinum and microscopically it may resemble amniotic cavity and yolk sac. β-HCG and αFP may be demonstrable. The gonadoblastoma is an intra-tubular neoplasm occurring in dysgenetic gonads, usually in patients under the age of 20. The karyotype of the patient is generally 46 XY (male pseudo-hermaphrotidism) or 46 XY 4/45 XO (mosaicism). This tumour is often found by chance on examination of a dysgenetic gonad at the time of surgery for other reasons and, generally, it behaves in a benign fashion. In about 20% of patients the tumour may contain malignant components. Microscopically, the tumour is composed of ovoid or irregular cell nests separated by connective tissue. Primordial germ cells and stromal cells resembling Sertoli cells are seen. Smaller stromal cells resembling Call-Extner bodies of the granulosa cell tumour are occasionally found (Takeda *et al.*, 1982; Scully 1970).

19.4 CLINICAL CHARACTERISTICS AND MANAGEMENT

The relative incidence, age and pathological subtypes of tumours at different sites are shown in Table 19.4.

19.4.1 SACROCOCCYGEAL TUMOUR

Of all germ cell tumours 40%, either malignant or benign, are found in the sacrococcygeal region. Half occur in neonates, mainly girls. Of these, 70% are benign, i.e. they have histological features of mature teratoma or immature teratoma without malignant components. A classification based on the anatomical location of sacrococcygeal tumours has been devised by Altman *et al.* (1974). In

Table 19.4 Relative incidence according to age, site and pathological subtype

Site	Relative incidence %	Age	Pathology
Sacrococcyx	41	Neonate	Mature 65%, immature 5%, malignant 30% (10% in <2/12)
Ovary	29	Early teens	Mature 65%, immature 5%, malignant 30%
Testis	7	Infant and adolescent	Mature 20%, malignant 80% – yolk sac 90% – germinoma 10% – embryonal carcinoma <1%
Cranial	6	Child	Embryonal carcinoma, germinoma, mature
Mediastinum	6	Adolescent	Mature 60%, mixed 20%, embryonal carcinoma 20%
Retroperitoneum	5	Infant < 2 years	Usually mature, immature – rarely malignant
Head/Neck	4	Infant & neonate	Usually mature, immature – rarely malignant
Vagina	2	Infant < 3 years	Usually yolk sac

80% of cases these tumours are either predominantly external or have an intrapelvic and external component. In 10% there is extensive intra-abdominal disease and this type is most likely to be malignant. A further 10% will have a presacral component alone. The histological subtype must be confirmed by pathological examination or markers, and as the anatomical classification does not correlate with subsequent neurological function it has little clinical application.

A tumour which is predominantly extra-abdominal will have few clinical signs, in contrast to a presacral lesion which may present with urinary frequency, lower extremity weakness, or constipation. Other diagnoses to be considered are listed in Table 19.5. An adequate rectal examination, if necessary under general anaesthetic, is essential to define any presacral mass. Ultrasound examination will be of benefit in defining abdominal disease and CT scans may also be helpful. Plain x-ray of the abdomen may show anterior displacement of a gas-filled rectum, and on lateral film a calcified soft tissue mass caudal to the sacrum may be found. Symptoms are suggestive of malignancy as benign tumours are almost invariably asymptomatic

(Valdiserri and Yunis, 1981; Whalen *et al.*, 1985).

For the majority of tumours, treatment is primarily surgical. The tumour should be excised as soon as the diagnosis is made and it is essential that the entire coccyx is removed. Failure to do this will result in a local recurrence rate of up to 40%. If the tumour appears difficult to resect, multiple biopsies should be done to determine the presence of any malignant elements. In the case of the latter, chemotherapy may be appropriate to produce tumour shrinkage and facilitate surgery. However, in the majority of tumours chemotherapy does not play a role as this highly differentiated tumour is usually chemo-resistant.

19.4.2 MEDIASTINAL TERATOMA

The differential diagnoses of an anterior mediastinal mass are listed in Table 19.5. These tumours are usually asymptomatic until they reach a considerable size and produce tracheal or bronchial compression. Coughing, wheezing or chest pain may result and haemoptysis has been described. Unusual presentations include hypogly-

Table 19.5 Differential diagnosis of sacrococcygeal, testicular and anterior mediastinal mass

Sacrococcygeal	Testicular	Anterior mediastinum
Meningomyelocoele	Torsion	Thymus
Imperforate anus	Infarct	Bronchogenic cyst
Pilonidal cyst	Epidydimo-orchitis	Goitre
Abscess	Haematoma	Enteric cyst
Lipoma	Hernia	Lipoma
Lymphangioma	Hydrocoele	Lymphangioma
Chondroma	Leukaemia/lymphoma	Thymoma
Giant cell tumour	Paratesticular rhabdomyosarcoma	T cell lymphoma
Neurogenic tumour		
Soft tissue sarcoma		

caemia and precocious puberty due to ectopic production of insulin or sex hormones.

Most teratomas in adolescent females are mature, cystic and benign. In males, however, there is a higher incidence of malignant teratomas at this site. Pericardial teratomas associated with cardiac failure have been described and intra-cardiac teratomas also occur.

On plain x-ray, a dense rounded opacity is evident with calcification evident in a third of cases; teeth may also be seen (Truong *et al.*, 1986; Carter *et al.*, 1982).

19.4.3 ABDOMINAL TUMOURS

Extragonadal abdominal teratomas are found in the retroperitoneal region, stomach, liver and almost any other organ. Retro-peritoneal primaries account for approximately 3% of tumours in childhood and occur predominantly under two years of age. They may present with vague abdominal pain or symptoms due to compression on bowel or urinary tract. Benign gastric teratoma usually occur in the first year of life, or occasionally, in the neonatal period.

Hepatic teratoma illustrates one important reason for performing biopsies in liver tumours even in the presence of a raised serum αFP. Only this will distinguish it from the more common hepatocellular carcinoma

or hepatoblastoma. Generally, this tumour occurs in the first few months of life and occupies all or part of one hepatic lobe.

Other less common sites of teratomas include abdominal wall, skin, placenta, prostate, bladder and uterus. Tumours presenting in the vagina may resemble the botryoid rhabdomyosarcoma with a polypoid friable mass. These are generally of yolk sac histology with raised serum αFP and are highly curable with chemotherapy. Conservative surgery, preserving normal genital structure, is usually possible (Lack *et al.*, 1985; Young and Scully, 1984; Witte *et al.*, 1983).

19.4.4 HEAD AND NECK TERATOMAS

Five per cent of teratomas arise in the head and neck with primaries in the nasopharynx, oral cavity, orbit and cervical region. These generally present at birth with extensive solid and cystic masses; respiratory or oral obstruction may result. These are generally benign tumours but, due to their site, may produce major management problems. Surgical excision is the only real option as the tumour is almost invariably chemo-resistant.

19.4.5 INTRACRANIAL TUMOURS

About 1% of all primary intracranial neoplasms are germ cell tumours. Most occur in the pineal area, suprasellar or infrasellar regions. Occasionally they are found in the cerebral hemisphere or spinal cord. Classically, these tumours cause third ventricular obstruction with secondary hydrocephalus and Perinaud's syndrome. With more extensive lesions a variety of neurological signs will be evident. Approximately a third of pineal region tumours will be of germ cell origin, either germinoma, embryonal carcinoma, or teratoma. If the tumour contains yolk sac or trophoblastic elements the CSF αFP or β-HCG will be elevated and these are useful for following response to treatment (Hisa *et al.*, 1985; Tavcar *et al.*, 1980; Packer *et al.*, 1984).

19.4.6. MANAGEMENT OF EXTRAGONADAL TUMOURS

A staging system for extra-gonadal tumours is shown in Table 19.6. If the mass is resectable, surgery is the treatment of choice. This will be curative in the case of benign tumours and will reveal any malignant component in the others. If complete excision has been achieved in the latter (Stages I & II), then this is all that is required provided tumour mar-

Table 19.6 Staging for extragonadal tumours

Stage I	Disease limited to one organ or structure and completely resected
Stage II	Disease extending to structures adjacent to the primary tumour but completely resected
Stage III	Tumours with microscopic residual following surgery, due to spillage or extension of tumour to resection margins or Tumours incompletely resected at surgery or biopsy only
Stage IV	Disseminated disease

kers return to normal with the anticipated half-life. If there is no tumour marker then close follow-up with ultrasound, CT or MRI scanning is mandatory to detect any local recurrence early as this may be susceptible to further surgery, chemotherapy or radiotherapy.

In the event of a more extensive primary or where there has been spillage at resection and there is evidence of a malignant component, systemic chemotherapy is mandatory (Stage III). Similarly, if there are distant metastases, usually involving lung, bone or bone marrow, chemotherapy is the first line treatment (Stage IV). Staging investigations should include chest x-ray and CT scan in all cases and bone scan with bone marrow aspirate and trephine in the case of more extensive or unresectable primary tumours.

In the case of mediastinal malignant germ cell tumour, if serum markers are elevated or biopsy shows malignant tumour, then attempts at radical surgery are unnecessary and dangerous. Where there is respiratory difficulty due to tumour obstruction at presentation, urgent measurement of serum markers may show elevated αFP or β-HCG which is sufficient evidence to commence chemotherapy without the hazard of biopsy.

19.4.7 GONADAL TUMOURS

About one-third of germ cell tumours arise in the ovary. The peak age incidence is around ten years of age and 70% are benign, mature cystic teratomas. A cystic mass replaces all or part of the ovary and may be bilateral in up to 5%. The tumour is often asymptomatic until it reaches a large size or may present with torsion, infarction or rupture. Occasionally, chronic abdominal pain or an acute abdomen resembling appendicitis may occur.

Detailed histological examination of any solid element in a teratoma is mandatory to exclude a malignant component. It should be noted that peritoneal 'spread' with mature neuroglial tissue (*gliomatosis peritonei*) does not influence prognosis and systemic chemotherapy is not required. With immature teratoma or tumours with malignant components the pattern of spread is usually that of ascites, peritoneal implants and distant metastasis to lymph nodes, liver and lung. Tumours with trophoblastic elements will produce β-HCG. Premature breast enlargement, pubic hair or menarche may be presenting features. Serum αFP will be elevated if there is any yolk sac component.

Plain abdominal x-rays often show calcification, particularly in the case of benign tumours. There may be urinary tract obstruction due to pressure or infiltration of the ureters and ultrasound is a useful imaging modality. Routine staging investigations in the case of advanced primary tumours should include CT scan of chest and abdomen, bone scan and bone marrow assessment. The staging system adapted from the FIGO (Federation of Gynaecology and Obstetrics) classification is shown in Table 19.7 (FIGO, 1987; Flamant *et al.*, 1978).

With localized tumour, complete surgical excision is curative even if malignant elements are found within the tumour, provided the serum markers fall at the expected rate. If there is no tumour marker, close

Table 19.7 Staging of ovarian tumours (Modified FIGO classification)

Stage I	Diseases limited to one or both ovaries; capsule intact; peritoneal fluid negative for malignant cells
Stage II	Disease including or beyond the ovarian capsule with local pelvic extension; retroperitoneal nodes and peritoneal fluid negative for malignant cells
Stage III	Positive retroperitoneal nodes, malignant cells in the peritoneal fluid, or abdominal extension
Stage IV	Extra-abdominal dissemination

surveillance with CT and ultrasound is required. At the time of laparotomy, the contralateral ovary must be examined and biopsied if appropriate.

With extensive, incompletely resected or unresectable primary tumours, chemotherapy is required and is usually highly effective. As modern regimens should not be sterilizing, bilateral oophorectomy is not necessary in the case of bilateral disease. Following maximum response to chemotherapy, excision of the primary tumour and localized excision of the contralateral lesion should enable maintenance of fertility and hormonal function. Extensive initial surgery with bilateral oophorectomy and hysterectomy is no longer acceptable in an era of effective chemotherapy (Smales and Peckham, 1987).

19.4.8 TESTICULAR TUMOURS

Teratoma of the testis represent about 10% of paediatric germ cell tumours. Most patients are less than four-years-old. Of these tumours, 20% are mature benign teratomas and 80% are malignant, the majority with yolk sac histology. Fewer than 5% are pure germinoma and only 0.1% embryonal carcinomas.

There is usually a solitary, multicystic and partially solid mass and, as with most mature teratomas, keratinous and differentiated bone or cartilage may be recognizable. The presence of malignant components is more common in the adolescent or young adult.

The differential diagnosis of a testicular mass is shown in Table 19.5. The incidence of malignant tumour *in situ* in the contralateral testis in adults with malignant germ cell tumours, suggests an inherent predisposition to malignancy in testicular tissue. The incidence of malignant change in an undescended testis is around thirty times higher than normal, justifying orchiopexy. The real value of the latter may in fact be to prevent late

Table 19.8 Classification according to the UKCCSG staging system

I.	Tumour confined to testis, completely resected, markers return to normal
II.	Tumour confined to testis and retroperitoneal/abdominal lymph nodes
III.	Supradiaphragmatic nodal disease (mediastinal and/or supraclavicular)
IV.	Extralymphatic spread (liver, lung, bone, brain, skin)

diagnosis in the event of an intra-abdominal testicular tumour. It is of note that testicular tumours are also more common in the descended testis of patients with cryptorchidism.

The UKCCSG (United Kingdom Children's Cancer Study Group) staging system is shown in Table 19.8. Lymph nodes are the usual site of tumour spread, but lung, bone, and bone marrow metastases should be sought at presentation in the case of a bulky tumour. Although there is still some controversy about the value of retroperitoneal lymphadenectomy in adults, there is no role for this procedure in children of any age. Refined CT scanning and MRI techniques should detect significant nodal involvement. Moreover, most patients will have tumour markers in the form of αFP and β-HCG and these can be used to confirm completeness of resection and absence of metastasis. In the small percentage of patients who are 'understaged', salvage chemotherapy is curable in the majority and therefore the potential sequelae of lymphadenectomy, such as impotence and retrograde ejaculation, cannot be justified.

Resection of testicular tumour should be by high inguinal orchiectomy. To avoid skin contamination with tumour, transcrotal biopsies are contraindicated. The inguinal approach is also necessary to ensure adequate excision of potentially infiltrated spermatic cord. The investigation of any child with a suspicious testicular mass should include pre-operative αFP

assessment which would prevent a number of inappropriate surgical interventions (Dewar *et al.*, 1987; MRC 1985; Fung *et al.*, 1988; Williams *et al.*, 1987a).

19.5 CHEMOTHERAPY

There is no role for chemotherapy in mature teratomas and surgical excision is usually curative. In children, tumours showing more aggressive behaviour with spread to nodes or other distant sites indicate mixed histology with malignant elements. For these patients chemotherapy is necessary.

The early demonstration of the dramatic effectiveness of methotrexate in gestational choriocarcinoma was followed by an evaluation of single agents and combined drug regimens in testicular germ cell tumours in adults. Actinomycin D, vinblastine and bleomycin were all found to be effective and the VAC regimen (vincristine, actinomycin, cyclophosphamide) came into standard use in paediatric germ cell tumours. Although this was comparatively effective for patients with extensive but non metastatic disease, overall cure rates remained poor. In adults, regimens such as VAB-cisplat (vinblastine, actinomycin D, bleomycin and cisplatin), produced complete response rates in excess of 60%. Subsequently, the PVB (cisplatin, vinblastine, bleomycin) regimen became the gold standard with an overall 100% response rate and 70–80% disease-free survival in advanced or metastatic testicular tumours (Williams *et al.*, 1987a; Bosl *et al.*, 1987; Peckman *et al.*, 1985; Pinkerton *et al.*, 1986; Garnick, 1985; Newlands *et al.*, 1983).

Unfortunately, many paediatric groups have lagged behind their non paediatric colleagues with regard to both the reduction of the number of drugs used and the duration of treatment. Despite demonstration in randomized trials that 'continuing' treatment was superfluous, regimens lasting up to two years have still not been abandoned by some. The approach of stopping chemotherapy after two courses beyond radiological CR or marker negativity has for a number of years been standard practice in adults. Moreover, it is clear that agents with significant late sequelae (such as the alkylating agents cyclophosphamide or ifosfamide and the anthracyclines) are unnecessary. The BEP regimen (bleomycin, etoposide and cisplatin) is a highly effective combination which should maintain fertility and minimize the risk of second tumours. Replacing cisplatin with the relatively non-nephrotoxic, non-ototoxic analogue carboplatin is currently under evaluation (JEB regimen: carboplatin (JM8); etoposide; bleomycin) (Pinkerton *et al.*, 1990). Randomized studies in adults suggest that bleomycin may not be necessary for low risk subgroups and its omission would further reduce the risk of late sequelae. Bleomycin-induced pneumonitis has been a significant complication of both the BEP and PVB regimens, where the drug is given weekly.

19.6 SURGERY

As already described, surgery is the mainstay of treatment for localized tumours. With bulky or infiltrative disease, biopsy only is usually appropriate as malignant germ cell tumours are highly chemosensitive and late, complete resection is therefore possible. There is some debate about the role of second look surgery (below). This may be of value with malignant tumours, both to confirm histological remission (where there is a residual imageable mass), and to achieve complete resection of any residual viable disease (Tait *et al.*, 1984; Jadvapour *et al.*, 1982; Pizzocaro *et al.*, 1985).

19.7 RADIOTHERAPY

Radiation has little role to play in germ cell tumours in children. The exception is in the case of an intracranial neoplasm. Despite the high chemosensitivity, most oncologists are reluctant to omit this treatment modality. In refractory or relapsed tumours there may be a role for consolidation radiotherapy after second line chemotherapy. Although in adults radiotherapy remains in use for pure germinomas (testicular seminoma with node involvement) this is not appropriate in children where this chemosensitive tumour should be managed as for any other malignant histological subtype (Read *et al.*, 1986; Mameghan *et al.*, 1985).

19.8 CURRENT CONTROVERSIES

19.8.1 IS TISSUE ALWAYS NEEDED AT PRESENTATION FOR DIAGNOSIS IN THE PRESENCE OF RAISED MARKERS?

Raised αFP or β-HCG levels in the presence of an anterior mediastinal mass or a testicular mass with node or lung metastases, are pathognomonic of malignant teratoma, either pure extraembryonal or of mixed histology. In such cases where initial curative surgery is not feasible the nature of the chemotherapy given is not dependant on histology. In metastatic neuroblastoma, elevated tumour markers (urinary catecholamines) in the presence of characteristic radiology, is often taken as diagnostic. Similarly, a large intrahepatic mass with raised αFP levels is almost certain to be either a hepatoblastoma or hepato-cellular carcinoma for which the pre-operative chemotherapy is the same. In these situations it may be argued that histological confirmation is not always necessary.

In general, however, it is desirable to obtain tissue unless the procedure itself is potentially hazardous. This is not only to confirm the diagnosis (for example the intrahepatic tumour could be an intrahepatic teratoma) but also to document histological subdivisions. Although treatment may at present be standard for the different histological sub-

403

types, this may not be the case in the future. Only prospective studies correlating outcome with histology will lead to refinement of treatment.

19.8.2 HOW MANY DRUGS ARE REQUIRED FOR CURE IN UNRESECTABLE OR METASTATIC TUMOURS?

Randomized studies in adults with testicular tumours have shown that the combination PVB is as effective as longer or more complex chemotherapy regimens (Williams *et al.*, 1987b). In children, the results with PVB or BEP are superior to VAC with high overall cure rates in both bulky and metastatic tumours (Mann *et al.*, 1989). The problem is the late morbidity of this regimen due to bleomycin lung toxicity and platinum-related ototoxicity and nephrotoxicity. Some adult studies have suggested that bleomycin contributes significantly to the efficacy of BEP (Brada *et al.*, 1987). However, this has been questioned and provisional results from randomized studies in low stage testicular tumours suggest that it is not the case (Levi *et al.*, 1986). In contrast, the results with etoposide and platinum alone in more bulky tumours have been disappointing and it seems likely that separate regimens are required based on risk factors at presentation. Various systems for the latter have been devised in adults but are difficult for children. It is not clear whether absolute bulk, i.e. volume of the tumour irrespective of the child's size, is of significance as seems the case in adults, where this is an indication for more intensive treatment (Raghavan *et al.*, 1982). The more complex POMB-ACE regimen (adding methotrexate, vincristine, adriamycin and cyclophosphamide) (Newlands *et al.*, 1983) is effective in high risk testicular tumours and a further modification with increased dose intensity is under evaluation (Rustin *et al.*, 1989).

Whether carboplatin can routinely replace cisplatin has been questioned (von Hoff, 1987) but it appears that, provided a sufficient dose is given and the inevitable myelosuppression accepted, comparable results should be obtained (Harland and Horwich, 1987; Pinkerton, 1990; Horwich *et al.*, 1991). The risk is that patients will be under-dosed due to concern about thrombocytopenia and neutropenia with an adverse effect on outcome (Edmonson *et al.*, 1988). Application of a dose formula based on renal function appears to be necessary for optimum use of this drug (Calvert *et al.*, 1990).

19.8.3 IS THERE A ROLE FOR MEGATHERAPY IN GERM CELL TUMOURS?

Patients who are refractory to initial chemotherapy or who relapse following treatment have in the past been difficult to salvage. The use of high dose cisplatin-etoposide or ifosamide-based regimens produce responses but usually only of short duration. As these are inherently highly chemosensitive tumours, dose escalation might be expected to have some value, as in the case of lymphomas. Very high dose carboplatin, etoposide and ifosamide combinations are under evaluation and have been reported to produce sustained remissions and possibly cures (Nichols *et al.*, 1988; Ozols *et al.*, 1983; Pico *et al.*, 1989).

19.8.4 IS RADIOTHERAPY NECESSARY IN INTRACRANIAL GERM CELL TUMOURS?

Because the overall cure rate for intracranial germinomas is high with chemotherapy and radiotherapy, clinicians are reluctant to leave out radiotherapy, although this tumour may, in fact, be chemocurable. There are small series of children who have been treated with chemotherapy alone in which there are long-term survivors. Whole brain and spinal irradiation continues to be given in most centres, although, in the absence of clear disease spread at presentation, the latter is probably not required and is a cause of significant adverse effects on growth. Elective omission of radiotherapy in the young child because of concern about toxicity may give a guide to the necessity or otherwise of this modality of treatment.

19.8.5 THE ROLE OF SECOND LOOK SURGERY OR METASTATECTOMY

In patients with advanced or metastatic disease following chemotherapy, there is often residual imageable disease on ultrasound, CT or MRI. Provided serum markers have fallen to normal, it is likely that this residual tissue is fibrosis or, more commonly, mature teratoma. Although it has been suggested that chemotherapy produces differentiation in immature teratoma, it seems probable that the mature component has always been present. Being chemo-resistant, however, it persists and even grows during chemotherapy. In the case of abdominal disease, second look laparotomy is justified both to confirm complete remission and to resect residual mature teratoma. The latter could either continue to grow, causing local problems, or undergo malignant change. The presence of viable malignant tumour in a residual mass correlates with adverse outcome. Failure to completely resect such residual tissue is an indication for external beam irradiation or further chemotherapy with dose escalation.

In the case of residual lesions on chest x-ray or chest CT scan, the same approach may apply although a reluctance to do bilateral thoracotomies in such patients has resulted in a number being followed without intervention. In many cases these lesions have persisted unchanged or resolved over the ensuing months or years. In no case is irradiation indicated for presumed residual thoracic disease and surgical confirmation is necessary before any active change of treatment.

19.8.6 SHOULD ELEVATED SERUM MARKERS DURING FOLLOW-UP BE AN INDICATION FOR RETREATMENT IN THE ABSENCE OF MEASURABLE DISEASE ELSEWHERE?

Serum αFP or β-HCG levels are routinely followed during the post-treatment period, usually up to 18 months beyond which the risk of relapse is very slim. In the event of a rising marker, it is essential to perform an exhaustive search for recurrent disease – either at the primary site or potential sites of metastases. CT scan, bone scan, MRI and ultrasound will reveal the site of recurrence in most cases. Radiolabelled αFP scans may have a role to play. Not infrequently, transient inexplicable elevations in tumour marker are seen with an αFP as high as 40 or 50 ng/ml. When repeated weekly, the level remains static or will decline. Precipitous action in this context is unnecessary and will lead to inappropriate treatment.

19.8.7 ARE PLATINUM-BASED REGIMENS STERILIZING?

It has been suggested that children treated with cisplatin-based regimens have impaired fertility. Studies in adults have shown that the risk of infertility is in fact very low with these regimens. Prospective sperm count evaluation shows that, although there may be a decline during treatment, almost invariably there is complete recovery within 6–12 months of cessation of treatment (Senturia *et al.*, 1985; Drasga *et al.*, 1983).

REFERENCES

Ablin, A.R. (1982) Malignant germ cell tumors in children. *Front. Radiat. Ther. Onc.*, **16**, 141–9.

Ablin, A. and Isaacs, H. (1989) Germ cell tumours, in *Principles and Practice of Paediatric Oncology* (eds P.A. Pizzo and D.G. Poplack) J.B. Lippincott, Philadelphia, pp. 713–32.

Altman, R.P. *et al.* (1974) Sacrococcygeal teratoma. *J. Pediatr. Surg.*, **9**, 389–98.

Bosl, G.J., Geller, N.L., Vogelzang, N.J. *et al.* (1987) Alternating cycles of etoposide plus cisplatin and VAB-6 in the treatment of poor-risk patients with germ cell tumors. *J. Clin. Oncol.*, **5** (3), 436–40.

Brada, M., Horwich, A. and Peckham, M.J. (1987) Treatment of favourable-prognosis nonseminomatous testicular germ cell tumors with etoposide, cisplatin, and reduced dose of bleomycin. *Cancer Treat. Rep.*, **71** (6), 655–6.

Calvert, A.H., Newell, D.R., Gumbrell, L.A. *et al.* (1989) Carboplatin dosage: Prospective evaluation of a simple formula based on renal function. *J. Clin. Oncol.*, **7**, 1748–56.

Carter, D., Bobro, M.C. and Touloukian, R.J. (1982) Benign clinical behavior of immature mediastinal teratoma in infancy and childhood. Report of two cases and review of the literature. *Cancer*, **49**, 398–402.

Castedo, S.M.M.J., de Jong, B., Oosterhuis, J.W. *et al.* (1989) Chromosomal changes in mature residual teratomas following polychemotherapy. *Cancer Res.*, **49**, 672–6

Dehner, L.P. (1986) Gonadal and extragonadal germ cell neoplasms-teratomas in childhood, in *Pathology of Neoplasia in Children and Adolescents.* (eds M. Finegold and V.L. Benington) Major Problems in Pathology, Vol. 18, W.B. Saunders, Philadelphia, pp. 282–312.

Dewar, J.M., Spagnolo, D.V., Jamrozik, K.D. *et al.* (1987) Predicting relapse in Stage I non-seminomatous germ cell tumours of the testis. *Lancet*, **i**, 454.

Drasga, R.E., Lawrence, H.E., Williams, S.D. *et al.* (1983) Fertility after chemotherapy for testicular cancer. *J. Clin. Oncol.*, **1** (3), 179–83.

Edmonson, J.H., McCormack, G.M., Wieand, H.S. *et al.* (1988) Comparison of cyclophosphamide + carboplatin vs cyclo + cisplatin in Stage III & IV ovarian carcinoma. *Proc. ASCO* **7**, 137.

Einhorn, L.H., Crawford, E.D., Shipley, W.U. *et al.* (1989) Cancer of the Testis, in *Cancer – Principles & Practice of Oncology*, (eds V.T. Devita, S. Hellman and S.A. Rosenberg) J.B. Lippincott, Philadelphia, pp. 1071–98.

Flamant, F., Caillou, B., Pejovic, M.-H. *et al.* (1978) Prognostic factors in malignant germ cell tumors of the ovary in children excluding pure dysgerminoma. *Eur. J. Cancer*, **14**, 901–6.

Flamant, F., Schwartz, L., Delons, E.*et al.* (1984) Nonseminomatous malignant germ cell tumors in children. *Cancer*, **54**, 1687–91.

Fung, C.J., Kalish, L.A., Brodsky, G.L. *et al.* (1988) Stage I nonseminomatous germ cell testicular tumor: Prediction of metastatic potential by primary histopathology. *J. Clin. Oncol.*, **6** (9), 1467–73.

Garnick, M.B. (1985) Advanced testicular cancer: treatment choices in the 'Land of Plenty'. *J. Clin. Oncol.*, **3** (3), 294–7.

Harland, S. and Horwich, A. (1987) What dose of carboplatin can be combined with etoposide and bleomycin in patients with testicular cancer? *Proc. ASCO* **6**, 48 (abstract 184).

Hisa, S., Morinaga, S., Kobayashi, Y. *et al.* (1985) Intramedullary spinal cord germinoma producing HCG and precocious puberty in a boy. *Cancer*, **55**, 2845–9.

Horwich, A., Dearnley, D.P., Nicholls, J., *et al.* (1991) Effectiveness of carboplatin, etoposide and bleomycin combination chemotherapy in good prognosis metastatic testicular nonseminomatous germ cell tumors. *J. Clin. Oncol.*, **9**, 62–9.

International Federation of Gynecology & Obstetrics (1987) Changes of definitions of clinical staging for carcinoma of cervix and ovary. *Am. J. Obstet. Gynecol.*, **156**, 236.

Javadpour, M., Ozols, R.F., Anderson, T. *et al.* (1982) Randomized trial of cytoreductive surgery followed by chemotherapy versus chemotherapy alone in bulky Stage III testicular cancer with poor prognosis features. *Cancer*, **50**, 2004–10.

Kurman, R.J. and Norris, H.J. (1976) Embryonal carcinoma of the ovary. A clinicopathologic entity distinct from endodermal sinus tumor resembling embryonal carcinoma of the adult testis. *Cancer*, **38**, 2420–33.

La Vecchia, C., Morris, H.B. and Draper, G.J. (1983) Malignant ovarian tumours in childhood in Britain, 1962–78. *Br. J. Cancer*, **48**, 363–74.

Lack, E.E., Travis, W.D. and Welch, K.J. (1985) Retroperitoneal germ cell tumors in childhood. *Cancer*, **56**, 602–8.

Levi, J., Raghavan, D., Harvey, V. *et al.* (1986) Deletion of bleomycin from therapy for good prognosis advanced testicular cancer. *Proc ASCO* **5**, 97 (Abstract 374).

Mameghan, H., Karolis, C., Kern, I. *et al.* (1985) Tumor control with ^{125}I seeds in childhood pelvic yolk sac tumor. *Radiat. Oncol. Biol. Phys.*, **11** (6), 1227–8.

Mann, J.R., Lakin, G.E., Leonard, J.C. *et al.* (1978) Clinical applications of serum carcinoembryonic antigen and alpha-fetoprotein levels in children with solid tumours. *Arch. Dis. Child.*, **53**, 366–74

Mann, J.R., Pearson, D., Barrett, A. *et al.* (1989) Results of the United Kingdom Children's Cancer Study Group's malignant germ cell tumor studies. *Cancer*, **63**, 1657–67.

Medical Research Council Working Party on Testicular Tumours. (1985) Prognostic factors in advanced non-seminomatous germ-cell testicular tumours: results of a multicentre study. *Lancet*, **i**, 8–11.

Newlands, E.S., Begent, R.H.J., Rustin, G.J.S. *et al.* (1983) Further advances in the management of malignant teratomas of the testis and other sites. *Lancet*, **i**, 948–51.

Nichols, C., Williams, S., Tricot, G. *et al.* (1988) Phase I study of high dose VP-16 plus carboplatin with autologous bone marrow rescue in refractory germ cell cancer. *Proc. ASCO* **7**, 118.

Ozols, R.F., Deisseroth, A.B., Javadpour, N. *et al.* (1983) Treatment of poor prognosis nonseminomatous testicular cancer with a 'high-dose' platinum combination chemotherapy regimen. *Cancer*, **51**, 1803–7.

Packer, R.J., Sutton, L.N., Rosenstock, J.G., *et al.* (1984) Pineal region tumors of childhood. *Pediatrics*, **74**, 97.

Peckham, M.J., Barrett, A., Husband, J.E. and Hendry, W.F. (1982) Orchidectomy alone in testicular Stage I non-seminomatous germ-cell tumours. *Lancet*, **i**, 678–80.

Peckham, M.J., Horwich, A., Blackmore, C. and Hendry, W.F. (1985) Etoposide and cisplatin with or without bleomycin as first-line chemotherapy for patients with small-volume metastases of testicular nonseminoma. *Cancer Treat. Rep.*, **69** (5), 483–8.

Pico, J.L., Droz, J.P., Ostronott, M. *et al.* (1989) High dose chemotherapy with ABMT for poor prognosis non-seminomatous germ cell tumours in *Autologous Bone Marrow Transplantation*, (eds K.A. Dicke, G. Spitzer, S. Jogonnoth and M. Evinger-Hodges) University of Texas Press, p.469.

Pinkerton, C.R., Broadbent, V., Horwich, A. *et al.* (1990) JEB – a carboplatin based regimen for malignant germ cell tumours in children. *Br. J. Cancer*, **62**, 257–62.

Pinkerton, C.R., Pritchard, J. and Spitz, L. (1986) High complete response rate in children with advanced germ cell tumors using cisplatin-containing combination chemotherapy. *J. Clin. Oncol.*, **4** (2), 194–9.

Pizzocaro, G., Salvioni, R., Pasi, M. *et al.* (1985) Early resection of residual tumor during cisplatin, vinblastine, bleomycin combination chemotherapy in Stage III and bulky Stage II nonseminomatous testicular cancer. *Cancer*, **56**, 249–55.

Raghavan, D., Vogelzang, N.J., Bosl, G.J. *et al.* (1982) Tumor classification and size in germ-cell testicular cancer. Influence on the occurrence of metastases. *Cancer*, **50**, 1591–5.

Read, G., Johnson, R.J. and Wilkinson, P.M. (1986) The role of radiotherapy after chemotherapy in the management of persistent para-aortic nodal disease in non-seminomatous germ cell tumours. *Br. J. Cancer*, **53**, 623–8.

Rustin, G.J.S., Newlands, E.S., Begent, R.H.J. *et al.* (1989) Weekly alternating etoposide, methotrexate, and actinomycin/vincristine and cyclophosphamide chemotherapy for the treatment of CNS metastases of choriocarcinoma. *J. Oncol.*, **7** (7), 900-3.

Scully, R.E. (1970) Gonadoblastoma. A review of 74 cases. *Cancer*, **25**, 1340–56.

Senturia, Y.D., Peckham, C.S. and Peckham, M.J. (1985) Children fathered by men treated for testicular cancer. *Lancet*, **i**, 766–9.

Smales, E. and Peckham, M.J. (1987) Chemotherapy of germ-cell ovarian tumours: First-line treatment with etoposide, bleomycin and cisplatin or carboplatin. *Eur. J. Cancer Clin. Oncol.*, **23** (5), 469–74.

Tait, D., Peckham, M.J., Hendry, W.F. and Goldstraw, P. (1984) Post-chemotherapy surgery in advanced non-seminomatous germ-cell testicular tumours: The significance of histology with particular reference to differentiated (mature) teratoma. *Br. J. Cancer*, **50**, 601–9.

Takeda, A., Ishizuka, T., Goto, T. *et al.* (1982) Polyembryoma of ovary alpha-fetoprotein and HCG: Immunoperoxidase and electron microscopy study. *Cancer*, **49**, 1878.

Tavcar, D., Robboy, S.J. and Chapman, P. (1980)

Endodermal sinus tumor of the pineal region. *Cancer*, **45**, 2646–51.

Truong, L.D., Harris, L. and Mattioli, C. (1986) Endodermal sinus tumor of the mediastinum: A report of seven cases and review of the literature. *Cancer*, **58**, 730–9.

Tsuchida, Y., Endo, Y., Saito, S. *et al.* (1978) Evaluation of alpha-fetoprotein in early infancy. *J. Ped. Surg.*, **13**, 155-6

Valdiserri, R.O. and Yunis, E.J. (1981) Sacrococcygeal teratomas: A review of 68 cases. *Cancer*, **48**, 217–21.

Vugrin, D., Friedman, A. and Whitmore, W.F. (1984) Correlation of serum tumor markers in advanced germ cell tumors with responses to chemotherapy and surgery. *Cancer*, **53**, 1440–5

von Hoff, D.D. (1987) Whither carboplatin? – A replacement for or an alternative to cisplatin? *J. Clin. Oncol.*, **5** (2), 169–71.

Weinblatt, M.E. and Ortega, J.A. (1982) Treatment of children with dysgerminoma of the ovary. *Cancer*, **49**, 2608–11.

Whalen, T., Mahour, G., Landing, B. and Wooleyt, M.M. (1985) Sacrococcygeal teratomas in infants and children. *Am. J. Surg.*, **150**, 373.

Williams, S.D., Birch, R., Einhorn, L.H. *et al.* (1987a) Treatment of disseminated germ-cell tumors with cisplatin, bleomycin, and either vinblastine or etoposide. *N. Engl. J. Med.*, **316**, 1435–40.

Williams, S.D., Stablein, D.M., Einhorn, L.H. *et al.* (1987b) Immediate adjuvant chemotherapy versus observation with treatment at relapse in pathological Stage II testicular cancer. *N. Engl. J. Med.* **317** (23), 1433–8.

Witte, D., Kissane, J. and Askin, F. (1983) Hepatic teratomas in children. *Pediatr. Pathol.*, **1**, 81.

Witzleben, C.L. and Bruninga, G. (1968) Infantile choriocarcinoma: A characteristic syndrome. *J. Pediat.*, **73**, 374–8.

Young, R. and Scully, R.E. (1984) Endodermal sinus tumor of the vagina: A report of nine cases and review of the literature. *Gynecol. Oncol.*, **18**, 380–92.

Chapter 20

Liver tumours

E.A. SHAFFORD AND J. PRITCHARD

20.1 INTRODUCTION

Primary malignant liver tumours account for only 1.2–5% of all paediatric neoplasms, but occur more frequently than benign tumours (Table 20.1; Ishak and Glunz, 1967; Exelby *et al.*, 1975). As in adults, hepatic secondaries are numerically more common than primary tumours. Neuroblastoma and nephroblastoma are the two paediatric tumours most likely to metastasize to the liver. However, since it is rare to encounter a child with a single or multiple liver metastases and an undetectable primary, there is hardly ever a problem in differential diagnosis.

There are two main types of malignant tumour, those of epithelial origin – hepato-blastoma and hepatocellular carcinoma – and the rarer mesenchymal tumours (relative frequency approximately 9:1).

20.2 HEPATOBLASTOMA AND HEPATOCELLULAR CARCINOMA

20.2.1 AETIOLOGY

Hepatoblastoma is classified as an 'embryonal' tumour of the liver. Embryonal tumours are thought to be the consequence of critical genetic changes (Knudson's 'two-hit hypo-

Table 20.1 Classification of liver tumours

Malignant	Benign
Epithelial	
Hepatoblastoma	Adenoma
Hepatocellular carcinoma	Focal nodular hyperplasia
Mesenchymal	
Mixed mesenchymal	Haemangioma
Rhabdomyosarcoma	Haemangioendothelioma
Angiosarcoma	Hamartoma
Undifferentiated sarcoma	

Table 20.2 Associated findings in hepatoblastoma and hepatocellular carcinoma (data from Ishak and Glunz, 1967 with the permission of the edition of *Cancer*; Mahour *et al.*, 1983, with the permission of the editor of *Amer. J. Surg.*; Fraumeni *et al.*, 1968 with the permission of the editor of *J. Natl. Cancer Inst.*)

Hepatoblastoma	Hepatocellular carcinoma
Hemi-hypertrophy	Cirrhosis
Beckwith-Wiedemann syndrome	Glycogen storage disease
Renal abnormalities	Tyrosinaemia
	De Toni Fanconi syndrome
Family history of FAP	Lipid storage disease

thesis') in tumour cells. The 'gene' for retino-blastoma is now known to be located on the long arm of chromosome 13 (13q) and one of the Wilms' tumour genes on the short arm of chromosome 11 (11p). Loss of constitutional heterozygosity, as detected by restriction enzyme digestion, Southern blotting and the appropriate DNA probes, can indicate the site(s) of the potential 'tumour genes' like these but, because of its rarity, little work has been carried out in hepatoblastoma. There is a report of loss of heterozygosity for parts of 11p in hepatoblastomas from two patients with the Beckwith-Wiedemann syndrome (Koufos *et al.*, 1985) but the molecular mechanism in these patients, who are predisposed to several kinds of paediatric tumours, may be different from that of tumours arising in otherwise normal patients.

The clear-cut association between familial adenomatous polyposis and hepatoblastoma may be the best clue to the location of a hepatoblastoma gene – one of the familial adenomatous polyposis genes has recently been located on chromosome 5q (Bodmer *et al.*, 1987). Kingston *et al.* (1983) noted the association between hepatoblastoma and a family history of familial adenomatous polyposis (FAP). They reported five such cases occurring during a 50-year period and calculated that familial adenomatous polyposis occurs 100 times more frequently in parents of children with hepatoblastoma than in the general population. Children cured of hepatoblastoma who have a parent with familial adenomatous polyposis have a 50% chance of developing this disease and must be screened regularly. Finally, hepatoblastomas almost always arise in an otherwise normal liver. Hepatocellular carcinoma, by contrast, is frequently associated with cirrhosis or other pre-existing parenchymal liver disorder (Table 20.2; Kasai and Watanabe, 1970; Mahour *et al.*, 1983).

Five of 32 children and adolescents with hepatocellular carcinoma studied by Lack *et al.* (1983) had cirrhosis, two had a hepatic adenoma, and one had previously been treated with orthovoltage radiation for a Wilms' tumour. Twenty of 28 Taiwanese children with hepatocellular carcinoma had cirrhosis (Chen *et al.*, 1988). The association of hepatitis B infection and hepatocellular carcinoma in adults has been well documented, and there are increasing numbers of reports of this association in children. Chen *et al.* (1988) for example, demonstrated 100% positivity for HBsAg in 25 children with hepatocellular carcinoma in Taiwan. Southeast Asia is, of course, a high prevalence area for hepatitis B virus infection, but HBsAg in association with hepatocellular carcinoma in children has also been reported in Europe (Leuschner *et al.*, 1988). The HBsAg status of 15 of the Taiwanese patients' families was ascertained. Fourteen of 15 mothers were HBsAg positive indicating that vertical transmission from the mother is a very important source of hepatitis B infection in children. Administration of hepatitis B immune globulin at birth to infants of HBsAg positive mothers, followed by hepatitis B vaccination, and vaccination of hepatitis B negative children in areas with a high incidence of hepatitis B infection should reduce the incidence of the chronic HBsAg carrier state and thus the incidence of hepatocellular carcinoma in children and in adults.

The incidence of hepatoblastoma throughout the world is fairly constant at 0.5–1.5 cases per million children (Parkin *et al.*, 1988). In most countries, hepatocellular carcinoma is less common than hepatoblastoma, but there is considerable geographic variation, with rates ranging from 0.2 per million in England and Wales to 2.1 per million children in Hong Kong. In some populations hepatocellular carcinoma occurs more frequently than hepatoblastoma, in, for example, Hong Kong and Taiwan (Chen *et al.*, 1988; Parkin *et al.*, 1988). Boys are more commonly affected than girls, especially in the case of hepatoblastoma (m:f approximately 2:1; Ishak and

Glunz, 1967; Kasai and Watanabe, 1970; Exelby *et al.*, 1975; Lack *et al.*, 1982; 1983). The vast majority of hepatoblastomas occur in children under the age of five years, with 50% in children less than 18 months of age. Occasionally the tumour may be detected (by ultrasound) prenatally or at birth. Hepatocellular carcinoma, by contrast, is a tumour of older children with a peak incidence between 10 and 14 years (Ishak and Glunz, 1967; Exelby *et al.*, 1975; Kasai and Watanabe, 1970; Lack *et al.*, 1982).

20.2.2 PATHOLOGY

(a) Hepatoblastoma

The majority of hepatoblastoma are unifocal and located in the right lobe of the liver. The macroscopic characteristics are variable. Tumours may be encapsulated or unencapsulated, nodular or smooth, firm, soft or friable. The cut surface varies in colour from greyish-white to tan. Areas of haemorrhage, calcification and necrosis may be seen (Ishak and Glunz, 1967).

Attempts have been made to divide hepatoblastoma into histopathological subtypes, and relate them to prognosis. Willis (1953) used the term hepatoblastoma for all embryonal tumours containing hepatic epithelial parenchyma, subdividing them into three types: (1) embryonal-pure epithelial; (2) mixed-epithelial and mesenchymal, and (3) rhabdomyoblastic mixed tumour. Ishak and Glunz (1967) modified this classification; they pre-

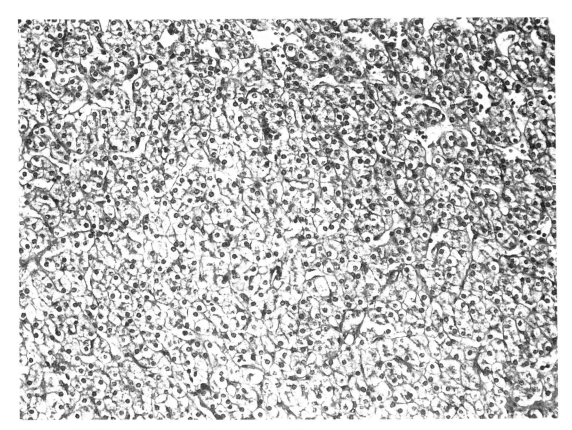

Fig. 20.1 Fetal hepatoblastoma showing glycogen-rich area.

411

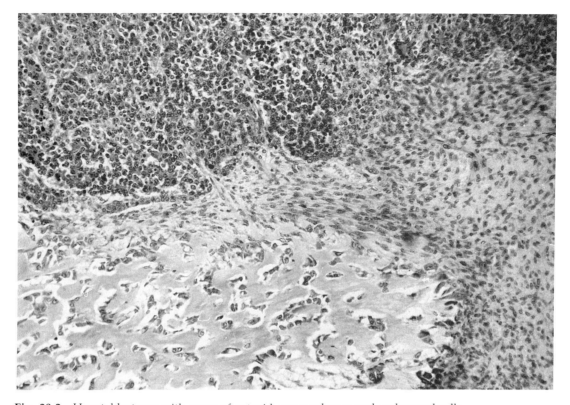

Fig. 20.2 Hepatoblastoma with areas of osteoid, mesenchyme and embryonal cells.

ferred two rather than three categories: (1) epithelial; (2) epithelial and mesenchymal. In the pure epithelial tumours, which were usually nodular and had a cut surface of uniform appearance, they recognized two types of cells. Fetal-type cells resemble the cells of the fetal liver and are usually arranged in irregular plates, two-cells thick. The cells vary in size but are smaller than normal hepatocytes, and have acidophilic cytoplasm containing glycogen (Fig. 20.1). Their nuclei are round or oval, and basophilic, with few mitotic figures. Embryonal type cells are less well differentiated, and arranged in sheets. The cells are small and darkly staining with scanty cytoplasm containing little or no glycogen. Nuclei are hyperchromatic and mitoses frequent. Mixed tumours have a lobulated cut surface appearance with bands of collagenous material separating the lobules. There are areas of fetal and embryonal type cells, as well as supporting reticulin fibres and blood vessels. Primitive mesenchyme, containing elongated spindle cells with scanty cytoplasm and areas of osteoid tissue, is another notable component of these tumours (Fig. 20.2). Kasai and Watanabe (1970) suggested an alternative sub-classification into: (1) fetal; (2) embryonal, and (3) anaplastic varieties. Anaplastic tumours consist of small cells with scanty cytoplasm, with no glycogen, resembling neuroblasts. Mitoses are uncommon. They found that the morphologically poorly differentiated tumours, i.e. embryonal and anaplastic subtypes had a worse prognosis than the better differentiated fetal tumours, a view supported by Lack *et al*. (1982).

412

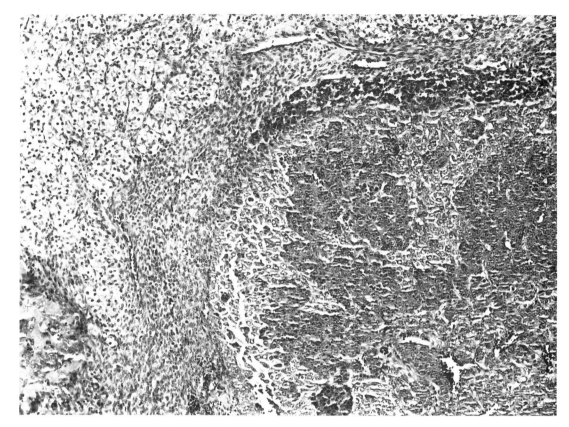

Fig. 20.3 Hepatoblastoma – juxtaposition of fetal, small cell and embryonal cell.

In a joint study by the Children's Cancer Study Group (CCSG), Southwest Oncology Group (SWOG), and Paediatric Oncology Group (POG) (Haas *et al.*, 1989) tumours were classified according to Weinberg and Finegold (1986), as: (1) fetal; (2) embryonal; (3) macrotrabecular; (4) small cell undifferentiated (anaplastic). Because of the morphological similarity of small cell undifferentiated tumours to neuroblastoma, lymphoma, and rhabdomyosarcoma, areas of epithelial (usually fetal) hepatoblastoma must be seen to confirm the diagnosis (Fig. 20.3). In the macrotrabecular sub-type, cells are arranged in trabeculae ten to 20 or more cells thick. Cells may be larger than the surrounding normal liver cells, and resemble hepato-cellular carcinoma, but fetal cells are always also present. Although there are overlaps between these classifications there are, at present, no internationally agreed histopathological criteria for subclassification of hepatoblastoma.

(b) Hepatocellular carcinoma

The majority of these tumours (70–80%) are either multifocal or involve both lobes at the time of diagnosis (Exelby *et al.*, 1975; Lack *et al.*, 1983; Chen *et al.*, 1988). Macroscopically, they are nodular and vary in consistency from soft to firm and in colour from yellow to green. Often there are areas of necrosis or haemorrhage. Microscopically, the tumours

413

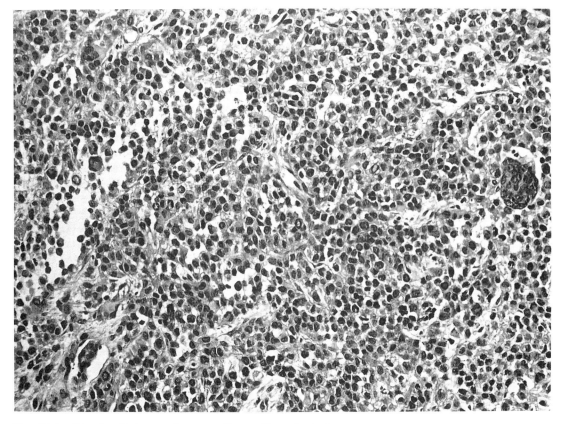

Fig. 20.4 Hepatocellular carcinoma with multi-nucleate forms.

resemble hepatocellular carcinoma in adults, with a trabecular pattern up to 20 layers of cells thick. The cells are usually larger than those of the surrounding liver, but vary markedly in size. Giant cells are common and mitoses frequent (Ishak and Glunz, 1967; Kasai and Watanabe, 1970; Fig. 20.4). Evidence of cirrhosis is seen in the non-tumorous liver in 10–70% of cases (Ishak and Glunz, 1967; Kasai and Watanabe, 1970; Lack *et al.*, 1983; Chen *et al.*, 1988).

The fibrolamellar variant of hepatocellular carcinoma, which is probably a distinct clinicopathological entity, invariably arises in a non-cirrhotic liver. The two distinctive features of this epithelial tumour are: (1) tumour cells with eosinophilic cytoplasm; and (2) broad fibrous septa dividing the hepatocytes into thin colums of cells or large nodules. Mitotic figures are rare (Fig. 20.5; Craig *et al.*, 1980).

20.2.3 CLINICAL PRESENTATION

The presenting symptoms of hepatoblastoma and hepatocellular carcinoma are similar. Abdominal mass and/or abdominal distension are the most common features. Anorexia and lethargy are also frequent. Jaundice and abdominal pain are unusual in patients with hepatoblastoma, but are more common (10–20% and 15–65% of patients respectively) in hepatocellular carcinoma, especially in patients with underlying liver disease. In rare cases,

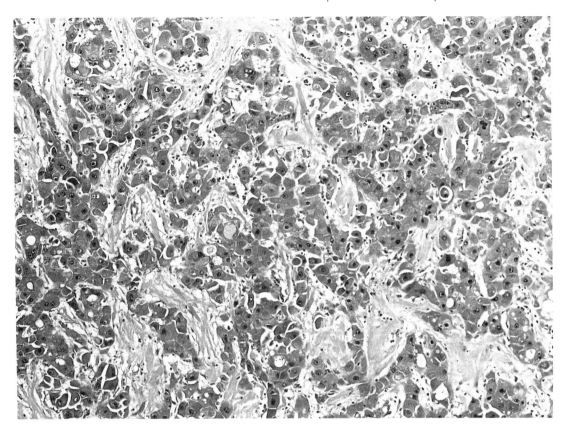

Fig. 20.5 Fibrolamellar hepatocellular carcinoma.

presentation is with an 'acute abdomen' due to tumour rupture or intra-tumoral haemorrhage (Ishak and Glunz, 1967; Exelby *et al.*, 1975; Lack *et al.*, 1982; Lack *et al.*, 1983). Precocious puberty is an unusual presentation of hepatoblastoma but has not been reported in hepatocellular carcinoma (Nakagawara *et al.*, 1985). Virilization is due to gonadotrophin production by the tumour, which stimulates testosterone secretion by the testes. Testicular biopsy shows Leydig cell hyperplasia with no spermatogenesis. Osteoporosis is present in about 20% of patients with hepatoblastoma (Lack *et al.*, 1982) and when severe may lead to multiple fractures and the suspicion of non accidental injury. Hepatomegaly, with or without a distinct hepatic mass, is almost always

present and pallor is common. There may be evidence of weight loss, dilated abdominal veins and jaundice. Features of the Beckwith-Wiedemann syndrome may be evident.

Enquiry should be made for a family history of familial adenomatous polyposis, for maternal ingestion of androgens during pregnancy, and a past history of hepatitis or other antecedent liver disease in the parents or the child. All of these factors may have aetiological implications (Fraumeni *et al.*, 1968).

20.2.4 INVESTIGATIONS

(a) **Laboratory**

Many patients are anaemic at diagnosis and

thrombocytosis is common, especially in hepatoblastoma (Lack *et al.*, 1982; Lack *et al.*, 1983). The platelet count may be $> 1,000 \times 10^9/l$, probably due to production by the tumour of a circulating 'thrombopoietin' (Nickerson *et al.*, 1980). Liver function tests in hepatoblastoma are usually normal, but in hepatocellular carcinoma, serum bilirubin, AST, ALT, and alkaline phosphatase levels may be elevated (Exelby *et al.*, 1975; Lack *et al.*, 1982; Lack *et al.*, 1983; Chen *et al.*, 1988). Alpha fetoprotein (αFP) is produced by the normal fetal liver and although present in decreasing amounts in the serum of babies up to six to nine months old, is not normally detected in the serum of older children and adults (Wu *et al.*, 1981). An elevated level of serum αFP is found in >90% of cases of hepatoblastoma, (Pierro *et al.*, 1989; Shafford *et al.*, 1989) and 60–90% of hepatocellular carcinomas (Perilongo *et al.* 1987a, Pierro *et al.*, 1989). It is a very sensitive 'tumour marker' but not specific to hepatoma as elevated levels are also found in patients with malignant germ cell tumours, especially those containing yolk sac elements. Serum αFP is normal in serum of patients with the fibrolamellar variant of hepatocellular carcinoma but unsaturated vitamin B_{12} binding capacity is a useful tumour marker (Paradinas *et al.*, 1982; Wheeler *et al.* 1986). Increased excretion of cystathionine may be detected in the urine of children with hepatoblastoma, but this amino acid is not a specific tumour product and is not useful in follow up.

(b) Imaging

In a child with a suspected hepatic tumour, imaging will confirm the intra-hepatic location, demonstrate the nature of the mass, identify metastases, and give an indication of resectability (de Campo and Phelan, 1988). In many cases hepatomegaly is evident on plain abdominal x-ray, and in 10–20% calcification is visible (Ishak and Glunz, 1967; Lack *et al.*, 1982; 1983; Dachman *et al.*, 1987). Calcification is

usually coarse and dense, contrasting with the fine granular calcification seen in haemangioendothelioma. Abdominal ultrasound helps define the site and the extent of tumour. The inferior vena cava, portal vein and hepatic veins and arteries can also be identified. The majority of hepatocellular tumours are hyperechoic whereas haemangioendotheliomas are usually hypoechoic, and mesenchymal hamartomas have large cystic areas (Dachman *et al.*, 1987). Abdominal CT scanning delineates the tumour which is characteristically of low attenuation compared to the surrounding liver. Involvement of the hepatic veins, inferior vena cava or portal vein is best seen after contrast enhancement. Failure to recognize invasion (intraluminal tumour/thrombus) of hepatic veins or inferior vena cava may lead to pulmonary embolization at the time of operation with a possible fatal outcome (Dorman *et al.*, 1985). MRI gives definition of tumour and hepatic veins without I.V. contrast and enables assessment of the segmental extent of the tumour to be made (Boechat *et al.*, 1988; Finn *et al.*, 1990). Angiography is considered useful in demonstrating the blood supply to the tumour as well as vascular anomalies, both of which may be important when assessing the resectability of the tumour. Some centres, however, feel that MRI or CT with I.V. enhancement is as useful in this respect as angiography. In around 10% of patients with hepatoblastoma, pulmonary metastases are visible

Table 20.3 Typical investigation of a patient with a suspected liver tumour

Mandatory	Optional
Abdominal x-ray	Angiography
Abdominal ultrasound	MRI scan
Abdominal CT scan	
Chest x-ray	
Lung CT scan if chest x-ray normal	Lung CT scan if chest x-ray shows metastases

on initial chest x-ray (Exelby *et al.*, 1975; Lack *et al.*, 1982). Lung CT scanning may reveal metastases not visible on chest x-ray.

Osteoporosis, detected by plain x-rays, is seen in some patients with hepatoblastoma (Lack *et al.*, 1982) and hepatocellular carcinoma (Fraumeni *et al.*, 1968). This is probably due to a circulating bone resorbing factor and when severe leads to fractures. Bone density returns to normal after successful treatment of the tumour. Because of the rarity of bone and brain secondaries at diagnosis, scanning of these organs is not justified without a specific clinical indication. All patients with a suspected liver tumour should be investigated as indicated in Table 20.3.

20.2.5 STAGING

Traditionally, a post surgical staging system is used, with stage related to the amount of tumour removed at initial surgery, as shown in Table 20.4 (Haas *et al.*, 1989). 'Local' staging, based on initial surgery, is dependant on: (1) the decision to attempt resection rather than give preoperative chemotherapy; and (2) the surgeon's expertise, which lessens the value of comparison of results from different studies.

In the current International Society of Paediatric Oncology (SIOP) liver tumour study 'SIOPEL I', a pre-operative grouping

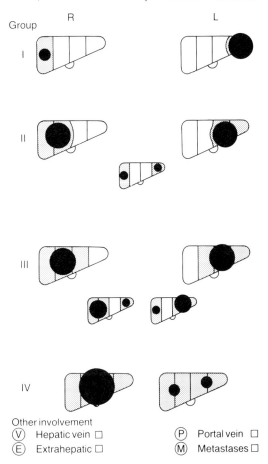

Fig. 20.6 SIOP pre-treatment grouping system describing extent of disease (by kind permission of Professor Anton Vos).

Table 20.4 Post surgical staging of hepatocellular tumours

Stage I – completely resected at initial surgery
Stage II – resection with localized disease at the margin
Stage III – unresectable or gross residual, but not metastatic
Stage IV – metastatic disease
Note: A distinction may be made between Stage IIIA – patients with a large unifocal unresectable tumour – and Stage IIIB – patients with multifocal disease involving both lobes.

system has been introduced (Vos *et al.*, 1989). This system describes the site and size of the tumour, invasion of vessels, and distant spread, as judged by pre-treatment imaging with ultrasound, CT scan and MRI (Fig. 20.6). Group indicates the number of sectors involved by tumour – i.e. Group II implies two sectors involved, and Group IV all four sectors involved. More universal use of this system should facilitate comparison of results from different studies.

20.2.6 TREATMENT

(a) Surgery

In a child with a liver mass and a markedly elevated serum αFP level for age, the diagnosis is almost certainly a hepatocellular tumour, but the distinction between hepatoblastoma or hepatocellular carcinoma and exclusion of malignant germ cell tumour can only be made on histology. Opinions differ, but if pre-operative chemotherapy is to be given, most would favour a pre treatment biopsy either by percutaneous needle biopsy (trucut or Menghini) or via mini-laparotomy so that several parts of the tumour may be sampled. Fine needle aspiration probably provides too little tissue to be of practical use.

Complete tumour resection is of paramount importance for cure but operative mortality, without prior chemotherapy, has been reported to be as high as 10–20% (Ishak and Glunz, 1967; Exelby *et al.*, 1975; Lack *et al.*, 1982; 1983). In addition, less than 50% of tumours are resectable at diagnosis (Ishak and Glunz, 1967; Kasai and Watanabe, 1970; Exelby *et al.*, 1975; Evans *et al.*, 1982; Mahour *et al.*, 1983; Haas *et al.*, 1989) and survival of patients with unresectable tumours is rare (Quinn *et al.*, 1985).

Prior to surgery, detailed imaging of the tumour is necessary. The liver is divided into a right and left lobe by the inferior vena cava and the gall bladder. The right lobe is subdivided into anterior and posterior lobes and the left, by the falciform ligament, into medial and lateral lobes. The hepatic artery, a branch of the coeliac axis, usually divides into a right and left branch, but variations occur in 25% of the population, with the right hepatic artery arising from the superior mesenteric artery and the left from the gastric artery. The portal vein supplies all four lobes of the liver. Venous drainage is via the three hepatic veins to the inferior vena cava. The branches of the biliary tree usually follow those of the hepatic artery and the portal vein.

Blood loss is a major factor in the high operative mortality associated with hepatic resection, but improvements in anaesthetic and surgical techniques during recent years have substantially reduced the risk (Brown *et al.*, 1988; Davidson and Auldist, 1988). Isolation of the liver from the systemic circulation – by vascular slings, hypothermia and hypotension – can be used to reduce and control haemorrhage. In addition, the use of an ultrasonic dissector will further reduce blood loss by permitting the surgeon to define and control the numerous vascular radicles in the raw surface of the liver at the line of resection. Resectability depends on the location and the vascular supply of the tumour, and, in some instances, this may only be determined at laparotomy. The usual types of resection are right lobectomy (anterior and posterior lobes), or left lobectomy (medial and lateral lobes) (Fig. 20.7). In children, because of the capacity of the remaining liver to regenerate, trisegmentectomy, e.g. an extended right hepatectomy, removing the left medial lobe as well as the right lobe, may be performed. Post operatively patients need careful moni-

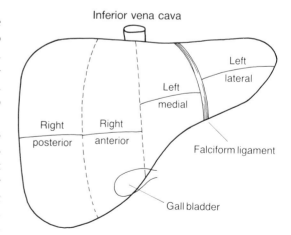

Fig. 20.7 Lobes of the liver showing usual resection types.

toring as they are at risk from hypogly-caemia, hypoproteinaemia, bleeding due to reduction in clotting factors, and infection. Damage to bile ducts during surgery may later cause stenosis and obstructive jaundice, or biliary fistula (Gauthier *et al.*, 1986; Davidson and Auldist, 1988).

Resection of pulmonary metastases is justi-fied in patients who have shown a response to chemotherapy with complete resection of their primary tumour, but incomplete resolu-tion of the secondaries. This kind of approach may be curative (Gauthier *et al.*, 1986).

(b) Chemotherapy

Most patients with hepatocellular tumours present with unresectable or metastatic dis-ease. The possibility that chemotherapy could convert unresectable to resectable disease was first appreciated by Hermann and Lonsdale (1970), who reported a child with hepatoblast-oma treated preoperatively with vincristine, cyclophosphamide and radiotherapy. Exelby *et al.* (1975) reported three patients respond-ing to vincristine, actinomycin D and cyclo-phosphamide, and Shafer and Selinkoff (1977) reported three patients who had complete re-section of hepatoblastoma after treatment with vincristine, actinomycin D and radiother-apy. Ikeda *et al.*'s two cases (1979) responded to preoperative vincristine and cyclophos-phamide. Response of lung metastases to chemotherapy was shown by Andrassy *et al.* (1980). They reported six cases of unresect-able hepatoblastoma treated with combination chemotherapy including cyclophosphamide, vincristine, 5-fluorouracil and adriamycin. Four patients, including two with pulmonary metastases, showed a response (complete disappearance of lung secondaries in one, and decrease in size by 90% in the other), and three had complete resection of their primary tumour. The fourth patient died from adriamycin cardiomyopathy.

Reports of hepatocellular carcinoma re-sponding to chemotherapy are few. This might be either because it is a very rare tumour and/or it really is less responsive to chemotherapy than hepatoblastoma. Weinblatt *et al.* (1982) reported preoperative chemotherapy in eight children with hepatic malignancies, includ-ing two with hepatocellular carcinoma. One, with an anaplastic hepatocellular carcinoma involving both lobes, was treated with chemo-therapy (vincristine, cyclophosphamide, 5-fluorouracil and adriamycin) alone and was alive with no evidence of disease 21 months from diagnosis. The second had resolution of 90% of pulmonary metastases and 75% re-gression of primary tumour sustained for four months. Perilongo *et al.* (1987a) treated one patient with hepatocellular carcinoma with preoperative cisplatin and etoposide with complete disappearance of lung metastases and more than 50% reduction of the primary tumour.

In those patients who have initial complete resection of hepatoblastoma (Stage I) survival with surgery alone is around 50% (Ishak and Glunz, 1967; Kasai and Watanabe, 1970; Lack *et al.*, 1982). Survival after surgery alone for hepatocellular carcinoma is poor. In Kasai and Watanabe's series (1970) only three of 13 patients had complete resection of tumour. Two died within 18 months and the other was lost to follow-up. Of 32 patients reported by Lack *et al.* (1983), seven were treated by surgery alone and only three survive.

In two studies of surgery then chemother-apy for children with hepatocellular tumours (Evans *et al.*, 1982), seven of 11 patients treated with surgery alone relapsed, com-pared to one of 16 given post operative chemo-therapy (vincristine, cyclophosphamide, adriamycin and 5-fluorouracil) after complete resection of tumour. Results of recent chemo-therapy studies are summarized in Table 20.5.

Adriamycin and cisplatin are acknowl-edged to be the most effective single agents for treating hepatoblastoma. The toxicity of both drugs is cumulative and dose related so

419

Table 20.5 Results of pre operative chemotherapy in hepatoblastoma

Author	Chemotherapy	N	Resectable	Metastases cleared
Douglass *et al.*, 1985	CDDP, VCR, 5FU	6	4	3/3
Gauthier *et al.*, 1986	VCR, CPM, ADR, 5FU/CDDP	13	7	no details
Ortega *et al.*, 1989	ADR, CDDP	10 Hbl. 5HCC	8 1	no details
Pierro *et al.*, 1989	ADR, CDDP, VBL BLEO, CPM, 5FU, VCR	11	8	2/3
Quinn *et al.*, 1985	ADR, CDDP	3	2	1/1
Shafford *et al.*, 1989	ADR, CDDP	14	10	4/5
	Total	62	40	10/12

CDDP = cisplatin; VCR = vincristine; 5FU = 5-fluorouracil; CPM = cyclophosphamide; ADR = adriamycin; VBL = vinblastine; BLEO = bleomycin.

careful monitoring of cardiac function (measurement of left ventricular ejection fraction), renal function (preferably measurement of glomerular filtration rate by isotope clearance), and serial audiometry are necessary during therapy with these drugs.

Cisplatin causes high frequency hearing loss. The median age at diagnosis for patients with hepatoblastoma is around 18 months, an age when children are developing language skills. Detection of high frequency hearing loss in young children is difficult, so assessment by an expert audiologist is desirable. Brock *et al.* (1988) have proposed a grading system for ototoxicity in children treated with cisplatin, which will facilitate comparison of toxicity of different regimes. There is evidence that continuous infusion of adriamycin is less cardiotoxic, and continuous infusion of cisplatin may be less ototoxic than bolus injection (Legha *et al.*, 1982). The place of epirubicin, carboplatin, etoposide and ifosfamide in the treatment of hepatocellular tumours is discussed in the current controversies section of this chapter.

In summary, surgery and chemotherapy is necessary in the treatment of most children with hepatoblastoma or hepatocellular carcinoma. Pre operative chemotherapy may convert unresectable to resectable disease and invariably makes the operation less hazardous. Post operative chemotherapy after initial complete resection is effective against micrometastases and considerably reduces the risk of metastatic relapse.

(c) Radiotherapy

The role of radiotherapy, if any, in the treatment of hepatoblastoma and hepatocellular carcinoma has not yet been clearly defined. The majority of patients who have radiotherapy also have chemotherapy, so it is difficult to attribute tumour shrinkage or cure to one or other modality (Habrand, 1991).

(i) Primary site

In a survey by Exelby *et al.* (1975) 27 of 129 patients with hepatoblastoma were treated with radiotherapy to the primary site at some stage during their treatment programme. Three patients had complete resection of an initially unresectable tumour after treatment with radiotherapy and combination chemotherapy, but no patient with an inoperable tumour was cured by radiotherapy and chemotherapy alone. In the same survey no patient with hepatocellular carcinoma treated with radiotherapy to the liver or whole abdomen survived. In a USA CCSG/SWOG study of combination chemotherapy in hepatoma (Evans *et al.*, 1982) seven of 27 patients had a complete or good partial response, four of whom were treated with chemotherapy and radiotherapy. In three patients, an initially unresectable tumour became resectable after chemotherapy and radiotherapy. Shafer and Selinkoff (1977) reported a similar finding. In a report by Quinn *et al.*, (1985) one patient whose tumour remained unresectable after treatment with adriamycin and cisplatin, was given 45 Gy to the tumour; afterwards, and without surgery, the serum αFP level fell to normal. Further chemotherapy was given and the child is alive and well over six years later. In the SIOPEL 1 study, patients who have 'miniscopic' (i.e. small volume macroscopic) residual disease have two further courses of chemotherapy and the option of small field radiotherapy.

(ii) Metastases

Radiotherapy has also been used, in combination with chemotherapy, to treat pulmonary metastatic disease. In our own series (Shafford *et al.*, 1989) four of five Stage IV patients with lung metastases received whole lung radiotherapy; three after complete radiological response to adriamycin and cisplatin and complete resection of primary tumour, and one at the time of metastatic relapse. The dose was 12–15 Gy in 8–10 fractions. Three are long-term survivors but the fourth died of metastatic disease. Another patient was treated with adriamycin, vincristine, and whole lung radiotherapy for pulmonary metastases which occurred 11 months after surgery, vincristine and cyclophosphamide treatment of a Stage I tumour. She is a long-term survivor (Pritchard *et al.*, 1982).

Given doubt about the value of adding lung radiotherapy, with its attendant late morbidity, to chemotherapy, patients with lung metastases at diagnosis entered into the current SIOP, GPO, and American studies, are not being given pulmonary radiation.

In summary, there are no randomized studies which are examining the value of radiotherapy in hepatoblastoma/hepatocellular carcinoma and no studies in which radiotherapy has been evaluated as a single agent. Most patients who 'respond' to radiotherapy also receive concomitant chemotherapy. There is a consensus view that radiotherapy is probably not valuable in the management of lung secondaries or gross primary disease. Its role in post operative residual disease is due to be evaluated in SIOPEL 1. As with most other paediatric tumours, radiotherapy may be useful as part of palliative care.

(d) Alternative therapy

For patients who do not respond to treatment with adriamycin and cisplatin-containing chemotherapy, or who relapse after treatment, alternatives are required. Hepatic artery embolization with gel foam has been used in the treatment of hepatocellular tumours to reduce vascularity and tumour size prior to surgery. It may also be used as palliative treatment for an inoperable tumour (Chaung and Wallace, 1981). Intra-arterial therapy with anti-tumour drugs dispersed in a lipid contrast medium has been shown to be effective in some unresectable hepatocellular tumours. When lipiodol is injected into the hepatic artery it selectively accumulates in hepatocellular tumour tissue and can act as a carrier for anti-tumour drugs. Ogita *et al.* (1987) treated two infants with unresectable hepatoblastoma with intra-arterial injection of adriamycin, cisplatin and 5-fluorouracil

421

dispersed in lipiodol. The anti-tumour drug complex selectively accumulated in the tumour tissue and was accompanied by marked tumour shrinkage. In one patient the tumour was completely resected, but resection was not attempted in the other patient because of pulmonary metastases. Sue *et al.* (1989) used intra-arterial injections of a cisplatin, 5-fluorouracil/lipiodol suspension together with systemic chemotherapy to treat two patients with unresectable hepatoblastoma. One child died of progressive disease but the other achieved a complete response after surgery and further intra-arterial chemotherapy. Kobayashi *et al.* (1986) used transarterial internal irradiation to treat adult patients with hepatocellular carcinoma using ^{131}I iodized oil. Of the seven patients treated (two of whom had received previous intra-arterial chemotherapy) six had a marked reduction in serum αFP level and all had a reduction in tumour size ranging from 30–80% over 5–25 weeks from the time of treatment.

Ferritin is found in high concentration in hepatocellular carcinoma. [131]I antiferritin antibodies have therefore been used in the treatment of these tumours. In a study by Order *et al.* (1985) 105 adults/teenagers with hepatoma (age range 15–82 years) were treated with external radiation and chemotherapy followed by ^{131}I anti ferritin. Of these patients, 7% achieved a complete response and 41% a partial response. Median survival was 5–7 months but the longest complete response lasted three years, six months. The major toxicity was thrombocytopenia. In Order's current studies, patients are treated with external beam radiation and chemotherapy then randomized to either further chemotherapy, or ^{131}I anti ferritin plus chemotherapy. De Kraker *et al.* (1989) used ^{131}I labelled Rose Bengal to treat an infant with an unresectable hepatoblastoma. There was a drop in serum αFP level but no other measurable response.

In many of these studies patients have received concurrent systemic chemotherapy which makes interpretation of the results and assessment of tumour response to the 'alternative' therapy difficult. Further studies of 'targeted' therapy for unresectable hepatocellular tumours is needed.

20.2.7 RESPONSE

Patients given preoperative chemotherapy are assessed for response by clinical examination, imaging, with measurement of tumour dimensions, and serial serum αFP levels. To evaluate the response of a tumour to preoperative chemotherapy, and to compare the results of different studies, response must be clearly defined. Complete response (CR), i.e. complete disappearance of all tumour; and no response (NR), i.e. no measurable regression of disease, are clear cut. The difficulty comes in defining partial response. Evans *et al.* (1982) used good partial response (GPR) – objective regression of disease of more than 50% (as measured by the sum of two diameters – and partial response (PR) – objective regression of disease of less than 50%. In the SIOPEL 1 study, the terms used to define response are as follows: complete response; partial response (any tumour shrinkage); no response; and progressive disease (unequivocal increase in one or more dimensions). For metastatic disease a fifth category is added, 'minimal residual disease', denoting complete clearing of PA and lateral chest x-ray with minimal residual change on lung CT scan. In multifocal or metastatic disease, these criteria are applied to each tumour, and the patient's response is classified according to the 'worst responding' tumour. Allowance is also made for the fact that in the early stages of chemotherapy, real or apparent size increase may be due to intratumoral haemorrhage or oedema.

To qualify for complete or partial response categories in the SIOPEL 1 study, the serum αFP level must have fallen from its initial elevated value. Patients with a good response to chemotherapy usually show a marked decrease in serum α FP level (Quinn *et al.*, 1985; Pierro *et al.*, 1989; Shafford *et al.*, 1989). A rising serum αFP level is often the first indication of relapse. In rare cases, relapse may be αFP negative.

In fibrolamellar hepatocellular carcinoma, serum transcobalamin I (TCI) level is a useful tumour marker and a rising level suggests disease recurrence (Wheeler *et al.*, 1986).

Patients suspected of relapse should be re-investigated with chest and abdominal imaging, as at the time of their initial presentation, to determine the extent of recurrence. Relapse may be local (in the remaining liver) or metastatic. The commonest sites for metastases are the lungs and abdominal lymph nodes. In rare cases, these tumours metastasize to brain or bone (Ishak and Glunz, 1967; Exelby *et al.*, 1975; Lack *et al.*, 1982; 1983).

20.2.8 SURVIVAL

The outlook for children with hepatocellular tumours in the past was poor, with an overall survival between 9% and 35% (Table 20.6). In these series, no child who had an initially unresectable tumour survived. In those patients who had initial complete resection of tumour, survival for hepatoblastoma was 40–

60%. Less than a third of patients with hepatocellular carcinoma had complete resection of tumour and survival was poor.

In a CCSG, SWOG study between 1976 and 1978, 62 patients with hepatocellular tumours (40 Hbl; 12 HCC) were treated with surgery and combination chemotherapy (vincristine, adriamycin, cyclophosphamide and 5-fluorouracil). Radiotherapy was given to patients with residual disease. Of these patients, 83% who had complete surgical resection of tumour survived at a median of 30 months (Evans *et al.*, 1982). In a more recent CCSG, POG study of 177 children, patients with Stage I or II tumours were treated with vincristine, cyclophosphamide, adriamycin, and 5-fluorouracil. Patients with more advanced disease were given bleomycin and *cis*platinum in addition. Stage for stage there was no significant difference in survival between patients with hepatoblastoma and those with hepatocellular carcinoma. The three-year disease-free survival was as follows: Stage I 67%; Stage II 60%; Stage III 22%; Stage IV 7% (Ablin *et al.*, 1988).

In all these studies, complete resection of tumour was a critical prognostic factor, but only 20–40% of all patients have complete surgical resection. To improve the survival of children with hepatocellular tumours, the percentage of tumours which can be resected must be increased. Recent reports have indi-

Table 20.6 Survival of children with hepatocellular tumours

Study		N	Overall survival	Patients having csr	Survival after csr
Ishak and Glunz, 1967	Hbl	35	28%	18	50%
	HCC	12	0	3	0
Kasai and Watanabe, 1970	Hbl	57	21%	24	50%
	HCC	13	0	3	0
Exelby *et al.*, 1975	Hbl	129	35%	78	58%
	HCC	98	12%	33	36%
Lack *et al.*, 1982; 1983	Hbl	54	24%	32	40%
	HCC	32	9%	7	42%

Hbl = Hepatoblastoma; HCC = Hepatocellular carcinoma; csr = complete surgical resection.

cated the responsiveness of hepatoblastoma to adriamycin and cisplatin chemotherapy, with some unresectable tumours becoming resectable, and promisingly low recurrence rate (Evans *et al.*, 1982; Douglass *et al.*, 1985; Ortega *et al.*, 1989).

In our series, 14 patients with unresectable hepatoblastoma have been treated. Two had initial surgery and 12 had pre-operative chemotherapy with adriamycin and cisplatin. Of these 14, 10 had complete resection of their tumour, and eight (80%) survive disease-free. The overall survival is 57% with a median follow-up of 21 months (Shafford *et al.*, 1989; ASCO 1989). Median follow-up is now 42 months. However, this regimen is potentially toxic. Two patients developed adriamycin cardiomyopathy (total doses 350 and 400 mg/m^2), one of whom died, and one patient has a moderate high tone hearing loss (Brock grade 3, Brock *et al.*, 1988). Pierro *et al.* (1989) also used pre-operative chemotherapy with adriamycin and cisplatin to treat 11 patients with unresectable hepatoblastoma. Overall survival was 63% (7/11) and 87% (7/8) for patients having a complete resection of their tumour. These figures indicate a marked improvement in overall survival for patients with Stage III and IV disease.

20.3 MALIGNANT MESENCHYMAL TUMOURS

These tumours comprise 9–15% of primary malignant liver tumours (Exelby *et al.*, 1975; Perilongo *et al.*, 1987b) and include rhabdomyosarcoma, angiosarcoma, fibrosarcoma, and undifferentiated (embryonal) sarcoma. The latter is the most common of the various types. Here, absence of differentiated components, e.g. rhabdomyoblasts, precludes diagnosis by cell type. Undifferentiated sarcomas occur most commonly in children between six and ten years old. In the largest series (Stocker and Ishak, 1978) the sex incidence was equal, but two smaller series (Perilongo

et al., 1987b; Horowitz *et al.*, 1987) report a male predominance. The commonest presenting symptoms are an abdominal mass, abdominal pain and fever. Jaundice is unusual. Full blood count and liver function tests are usually normal, and serum αFP is never elevated. Imaging studies show a space-occupying lesion which may be solid or cystic, hypervascular or avascular. Tumours are well demarcated from the surrounding liver but are not encapsulated. The cut surface is gelatinous or glistening and yellowish-grey to tan in colour. Half the tumours have multiple cystic areas. The majority of the tumour is made up of sarcomatous elements. The cells are stellate or spindle shaped with round, elongated or irregular shaped nuclei, and may be closely packed or scattered loosely in an acid mucopolysaccharide material. Reticulin and collagen fibres may also be present. Multinucleate giant cells are seen and mitoses are frequent. Clusters of hepatocytes and bile duct-like structures may be found at the periphery of the tumour (Stocker and Ishak, 1978).

The prognosis of these tumours to date has been poor. In a retrospective study of 31 undifferentiated sarcomas diagnosed between 1955 and 1975 partial or complete resection was attempted in 23 patients; nine had chemotherapy, seven chemotherapy and radiotherapy, and three radiotherapy alone (Stocker and Ishak, 1978). Only six patients survived, with a median survival of nine months (range 2–52 months). In an Italian study of eight patients diagnosed between 1975 and 1981 and treated with surgery and chemotherapy, two had initial complete resection, and a third patient had complete resection after chemotherapy (adriamycin, cyclophosphamide, vincristine, and 5-fluorouracil) followed by radiotherapy to microscopic residual disease (Perilongo *et al.*, 1987b). Two patients survive at 14 and 60 months. There were no survivors of unresectable disease. In a more recent study by Horowitz *et al.* (1987) five patients with undifferentiated sarcoma and three with embryonal rhabdomyosarcoma (without involvement of bile ducts) were treated with surgery and chemotherapy (vincristine, adriamycin, actinomycin, cyclophosphamide ± DTIC). Six had measurable disease after surgery. Two had a complete response, two a partial response, one an objective response to chemotherapy, and one a partial response to chemotherapy and radiotherapy. Median survival was 19.5 months (range 6–73+ months). Two patients who had lung metastases at diagnosis had metastases to brain or bone at death. Treatment of these tumours with surgery and appropriate (sarcoma-type) multiagent chemotherapy may be curative. We have 3/3 survivors of ten, three and one year following treatment with vincristine, actinomycin D, cyclophosphamide and surgery. The role of radiotherapy has not yet been defined.

20.4 BENIGN TUMOURS

Benign tumours account for 33% of primary liver tumours in children (Exelby *et al.*, 1975) see Table 20.1, above. The most common (40–60%) are the vascular tumours haemangioma and haemangioendothelioma, although the distinction between the two is not always made in published reports (Exelby *et al.*, 1975; Ehren *et al.*, 1983). Microscopically, haemangiomas are composed of dilated vascular spaces lined by one or more layers of endothelium, separated by connective tissue-containing fibroblasts. Areas of thrombus, haemorrhage and calcification may be seen. Haemangioendotheliomas are composed of vascular channels lined by endothelial cells. Tumours may be single or multiple and the majority present within the first six months of life. Presenting symptoms are abdominal distension and congestive cardiac failure. Cutaneous haemangiomata may be present. Stippled calcification may be seen on plain abdominal x-ray. CT scanning with rapid scanning technique will demonstrate abnormal flow patterns. Abnormal vascular lesions retain contrast and appear brighter than the surrounding normal liver. Angiography demonstrates the highly vascular nature of the tumour. Tumours commonly undergo spontaneous regression after the age of 12 months but treatment may be necessary prior to this because of intractable cardiac failure. Treatment options include steroids, hepatic artery embolization or ligation, or cytotoxic drugs, e.g. cyclophosphamide or radiotherapy, but none is reliable and it is hard to be sure whether tumour regression is spontaneous or treatment-induced (Ehren *et al.*, 1983; Cornelius *et al.*, 1989).

Mesenchymal hamartoma is the second most common benign tumour (30%) and usually occurs in children under two years old. The commonest presenting symptom is abdominal distension, shown on imaging to be due to a solitary cystic avascular mass. Serum αFP level may be elevated due to production by proliferating hepatocytes (Ito *et al.*, 1984). Tumours are well demarcated and composed of cysts of various sizes filled with clear fluid or mucoid material. Treatment is by resection or ennucleation.

Focal nodular hyperplasia and adenoma are both extremely rare, accounting for only 9% of benign tumours (Exelby *et al.*, 1975) and usually present as asymptomatic hepatomegaly. Focal nodular hyperplasia is a solitary lesion which on angiography is highly vascular, in 10-15% of cases resembling haemangioma. Microscopically, the tumour has a nodular appearance with aggregates of hepatocytes and stellate fibrous tissue. No treatment is necessary unless the patient is symptomatic, or the diagnosis is in doubt, when resection of the lesion should be performed. Adenoma may be associated with glycogen storage disease or androgen therapy. Tumours are usually multiple, may be vascular, and are composed of cords of hepatocytes several cells thick. Differentiation from a well differentiated hepatocellular carcinoma may be difficult so resection of the tumour and careful follow-up is advised. There are no reports of

425

serum αFP levels in adenoma patients. A rising αFP may indicate transformation of adenoma to hepatocellular carcinoma.

20.5 CURRENT CONTROVERSIES

20.5.1 THE CASE FOR PREOPERATIVE CHEMOTHERAPY VERSUS INITIAL SURGERY

In each of three major current studies of treatment for hepatocellular tumours there is a different emphasis. In the SIOPEL 1 study most patients receive preoperative chemotherapy using three weekly courses of cisplatin and adriamycin (PLADO), both given by continuous infusion over a total of 72 hours. Surgery is delayed until after four or six courses of chemotherapy. The rationale for this is as follows: (a) children are cured of hepatoblastoma/hepatocellular carcinoma only if complete resection can be achieved; (b) preoperative chemotherapy increases the resection rate; (c) the operation becomes safer and easier after preoperative chemotherapy; and (d) there is no delay in treating micro metastases. As some patients have been cured by surgery alone (Ishak and Glunz, 1967; Lack *et al.*, 1982; 1983) patients who have a 'small' easily resectable tumour (i.e. tumour clearly limited to either left lateral or right posterior sector) at diagnosis, are treated with surgery alone. These tumours are designated Group Is. What is a 'small' tumour? Because opinion about resectability is so subjective the 'small' Group Is tumour has been very clearly but conservatively defined as a tumour with a tumour index ≤0.05. Tumour index (TI) gives a ratio of the size of the tumour in relation to the cross section of the body (on CT scan or MRI) at the level of the liver hilus (Fig. 20.8).

$$TI = \frac{T_1 \times T_2}{B_1 \times B_2}$$

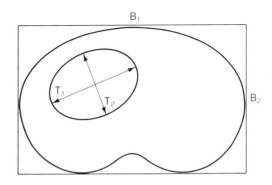

Fig. 20.8 Measurement of tumour index according to the SIOPEL 1 study: T_1 and T_2 are chosen at the largest diameter of the tumour; B_1 and B_2 are sections containing the liver hilus.

This definition may need to be amended as results from these studies become available.

By contrast, both the German Society for Paediatric Oncology (GPO) study and the Intergroup USA study advocate primary resection of the tumour where feasible, followed by chemotherapy. In the GPO study, HB 89, patients receive adriamycin, carboplatin, and ifosfamide. In the Intergroup study a short course of adriamycin only is given to patients who have complete resection of tumour with pure fetal histology. Patients with completely resected tumours with histology other than purely fetal, and incompletely resected or unresectable tumours, are randomized to receive either adriamycin and cisplatin, or cisplatin, vincristine and 5-fluorouracil. In the GPO and Intergroup studies, all patients have an initial laparotomy, and biopsy if the tumour is unresectable to provide a histological diagnosis. Open biopsy allows several areas of the tumour to be biopsied and reduces the risk of uncontrollable bleeding. In the SIOPEL 1 study, biopsy prior to chemotherapy is strongly recommended. It could be argued that in a child with a hepatic mass and a raised serum αFP level for age, biopsy is not justified because the diagnosis of a hepatocellular tumour is hardly in doubt. Also liver biopsy is not without risk, and a single needle biopsy may not be representative of the tumour. However, the distinction between hepatoblastoma, hepatocellular carcinoma and the rare hepatic germ cell tumour (Mann *et al.*, 1989) can only be made on histology. It is recommended that needle biopsy (preferably using a Menghini or Trucut needle) via a mini laparotomy should be done so that several parts of the tumour may be sampled and the risk of bleeding reduced. If a biopsy is not done there may never be histological confirmation of the diagnosis as in a proportion of patients (1 in 10; Shafford *et al.*, 1989) tumour is completely necrotic after pre operative chemotherapy. However, the limitations of biopsy must be recognized. It may not be possible, on a small tissue sample, to differentiate between hepatoblastoma and hepatocellular carcinoma, nor to classify hepatoblastoma by histological subtype, as its histological appearance may vary from area to area.

20.5.2 WHAT IS 'GOOD' HISTOLOGY IN HEPATOBLASTOMA?

Weinberg and Finegold (1986) report an improved prognosis for patients with hepatoblastoma of pure fetal histology. A joint study by the CCSG, SWOG, and POG (Haas *et al.*, 1989) of 168 patients with hepatoblastoma demonstrated an improved prognosis for patients with tumours of pure fetal histology, although only in Stage I disease. The proportion of patients with pure fetal histology was similar for Stage I (28/55) and those with more advanced disease (60/113), indicating that the improved prognosis was not due to the fact that patients with this type of histology have less aggressive tumour. Absence of mitotic figures was a good prognostic factor whatever the tumour stage. Patients with advanced disease but with chondroid or squamous epithelial metaplasia had a better

prognosis than those whose tumours lacked this type of differentiation. Patients with a small cell undifferentiated tumour, described by others as 'anaplastic' tumour had a poorer prognosis for survival (Kasai and Watanabe, 1970).

In the current Intergroup study, treatment of patients with Stage I tumours is dependant on histology, as already explained. In the SIOPEL 1 and GPO studies, no such distinction is made. In SIOPEL 1, no chemotherapy is given after complete resection of a Group Is tumour, and in the GPO study, all patients receive the same chemotherapy. Both these studies should provide more information on the influence (if any) of histology on prognosis.

20.5.3 SHOULD HEPATOCELLULAR CARCINOMA AND HEPATOBLASTOMA BE TREATED THE SAME?

In all three studies previously mentioned, hepatoblastoma and hepatocellular carcinoma are treated in the same way. Information about hepatocellular carcinoma in children is scanty at present and insufficient to warrant a different strategy. There are well documented prolonged responses of hepatocellular carcinoma in children to cisplatin-containing chemotherapy. Prospective studies such as SIOPEL 1, GPO, and Intergroup will provide crucial information on this point. Fibrolamellar carcinoma, however, is resistant to currently available drugs and therefore still constitutes 'surgical disease'.

20.5.4 THE ROLE OF TRANSPLANTATION

The child with a multifocal primary tumour (more commonly hepatocellular carcinoma than hepatoblastoma) involving both lobes of the liver, presents a particular therapeutic problem. Complete resection of tumour is only possible if liver transplantation is performed. These patients account for only a small percentage (4–12%) of liver transplants in children (Bismuth *et al.*, 1987). The results of transplantation for primary liver cancer in adults are poor and relatively few transplants have been carried out in children. However, greatly improved chemotherapy means that metastases can be eradicated in at least 50% of patients with advanced disease. As a consequence, liver transplantation, albeit still experimental, is now a serious treatment option. Patients must be selected with extreme care and should probably be responding to chemotherapy at the time the transplant is carried out.

20.5.5 INTRODUCING NEW DRUGS

Adriamycin and cisplatin are recognized as the best two single agents for hepatoblastoma, but may cause acute and chronic toxicity. Are there any other drugs which are equally effective and less toxic? Carboplatin and epirubicin are chemically similar to cisplatin and adriamycin but less toxic to ears and kidneys, and heart respectively, although carboplatin is more myelotoxic than cisplatin. As yet, however, there are few reports giving data on their efficacy in the treatment of hepatoblastoma (van den Berg *et al.*, 1989). Further studies are necessary before these drugs replace adriamycin and cisplatin in the treatment of hepatocellular tumours.

In two studies ifosfamide was given to patients relapsing after standard chemotherapy for various tumours; there was no response to treatment in four out of four patients with hepatocellular tumours (Pinkerton and Pritchard, 1989; Pratt *et al.*, 1989). Of 16 adults with unresectable hepatocellular carcinoma in a phase II study of ifosfamide, three showed a partial response lasting four, ten and 11 months (Thongprasert *et al*, 1988). Ifosfamide is nephrotoxic and should be used with caution in patients previously treated with cisplatin. Neurotoxicity has also been noted in patients previously treated with cis-

platin (Pratt *et al.*, 1989). Etoposide, in moderate dosage, has also been used in the treatment of adult hepatocellular carcinoma, but results are not encouraging. Three of 24 patients (Cavalli *et al.*, 1981) and one of 21 patients (Yoshino *et al.*, 1989) with unresectable hepatocellular carcinoma achieved a partial response lasting 8–35 weeks. Melia *et al.* (1983) compared the efficacy of etoposide and adriamycin in adults with unresectable hepatocellular carcinoma. For patients who had not received prior treatment there was no significant difference in the response rate achieved with etoposide (18%) or adriamycin (25%), but the duration of remission with adriamycin was significantly longer. Further studies of ifosfamide and etoposide in paediatric hepatocellular tumours, including hepatoblastoma, are required. Ifosfamide is included in the GPO study in combination with adriamycin and carboplatin. Etoposide is being used in the SIOPEL 1 study for patients who do not respond to, or relapse after, treatment with adriamycin and cisplatin.

20.5.6 TOWARDS A COMMON LANGUAGE

In order that meaningful comparison may be made of present and future studies there needs to be agreement on the following:

(a) pathological subclassification of hepatocellular tumours;
(b) staging of tumours;
   (i) clinically by specified imaging investigations
   (ii) at surgery
(c) definitions of response;
(d) assessment of treatment toxicity;

To this end, a group has been formed with representatives from CCSG, GPO, POG, SIOP, and Japan to develop a common language for hepatocellular tumours (Plaschkes *et al.* 1991).

The authors acknowledge the contribution of Professor Spitz and Dr Keeling.

REFERENCES

Ablin, A., Krailo, M., Haas, J. *et al.* (1988) Hepatoblastoma and hepatocellular carcinoma in children: a report from the Children's Cancer Study Group (CCSG) and the Pediatric Oncology Group (POG). *Med. Pediatr. Oncol.*, **16**, 417.

Andrassy, R.J., Brennan, L.P., Siegel, M.M. *et al.* (1980) Preoperative chemotherapy for hepatoblastoma in children: report of six cases. *J. Pediatr. Surg.*, **15**, 517–22.

Bismuth, H., Castaing, D., Ericzon, B.G. *et al.* (1987) Hepatic transplantation in Europe. First Report of the European Liver Transplant Registry. *Lancet*, **ii**, 674–76.

Bodmer, W.F., Bailey, C.J., Bodmer, J. *et al.* (1987) Localisation of the gene for familial adenomatous polyposis on chromosome 5. *Nature*, **328**, 614–16.

Boechat, M.I., Kangarloo, H., Ortega, J. *et al.* (1988) Primary liver tumours in children: comparison of CT and MRI. *Radiology*, **169**, 727–32.

Brock, P., Pritchard, J., Bellman, S. and Pinkerton, C.R. (1988) Ototoxicity of high-dose cis platinum in children. *Med. Pediatr. Oncol.*, **16**, 368–9 (letter).

Brown, T.C.K., Davidson, P.D. and Auldist, A.W. (1988) Anaesthetic considerations in liver tumour resection in children. *Pediatr. Surg. Int.*, **4**, 11–15.

Cavalli, F., Rozencweig, M., Renard, J. *et al.* (1981) Phase II study of oral VP-16-213 in hepatocellular carcinoma. *Eur. J. Cancer Clin. Oncol.*, **17**, 1079–82.

Chaung, V.P. and Wallace, S. (1981) Hepatic artery embolisation in the treatment of hepatic neoplasms. *Radiology*, **140**, 51–8.

Chen, W.J., Lee, J.C. and Hung, W.T. (1988) Primary malignant tumour of liver in infants and children in Taiwan. *J. Pediatr. Surg.*, **23**, 457–61.

Cornelius, A.S., Womer, R.B. and Jakacki, R. (1989) Multiple hemangioendotheliomas of the liver. *Med. Pediatr. Oncol.*, **17**, 501–4.

Craig, J.R., Peters, R.L., Edmonson, H.A. and Omata, M. (1980) Fibrolamellar carcinoma of the liver. *Cancer*, **46**, 372–9.

Dachman, A.H., Pakter, R.L., Ros, P.R. *et al.* (1987) Hepatoblastoma: Radiologic-pathologic correlation in 50 cases. *Radiology*, **164**, 15–19.

Davidson, P.M. and Auldist, A.W. (1988) Surgical anatomy and operative techniques for elective hepatic resection in children. *Pediatr. Surg. Int.*, **4**, 7–10.

Dorman, F., Sumner, E. and Spitz, L. (1985) Fatal intraoperative tumour embolism in a child with hepatoblastoma. *Anaesthesiology*, **63**, 692–3.

Douglass, E.C., Green, A.A., Wrenn, E. *et al.* (1985) Effective cisplatin (DDP) based chemotherapy in the treatment of hepatoblastoma. *Med. Pediatr. Oncol.*, **13**, 187–90.

de Campo, J. and Phelan, E. (1988) Imaging of liver tumours in childhood. *Pediatr. Surg. Int.*, **4**, 1–6.

de Kraker, J., Hoefnagel, C.A. and Voûte, P.A. (1989) I^{131} Rose Bengal therapy in inoperable hepatoblastoma. *Med. Pediatr. Oncol.*, **17**, 278 SIOP XXI Meeting abstract.

Ehren, H., Mahour, G.H. and Isaacs, H. (1983) Benign liver tumours in infancy and childhood: report of 48 cases. *Am. J. Surg.*, **145**, 325–9.

Evans, A.E., Land, V.J., Newton, W.A. *et al.* (1982) Combination chemotherapy (vincristine, adriamycin, cyclophosphamide, and 5-fluorouracil) in the treatment of children with malignant hepatoma. *Cancer*, **50**, 821–6.

Exelby, P.R., Filler, R.M. and Grosfeld, J.L. (1975) Liver tumours in children with particular reference to hepatoblastoma and hepatocellular carcinoma: American Academy of Pediatrics Surgical Section Survey–1974. *J. Pediatr. Surg.*, **10**, 329–37.

Finn, J.P., Hall-Craggs, M.A., Dicks-Mireaux, C. *et al.* (1990) Primary malignant liver tumours in childhood: assessment of resectability with high-field MR and comparison with CT. *Paediatr. Radiology.*, **21**, 34–8.

Fraumeni, J.F., Miller, R.W. and Hill, J.A. (1968) Primary carcinoma of the liver in childhood: an epidemiologic study. *J. Natl. Cancer Inst.*, **40**, 1087–99.

Gauthier, F., Valayer, J., Le Thai, B. *et al.* (1986)

Hepatoblastoma and hepatocarcinoma in children: analysis of a series of 29 cases. *J. Pediatr. Surg*, **21**, 424–9.

Haas, J.E., Muczynski, K.A., Krailo, M. *et al.* (1989) Histopathology and prognosis in childhood hepatoblastoma and hepatocarcinoma. *Cancer*, **64**, 1082–95.

Habrand, J.L. (1991) Role of radiotherapy in hepatoblastoma and hepatocellular carcinoma in children and adolescents: results of survey conducted by the SIOP Liver Tumour Group. *Med. Ped. Oncol.*, **19**, 208.

Hermann, R.E. and Lonsdale, D. (1970) Chemotherapy, radiotherapy, and hepatic lobectomy for hepatoblastoma in an infant: report of a survival. *Surgery*, **68**, 383–8.

Horowitz, M.E., Etcubanas, E., Webber, B.L. *et al.* (1987) Hepatic undifferentiated (embryonal) sarcoma and rhabdomyosarcoma in children: results of therapy. *Cancer*, **59**, 396–402.

Ikeda, K., Suita, S., Nakagawara, A. and Takabayashi, K. (1979) Preoperative chemotherapy for initially unresectable hepatoblastoma in children *Arch. Surg.*, **114**, 203–7.

Ishak, K.G. and Glunz, P.R. (1967) Hepatoblastoma and hepatocarcinoma in infancy and childhood. *Cancer*, **20**, 396–422.

Ito, H., Kishikawa, T., Toda, T. *et al.* (1984) Hepatic mesenchymal hamartoma of an infant. *J. Pediatr. Surg.*, **19**, 315–17.

Kasai, M. and Watanabe, I. (1970) Histological classification of liver cell carcinoma in infancy and childhood and its clinical evaluation. *Cancer*, **24**, 551–63.

Kingston, J.E., Herbert, A., Draper, G.J. and Mann, J.R. (1983) Association between hepatoblastoma and polyposis coli. *Arch. Dis. Child.*, **58**, 959–62.

Kobayashi, H., Hidaka, H., Kajiya, Y. *et al.* (1986) Treatment of hepatocellular carcinoma by transarterial injection of anticancer agents in iodized oil suspension or of radioactive iodized oil solution. *Acta. Radiol. Diag.*, **27**, 139–47.

Koufos, A., Hansen, M.F., Copeland, N.G. *et al.* (1985) Loss of heterozygosity in three embryonal tumours suggests a common pathogenetic mechanism. *Nature*, **316**, 330–4.

Lack, E.E., Neave, C. and Vawter, G.F. (1982) Hepatoblastoma – a clinical and pathologic study of 54 cases. *Am. J. Surg. Pathol.*, **6**, 693–705.

Lack, E.E., Neave, C. and Vawter, G.F. (1983) Hepatocellular carcinoma. Review of 32 cases in childhood and adolescence. *Cancer*, **50**, 1500–15.

Legha, S.S., Benjamin, R.S., Mackay, B. *et al.* (1982) Reduction of doxorubicin cardiotoxicity by prolonged continuous intravenous infusion. *Ann. Int. Med.*, **96**, 133–9.

Leuschner, I., Harms, D. and Schmidt, D. (1988) The association of hepatocellular carcinoma in childhood with hepatitis B infection. *Cancer*, **62**, 2363–9.

Mahour, G.H., Wogu, G.U., Siegel, S.E. and Isaacs, H. (1983) Improved survival in infants and children with primary malignant liver tumours. *Amer. J. Surg.*, **146**, 236–40.

Mann, J.R., Kasthuri, N., Raafat, F. *et al.* (1989) Malignant tumours of the liver in children: a population-based study of incidence and associated features. *Med. Pediatr. Oncol.*, **17**, 277.

Melia, W.M., Johnson, P.J. and Williams, R. (1983) Induction remission in hepatocellular carcinoma: a comparison of VP16 with adriamycin. *Cancer*, **51**, 206–10.

Nakagawara, A., Ikeda, K., Tsureyoshi, M. *et al.* (1985) Hepatoblastoma producing both fetoprotein and human chorionic gonadotrophin. *Cancer*, **56**, 1636–49.

Nickerson, H.J., Silberman, T.L. and McDonald, T.P. (1980) Hepatoblastoma, thrombocytosis and increased thrombopoietin. *Cancer*, **45**, 315–17.

Ogita, S., Tokiwa, K., Taniguchi, H. and Takahashi, T. (1987) Intraarterial chemotherapy with lipid contrast medium for hepatic malignancies in infants. *Cancer*, **60**, 2886–90.

Order, S.E., Stillwagon, G.B., Klein, J.L. *et al.* (1985) Iodine 131 antiferritin, a new treatment modality in hepatoma: a radiation therapy oncology group study. *J. Clin. Oncol.*, **3** 1573–82.

Ortega, J.A., Ablin, A., Haas, J. *et al.* (1989) Successful surgical resectability of liver tumours following continuous infusion chemotherapy with adriamycin cisplatin. *Med. Pediatr. Oncol.*, **17**, 277.

Paradinas, F.J., Melia, W.M., Wilkinson, M.L. *et al.* (1982) High serum vitamin B12 binding capacity as a marker of the fibrolamellar variant of hepatocellular carcinoma. *Br. Med. J.*, **285**, 840–2.

Parkin, D.M., Stiller, C.A., Draper, G.J. and Bieber,

C.A. (1988) The international incidence of childhood cancer. *Int. J. Cancer*, **42**, 511–20.

Perilongo, G., Carli, M., Guglielmi, M. *et al.* (1987a) Therapeutic approach to primary malignant epithelial tumours of the liver in childhood. *Pediatr. Hematol. Oncol.*, **4**, 179–88.

Perilongo, G., Carli, M., Sainati, L. *et al.* (1987b) Undifferentiated (embryonal) sarcoma of the liver in childhood: results of a retrospective Italian study. *Tumori*, **73**, 213–17.

Pierro, A., Langevin, A.M., Filler, R.M. *et al.* (1989) Preoperative chemotherapy in 'unresectable' hepatoblastoma. *J. Pediatr. Surg.*, **24**, 24–9.

Pinkerton, C.R. and Pritchard, J. (1989) A phase II study of ifosfamide in paediatric solid tumours. *Cancer Chemother. Pharmacol.*, **24**, S13–S15.

Plaschkes, J., Ablin, A., Jones, M. *et al.* (1991) A common language for hepatocellular tumours. *Med. Pediatr. Oncol.*, **19**, 149–50.

Pratt, C.B., Douglass, E.C., Etcubanas, E.L. *et al.* (1989) Ifosfamide in pediatric malignant solid tumours. *Cancer Chemother. Pharmacol.*, **24**, S24–S27.

Pritchard, J., da Cunha, A., Cornbleet, M.A. and Carter, C.J. (1982) Alpha feto protein monitoring of response to adriamycin in hepatoblastoma. *J. Pediatr. Surg.*, **17**, 429–30.

Quinn, J.J., Altman, A.J., Robinson, T. *et al.* (1985) Adriamycin and cisplatin for hepatoblastoma. *Cancer*, **56**, 1926–9.

Shafer, A.D. and Selinkoff, P.M. (1977) Preoperative irradiation and chemotherapy for initially unresectable hepatoblastoma. *J. Pediatr. Surg.*, **12**, 1001–7.

Shafford, E.A., Pritchard, J., Spitz, L. *et al.* (1989) Cis platinum doxorubicin and surgery for advanced hepatoblastoma; a real chance for cure? *ASCO Proc.*, 298.

Stocker, J.T. and Ishak, K.G. (1978) Undifferentiated (embryonal) sarcoma of the liver: report of 31 cases. *Cancer*, **42**, 336–48.

Sue, K., Ikeda, K., Nakagawara, A. *et al.* (1989) Intrahepatic arterial injections of cisplatin-phosphatidylcholine-lipiodol suspension in two unresectable hepatoblastoma cases. *Med. Pediatr. Oncol.*, **17**, 496–500.

Thongprasert, S., Klunklin, K., Phornphutkul, K. *et al.* (1988) Phase II study of ifosfamide (Holoxan) in hepatoma. *Eur. J. Cancer Clin. Oncol.*, **24**, 1795–6.

Vos, A., Gauthier, F., MacKinley, G. *et al.* (1989) Pre-operative surgical staging in hepatoblastoma. *Med. Pediatr. Oncol.*, **17**, (4) 278.

van den Berg, H.M., de Waal, F.C. and Veerman, A.J.P. (1989) Carboplatin and epirubicin in the treatment of hepatoblastoma. *Med. Pediatr. Oncol.*, **17**, (4) 281 SIOP XXI Meeting abstract.

Weinberg, A.G. and Finegold, M.J. (1986) Primary hepatic tumours in childhood, in *Pathology of Neoplasia in Children and Adolescents: Major Problems in Pathology.* (ed. M. Finegold) W.B. Saunders, Philadelphia, pp. 333–72.

Weinblatt, M.E., Siegel, S.E., Siegel, M.M. *et al.* (1982) Preoperative chemotherapy for unresectable primary hepatic malignancies in children. *Cancer*, **50**, 1061–4.

Wheeler, K., Pritchard, J., Luck, W. and Rossiter, M. (1986) Transcobalamin I as a 'marker' for fibrolamellar hepatoma. *Med. Pediatr. Oncol.*, **14**, 227–9.

Willis, R.A. (1953) *Pathology of Tumours* 2nd edn, C.V. Mosby, St Louis.

Wu, J.T., Book, L. and Sudar K. (1981) Serum alpha fetoprotein (αFP) levels in normal infants. *Pediatr. Res.*, **15**, 50–2.

Yoshino, M., Okazaki, N., Yoshida, T. *et al.* (1989) A phase II study of etoposide in patients with hepatocellular carcinoma by the Tokyo Liver Cancer Chemotherapy Study Group. *Jpn. J. Clin. Oncol.*, **19**, 120–2.

431

Chapter 21

Langerhans cell histiocytosis

V. BROADBENT and A.C. CHU

21.1 DEFINITION AND PATHOGENESIS

Langerhans cell histiocytosis (LCH) is a reactive disorder (Chu *et al.*, 1987) in which cells having the phenotypic markers of epidermal Langerhans cells are found in skin and other organs where they cause tissue damage by excessive production of cytokines and prostaglandins (Arenzana-Seisedos *et al.*, 1986)

The pathogenesis of LCH is unknown, but as with many diseases, a large number of possible aetiological agents have been suggested. In his original description of the disease in 1893, Hand suggested that the disease was due to tuberculosis. In the 1920s, many considered that a metabolic defect could be the underlying abnormality with accumulation of cholesterol in tissues (Rowland, 1928). This hypothesis lost favour when serum lipids were found to be normal (Thannhauser, 1947).

With the identification of the Birbeck granule, Nezelof and co-workers suggested that these could be viral inclusion bodies and considered that the natural history of the disease would fit with a viral aetiology (Nezelof *et al.*, 1973). A large epidemiological study of Letterer-Siwe disease in the USA between 1960 to 1964 showed a random geographical distribution and little month to month variation in incidence and this mitigates against a

conventional viral cause (Glass and Miller, 1986).

Until recently, the more fulminant forms of LCH have been considered to behave like a malignant process and to be invariably fatal (Aronson, 1951); this has resulted in the disease being classified as a form of cancer and treated as such by paediatric oncologists. Experience has now shown that many children spontaneously remit and this has led to a major rethink. Most now consider LCH to be a reactive disease which may run a chronic relapsing course. This has been supported by recent scientific research using flow cytometry, in which the lesional cells in LCH have been shown to be diploid with no evidence of aneuploidy (McLelland *et al.*, 1989). However, a study reported by Goldberg *et al.* (1986) on an elderly patient with clinically atypical LCH did show an aneuploid peak on flow cytometry. It was unclear from the report whether the patient had the rare malignant histiocytosis of Langerhans cell origin, or whether this report indicates that one part of the disease spectrum of LCH is malignant.

At one time, an immunological hypothesis for diseases of unknown aetiology was popular. LCH was one such disease and was extensively investigated for immunological abnormalities; a trial of immunotherapy was

also performed. The evidence for an immunological basis for the disease will be discussed
below, but current thinking is that the immunological abnormalities seen in LCH are
epiphenomena.

A number of studies have addressed the
possibility that LCH is genetically determined.
However, until the Histiocyte Society published the criteria for the diagnosis of LCH
(Chu et al., 1987) there was no uniformity in
diagnosis and many patients with other histi-
ocytoses (familial haemophagocytic lymphohistiocytosis and viral associated lymphohistiocytosis) were included in reports on
LCH. The genetic link reported by Juberg *et al.*
(1970) should thus best be ascribed to a case
of mistaken identity, and there is no good
evidence for such a link. Although the pathogenesis of LCH is unknown then, a number of
tantalizing observations have given us clues as
to the possible aetiological factors in this disease.

Morphological and immunocytochemical
studies have identified the predominant
lesional cell in LCH as showing many of the
characteristics of the epidermal Langerhans cell

Table 21.1 Comparison of the characteristics of
epidermal Langerhans cells and LCH cells

Marker	Langerhans cell	LCH cell
Acid phosphatase	+	+
ATP-ase	+	+
-naphthyl acetate esterase	+	+
Alkaline phosphatase	−	−
Peroxidase	−	−
-mannosidase	+	+
HLA DR	+	+
S100 protein	+	+
CD1a	+	+
Peanut agglutinin	−	+
IL2 receptor	±	+
CD4	+ (activated)	+
Birbeck granules	+	+

(Chu *et al.*, 1987; Table 21.1). The LCH cell
certainly exhibits the phenotype of an activated
Langerhans cell – but is this the primary cell in
LCH?

Langerhans cells are bone marrow-derived
cells of the macrophage/monocyte series which
migrate to the epidermis where they function
as potent antigen presenting cells (Stingl *et al.*,
1977; Pelletier *et al.*, 1984). Langerhans cells are
thus susceptible to control by cytokines such as
GM CSF, which will affect division and trop-
ism of the cell, and are capable of producing a
number of cytokines such as ILI, TNF and
prostaglandins, which can influence other
immunologically active cells and can cause
local and systemic disturbances.

Two possible scenarios could thus explain
the clinicopathological entity of LCH:

1. That Langerhans cells – probably at an early
   stage in their bone marrow development –
   are altered by a viral infection which leads
   to their abnormal accumulation in physiological and non-physiological sites, where
   they produce cytokines which cause local
   tissue damage and systemic symptoms of
   fever and weight loss.
2. That the Langerhans cells are bystander
   cells which are induced to the sites of involvement in LCH by trophic cytokines produced by an abnormal cell, possibly a T
   cell, and that the local production of cytokines by the Langerhans cells leads to the
   symptoms of LCH.

Both these possibilities have some supportive circumstantial data but definitive studies
are needed to examine these two hypotheses.

21.2 IMMUNOLOGY

The Langerhans cell is an important immunologically active cell and changes in the immune
system are bound to be present in patients
with LCH. A number of immunological abnormalities have been identified affecting T cells,

B cells and monocyte function, but none are consistent features of this disease and most must now be regarded as epiphenomena rather than being primary abnormalities.

21.2.1 B CELL FUNCTION

Studies have examined the immunoglobulin levels in LCH and have reported divergent and conflicting data. IgG and IgA levels have been shown to be depressed in some patients, elevated in others, and normal in some (Leiken *et al.*, 1973; Thommesen *et al.*, 1979; Nesbit *et al.*, 1981). The commonest feature is of reduced IgG and IgA levels. IgM and IgE levels are generally normal but isolated reports have shown increases in IgM and IgE levels.

There is no good explanation for the immunoglobulin disturbances observed, as the commonest B cell abnormality seen in LCH would theoretically lead to a hypergammaglobulinaemia. The fact that these abnormalities are not consistent strongly suggests that they are of no pathogeneic importance.

21.2.2 T CELL FUNCTION

As with B cell function, a variety of T cell functional abnormalities have been identified in LCH but none of these are consistent findings. Some patients show cutaneous anergy (Nesbit *et al.*, 1981), and some show reduced mitogenic, antigenic or alloantigenic responses (Leiken *et al.*, 1973; Thommesen *et al.*, 1979; Nesbit *et al.*, 1981). In some patients treated with cytotoxic drugs the T cell functional abnormality returned to normal following treatment (Leiken *et al.*, 1973). A fairly consistent feature in three reported series is a reduction in the CD8 positive T cell population in the blood of patients with LCH, associated with a normal or reduced total T cell number (Torok *et al.*, 1984; Eckstein *et al.*, 1984; Shannon and Newton, 1986). In one study, this phenotypic abnormality was associated with a reduced *in vitro* suppressor T cell activ-

ity (Shannon and Newton, 1986). Attempts to correct this abnormality have included the use of thymic extracts and TP5, the synthetic active pentapeptide of thymopoeitin (Osband *et al.*, 1981). Treatment of cells from patients with LCH *in vitro* and *in vivo* with these agents lead to a normalization of the T cell subpopulations but in one series the disease became more active after treatment in three patients.

The pathogeneic importance of the depressed CD8 positive T cell population is difficult to assess. This could easily be the result of cytokine production by the LCH cells, and the finding by Broadbent *et al.* (1984) that in two patients with LCH and low CD8 cell counts, spontaneous remission was associated with a normalization of the CD8 count, would support this.

Thymic abnormalities have been described in LCH and these appear to be related to the disease rather than to the cytotoxic treatment used in these children. Osband *et al.* (1981) showed thymic abnormalities in five out of seven children biopsied prior to treatment, and Hamoudi *et al.* (1982) showed thymic abnormalities in 23 of 28 patients with disseminated LCH. Histologically, the involved thymuses show loss of demarcation between the cortex and medulla, and epithelial cell damage with loss of Hassal's corpuscles. Fibrosis is the end result.

21.2.3 MONOCYTE/MACROPHAGE FUNCTION

Considering that the Langerhans cell is a member of the mononuclear phagocytic system, there are few reported abnormalities of the circulating monocytes and little data about the function of the mononuclear phagocytic system in LCH. Kragballe *et al.* (1981) showed reduced antibody-dependent cytotoxicity in six patients with LCH remission. Meacham *et al.* (1985) reported that LCH cells did not show the functional activity of Langerhans cells and they were inhibitory to normal T cell responses induced by mitogens. There is, however, no direct evidence for a general activation of the mononuclear phagocytic system which suggests that if LCH were due to cytokine production by a cell which induced the Langerhans cell response seen in LCH, the cytokine must have a very restricted target cell specificity.

21.3 HISTOPATHOLOGY

The diagnostic criteria for LCH have now been reviewed and modified by the Histiocyte Society (Chu *et al.*, 1987). A presumptive diagnosis is made by light microscopic examination of haematoxylin-eosin stained sections which show infiltrates of pink staining histiocytic cells surrounded by lymphocytes, plasma cells, eosinophils and occasional giant cells. The

diagnostic confidence increases if additional special stains are used, and a diagnosis is made if the histology is complemented by one of the following stains: surface ATP-ase, S 100, alpha D-mannosidase or peanut agglutinin. A definitive diagnosis is made when the histology is supported by staining of lesional cells with an anti-CDI marker or the finding of Birbeck granules on electron microscopy (Fig. 21.1).

21.4 EPIDEMIOLOGY

Between 15 and 20 cases of LCH are reported to the United Kingdom Children's Cancer Study Group register each year but this is almost certainly an underestimate for several reasons. Firstly, the disease is underdiagnosed, mild skin disease being mistaken for

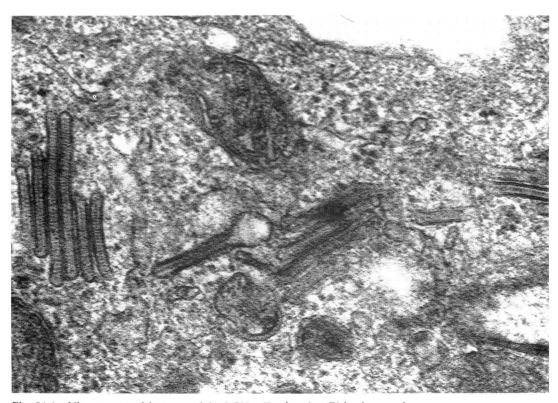

Fig. 21.1 Ultrastructural features of the LCH cells showing Birbeck granules.

seborrhoeic eczema or solitary bony scalp lumps for trauma. Secondly, the disease has a wide clinical spectrum and may present to a variety of specialists (orthopaedic, ENT, dermatology) who would not necessarily notify it to a cancer registry. The incidence in the paediatric age range is probably more likely to be 3–4 per million children under the age of 15 years (Swiss, USA personal communications) and we would expect the true incidence in the United Kingdom to be 40–50 cases annually. Boys are affected twice as commonly as girls and the peak age of presentation is between one to two years with a range from birth to old age. There is no recognized familial incidence although the disease has been reported in twins (Jakobson *et al.*, 1987).

21.5 CLINICAL FEATURES

21.5.1 GENERAL
The disease has a wide clinical spectrum as it can affect many different organs. In the very young it commonly occurs as multisystem disease accompanied by fever, failure to thrive, and constitutional upset. Vital organ failure (lung, liver and bone marrow) is more likely to occur in this group and is associated with a high mortality. Single system disease is usually

Table 21.2 Presenting symptoms of 30 children with LCH

Symptom	N
Skin rash	15
Recurrent aural discharge	8
Bone pain	5
Scalp lump(s)	5
Proptosis	4
Failure to thrive	3
Breathlessness	3
Lymphadenopathy	2
Hepatosplenomegaly	1
Spinal cord compression	1

Note: numbers add up to more than 30 as some children had multiple symptoms.

confined to bone and may be mono or polyostotic. It occurs more frequently in the older age group.

In a series of 58 patients seen over a seven-year period at a large referral centre, 14 had single system disease (13 bone and one skin) and 44 had multisystem disease, of whom 22 had vital organ dysfunction (McLelland *et al.*, 1990).

Failure to thrive is a common finding and is probably the result of many factors such as: (1) the chronic disease process; (2) loss of vertebral height due to disease; (3) corticosteroid treatment; (4) growth hormone deficiency in 30% of patients with diabetes insipidus (see below); (5) occult gut involvement. Symptom frequency according to specific organs is shown in Table 21.2.

21.5.2 BONE

Almost any bone may be affected, disease usually presenting with a bony lump or pain. The skull vault is the most common site (Fig. 21.2) followed by the proximal long bones and axial skeleton. The bones of the hands and feet are rarely affected. Orbital disease may give rise to proptosis and in rare cases compromize visual acuity by compressing the optic nerve. Vertebral collapse can cause spinal cord compression. There may be a soft tissue swelling or ulceration adjacent to the site of bony disease. The usual x-ray findings are of a circumscribed osteolytic area but periosteal reaction can mimic the appearances of Ewing's Sarcoma. Fracture through the lesion, especially in weight bearing bones, is not uncommon. Skeletal survey is a mandatory investigation in the primary evaluation of the patient and is superior to bone scan in picking up bony lesions.

21.5.3 SKIN

Skin involvement can be of a variety of types

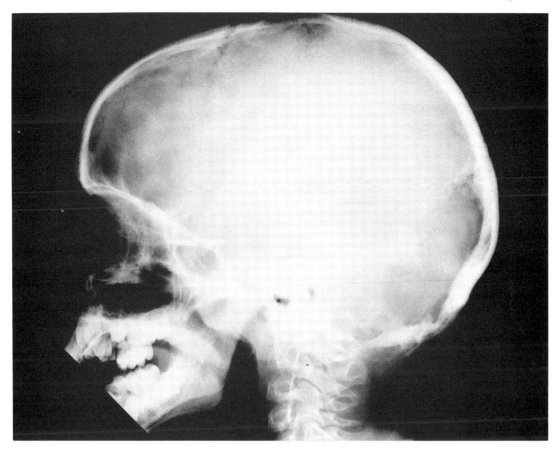

Fig. 21.2 Osteolytic lesions of the skull (occiput, frontal bones and vertex) in a 6-year-old child presenting with aural discharge.

and may be the sole site of disease. In the neonate it can present as the Hashimoto-Pritzker type of lesion (Hashimoto and Pritzker, 1973) which looks not unlike healing chickenpox. The lesions are discrete purple/brown nodules which are found all over the body including the palms of hands and soles of feet. It is a self-limiting disease which heals spontaneously over a few weeks. The most common presentation is a seborrhoeic rash involving the skin folds – groins, axillae and necklace area with more discrete brownish pink papules on the trunk and particularly over the sacral area. An extensive rash may involve the perineum, vulva and perianal region. The rash may be purpuric, especially if associated with bone marrow involvement and thrombocytopaenia. The scalp may be involved with a rash similar to severe cradle cap.

21.5.4 EARS

The disease may present with persistent aural discharge caused by extension of skin disease into the aural canal or from polypoid histiocytic tissue growing into the auditory canal from adjacent bony disease. The middle ear may be involved and disease in the mastoid can mimic mastoiditis.

21.5.5 BONE MARROW

Severe involvement is usually accompanied by dysfunction giving rise to leucopaenia, anaemia and thrombocytopaenia. Bone marrow aspirate shows infiltration of cells which mark as Langerhans cells and phagocytosis may be obvious. Splenomegaly is usually present in these circumstances and is often massive. Occult bone marrow disease can occur without dysfunction, a positive trephine biopsy being the only abnormality.

21.5.6 LUNGS

Lung involvement is not uncommon if lung function tests showing small stiff lungs with reduced total gas volume, decreased compliance, and increased resistance are used as criteria (Broadbent *et al.*, 1986). Pulmonary symptoms and signs, however, only occur when there is dysfunction. These are dyspnoea with tachypnoea and subcostal and/or suprasternal recession. X-ray changes due to interstitial alveolar infiltration by Langerhans cells show as fluffy shadowing in these circumstances. Another typical x-ray appearance is of honeycomb lung or pneumothorax due to rupture of peripheral bullae. Differentiation between opportunistic infections with organisms such as pneumocystis, measles and cytomegalovirus, and infiltration by Langerhans cells, may be difficult and may co-exist. The diagnosis is made by lung biopsy or bronchial washings.

21.5.7 LIVER

The commonest presenting sign is of hepatomegaly with ascites due to hypoalbuminaemia. In these cases there is usually periportal infiltration by histiocytes, not parenchymal infiltration, the hepatocyte dysfunction possibly being caused by the excessive production of cytokines and prostaglandin by the periportal Langerhans cells. Another common presentation is with jaundice, liver function tests suggesting an obstructive picture, and histology resembling sclerosing cholangitis (Leblanc *et al.*, 1981). Rarely, an isolated eosinophilic granuloma occurs in the liver and presents as a lump, or a filling defect on imaging. Histologically, Birkbeck granules are rarely found in hepatic Langerhans cells.

21.5.8 SPLEEN

Gross splenomegaly is usually associated with bone marrow involvement and dysfunction. In these circumstances it may be the site of extra medullary haemopoesis or haemophagocytosis. It may be infiltrated by Langerhans cells or may be enlarged due to portal hypertension in association with liver disease.

21.5.9 LYMPH NODES

Cervical lymphadenopathy which may be gross and cause respiratory obstruction may occur, or the disease may present as solitary nodal enlargement. Occasionally, suppuration mimicking infection occurs and the discharging necrotic material is often mistaken for pus due to its yellow hue. However, culture is negative but histology may show degenerate Langerhans cells.

21.5.10 CNS

The favoured site for involvement is the posterior pituitary presenting as diabetes insipidus. This may predate the diagnosis of LCH. The next most common site is the cerebellum, presenting as ataxia, dysarthria and nystagmus. Meningeal disease does occur as does direct intracranial extension from bony skull disease. Solitary intracerebral deposits may present with signs of a space-occupying lesion and symptoms of raised intracranial pressure or cranial nerve palsies.

21.5.11 ENDOCRINE

Diabetes insipidus may predate the diagnosis of LCH and is most likely to occur in the first four years after diagnosis. The incidence in our series was 23% with a cumulative risk of development of 42% in the first four years (Dungar *et al.*, 1989). Partial diabetes insipidus does occur and may spontaneously resolve. Growth hormone failure occurs in 30–50% of children with diabetes insipidus. Panhypopituitarism occasionally occurs and may be associated with a solid deposit in the hypothalamus (Fig. 21.3). Thyroid infiltration but not gonadal involvement has been reported (Lahey *et al.*, 1986).

21.5.12 GASTROINTESTINAL TRACT

Infiltration of the mucosa of the hard palate is a common site, giving it a granular appearance with widening of the palatal ridges. Thickening of gingivae due to soft tissue may be present and, in severe cases, cause gum retraction and loosening of teeth. Ulceration of the palate due to underlying bony disease may occur and bony lesions in the mandible or maxilla may protrude into the mouth.

Involvement of the lower gastrointestinal tract is probably underestimated as symptoms of malabsorption are rare. However, occult gastrointestinal disease may be responsible for failure to thrive in some patients.

21.6 INVESTIGATIONS

Diagnosis is made on tissue biopsy followed by evaluation of disease extent. The Histiocyte Society (Broadbent *et al.*, 1989a) has recommended mandatory initial evaluation with full blood count and differential liver function tests, coagulation studies, skeletal

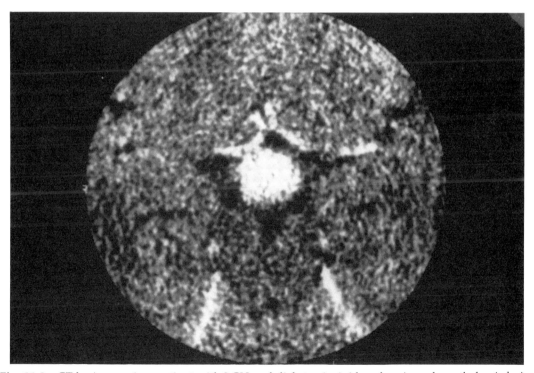

Fig. 21.3 CT brain scan in a patient with LCH and diabetes insipidus showing a hypothalamic lesion.

439

Table 21.3 Required laboratory and radiographic evaluation of new patients with LCH

	Follow-up test interval when organ system is:		
Test	*Involved*	*Not involved*	*Single bone lesion*
Haemoglobin and/or haematocrit	Monthly	6 months	None
White blood cell count and differential	Monthly	6 months	None
Platelet count	Monthly	6 months	None
Liver-function tests (SGOT, SGPT, alkaline phosphatase, bilirubin, total protein, and albumin)	Monthly	6 months	None
Coagulation studies (PT, PTT, fibrinogen)	Monthly	6 months	None
Chest radiograph, PA and lateral	Monthly	6 months	None
Skeletal radiograph survey*	6 months	None	Once, at 6 months
Urine osmolality measurement after overnight water deprivation	6 months	6 months	None

* Radionuclide bone scan is not as sensitive as the skeletal radiograph survey in most patients (Arenzana-Seisedos *et al.* 1986). It may be performed optionally but should not replace the skeletal survey.

survey and chest x-ray, together with urine osmolarity after overnight water deprivation (Table 21.3). Further evaluation will depend on specific indication (Table 21.4).

After evaluation, grouping of patients into those with single or multisystem disease and those with organ dysfunction is possible and may be important in assigning treatment and prognosis. An internationally acceptable clinical classification or grouping is currently under discussion by the Histiocyte Society.

21.7 TREATMENT

Ignorance of the pathogenesis of LCH inhibits a rational treatment policy. However, some general principles have emerged from clinical observation. It is generally agreed that patients with single system disease (usually bone, skin or lymph node) have a good prognosis with a high chance of spontaneous remission and favourable outcome. Eight of 14 patients with single system disease in McLelland's series (1990) required no treatment other than curettage at the time of initial biopsy. Bony lesions in weight bearing

bones with the risk of spontaneous fracture and those causing pain or disfigurement usually respond to intralesional steroid injection using 40–120 mg depomedrone (Broadbent and Pritchard, 1985). Those surrounding vital structures such as optic nerve and spinal cord which are inaccessible to injection may require urgent treatment with low dose (700–1000 cGy) radiotherapy. The 5% risk of second tumour developing after this form of treatment makes it unacceptable except in these circumstances now that the disease is known to be a 'reactive' disorder not a malignancy (Greenberger *et al.*, 1981).

Single system skin disease may need treatment if there are widespread areas of crusting and excoriation. Topical application of a 20% solution of nitrogen mustard is useful in these circumstances (Wong *et al.*, 1986).

The management of the child with multisystem disease is much more controversial. Spontaneous remission may occur (Broadbent *et al.*, 1984) and in the series reported by McLelland (1990) 8/44 with multisystem disease required no treatment. Historically, the disease has been treated as a malignancy and

Table 21.4 Evaluation of patients with LCH

Test	Indications	Follow-up test
Bone marrow aspirate and trephine biopsy	Anaemia, leukopenia, or thrombocytopenia	6 months
Pulmonary function tests	Abnormal chest, radiograph, tachypnea, intercostal retractions	Every 6 months
Lung biopsy, preceded by bronchoalveolar lavage, when available; when diagnostic, obviates the lung biopsy	Patients with abnormal chest radiograph in whom chemotherapy is being considered, to exclude opportunistic infection	None
Small bowel series and biopsy	Unexplained chronic diarrhoea or failure to thrive, evidence of malabsorption	None
Liver biopsy	Liver dysfunction, including hypoproteinaemia not due to protein-losing enteropathy, to differentiate active LCH of the liver from cirrhosis	To be performed if and when all other disease has resolved but liver dysfunction persists, to distinguish cirrhosis from continuing LCH
CT of brain/hypothalamic–pituitary axis, with IV contrast enhancement (MRI preferable, if available)	Hormonal, visual, or neurological abnormalities	Every 6 months
Panoramic dental radiography of mandible and maxilla; oral surgery consultation	Oral involvement	Every 6 months
Endocrine evaluation	Short stature, growth failure, diabetes insipidus, hypothalamic syndromes, galactorrhoea, precocious or delayed puberty; CT or MRI abnormality of hypothalamus/pituitary	None
Otolaryngology consultation and audiogram	Aural discharge, deafness	Every 6 months

* CT = computed tomography; MRI = magnetic resonance imaging

a wide variety of cytotoxic drugs used singly or in combination. Whatever regimen is used, the total response rate is between 50–70% (Pritchard, 1979) and the mortality in severe multisystem disease has declined only marginally since the advent of chemotherapy. Pulsed high dose prednisolone (2 mg/kg) in historical series and confirmed in a recent published series (McLelland *et al.*, 1990) is as effective as a combination of cytotoxic drugs. Etoposide is the drug of choice for those who fail to respond to steroids (Broadbent *et al.*, 1989b). There is no evidence to date that pulsed therapy is less effective than 'maintenance' therapy in preventing sequelae, although the higher incidence of diabetes insipidus in McLelland's conservatively treated patients (1990) as compared with the Austro/German DALHX83 (Gadner *et al.*, 1987) and AEIOP (Ceci; personal communication) series, in which 'maintenance' treatment was given, needs to be investigated.

The group which fare badly are those under the age of two years with vital organ (lung, liver or bone marrow) dysfunction. There is a 50% mortality in this group whatever treatment is given. A variety of experimental treatments have been investigated including thymic hormone (Osband *et al.*, 1981), interferon (Jakobson *et al.*, 1987), allogenic bone marrow transplant (Ringden *et al.*, 1987) and cyclosporin and have yet to be fully evaluated.

The role of radiotherapy in this disease is receding although it remains the treatment of choice in specific conditions such as bony disease in inaccessible sites with soft tissue extension compromising vital structures such as spinal cord or optic nerve or where there is intractable ulceration overlying a bony lesion of a chronically discharging sinus. Its role in the treatment of diabetes insipidus is more controversial. In Greenberger's series (1979) there were responses in 4/21 patients given pituitary irradiation within a few weeks of developing thirst and polyuria but there has been no response in our unpublished series of six patients in whom diabetes insipidus was fully documented by measurement of urinary vasopressin after a seven-hour period of water deprivation.

21.8 OUTCOME

The changing concept from a malignant disease to a reactive one has altered the perception of treatment objectives. The fulminant form of the disease which usually occurs in young children with soft tissue involvement and organ dysfunction is rapidly progressive

and is associated with a high mortality whatever treatment option is chosen. At the other end of the scale is localized disease which requires minimal treatment and rarely causes sequelae. The vast majority of patients will run a chronically recurring or recrudescent course and the treatment objective in these cases is prevention of long-term sequelae while the disease runs its course. There is no firm evidence to date that 'maintenance' as opposed to pulsed therapy has any effect on the development of long-term sequelae or length of course. After treatment 50% of patients in most large series (Sims, 1977; Komp *et al.*, 1980) will have sequelae. These range from minor facial deformity to more severe problems, diabetes insipidus, or other endocrine dysfunction, respiratory insufficiency, cirrhosis and neurological dysfunction.

21.9 CURRENT CONTROVERSIES

Most of the controversies in this disease have already been mentioned in the preceding sections, but some are worth highlighting.

21.9.1 NOMENCLATURE

As with many diseases of unknown cause, a large number of eponymous and 'descriptive' names have been adopted. Letterer-Siwe disease, Hand-Schuller-Christian disease, eosinophilic granuloma and histiocytosis-X are all still in common usage and serve to perpetuate the misinformation prevalent in this disease by such means as: 'Letterer-Siwe is universally fatal', 'Letterer-Siwe is an autosomal dominant disease'. These terms are also being used to describe different clinical manifestations of this disease by different groups involved in the management of these patients. At the inaugural meeting of the Histiocyte Society in 1985, the term first used by the Minnesota group to describe this group of diseases, Langerhans cell histiocytosis, was formally adopted (Risdall *et al.*, 1983). This term identifies the pathognomic cell in this disease as a cell indistinguishable from the epidermal Langerhans cell and highlights the importance of this cell in the diagnosis of the disease. It is, however, recognized that the Langerhans cell may not be the primary cell in this disorder.

21.9.2 DIAGNOSIS

A major factor that has inhibited our understanding of this disease has been the lack of commonly agreed diagnostic criteria for LCH. This has almost certainly led to a number of similar conditions, but ones with different pathogeneses and outcomes, to be included in series of LCH patients. Such diseases include the familial erythrophagocytic lymphohistiocytosis and viral associated haemophagocytic syndromes.

Uniformity of diagnostic tests is an absolute necessity in a rare disease where the clinical presentation can be so varied. For this reason, the writing group of the Histiocyte Society published a reclassification of the histiocytic conditions in childhood, and produced a new case definition of LCH based on pathological assessment of involved tissue (Chu *et al.*, 1987).

21.9.3 STAGING SYSTEMS

The current belief that LCH is a reactive rather than malignant condition has necessarily led to a major change in the way we assess and treat patients with LCH. Staging – with its connotation of malignant disease – is thus an inappropriate term when dealing with LCH. A scoring or simple disease assessment system would be more appropriate.

It is hoped that the internationally collaborative spirit fostered by the Histiocyte Society will permit a worldwide databank to be formed which will ultimately allow clinicians to devise an assessment of LCH based on morbidity and mortality and which will identify those patients in whom more intensive treatment may prevent the long-term sequaelae of this chronic disease.

21.9.4 RESPONSE CRITERIA

In a disease in which spontaneous regression is a common occurrence and the disease has a chronic and relapsing nature, assessment of response is very difficult. When LCH was considered a malignancy, the main therapeutic aim was disease irradication and optimal response was cure. In a chronic reactive disease, this is probably not acheivable and may not be advisable given the possible side effects of the therapeutic agents used. It is almost certain that some of the mortality seen in this disease is treatment-related.

Response can be measured as resolution of acute symptoms of specific organ disease – resolution of the skin eruption, normalization of the liver biochemistry, etc. – or the prevention of long-term sequaelae. In LCH, the response of acute symptoms of the disease to chemotherapy is generally good, but there is no good evidence that current therapeutic agents prevent the long-term morbidity or reduce the lifespan of the disease.

Good comparative, multicentre, randomized studies are needed to properly evaluate therapy in this disease and to specifically address the issue of long-term sequaelae and the effects of therapy on their incidence.

REFERENCES

Arenzana-Seisedos, F., Barby, S., Virelizier, J.L. *et al.* (1986) Histiocytosis X: purified (T6+) cells from bone granuloma produce interleukin 1 and prostaglandin E2 in culture. *J. Clin. Invest.*, **77**, 326–9

Aronson, R.P. (1951) Streptomycin in Letterer-Siwe disease. *Lancet*, **1**, 889.

Broadbent, V., Helms, P., Heaf, D. and Pritchard,

J. (1986) Respiratory function in infants with histiocytosis X. Abs. *Med. Pediatr. Oncol.* **7**, 29.

Broadbent, V., Davies, E.G., Heaf, D. *et al.* (1984) Spontaneous remission of multisystem histiocytosis X. *Lancet* **1**, 253–4

Broadbent, V., Pritchard, J. and Yeoman, E. (1989b) Etoposide (VP16) in the treatment of multisystem Langerhans cell histiocytosis. *Med. Pediatr. Oncol.* **17**, 97–100.

Broadbent, V. and Pritchard, J. (1985) Histiocytosis X – current controversies. *Arch. Dis. Child.*, **60**, 605–7.

Broadbent, V., Gadner, H., Komp, D. and Ladisch, S. (1989a) Histiocytosis syndromes in children II. Approach to the complete clinical and laboratory evaluation of children with Langerhans cell histiocytosis. *Med. Ped. Oncol.*, **17**, 492–5.

Chu, A., D'Angio, D.J., Favara, B. *et al.* (1987) Histiocytosis syndromes in children. *Lancet*, **i**, 208–9.

Davies, E.G., Levinsky, R.J., Butler, M., *et al.* (1983) Thymic hormone therapy for histiocytosis X. *N. Engl. J. Med.*, **309**, 493.

Dungar, D., Broadbent, V., Yeoman, E. *et al.* (1989) The frequency and natural history of diabetes insipidus in children with Langerhans cell histiocytosis. *N. Engl. J. Med.*, **321**, 157–62.

Eckstein, R., Huhn, D., Schneider D. *et al.* (1984) Influence on immune function parameters in histiocytosis X of thymostimulin. *Arzneimittelforsch*, **125**, 2611–14.

Gadner, H., Heitger, A., Ritter, J. *et al.* (1987) Langerhanszell-Histiozytose im kindersalter – Ergebniss der DALHX 83 studie. *Klin. Pediat.*, **199**, 173–82.

Glass, A.G. and Miller, R.W. (1986) US mortality from Letterer-Siwe disease, 1960-1964. *Pediatrics*, **42**, 112.

Goldberg, N.S., Bauer, K., Rosen, S.T. *et al.* (1986) Histiocytosis X. Flow cytometric DNA-content and immunohistochemical and ultrastructural analysis. *Arch. Dermatol.*, **122**, 446.

Greenberger, J.S., Cassady, J.R., Jaffe, N. *et al.* (1979) Radiation therapy in patients with histiocytosis: Management of diabetes insipidus and bone lesions. *Radiol. Oncol. Biol. Phys.*, **5**, 1749–55.

Greenberger, J.S., Crocker, A.C., Vawter, G. *et al.* (1981) Results of treatment of 127 patients with systematic histiocytosis. *Medicine* **60**, 331–8.

Hamoudi, A.B., Newton, W.H., Mancer, K. *et al.* (1982) Thymic changes in histiocytosis. *Am. J. Clin. Pathol.*, **77**, 169.

Hand, A. Polyuria and tuberculosis. (1893) *Arch. Pediatr.*, **10**, 673.

Hashimoto, K. and Pritzker, M.S. (1973) Electron microscopic study of reticulohistiocytoma. An unusual case of congenital, self-healing reticulohistiocytosis. *Arch. Dermatol.*, **107**, 263–9.

Jakobson, A.M., Kreuger, A., Hapberg, H. and Sundstrom, C. (1987) Treatment of Langerhans cell histiocytosis with alpha interferon. *Lancet*, **2**, 1520–1.

Juberg, R.C., Kloepfer, H.W. and Oberman, H.A. (1970) Genetic determination of acute disseminated histiocytosis-X (Letterer-Siwe syndrome). *Pediatrics*, **45**, 753.

Komp, D., El Mahdi, A., Starling K. *et al.* (1980) Quality of survival in histiocytosis X. A Southwest Oncology Group Study. *Med. Pediatr. Oncol.*, **8**, 35–40.

Kragballe, K., Zachariae, H., Herlin, T. *et al.* (1981) Histiocytosis X – an immune deficiency disease? Studies on antibody dependent monocyte mediated cytotoxicity. *Br. J. Dermatol.*, **105**, 13.

Lahey, M.E., Rallison, M.L., Hilding, D.A. and Ater J. (1986) Involvement of the thyroid in histiocytosis X. *Am. J. Pediatr. Hematol. Oncol.*, **8**, 257–9.

Leblanc, A., Hadchouel, M., Jehan, P. *et al.* (1981) Obstructive jaundice in children with histiocytosis X. *Gastroenterology*, **80**, 134–9.

Leikin, S., Puruganan, G., Frankel, A. *et al.* (1973) Immunologic parameters in Histiocytosis X. *Cancer*, **32**, 796–802.

McLelland, J., Newton, J.A., Malone, M. *et al.* (1989). A flow cytometric study of Langerhans cell histiocytosis. *Br. J. Dermatol.*, **120** 485–91.

McLelland, J., Broadbent, V., Yeoman, E. *et al.* (1990) Langerhans cell histiocytosis; A conservative approach to treatment. *Arch. Dis. Child.*, **65**, 301–3.

Meacham, R., Morris, J. and Chu, A.C. (1985) Morphological and immunological characteristics of histiocytosis X (HX) cells. *J. Invest. Dermatol.*, **84**, 440.

Nesbit, M.E. Jr., O'Leary, M., Dehner, L.P. *et al.* (1981). The immune system and the histiocytosis syndromes. *Am. J. Pediatr. Haematol./Oncol.*, **3**, 141–9.

Nezelof, C., Basset, F., Rousseau, M.F., (1973) Histiocytosis X: Histogenic arguments for a Langerhans cell origin. *Biomedicine*, **18**, 365.

Osband, M.E., Lipton, J.M., Lavin, P. *et al.* (1981) Histiocytosis X: Demonstration of abnormal immunity, T-cell histamine-H2-receptor deficiency and successful treatment with thymic extract. *N. Engl. J. Med..*, **304**, 146–53.

Pelletier, M., Perreault, C., Landry, D. *et al.* (1984) Ontogeny of human epidermal Langerhans cells. *Transplantation*, **38**, 475.

Pritchard, J. (1979) Histiocytosis X, Natural history and management in childhood. *Clin. Exp. Dermatol.*, **4**, 421–33.

Ringden, O. and Ahstrom, L. (1987) Allogeneic bone marrow transplantation in a patient with chemotherapy-resistant progressive histiocytosis X. *N. Engl. J. Med.*, **316**, 733–5.

Risdall, A.J., Dehner, L.P., Duray P. *et al.* (1983) Histiocytosis X (LC histiocytosis). Prognostic role of histopathology. *Arch. Pathol. Lab. Med.*, **107**, 59.

Rowland, R.S., (1928) Xanthomatosis and the reticuloendothelial system. *Arch. Intern. Med.*, **42**, 611.

Shannon, B.T. and Newton, W.A. (1986). Suppressor cell dysfunction in children with histiocytosis X. *J. Clin. Immunol.*, **6**, 1–9.

Sims, D.G. (1977) Histiocytosis X. A follow up of 43 cases. *Arch. Dis. Child.* **52**, 433–40.

Stingl, G. Wolff-Schreiner, E.C., Pichler, W.J. *et al.* (1977) Epidermal Langerhans cells bear Fc and C3 receptors. *Nature*, **266**, 245–6.

Thannhauser, S.J. (1947) Serum lipids and their value in diagnosis. *N. Engl. J. Med.*, **237**, 546.

Thommesen, P., Frederiksen, P. and Jorgensen, F. (1979) Immunologic response assessed by lymphocyte transformation tests. *Acta Radiol. Oncol.*, **17**, 524–8.

Torok, E., Laszlo, K and Erzsebet, E.W. (1984) Secsemokori histiocytosis syndroma (Histiocytosis X). *Orvosi Hetilsp.*, **125**, 2611–14.

Wong, E., Holden, C.A., Broadbent, V. and Atherton, D. (1986) Histiocytosis X presenting as intertrigo and responding to topical nitrogen mustard. *Clin. Exp. Dermatol.*, **11**, 183–7.

Chapter 22

Rare tumours

P.N. PLOWMAN

22.1 INTRODUCTION

The previous thirteen chapters in Part Two of this book have reviewed the management of specific tumours. There remains a heterogeneous group of tumours that are rarely encountered, and a selection of these merit review in some detail.

Paediatric oncologists will occasionally encounter squamous cancer of the tongue, granulosa cell tumour of the ovary, malignant melanoma, pulmonary blastoma and pulmonary carcinoid tumour, all in children. Reviews of these conditions have not been included here, however, as the management is identical to that in adults. Similar remarks apply to breast cancer and gastrointestinal tract cancers. We have therefore chosen to concentrate on tumours which are perhaps no more common than those just cited, but whose management contains an element of controversy in the paediatric versus the adult patient population.

22.2 THYROID CARCINOMA

Thyroid carcinoma is rare in childhood and afflicts girls more than boys. Of 59 paediatric cases presenting to the Mayo Clinic, 56 were papillary and only three were follicular carcinoma: a much higher proportion of papillary to follicular than is encountered in the adult

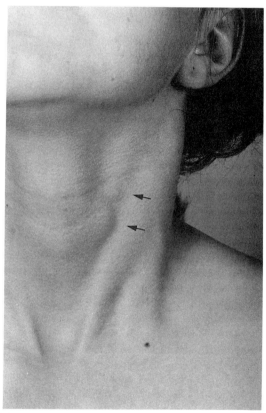

Fig. 22.1 Thyroid cancer presenting with cervical lymphadenopathy (arrow) in a teenage girl.

population (Woolner *er al.*, 1961). Of 576 cases of papillary thyroid carcinoma presenting to the Armed Forces Institute of Pathology (AFIP), approximately 7% occurred in patients aged 6–19 years (Mazzaferri *et al.*, 1977). Older children are more frequently afflicted.

Thyroid cancer usually presents in children, as in adults, in the form of a painless, discrete thyroid mass, or, less commonly, as a deep cervical chain lymph node mass (the 'lateral aberrant thyroid'; Fig. 22.1). Treatment recommendations are broadly similar to those applied to young adults: following histological diagnosis by biopsy, radical thyroidectomy – preserving recurrent laryngeal nerve function and parathyroid glands – is the preferred first therapeutic procedure. (This surgical approach is also indicated in patients presenting with lung metastases, in order to ablate most easily the highly iodine-avid normal thyroid tissue prior to radio-iodine therapy of the tumour.)

All involved lymph nodes must be excised from one or both deep cervical chains, and if computerized tomography shows that mediastinal nodes are involved, mediastinal exploration to clear such nodes is also indicated. Formal block dissection of the deep cervical chain is not routinely recommended but is occasionally necessary.

Following surgery, a normal thyroid remnant is invariably demonstrable on radio-iodine scanning, and as this iodine-avid normal remnant prevents the demonstration of less iodine-avid residual tumour deposits, an ablation dose of radioiodine (^{131}I) is given in the postoperative period before commencing liothyronine replacement therapy in TSH suppressive dosage. After three months, liothyronine is stopped eight days before performing a ^{131}I radioiodine profile scan; this provides the first opportunity to demonstrate tumour concentrating iodine without confounding high avidity normal thyroid tissue.

In recent years, serum thyroglobulin estimates have been helpful in the follow-up of patients with differentiated thyroid cancer. Serum thyroglobulin is secreted in small quantities by the cells of many cancers of follicular cell origin (including both papillary and follicular thyroid cancers). Black and colleagues reported in 1981 that, in radically ablated patients or those on fully TSH-suppressive doses of thyroid hormone, serum thyroglobulin estimations provided a marker for relapse detection. Recent studies by our group have confirmed the usefulness of serum thyroglobulin estimations as a marker in paediatric thyroid cancer (Kirk *et al.*, 1991).

Although not an infallible marker (Grant *et al.*, 1984), serum thyroglobulin estimations complement radioiodine scanning in the follow-up assessment of children with thyroid cancer, and may substitute for ^{131}I scanning in the lowest risk cases (see below).

Papillary thyroid carcinoma in young patients is very slow-growing, and relapse may occur ten to 20 years after a diagnosis is made. The initial site of recurrence is most commonly in the deep cervical node chains, followed by the mediastinal nodes, and lung metastases.

The incidence of nodal metastases in the Mayo Clinic papillary carcinoma series (all ages) was 39%, but the histological findings in the radical thyroidectomy specimen proved a strong prognostic factor for subsequent nodal relapse. Thus, 32% of those patients with intrathyroidal disease later developed nodal disease, whereas 57% of those with extrathyroidal disease at presentation later developed further nodal metastases (Woolner *et al.*, 1961).

The overall prognosis for young patients with papillary carcinoma of the thyroid is good. In a predominantly young adult population analysed by the AFIP, ten-year survival was 95% (Mazzaferri *et al.*, 1977). Particularly noteworthy from this careful analysis was the apparently paradoxical finding of a higher incidence of neck nodal recurrences in young patients than in older patients, and yet the better survival among younger patients. This

447

could be due to the high curability by surgery and radioiodine of neck node recurrences.

Mazzaferri and colleagues (1977) also demonstrated a significant survival advantage among patients undergoing radical thyroidectomy, radioiodine ablation and fully TSH-suppressive doses of thyroid hormone replacement compared with patients undergoing subtotal thyroidectomy.

In a series of 38 children presenting with differentiated thyroid cancer to the Gustav Roussy Institute, Tubiana *et al.* (1985) found an 88% survival at 15 years. However, it should be noted that there were two late deaths from thyroid cancer after 20 years of follow-up, demonstrating the long natural history of the disease. These workers therefore concluded that there was justification for a treatment programme similar to that used in adults.

At the Great Ormond Street Hospital for Sick Children, London, and St. Bartholomew's Hospital, London, recommendations have been the same for all patients presenting with large intrathyroidal papillary tumours, all extrathyroidal papillary tumours and all follicular carcinomas. This policy includes radical thyroidectomy, radioiodine ablation of the remnant thyroid, and assiduous follow-up with clinical examination (with particularly careful palpation of the neck), augmented by chest radiography, serum thyroglobulin measurements, and iodine profile scans – decreasing in frequency with time.

Between radioiodine profile scans, the patient is placed on fully TSH-suppressive doses of thyroid hormone. Our recommendations for serial iodine profile scans in papillary tumour patients have been based on the extensive studies of Pochin (1967), who found that over 80% of differentiated thyroid cancer concentrated radioiodine, and that tumours of predominantly papillary structure were equally likely to uptake, although histologically the amount of colloid/follicular structure allowed a fair prediction of this.

This has also been our experience; we have observed children with iodine-avid papillary carcinoma in the lungs, who achieved complete remissions with ^{131}I therapy. (It should be noted that a child relapsing in the neck nodes should always have a preoperative iodine profile scan to assess uptake, and hence the role of postoperative ^{131}I therapy.) Our algorithm of follow-up care has been published (Plowman, 1986).

Recently, despite Tubiana's warnings, we have been persuaded to treat children presenting with less than 2 cm diameter, histologically intrathyroidal papillary carcinomas by radical thyroidectomy, *no* radioiodine ablation, and careful clinical follow-up with serum thyroglobulin estimations (upon thyroid replacement). Time will tell whether this reduction in first therapy for the best prognostic group is as safe as the full ablation and iodine scanning programme, but all such children are at present under careful review.

Survivors of thyroid carcinoma, developing during childhood and treated by radioiodine, appear to suffer no discernible infertility or genetic damage (Sarkar *et al.*, 1976).

22.3 NASOPHARYNGEAL CARCINOMA

In a series of 248 patients presenting to the Royal Marsden Hospital, London with nasopharyngeal carcinoma, six patients (2.4%) were under 15 years of age; ten (4%) were under 20 years; and 28 (11%) were under 30 years of age (Lederman, 1961). In North America, the age incidence graph for this disease is bimodal, with a first small peak of incidence between 15 and 25 years (Greene *et al.*, 1971); this early small peak in incidence in youngsters has also been observed in Puerto Rico (Morales *et al.*, 1984), and in several other countries (India, Israel, Tunisia, Greece, Kuwait), but not in China where the overall incidence of the disease is greatest.

The male predominance of nasopharyngeal carcinoma, so obvious in the adult popula-

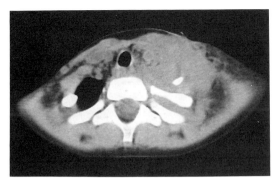

Fig. 22.2 Nasopharyngeal carcinoma presenting as massive low neck lymphadenopathy, demonstrated here on transaxial CT scan.

tion, is much less apparent in childhood. With regard to the epidemiology of the adult disease, the very much higher incidence of nasopharyngeal carcinoma in Hong Kong Chinese, Southern China and South East Asian countries, compared to Western countries, is attributed to racial predisposition, the intake of smoked and dietary salted fish, and Epstein-Barr virus infection (Ho, 1978).

Jenkin *et al.* (1981) suggested that the aetiology of the disease in children and young adults might be different from that encountered in later life. However, Naegele *et al.* (1982) demonstrated Epstein-Barr virus antibody titres suggestive of infection, and Epstein-Barr nuclear antigen positive carcinoma cells in seven American children with nasopharyngeal carcinoma. Furthermore, the clinical presentation, pattern of spread and prognosis of nasopharyngeal carcinoma in children and adults appear to be similar.

The primary nasopharyngeal carcinoma may in fact be 'silent', and the disease may then present clinically with cervical lymphadenopathy (Fig. 22.2); mirror examination of the nasopharynx may even be negative at this time.

Symptoms attributable to the primary tumour depend on its situation: tumours of the lateral nasopharynx wall may be associated with Trotter's triad of symptoms:

1. hypoacusia;
2. paresis of soft palate;
3. pain in the territory of the mandibular division of the mandibular nerve.

Larger growths may produce nasal obstruction or bleeding and a 'nasal twang' to the voice. Invasion of the skull base leads to severe pain and presages cranial nerve pareses.

The diagnosis is made by biopsy under general anaesthesia, at which time the palpable extent of the primary tumour is assessed. Histologically, the carcinoma is often poorly differentiated to undifferentiated (squamous). Tumours previously described as lymphoepitheliomas are now recognized as poorly differentiated squamous carcinomas. Blind adenoidal biopsy may be positive in occult cases presenting with cervical adenopathy. The differential diagnosis is from nasopharyngeal angiofibroma and parameningeal rhabdomyosarcoma.

The TNM staging system for nasopharynx carcinoma is as follows:

T0: no evidence of primary tumour;
T1: tumour limited to one region;
T2: tumour extending to two regions;
T3: tumour extending beyond the nasopharynx but without bone involvement;
T4: tumour extending beyond the nasopharynx, with bone or cartilaginous eustachean tube involvement.

The traditional N staging classification is relevant to conclusions on the prognosis which are drawn below, and is as follows:

N0: no palpable cervical nodes;
N1: mobile ipsilateral cervical adenopathy;
N2: mobile bilateral cervical adenopathy;
N3: fixed cervical adenopathy;
MO/M: absence/presence of distant metastases.

Plain skull radiology, including a submentoventrical view, and computerized tomography of the head and neck are essential staging procedures. Magnetic resonance imaging with gadolinium may give the best indication of skull base invasion.

In the Children's Cancer Study Group (CCSG) analysis, 41 children presented with T1 or T2 lesions, 19 presented with T3 lesions, and 43 presented with T4 lesions. This indicates a high frequency of skull base invasion at presentation, and is of great prognostic importance.

In the same CCSG series, 14 cases were N0, 9 were N1, 42 were N2 and 49 were N3, underlining the high frequency of clinically obvious nodal metastases at presentation (Jenkin *et al.*, 1981). Distant metastases are present at diagnosis in less than 5% of cases, most frequently seen in lungs and bone.

22.3.1 MANAGEMENT

(a) Radiotherapy

Nasopharyngeal carcinoma is not amenable to surgical attack, but as the lesion is radiosensitive, treatment is based on high dose, megavoltage radiotherapy. Our group's radiation technique commences with the child lying supine in an individually made perspex mask, with a dental splint keeping the tongue and floor of the mouth out of the radiation portals. The orbitomeatal line (Reid's baseline) is vertical and all planning (including field junctions) is parallel or perpendicular to this plane. Planning and treatment then continue in a fashion similar to a previously published technique (Lederman and Mould, 1968).

The recommended tumour dose to the nasopharynx primary is 50 Gy (for small tumours in young children), to 60 Gy (for large tumours invading the skull base in

older children), in conventionally fractionated 175–185 cGy daily fractions. We do not deliver doses of 65–70 Gy to children, as opposed to our adult practice.

By using a three-field boost to the nasopharynx, the incidence of treatment-induced late trismus is low. Even if clinically normal, the neck nodes down to the clavicles receive a conventionally fractionated dose of 45–50 Gy. A good, reproducible radiation technique for nasopharyngeal carcinoma is a technically demanding exercise.

The careful study of adults by Ho in 1978 established a prognosis related to the stage of the primary tumour (invasion of the base of the skull being a particularly bad prognostic sign), and to neck node stage (fixed, bilateral and low cervical neck nodes carrying a worse outlook than high mobile and unilateral cervical nodes). Distant metastases are almost invariably fatal.

For tumours confined to the nasopharynx, the five-year survival was 84%, and for large primaries without base of skull invasion and/or mobile, high unilateral cervical nodes, the survival was 62%. However, where there was more extensive nodal involvement, the five-year survival dropped to 40%. Failure at the primary site is particularly common where there is invasion of the base of the skull at presentation (Petrovitch *et al.*, 1985).

Jenkin and colleagues (1981) analysed the results of treatment in 119 patients under 30 years of age at diagnosis, and found the five-year relapse-free and overall survival rates to be 36% and 51% respectively. Where the primary tumour was initially staged as T1/T2, the five-year survival figure was 75%.

These figures are similar to those reported for adults (Ho, 1978). Jenkin *et al.* (1981) also analysed patterns of relapse in patients with initially localized disease. In approximately one-third of relapsing patients there was only local recurrence, whilst in the remaining patients recurrence was outside the irradiation field, particularly in the lungs and liver.

(b) Chemotherapy

In view of the imperfect control rates by radiotherapy alone, chemoradiotherapy is being actively explored. There is no doubt that nasophayngeal carcinoma will respond to single chemotherapeutic agents and, better still, to several varied multidrug combinations; for example, VAC (vincristine, actinomycin, cyclophosphamide) or BEP (bleomycin, etoposide, platinum). Although neoadjuvant (preradiation) chemotherapy studies in squamous head and neck cancer have not shown definite advantages over radiation alone (Brady, 1988), such promise as there is may probably be best demonstrated in nasopharyngeal carcinoma in young patients.

For four to six children with marker disease in the neck, and for several years, we employed a strategy of two to three cycles of BEP chemotherapy prior to radiotherapy. We observed excellent initial shrinkage of the tumour with chemotherapy, and good local control with dosages of radiotherapy (50–55 Gy) to the primary tumour, lower than we had previously been prescribing in this small cohort of patients. However, we encountered toxicity, some of which was predicted (for example, apical lung fibrosis, mucositis) and some which was not – for instance, high tone hearing loss due to synergistic ototoxicity caused by cisplatin and radiation (Kirkbride and Plowman, 1989).

Since that time, we have attempted cochlear shielding during radiotherapy, where safe (Kirkbride and Plowman, 1989). We also abandoned the BEP regimen in favour of cisplatin or carboplatin (where cochlea shielding is not possible) and 5-fluorouracil/folinic acid combination. We have observed excellent regression of cervical lymph node metastases and reduced symptoms from primary tumour invasion following such therapy.

Our present policy is to 'pack in' one to two courses of this alternative chemotherapy as rapidly as possible before progressing to radiotherapy by the third to fifth week. Dental checks and moulding of a radiotherapy mask are carried out during the chemotherapy stage. Admittedly, however, it still has to be proved whether neoadjuvant therapy increases the overall survival.

22.4 SALIVARY GLAND TUMOURS

Of all salivary gland tumours, 2–4% occur in patients under 16 years of age (Castro *et al.*, 1972; Krolls *et al.*, 1972). Fortunately, the majority of these are not true neoplasms, and those that are neoplastic are usually benign.

There were 430 paediatric cases in the series of salivary swellings analysed by the American Armed Forces Institute of Pathology (Krolls *et al.*, 1972). Of these cases (of which mumps was virtually excluded), 262 were non-neoplastic and, amongst those, mucucoeles comprised the majority (185 cases). However, there were 168 true neoplasms of the salivary glands. The majority (124 cases) occurred in the parotid gland, and 124 of those were benign (45 pleomorphic adenomas and 40 vascular tumours).

Pleomorphic adenoma in children, as in adults, occurs predominantly in the parotid gland. It is more common in females, the sex ratio being 2:1 in one series (Malone and Baker, 1984). Teenagers are more commonly affected than younger children. Presentation is with a slowly enlarging, smooth mass.

The treatment of choice is parotidectomy with preservation of the facial nerve. Tumours lateral to the facial nerve or in the tail of the parotid gland are managed by a lateral (superficial) parotidectomy, whilst deep seated tumours are managed by total parotidectomy with preservation of the nerve. Local excision alone or with radiotherapy can be regarded as inferior management schemes.

In the Ann Arbor experience, 18 previously

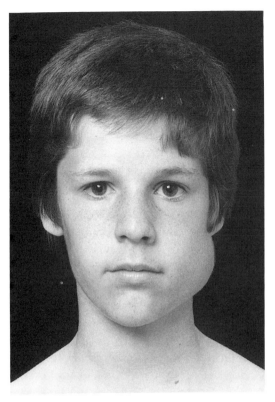

Fig. 22.3 Haemangioma of the parotid gland (courtesy of Professor L. Spitz).

untreated patients underwent conservation parotidectomy with preservation of the facial nerve. All patients remained free of disease at the time of reporting. However, these authors also reported 12 children referred to them with recurrent tumour following surgery at other institutions, and only one of those patients had had surgery as major as superficial parotidectomy (Malone and Baker, 1984). The authors point out that not only does local excision carry a risk of a high local recurrence rate, but that with further surgery it is less easy to preserve the facial nerve. Moreover, there is a risk of true malignancy (carcinoma ex-pleomorphic adenoma): two of the twelve children referred

with local recurrence developed distant metastases.

Of salivary gland tumours the group of vascular tumours comprises: juvenile cellular haemangioendotheliomata (in infants), haemangiomata, and lymphangiomata. The parotid is the most common site of occurrence, and females are more often affected. These lesions give rise to smooth, soft, slowly enlarging (to a plateau size) masses that fluctuate (Fig. 22.3). Surgical excision of large masses, or radiotherapy in exceptional circumstances (see below), is the treatment of choice.

Of 168 paediatric true salivary neoplasms assimilated by the AFIP, 54 were malignant epithelial tumours and the remaining 19 cases were a heterogeneous collection of primary and secondary sarcomas (rhabdomyosarcoma, fibrosarcoma, anaplastic tumours). From the Memorial Hospital series, it seems likely that undiagnosed neoplasms in the submandibular gland are more likely to be malignant than those in the parotid. The rare neoplasms in the sublingual gland were all malignant (Castro *et al.*, 1972).

Mucoepidermoid carcinoma, the most common salivary carcinoma, accounted for 20 out of 35 malignant epithelial cancers in the AFIP series (14 out of 20 cases in the parotid). The majority of patients presented only because of swelling, and pain or facial nerve paresis was rare. A histological grading system (grades I–III) was found to be prognostically useful, and patients with facial nerve dysfunction or positive cervical nodes were more likely to have low grade (I) histology. However, although these tumours were often felt to be clinically mobile and discrete, histologically, they had no true capsule. In this large study, embracing all age groups, prognosis was clearly better in younger patients (Spiro *et al.*, 1975).

Treatment recommendations for childhood mucoepidermoid carcinoma are the same as in adult practice. The recommended surgical strategy is complete removal of the neoplasm with minimum morbidity of normal tissue. The type of operation depends on the extent of the lesion. A subtotal parotidectomy with sparing of the facial nerve is optimal if it complies with this strategy, but for more extensive growths, total parotidectomy with nerve sacrifice and postoperative radiotherapy may be necessary.

Limited surgery, where histology shows disease at or close to the margins, and postoperative radiotherapy probably represent an inferior treatment strategy. However, postoperative radiotherapy does decrease the local relapse rate in higher risk patients (Imperato *et al.*, 1984).

Mucoepidermoid carcinoma of submandibular and sublingual glands is treated by radical gland resection. Block dissection of cervical lymph nodes is indicated either at presentation or at relapse when these nodes are clinically involved. Overall, with optimal management, the expected survival rate for children with salivary mucoepidermoid carcinoma should exceed 90%.

Three very rare malignant epithelial salivary tumours, in decreasing incidence and worsening prognosis, are actinic cell carcinoma, adenoid cystic carcinoma, and adenocarcinoma. The clinical presentation and principles of therapy are exactly as for mucoepidermoid carcinoma.

True neoplasms of the minor salivary glands are extremely rare in childhood, but they comprise the same tumours with similar relative incidence as discussed above (Buduick, 1984). Treatment principles are also similar.

22.5 AMELOBLASTOMA

The ameloblastoma is a rare tumour of the enamel organ stem cells. It usually presents as a cystic mass, much more commonly in the mandible (85% of cases) than in the maxilla. On section, there may be both cystic and solid components. Surgical resection is the treatment of choice, but incomplete excision frequently leads to local recurrence. Thus, wide surgical clearance is the optimal treatment, with radiotherapy reserved only for failure to achieve microscopically clear margins. Metastatic spread is extremely rare.

22.6 CHORDOMA

Chordomata are rare malignant tumours developing from the vestigeal remnants of the notochord. Although they most commonly occur in the sacroccygeal region, 39% of cases occur in the cranial region, particularly arising in the clivus (Utne and Pugh, 1955). Interestingly, there is a tendency for cranial cases to occur in younger age groups, and there is a male predominance.

Macroscopically, chordomata are lobulated, apparently encapsulated growths, of mucoid appearance. Microscopically, large,

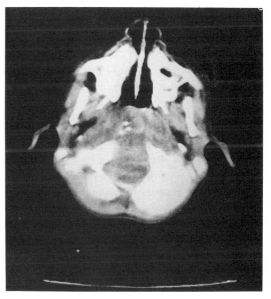

Fig. 22.4 Chordoma of the clivus. Soft tissue tumour mass eroding the base of skull, shown here on transaxial CT scan.

453

vacuolated (physaliferous) cells are often arranged in chords in a background of mucus. Mitotic figures are sparse.

Clival chordomata usually present with a lengthy history of headaches, or with focal neurological signs. Posterior extension leads to brainstem pressure, whilst anterior extension will lead to obstruction of the nasopharynx or bleeding.

Plain radiographs of the skull usually show destruction of the clivus, perhaps extending rostrally to involve the *sella turcica* or laterally to involve the sphenoid or petrous temporal bones. Computerized tomography and magnetic resonance imaging will delineate the tumour extent more accurately (Fig. 22.4).

While radical surgical excision is the treatment of choice, surgical access for radical excision has, until recently, been a major problem. However, a new surgical approach via an anterior Le Fort I osteotomy/maxillotomy gives improved access for clinical resection, and represents an advance in the treatment of clival tumours (Uttley *et al.*, 1989). It is hoped that improved resectability rates will ensue.

High dose radiotherapy is certainly palliative and capable of causing tumour regression (Phillips and Newman, 1974). There does appear to be a radiation dose-effect relationship; in their series, these authors observed tumour control only in patients receiving a high total dose (60 Gy, conventionally fractionated).

Owing to the proximity of the brainstem, the delivery of such doses of radiotherapy has been problematic. However, in this area too there have been advances. Focal radiotherapy methods, notably by the photon beam, have allowed the Boston group to successfully treat a large number of clivus chordomata by 'Bragg peak' delivery of a high radiation dose to the clivus alone and sparing the brainstem (Austin-Seymour *et al.*, 1985). Recently, other focal radiation methods have become available (Plowman, 1990), and

this facility may have more widespread usage.

22.7 ADRENAL CARCINOMA

Adrenal carcinoma is one of the few carcinomas with an age prevalence peak in young to middle age adults; children with this disease are also encountered in the busy paediatric oncology practice. Females are 2.5 times more likely to develop this disease than males, and their age at presentation appears to be younger than in males. For example, in one study, the average age at presentation in females was 37 years, and in males it was 48 years (Nader *et al.*, 1983).

Children with adenocortical carcinoma are at greater risk of developing other tumours, such as brain tumours, melanomas and sarcomas (Levine, 1978), and there is an association with developmental defects, for example hemihypertrophy.

Approximately 80% of patients have functioning tumours, and at presentation 68% of patients have signs and symptoms of hormonal excess – more commonly Cushing's syndrome than virilization, but a combination of both is also common (Luton *et al.*, 1990). Other presenting clinical features include abdominal pain, weight loss, anorexia, fever, lassitude and abdominal mass.

Histologically, adrenal cortical carcinoma may be a differentiated or anaplastic carcinoma. In the differentiated tumours the cells are often polygonal, and ultrastructural studies may show features of steroid forming cells (for example, prominent endoplasmic reticulum and mitochondrial cristae). Some adrenal carcinomas may contain glycogen and appear as 'clear cells' on haematoxylin and eosin staining; they must then be distinguished from renal carcinomas.

Clinically, adrenal carcinoma behaves as an aggressive tumour with a propensity to early infiltration and venous invasion; the most common sites of metastases are regional nodes (paraaortic and paraclaval), peritoneal surfaces, liver and lungs; the proclivity for spread to bone and brain differs in various reported series. Iodocholesterol scanning is based on the high metabolic rate of cholesterol in functional adrenal tissue, but the technique has proved disappointing for the detection of metastases.

For apparently localized tumours, radical surgical resection with or without nephrectomy is the recommended treatment of choice. Although there is little documented evidence in favour of the practice, it has been our policy to deliver postoperative radiotherapy to the flank in higher risk cases (for example, disease at the margins of resection); this is less easy where nephrectomy has not been performed. There is no evidence that other adjuvant therapy at this time prolongs survival.

In relapsing patients, both specific systemic therapy and endocrine blockade need to be considered. O'p'DDD (1,1-dichlorodiphenyl-dichloroethane or mitotane) is an agent that causes necrosis and atrophy of normal adrenal tissue and also of differentiated adrenal carcinoma cells. Hutter and Kayhoe reported in 1966 a steroid response rate of 72% and an objective regression of tumour bulk in 34% of patients. Other workers have subsequently confirmed the usefulness of this agent in adrenal carcinoma (Luton *et al.*, 1990), but responses may be slow (months) and there may be associated gastrointestinal (vomiting and diarrhoea) and neuromuscular (lethargy and weakness) side effects.

However, some recent work in France has suggested that the poor side effect profile of O'p'DDD is due to impurities, such as DDT. Highly purified O'p'DDD is available from French sources and in our experience is much better tolerated, even in high doses. As the compound is explosive, great care is required in its preparation and storage. O'p'DDD is not myelosuppressive. Glucocorticoid and mineralocorticoid cover is essential for patients receiving this therapy.

Cushing's syndrome due to adrenal carcinoma may be palliated by metyrapone therapy (250 mg to 1 g, four times daily, commencing at the lower dose). Metyrapone inhibits 11-beta-hydroxylase (the enzyme converting the metabolically inactive 11-deoxycortisol to cortisol); dose adjustment to prevent Addisonian crisis is necessary, otherwise cortisol cover should be given.

Metyrapone may cause gastrointestinal upset and allergic reactions. Furthermore, the drug shunts steroid precursors into androgen precursors, and may cause or augment virilism. Aminoglutethimide, an inhibitor of the desmolase-mediated cholesterol to pregnenolone conversion, may be added usefully to metyrapone where the latter is not tolerated or is incompletely effective.

Unfortunately, despite radical surgery and early use of O'p'DDD, the prognosis is still poor. In the recent French analysis, the median survival was 14.5 months, and the five-year survival was 22%. Age over 40 years and presence of metastases at presentation were bad prognostic signs.

22.8 FIBROMATOSIS

The fibromatoses are a heterogeneous collection of clinical conditions, with similar histopathological appearances, which are difficult to distinguish from fibrosarcoma (Stout and Lattes, 1967). Aggressive fibromatosis (desmoid tumour) is a fibroblastic condition behaving like a locally invasive tumour, but rarely metastasizing, and it may occur in any musculoaponeurotic structure – head and neck, trunk and limb tumours are all encountered. The condition tends to affect younger age groups. For example, of 25 patients presenting to Massachusetts General Hospital (MGH), 76% were under 40 years of age.

Radical surgical excision is curative, but if these dense growths tie in vital structures such surgery may not be possible. In 1977, Stein reported that aggressive fibromatoses responded to VAC chemotherapy, and more recently we have observed responses in paediatric patients to vincristine and actinomycin chemotherapy given without the alkylating agent.

Radiotherapy is also an effective form of therapy. In the MGH experience, eight out of ten patients treated primarily by radiotherapy achieved complete remission without an attempt at resection (five cases), or achieved stabilization (three cases) of their disease after some regression. Regression post-radiotherapy was slow (Kiel and Suit, 1984). Kiel and Suit recommend radiotherapy where wide field resection is not possible.

The observation that desmoids occurred in Caesarian section scars led to the discovery of sex steroid receptors in these tumours, and subsequently to case reports of regression with tamoxifen therapy. More recently, endocrine inactive derivatives of tamoxifen have caused major regressions in patients with aggressive fibromatoses (Baum, personal communication). This area requires further research.

22.9 COMPLICATED ANGIOMAS

There are several types of angiomas seen in infancy and childhood. The 'neonatal stain' on the head and neck fades spontaneously, whilst the 'salmon patch' remains unchanged. The 'port wine' stain is a sharply defined area of intense intradermal erythema which persists throughout life.

The 'strawberry' (capillary) haemangioma presents at birth or soon afterwards, most commonly in the head and neck region. Initially, this lesion may grow rapidly, and the fast response to low doses of radiotherapy led to widespread application of this method in the past. However, after the age of nine months, most lesions involute spontaneously, and it is only those lesions threatening severe

complications (for example, amblyopia) that justify active therapy.

Cavernous haemangiomas are subcutaneous lesions with less easily distinguishable margins on the skin. They are present at birth or appear in the first six months of life, and may occur anywhere in the body (vertebrae, liver, pericardium, orbit, subglottis, etc.). Cavernous haemangiomas may also be complicated by thrombocytopenia and consumption coagulopathy due to sequestration within the lesion (Kasabach-Merritt syndrome).

The natural history of cavernous haemangiomas is similar to that of 'strawberry' naevi, with a growth phase, plateau phase and subsequent involution phase. During the growth phase, the haemangioma may reach giant dimensions with major clinical repercussions, such as stridor and strangulation due to tracheal compression, high output heart failure due to blood shunting, and bleeding due to thrombocytopenia (for example, retinal detachment). It is these examples of compli-

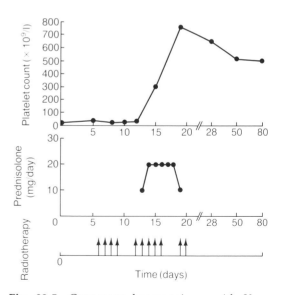

Fig. 22.5 Cavernous haemangioma with Kasabach-Merritt syndrome; response of platelet count to steroid therapy.

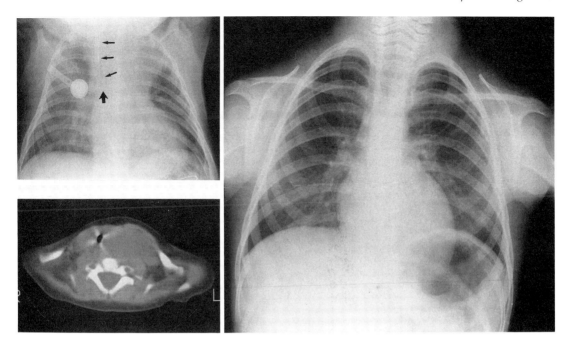

Fig. 22.6 Massive cavernous haemangioma of the thoracic inlet with tracheal compression. Left: plain chest radiography and transaxial CT scan-ning at this level. Following low dose radiother-apy, an excellent response rapidly occurred. Right: chest x-ray three years later.

cated cavernous haemangiomas that are most likely to present to the oncologist.

Treatment of complicated haemangiomas depends on the site, size and complicating factors. For instance, steroid therapy may raise the platelet count in Kasabach-Merritt syndrome (Fig. 22.5), although it does not significantly alter the size of the underlying haemangioma. Surgical excision of a cavernous haemangioma may offer cure but can be hazardous. Embolization may also be effec-tive but also carries risks; one child presented

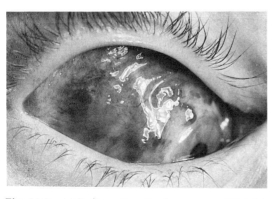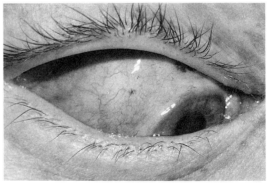

Fig. 22.7 (a) Left: conjunctival angioma; (b) right: after strontium plaque beta radiotherapy.

457

to us recently with infarction and gangrene of the arm, following unsuccessful embolization attempts for an upper thoracic giant cavernous haemangioma.

Low dose radiotherapy remains an important therapeutic weapon against haemangiomas presenting with complications. Where steroid therapy is not able to control an inoperable lesion, radiotherapy can be highly effective (Figs 22.6 and 22.7); (Plowman and Harnett, 1986; Dutton and Plowman, 1991). Focal stereotactic radiotherapy now has an established place in the management of inoperable cerebral arteriovenous malformations (Plowman, 1990).

REFERENCES

Austin-Seymour, M., Munzenrider, J.E., Goiten, M. and Suit, H. (1985) Progress in low LET heavy particle therapy: intracranial and paracranial tumours and uveal melanomas. *Paediat. Res.*, **104**, 5219–26.

Black, E.G., Cassoni, A., Gimlette, T.M.D. *et al.* (1981) Serum, thyroglobulin in thyroid cancer. *Lancet*, **2**, 443–5.

Brady, L.C.O. (1988) Head and Neck Cancer. *Seminars in Oncology*, **15**.

Buduick, S.D. (1984) Minor salivary gland tumours in children. *J. Dent. for Children*, **49**, 44–7.

Castro, E.D., Huvos, A.G., Strong, E.W. and Foote, F.W. (1972) Tumours of the major salivary glands in children. *Cancer*, **29**, 312–17.

Dutton, S.C. and Plowman, P.N. (1991) Paediatric haemangiomas: the role of radiotherapy *Br. J. Radiol.*, **64**, 261–9.

Grant, S., Lattrell, B., Reeve, T. *et al.* (1984) Thyroglobulin may be undetectable in the serum of patients with metastic disease secondary to differentiated thyroid carcinoma. *Cancer*, **54**, 1625–8.

Greene, M., Fraumeni, J.F., Hoover, R. (1971) Nasopharyngeal cancer among young people in the United States: racial variations in cell type. *J. Nat. Canc. Inst.*, **58**, 1267–70.

Ho, J.H.C. (1978) An epidemiologic and clinical study of nasopharyngeal carcinoma. *Int. J. Radiat. Oncol. Biol. Phys.*, **4**, 183–98.

Hutter, A.M. and Kayhoe, D.E. (1966) Adrenal cortical carcinoma. Results with O'p'DDD in 138 patients. *Am. J. Med.*, **41**, 581–6.

Imperato, J.P., Weichselbaum, R.R. and Ervin, T.J. (1984) The role of post-operative radiation therapy in the treatment of malignant tumours of the parotid gland. *J. Surg. Oncol.*, **27**, 163–7.

Jenkin, R.D.T., Anderson, J.R., Jereb, B. *et al.* (1981) Nasopharyngeal carcinoma – a retrospective review of patients less than 30 years of age. *Cancer*, **47**, 360–6.

Kiel, K.D., Suit, H.D. (1984) Radiation therapy in the treatment of aggressive fibromatosis (desmoid tumour). *Cancer*, **54**, 2051–5.

Kirk, J., Mort, C., Grant, D. *et al.* (1991) The usefulness of serum thyroglobulin in the follow-up of differentiated thyroid carcinoma in children. *Med. Ped. Oncol.* (In press).

Kirkbride, P. and Plowman, P.N. (1989) Platinum chemotherapy, radiotherapy and the inner ear: implications for standard radiation portals. *Br. J. Radiol.*, **62**, 457–62.

Krolls, S.O., Trodahl, J.N. and Boyers, R.C. (1972) Salivary gland lesions in children. *Cancer*, **30**, 459–69.

Lederman, M. (1961) *Cancer of the Nasopharynx: Its Natural History and Treatment*. C.C. Thomas, Springfield, IL.

Lederman, M. and Mould, R.F. (1968) Radiation treatment of cancer of the pharynx with special reference to telecobalt therapy. *Br. J. Radiol.*, **41**, 251–74.

Levine, G.W. (1978) Adrenocortical carcinoma in two children with subsequent primary tumours. *Am. J. Dis. Child.*, **132**, 238–40.

Luton, J., Cerdas, S., Billand, L. *et al.* (1990) Clinical features of adrenocortical carcinoma, prognostic factors and the effect of mitotane therapy. *N. Engl. J. Med.*, **322**, 1195–201.

Malone, B. and Baker, S.R. (1984) Benign pleomorphic adenomas in children. *Ann in Otol, Rhinol. and Laryngol.*, **93**, 210–14.

Mazzaferri, E.L., Young, R.L., Oertel, J.E. *et al.* (1977) Papillary thyroid carcinoma: the impact of therapy in 576 patients. *Medicine* (Baltimore), **56**, 171–96.

Morales, P., Bosch, A., Salaverry, S. *et al.* (1984) Cancer of the nasopharynx in young patients. *J. Surg. Oncol.* **27**, 181–5.

Nader, S., Hickey, R.C., Sellin, R.V. and Samaan,

N.A. (1983) Adrenal cortical carcinoma: a study of 77 cases. *Cancer*, **52**, 707–11.

Naegele, R.F., Champion, J., Murphy, S. *et al.* (1982) Nasopharyngeal carcinoma in American children, Epstein-Barr virus specific antibody titers and prognosis. *Int. J. Cancer*, **29**, 209–12.

Petrovitch, Z., Cox, J.D., Middleton, R. *et al.* (1985) Advanced carcinoma of the nasopharynx. Pattern of failure in 256 patients. *Radiother. and Oncol.*, **4**, 15–20.

Phillips, T.L., and Newman, H. (1974) Chordomas, in *Modern Radiotherapy and Oncology*. Central Nervous System Tumours (ed T.J. Dealey). Butterworths, London, pp. 184–203.

Plowman, P.N. (1986) Endocrine cancer, in *Radiotherapy in Clinical Practice* (ed. H. Hope-Stone) Butterworths, London, pp. 300–15.

Plowman, P.N. (1990) Focal Brain Radiotherapy. *J. Neurol. Neurosurg. Psychiat.*, **53**, 541.

Plowman, P.N. and Harnett, A.N. (1986) Radiotherapy in benign orbital disease 1: Complicated ocular angiomas. *Br. J. Ophthalmol.*, **72**, 286–8.

Pochin, E.E. (1967) Prospects for the treatment of thyroid carcinoma with radio-iodine. *Clin. Radiol.*, **18**. 113–15.

Sarkar, S.D., Beikrwaltes, W.H., Gill, S.P. and Cowley, P.J. (1976) Subsequent fertility and birth histories of children and adolescents treated with ^{131}I for thyroid cancer. *J. Nuclear Med.*, **17**, 460–4.

Spiro, R.H. Huvos A.G. and Strong, E.W. (1975) Cancer of the parotid gland. A clinicopathological study of 288 primary cases. *Am. J. Surg.*, **130**, 452–9.

Stein, R. (1977) Chemotherapeutic response in fibromatosis of the neck. *J. Paediatr.*, **90**, 482–3.

Stout, A.P. and Lattes, R. (1967) Tumours of the soft tissues. Atlas of Tumour Pathology. Second Series Armed Forces Institute of Pathology. *Fascicle* I, 17–30.

Tubiana, M., Schlumberger, M. and Rougier, P. (1985) Long-term results and prognostic factors in patients with differentiated thyroid carcinoma. *Cancer*, **55**, 794–804.

Utne, J.R. and Pugh, D.G. (1955) The roentgenologic aspects of chordoma. *Am. J. Roentgenol.*, **74**, 595–602.

Uttley, D., Moore, A. and Archer, D.J. (1989) Surgical management of midline skull base tumours: a new approach. *J. Neurosurg.*, **71**, 705–10.

Woolner, L.B., Beahrs, O.H., Black, B.M. *et al.* (1961) Classification and prognosis of thyroid carcinoma. *Am. J. Surg.*, **102**, 354–88.

Part Three

Late Effects, Supportive Care and Advances in Therapy

Chapter 23

Megatherapy and immunotherapy in paediatric solid tumours

R. LADENSTEIN and T. PHILIP

23.1 THE ROLE OF MEGATHERAPY

23.1.1 INTRODUCTION

Paediatric solid tumours comprise a variety of malignancies with different tumour cell characteristics as well as different responses to conventional drug combinations. In contrast to most adult malignancies, they are notable for the markedly high in response rates. The value of chemotherapy is proven by the progress achieved during the last decades. It is now clear that dose and delivery time are fundamental factors in drug efficacy. This has led to the introduction of megatherapy followed by bone marrow (BM) rescue for bad prognosis childhood solid tumours. Massive chemotherapy and radiotherapy regimens are presently widely used with more than 2000 children already being treated in such a way. Several extensive reviews (Philip and Pinkerton, 1989a; 1989b; Armitage and Gale, 1989; Armitage 1989; Cheson *et al.*, 1989; Yaniv *et al.*, 1990) reflect the persistent effort to establish more successful drug combinations in terms of response and survival. For some diseases such as lymphomas this

treatment modality has proven curative value. However, for the majority of bad prognosis solid tumours of childhood, we are still in the phase of pilot studies and pragmatic recommendations only can be given at this time. With the availability of growth factors, a new tool in oncology was gained and this probably will enable us to apply megatherapy without consecutive BM rescue in the near future. Nevertheless, we are now approaching the limits of the dose response concept in clinical practice and will have to progress to new ideas to improve prognosis in children with bad prognosis malignancies. New therapeutic strategies should be based on different mechanisms of anti-tumour activity and immunotherapy may be such an approach.

23.1.2 DOSE-EFFECT RELATIONSHIP

Clinical observations such as the prognostic significance of initial tumour bulk or disease progression occurring during treatment after an initial impressive clinical response, have been explained by the theories postulated by Goldie and Coldman (1979; 1983; 1985). They have suggested that mutations occurring stochastically during the tumoral development favour the selection of resistant clones and the emergence of metastatic phenotypes. The probability of a tumour developing a drug resistant clone follows Poisson's law and is an inherent feature of any cell population capable of spontaneous mutation. The appearance of resistance is therefore independent of prior drug exposure and relates simply to the nature of the population dynamics. Thus, a large tumour with a high growth fraction and rapid tumour cell turnover is more likely statistically to develop subpopulations that are drug resistant. Moreover, as the tumour grows, this likelihood increases.

This fact has been the basis for the design of non crossresistant drug regimens aiming for a maximum of tumour cell kill by affecting different subpopulations. Re-emergence of partially treated populations and development of new resistant cell clones might be prevented by a minimum of delay between treatment courses. Thus, the most important factors for drug efficacy are dose and frequency of administration as highlighted in the review of Frei *et al.* (1980).

Dose escalation, either of single agents or of drug combinations, is assumed to be a key factor in the attempt to convert response into cure. Studies in the Ridgeway sarcoma model in dogs have shown that the dose-response curve is steep and that small modifications of dose intensity and/or dose rate of many cytostatics can modify tumour response from partial response to complete regression or cure (Skipper *et al.*, 1964). However, doses used in clinical practice reflect the limitations imposed by toxicity rather than the ideal dose to achieve maximum antitumor activity (Gehan, 1984).

To conclude this section, the Goldie and Coldman argument supports multimodality treatment including stepwise chemotherapy, radiotherapy, and delayed surgery to excise

a residual, chemoresistant tumour mass. These latter modalities are not limited by the same cellular heterogeneity that applies to drugs. For the above reasons, single dose high dose chemotherapy should be applied in a situation of minimal residual disease (Goldie and Coldman, 1983). This is also in agreement with other theories of the dose-effect relationship (Norton and Simon, 1977; Norton, 1985).

23.1.3 HIGH DOSE THERAPY WITH BONE MARROW RESCUE

Autologous BMT rescue in solid tumours permits the selection of the most active agents for use in combination at doses limited only by extramedullary toxicity. Thus drug dosages are able to be increased three- to tenfold above levels normally used in cancer treatment (De Vita, 1986). Toxicities involve those tissues which share a rapid cellular proliferation rate (Table 23.1).

The essential problem to overcome mechanisms of drug resistance is a complex one as are the mechanisms of drug action, with most of them still poorly understood *in vivo*. Culture assays of tumour cells have shown cell adaptations such as alterations in the transport system, changes in activation and inactivation, alterations in the structures and genetic modifications (Goldie and Coldman, 1983; 1985; Waxman, 1988; Philip *et al.*, 1989a; Ivy *et al.*, 1989; Rothenberg and Ling, 1989; Chabner and Fojo, 1989; Goldstein *et al.*, 1990). The strategy for bypassing resistance is to increase the dose of drug as postulated by Goldie and Coldman (1983; 1985). Alkylating agents may overcome resistance when applied in high doses and may act synergistically (Frei *et al.*, 1988). For example, high dose cisplatin can bypass inadequate membrane transport and saturate other mechanisms, such as detoxification and DNA repair (Scanlon *et al.*, 1989; Canon *et al.*, 1990).

The potential of allogenic BMT to induce a

461

Table 23.1 Toxicity related to megatherapy

Drugs	Related toxicity					
	CMP	Pneumonitis	VOD	ARF	Haemorrhagic cystitis	Leukoencephalopathy
Bleomycin		+				
Cytosine arabinoside			+			+
Carmustine		+	+			
Cisplatin				+		+
Carboplatin				+		+
Cyclophosphamide	+		+		+	
Doxorubicin	+					
Etoposide				+		
Melphalan		+	+	+		
Methotrexate		+		+		+
Thiotepa			+			+
TBI		+	+	+		+

CNS = central nervous system; CMP = cardiomyopathy; VOD = veno-occlusive disease; ARF = acute renal failure.

graft versus tumour effect has been recently reported by Jones (1990) for both Hodgkin's disease and non Hodgkin's lymphoma, demonstrating a 18% actual relapse rate for the allogeneic group versus 45% for the autologous group. Nevertheless, autologous BMT (ABMT) has become the method of choice in solid tumours because of its practicality and the fact that only 25% of patients have HLA and DR matched donors. It is used either to shorten the period of aplasia after non-ablative high-dose chemotherapy, or as a rescue after massive, presumptively lethal myeloablative chemotherapy, often with total body irradiation (TBI). There are several critical problems to be faced along with ABMT: the best induction regimen to achieve a good quality remission marrow where it has been initially involved, the ideal timing for harvesting, and the real significance of minimal residual bone marrow disease.

Several questions are of interest and still require to be answered concerning solid tumours. In the majority of phase II studies, impressive response rates are observed in progressive disease resistant to conventional

drug doses. Thus there is clinical confirmation of a dose-effect relationship in solid tumours. In contrast to leukaemia or lymphoma, where responses are usually complete even in disease resistant to conventional chemotherapy, in the majority of cases with solid tumours only incomplete remissions are achieved in a similar situation. Thus, there is still need to establish better treatment strategies to produce cure. Multiagent regimen phase II studies have been reviewed by Appelbaum and Buckner (1986) and Pinkerton *et al.* (1986). Examples of the different high dose regimens reported in childhood solid tumours are shown in Tables 23.4–23.10.

23.1.4 PURGING

A possible limitation of ABMT after supra-lethal treatment with high-dose chemotherapy and TBI is the potential contamination of the transplanted bone marrow or peripheral blood stem cells (PBSC) by malignant cells. Considerable efforts have consequently been made to remove tumour cells from the BM before reinjection.

Techniques such as percoll or bovine serum albumin (BSA) gradients were the first methods described and more recently counterflow centrifugation has been reported (De Witte *et al.*, 1986). Sheep red blood rosetting or soybean lectin separation have more restricted applications in T-cell depletion (Reisner *et al.*, 1983). Chemotherapeutic agents may destroy malignant cells with at least a partial preservation of normal haematopoietic progenitors (Korbling *et al.*, 1987). Active derivatives of cyclophosphamide, either 4-hydroperoxycyclophosphamide (4-HC) or mafosfamide (ASTA Z 7557), are now extensively used in clinical trials of autografting in ALL, AML, NHL and neuroblastoma (Hervé *et al.*, 1984; Kaizer *et al.*, 1985; Hartmann *et al.*, 1985; Yeager *et al.*, 1986; Gorin *et al.*, 1986). Some non-chemotherapeutic agents are of potential interest. For example, merocyanine 540, a DNA dye with lytic activity after photoactivation (Sieber *et al.*, 1984) and 6-hydroxydopamine (Reynolds *et al.*, 1982). Immunomagnetic depletion involves targeting small magnetic beads on tumour cells by means of specific monoclonal antibodies (MoAbs) and then removing the coated tumour cells from the bone marrow through a flow system using permanent samarium cobalt magnets. The procedure produces a significant loss of mononuclear cells but it is not toxic for stem cells (Poynton *et al.*, 1983; Treleaven *et al.*, 1984; Reynolds *et al.*, 1986; Favrot *et al.*, 1987; Kemshead, 1988; Combaret *et al.*, 1987; 1989a). The same principle is used when malignant cells are adsorbed in a column via MoAbs attached to a solid phase through avidin biotin linkages (Berenson *et al.*, 1986; Favrot and Philip, 1989a). Another possibility to eliminate targeted cells is complement lysis. MoAbs (IgM or IgG2a isotypes) lyse targeted cells in the presence of rabbit complement (Lebein *et al.*, 1985; Favrot *et al.*, 1986) or human complement (Stepan *et al.*, 1984; Bast *et al.*, 1985; Janossy *et al.*, 1987). Finally, MoAbs can also be conjugated to various plant toxins. Ricin is the one most commonly used in clinical trials (Filipovich *et al.*, 1984).

Reasons for observed delays in grafting are difficult to assess but often previous damage to the BM microenvironment by heavy and prolonged pretreatment or by double BMT programmes is more likely to be the cause than toxic stem cell damage by purging procedures. In a recent analysis of autologous BMT performed in the Centre Léon Bérard, qualitative parameters of the bone marrow infused were predictive factors of BM recovery and suggested a minimal count of 0.5×10^8 mononuclear cells/kg with a minimum of GMCFU activity of 3×10^4/kg to be necessary (Bouffet *et al.*, 1990a).

The role of purging procedures was first evaluated when it was demonstrated that Asta Z was able to clear the marrow in adult acute leukaemia. This was of little benefit for high risk patients but in standard risk patients it produced some improvement in survival (Gorin *et al.*, 1986). Bad prognosis Burkitt's Lymphoma (BL) has also been studied (Favrot *et al.*, 1989a). The use of a liquid cell culture assay demonstrates the presence of residual BL cells in the BM (Philip I, *et al.*, 1987) and their elimination by purging procedures (Favrot *et al.*, 1987). BM contamination of neuroblastoma cells before and eventually after the purging procedure can be demonstrated by dual immunofluorescence staining for quality control (Beck *et al.*, 1988; Combaret *et al.*, 1989b; 1990; Bowman *et al.*, 1990a). Five different monoclonal antibodies (HLA.ABC, UJ13A, LEU 7, NKH 1, ANTI-GD2) are currently used for the detection of neuroblastoma micrometastases in the bone marrow in our centre with a limit of detection of 10^{-5} malignant cells.

The basic discussion as to whether or not purging is necessary is still not settled. In neuroblastoma, for example, clinical observations demonstrate that relapses emerge from residual tumour sites rather than from reinfused malignant cells in the BM. In practice, the need for purging procedures remains a controversial issue as the clonogenic potential of reinfused tumour cells is difficult to demonstrate (Favrot *et al.*, 1989c) and there is no substantial data in solid tumours so far to prove a positive impact on patient survival. The outcome of 34 neuroblastoma patients grafted with unpurged marrows was reported to be identical to that in patients receiving purged marrows after the same megatherapy (Dini *et al.*, 1990). To prove the necessity of this sophisticated procedure, the BM should be assayed with very sensitive methods to detect the presence or absence of residual malignant cells to allow a conclusion regarding efficiency to be made in each particular case. Purging procedures should ideally be compared with non-purged marrows in cases with residual disease.

23.1.5 THE ROLE OF HAEMOPOIETIC GROWTH FACTORS

The advances of recombinant technology have permitted the generation of haemopoietic growth factors (Mauch *et al.*, 1989a). The colony-stimulating factors GM-CSF and G-CSF are under trial for stimulation of progenitors to increase the number and activity of leukocytes as well as to increase the population of marrow and peripheral blood stem cells before harvesting. The use of growth factors (GF) will eventually reduce the need for the difficult and costly procedure of autologous BMT. The *in vivo* effects of haemopoietins (with the exception of erythropoietin) are still not well defined. Furthermore, the risks of depleting the stem cell pool (Mauch *et al.*, 1989b; Lord *et al.*, 1989; Ho *et al.*, 1990) and eventually stimulating neoplastic residual cells are worth considering (Dexter and White, 1990). It has also been shown that GF can prevent fragmentation of stem cells (Williams *et al.*, 1990). The normal steady state haemopoiesis is locally regulated by the specific microenvironment in the bone marrow. The stromal cells have a critical role and secrete GF (GM-CSF, G-CSF, M-CSF, IL-1, IL-3, IL-5, IL-6) and also can bind exogenous GM-CSF and IL-3 thus supplying them to stem cells and committed precursors (Daniel and Dexter, 1989; Graham *et al.*, 1990; Athanasou *et al.*, 1990). After BMT, stromal cells have a reduced capacity to produce G-CSF and probably other growth factors as well (Cayeux *et al.*, 1989a; Migliaccio *et al.*, 1990). The insufficient production and response of T cells to IL-2 is well documented. There are also data indicating that overactive mononuclear cells express Leu 7 and CD 8 in some cases of delayed engraftment after autologous BMT (Favrot *et al.*, 1990e).

Timed administration of GF could help obtain a better stem cell harvest from either BM or peripheral blood for autografts. Moreover, they may improve the safety of BMT procedures when used to shorten the aplastic period after megatherapy and marrow infusions. Finally, they are a potential key to the use of megatherapy without marrow rescue thus simplifying the approach.

23.1.6 TOTAL BODY IRRADIATION

Historically, the use of TBI has evolved from its role in leukaemia. Up to 1989 there was general consensus that patients treated with cyclophosphamide and total body irradiation did better than those without (Bouffet *et al.*, 1990b; Cabanillas *et al.*, 1990). Since the introduction of busulphan and cyclophosphamide for leukaemia and lymphoma, equivalent results have been observed and thus the role of TBI has been questioned for these diseases (Philip *et al.*, 1987a; Armitage and Bierman, 1989; Phillips *et al.*, 1989; Colombat *et al.*, 1989).

Many conventional treatment regimens take advantage of the radiosensitivity of most solid tumours for local treatment. For this reason TBI seemed to be an appealing means as part of treatment regimens for solid tumours. Basic radiobiological response studies for neuroblastoma were outlined by Deacon (1985). The human neuroblastoma cell line HX 138 in different experimental systems behaved in keeping with the clinical radio-responsiveness of neuroblastoma. The capacity to repair potentially lethal damage is a significant factor for the underlying differences in clinical radioresponsiveness of human tumours (Weichselbaum *et al.*, 1982). The above studies were able to demonstrate the radiosensitivity of NBL to the fairly low irradiation dose of 2 Gy. Furthermore, the rationale to irradiate small bulk residual tumour was supported since increasing radioresistance was observed under hypoxic conditions. The latter strongly correlates with greater tumour volumes as previously shown in V79 Chinese Hamster cells (West *et al.*, 1984). Studies on the molecular basis of radiosensitivity such as experiments on transfection of DNA repair genes, are under way. Characterization of the genetic control of radiation damage repair may have far reaching implications for radiation-related carcinogenesis as well as therapy.

Nevertheless, the need for TBI in massive chemotherapy regimens for solid tumours remains an area of debate. There is an understandable reluctance to use such therapy in young children because of the considerable early, and as yet ill-defined long-term toxicity. Similarly, the advantages of fractionated TBI remains controversial although pulmonary toxicity has been reduced (Pino *et al.*, 1982). The relative cytotoxic effect in tumours with shouldered response curves remains to be clarified (Kinsella *et al.*, 1983). If these treatment approaches should progress beyond the phase II level and are offered to patients in 1st CR as consolidation treatment, further aspects such as late effects, e.g. growth disturbances, sterility, hormone imbalances and potential second malignancies, assume great importance.

23.2 NEUROBLASTOMA

23.2.1 INTRODUCTION

The outcome with surgery alone is good in the (rare) Stage 1 patient, as well as patients in Stage 2 in whom there is no associated lymph node involvement. Chemotherapy, given either alone or combined with radiation therapy, is highly effective in the remaining Stage 2 patients, resulting in long-term survival in more than 75% of cases (Rosen *et al.*, 1984). With more advanced, initially unresectable disease (Stage 3) the outcome appears to depend, at least to some extent, upon the completeness of eventual surgical resection following primary chemotherapy (Le Tourneau *et al.*, 1985). Thus, the wide variation in long-term survival for this stage (40% to 70%) reflects variable effectiveness of chemotherapy and variations in surgical expertise.

In Stage 4 patients, age remains an important prognostic factor. For patients under one year, even in those with metastatic disease, cure rates may exceed 50%. For children between one and two years of age, the prognosis is intermediate. However, for patients older than two years at diagnosis, the likelihood of long-term survival with standard chemotherapy is only about 10%. The rapid initial response to chemotherapy may arouse false optimism, since with most modern treatment regimens up to 80% to 90% of patients achieve at least a partial response, with disappearance or shrinkage of metastases. Unfortunately, even with use of aggressive surgery and intensive radiotherapy, this improvement is rarely converted to a complete remission and progression of the disease usually occurs within the following year.

Apart from clinical staging, a number of other parameters have been introduced which may aid in assessing prognosis. A summary of these risk factors is outlined in detail in Table 23.2. Elevated serum neurone-

465

Table 23.2 Prognostic factors in neuroblastoma

Prognostic factor		Reported prognosis (two-year survival)	Authors
Stage of disease	Stage 1	100%[+]	Stephenson, 1986
	Stage 2	82%[+]	Carlsen, 1986
	Stage 3	42%[+]	Evans, 1987
	Stage 4	30%[+]	Brodeur, 1988
	Stage 4s	80%[+]	
Age	<2 years	77%[+]	Carlsen, 1986
	>2 years	38%[+]	Evans, 1987
			Philip, 1987b
Ferritin	0–150 ng/ml	83%[+]	Evans, 1987
	>150 ng/ml	17%[+]	Imashuku, 1988
			Hann, 1985
NSE (neurone-specific enolase)	1–100 ng/ml	76%[+]	Zeltzer, 1986
	>100 ng/ml	17%[+]	Evans, 1987[+]
			Tsuchida, 1987
GD2 (circulating) (diganglioside)	>50 pmol/ml	(−)	Ladisch, 1987
NPY-LI	>200 pmol/L	(−)	Kogner, 1990
(neuropeptide-like immunoreactivity)	<200pmol/L	(+)	
VMA/HVA ratio	>1	84%[+]	Evans, 1987[+]
	<1	44%[+]	
Dopaminergic NBL		(−)	Nakagawara, 1988
Shimada criteria	Favourable	94%	Shimada, 1984, 1985
	Unfavourable	39%	
Marker Chromosome 1	+	10%	Christiansen, 1988
	−	90%	Schwab, 1990
Double minutes homogenously staining regions		(−) (−)	Hayashi, 1989
Numerical abnormalities	Diploid,	(−)	Christiansen, 1988
	Hypotetraploid	(−)	Hayashi, 1989
	Hyperdiploid,	(+)	
	Triploid	(+)	
DNA index	>1.0	RFS:96%°	Bowman, 1990b
	=1.0	RFS:29%°	
n-*myc* oncogene amplification	Yes	DFS:0%°	Bourhis, 1990
	No	DFS:>90%°	Seeger, 1985
			Nakagawara, 1987
			Combaret, 1989c
			Tsuda, 1987

(−) = adverse
(+) = good

specific enolase (NSE), raised ferritin, and high copy number of the N-*myc* oncogene in tumour tissue all correlate with an unfavourable prognosis. The Shimada histopathological classification, based upon details of stromal elements, cell differentiation, mitotic

Table 23.3 Grouping of clinical and genetic types of neuroblastoma as related to prognosis

Features	Type 1	Type 2	Type 3
Karyotype and ploidy	Hyperdiploid near triploid	Diploid/tetraploid	Tetraploid
Chromosome 1p	Normal	Normal	Deleted
N-*myc* copy	Normal	Normal	Amplified
LDH	Normal	<5 times elevated	Increased
Ferritin	Normal	<150 mg/ml	>150 mg/ml
Age	<12 months	Any	Any age
Stage	1, 2, 4s	3, 4	Any stage
Shimada	Good	Any	Bad
Outcome	Good	Intermediate	Bad

(modified according to Brodeur as presented at the XIIth SIOP meeting, Rome, 1990).

index, and age, has been shown to accurately identify poor prognosis subgroups within clinical stages (Table 23.3).

Use of *meta*-iodobenzylguanidine (MIBG) scintigraphy (Moyes *et al.*, 1989) and magnetic resonance imaging (MRI) (Couanet and Geoffray, 1988) have thrown the classical staging systems for neuroblastoma somewhat into disarray. The International Staging System Working Party is currently engaged in keeping up with these changes and has produced an interim working system (Brodeur *et al.*, 1988). The parameters in Table 23.3 are helpful in making treatment decisions for the lower stages (such as Stage 2 and 3) when more aggressive approaches may be warranted. However, in Stage 4 disease, the outlook is so poor that there is little indication at the moment for a reduction in treatment intensity. Nonetheless, such subclassification does permit better characterization of the small group of survivors. The improvement of therapy in Stage 4 remains the major goal of the treatment of neuroblastoma (Graham-Pole *et al.*, 1989; Michon *et al.*, 1989; Vossen, 1990; Pinkerton, 1990).

Because of the limited availability of matched, related donors in this very young group of patients, experience with autologous marrow transplants is greater than

with allogeneic transplants. Moreover, unlike leukaemia, neuroblastoma only secondarily involves the bone marrow, which may be cleared of visible tumour cells by effective chemotherapy prior to marrow harvest. The need for such purging procedures in practice remains a contentious issue as already outlined (Favrot and Philip, 1989a). The main limiting effect in the use of megadosage therapy remains the ability of such therapy to completely ablate the malignant cells.

23.2.2 THE ROLE OF TOTAL BODY IRRADIATION

The potential value of total body irradiation was suggested by the finding of 20% progression-free survival at two years in a group of highly selected patients with recurrent neuroblastoma when TBI was used in the regimen. No progression-free survivors were reported when TBI conditioning was not included (Philip and Pinkerton, 1989a; 1989b). With or without TBI, with single or two sequential graft procedures, 40% to 45% progression-free survivors at two years were reported in patients grafted either in complete or partial remission (Philip *et al.*, 1987c; 1987d; Hartmann *et al.*, 1987). No advantage was shown at two years in the

467

Table 23.4 Development of megatherapy regimens reported for neuroblastoma phase II studies

Year	Author	Drug	Dose/day	-10	-9	-8	-7	-6	-5	-4	-3	-2	-1	0
1982	Pritchard	L-PAM	140 mg/m²										X	
1984	August	DXR	45 mg/m²				X		X					
		VM26	180 mg/m²				X		X					
		L-PAM	140 mg/m²					X						
			70 mg/m²							X				
		TBI	333 rad									X	X	X
1984	Kingston	CYC	300 mg/m²				X							
		L-PAM	180–220 mg/m²										X	
1986	Hartmann	BU	4×1 mg/kg p.o.			X	X	X	X					
		CYC	50 mg/kg							X	X	X	X	
1985	Philip	VCR	1.5 mg/m² bolus				X							
			0.5 mg/m² ctn				X	X	X	X	X			
		L-PAM	180 mg/m²										X	
		TBI	2×2 Gy							X	X	X		
1987	Hartmann	BCNU	300 mg/m²				X							
		VM26	250 mg/m²				X	X	X	X				
		L-PAM	180 mg/m²								X			
1987c	Philip	1st: BCNU	300 mg/m²				X							
		VM26	250 mg/m²						X	X	X	X	X	
		CDDP	40 mg/m²						X	X	X	X	X	
		(or CBDCA	250 mg/m²)											
		2nd: see Philip 1985												
1988	Graham-Pole	L-PAM	60 mg/m²						X	X	X			
		TBI	2×2 Gy									X	X	X
1989	Reynolds	CDDP	90 mg/m²		X									
		VP16	150 mg/m²				X		X					
		DXR	45 mg/m²				X							
		L-PAM	140 mg/m²					X						
			70 mg/m²							X				
		TBI	3.33 Gy									X	X	X
1989	Michon	L-PAM	140 mg/m²	X										
		BU	150 mg/m²			X	X	X	X					
		CYC	2.2 g/m²							X	X			
		1st:VM26	250 mg/m²					X	X	X	X			
		L-PAM	180 mg/m²								X			
		2nd: BU	150 mg/m²			X	X	X	X					
		CYC	2.2 g/m²							X	X			
1989	Pinkerton	VCR	1.5 mg/m² bolus				X							
			0.5 mg/m² ctn				X	X	X	X	X			
		L-PAM	180 mg/m²											X
		VP16	200 mg/m²						X	X	X	X	X	
		CBDCA	200 mg/m²						X	X	X	X	X	
1990	Hartmann	1st: VM26	250 mg/m²					X	X	X	X			
		L-PAM	180 mg/m²									X		
		2nd: BU	150 mg/m²			X	X	X	X					
		CYC	2.2 g/m²							X	X			
		L-PAM	140 mg/m²	X										
		BU	150 mg/m²			X	X	X	X					
		CYC	2.2 g/m²							X	X			

L-PAM = melphalan, DXR = doxorubicin; VM26 = teniposide; CYC = cyclophosphamide; BU = busulfan; VCR = vincristine; BCNU = carmustine; CDDP = cisplatin; CBDCA = carboplatin; 1st/2nd: refers to double graft programmes for first and second graft; ctn = continuous infusion.

group given the TBI-containing regimen. The mortality rate is similar with use of either regimen.

It is clear that in all studies no plateau has yet been reached in the survival curves at or beyond two years. Survival of approximately 20% at five years and 15% at six to seven years are expected. However, a 40% survival rate at five years with no late relapse was recently observed in a small subgroup of patients in whom there was complete remission for bone, bone marrow and urinary catecholamines before surgery. Similar findings were also shown in two other studies (Philip *et al.*, 1991).

Interest in the concept of a double graft procedure in neuroblastoma has been kindled by the frequency of early relapse following bone marrow transplantation, occurring three to 12 months post-graft in the majority of the cases. Among selected patients in partial remission after induction therapy, who received a double graft without TBI, there were no survivors at two years (Hartmann *et al.*, 1987). This differs from a current pilot study in which a double graft and TBI were used instead of a single graft, with survivors up to five years (Philip *et al.*, 1989b).

A prospective randomized study of high dose melphalan was carried out in patients with Stage 3 and 4 neuroblastoma who achieved at least partial remission after a standardized cisplatin-containing induction regimen. There was a significant advantage at two years for the melphalan group, both in terms of median survival and length of the progression-free interval. The results of the study provide a rational basis for inclusion of melphalan at high dose in future protocols (Pritchard *et al.*, 1986). A summary of the high dose therapy approaches for neuroblastoma is given in Table 23.4. TBI is still included in many pretransplant regimens because of *in vitro* radiosensitivity findings and early clinical experience.

However, because of concern about the contribution of TBI to both short- and long-term morbidity, its inclusion requires prospective evaluation. It is possible that the substitution of other drugs at high dose might provide a better therapeutic index. Late effects of radiation such as second malignancies are beginning to appear in the literature and avoidance, if possible, of this risk must be a consideration in the design of new regimens. However, for the present, the first concern is to achieve prolonged good quality remission in patients with neuroblastoma.

More than 400 autologous bone marrow transplants have been performed in Europe, more than 200 in the USA, and approximately 200 in other countries (Shimada *et al.*, 1985; Graham-Pole, 1989; Dini *et al.*, 1989a; Hartmann *et al.*, 1987; August and Auble, 1989; Reynolds *et al.*, 1989). From the 439 procedures included in the review by the European Bone Marrow Transplantation Group, 385 were a consolidation of first line therapy (complete remission and very good partial remission in 212; partial remission in 173) and 50 after relapse or progression (including 35 sensitivity relapses). In 80% of patients the marrow was purged using immunomagnetic beads (40%) or mafosfamide (40%). (EBMT database, Lyon.)

The following conclusions may be drawn from this large review (Figs. 23.1 and 23.2):

1. It is not worthwhile to treat patients with resistant relapses with such a therapy. None of the children are alive progression-free at two years.
2. Of the patients grafted as a consolidation of first line therapy, 40% are alive without progression two years after bone marrow transplantation. Regimens with or without TBI produced equivalent results. Such is the case also for one versus two autologous bone marrow transplants, as well as for use of purged versus unpurged marrow with at least a two-year median follow-up. Patients showing only partial

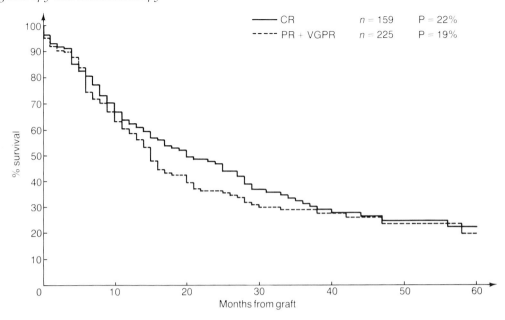

Fig. 23.1 EBMT 90 Neuroblastoma: Consolidation of CR versus VGPR+PR.

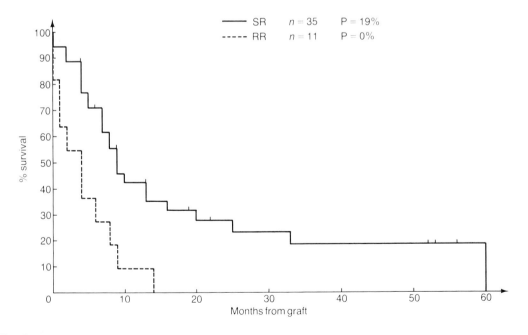

Fig. 23.2 EBMT 90 Neuroblastoma: Sensitive versus resistance relapses.

470

response did as well as those who had complete remissions or very good partial remissions before ABMT, and quality of surgical excision and age also did not contribute to improving survival. Patients with negative *m*IBG bone scans at the time of bone marrow transplantation did better than all the other patients.

3. Patients alive and without progression at two years are not cured, and no more than 20% are still alive at five years. Patients with no bone marrow involvement at diagnosis did better, with a survival of 50% at five years.
4. Patients with relapse whose tumours were sensitive to therapy were alive without progression in 30% of cases after two years. Additional studies in this group of patients are warranted.
5. Toxic death rate is 18% for relapses and 11% for consolidation. No difference is found between programmes including one or two grafts. However, total body irradiation is more toxic with toxic death in 16% of those given TBI as compared to 8% in those given chemotherapy alone.

In the USA, during 1984–1989, 74 patients with disseminated neuroblastoma between one and 15 years of age (median four), were enrolled in a collaborative study. Seven additional patients had allogeneic bone marrow transplants. The myelo-ablative treatment consisted of melphalan and TBI, and immuno-magnetic purging of the marrow was used. Of the 81 patients who were engrafted, 37 (46%) relapsed at one to 21 months (median six months), while 12 (15%) died of treatment-related toxicity. Thirty-two (31.8%) children are in continuous complete remission (CCR) with a short median follow-up of 14 months (Graham-Pole, 1989). Another study presented similar results in 28 patients, aged from two to 30 years; 35% are in CCR at nine to 90 months (August 1989). Finally, 31 patients in Stages 2 to 4 with poor prognosis

were entered in a limited pilot study. The regimen included cisplatin, etoposide, adriamycin and melphalan plus TBI. At 23 months, the overall survival probability is near 50% (Reynolds *et al.*, 1989).

A review by the International Bone Marrow Transplant Registry showed a similar relapse rate with use of allogenic bone marrow transplantation as compared to autologous bone marrow transplantation. At 17 months, there were 29 patients with CCR out of 92 patients (Graham-Pole, 1989).

In a recent review of 62 patients treated by the LMCE group in France, the median follow-up was 59 months after autologous bone marrow transplantation. The rate of continuous complete remission was 40% at two years; 25% at five years, and 13% at seven years. For a subgroup of 19 children who showed complete regression of metastases, the disease-free survival rate is 37% at four years with no relapses up to five years after autologous bone marrow transplantation. Thus, a small group of Stage 4 neuroblastoma patients can be cured with this modality of therapy.

23.2.3 CONCLUSION

The following conclusions may be drawn regarding treatment of advanced neuroblastoma:

1. the most effective first-line chemotherapy should include a large number of non cross-resistant drugs despite the fact that the Goldie-Coldman concept has not demonstrated in practice for this disease;
2. prognosis improves if patients receive early high dose consolidation therapy;
3. autologous and allogenic BMT result in similar relapse rates;
4. purging seems not to be critical at this point;
5. TBI does not produce major advantages for survival at two years;

6. double procedures do not improve survival rates at two years.

23.3 SARCOMAS

23.3.1 SOFT TISSUE SARCOMAS

For non-metastatic rhabdomyosarcoma, treated with current regimens, the cure rates are at least 50%. In contrast, long-term survival decreases to 20% when patients present with metastases, usually to the lung or bone, often with the unfavourable alveolar histology. This is the same despite the use of any of several new protocols including platinum derivates, etoposide and ifosfamide.

Melphalan has found a place in most megatherapy regimens for rhabdomyosarcoma. High dose chemotherapy protocols either use melphalan alone within a dose range of 180–220 mg/m², sometimes preceded by a priming cycle of low dose cyclophosphamide, or are intensified with carboplatin. Other groups have chosen TBI containing regimens in combination with melphalan or the high dose VACA strategy as reported by Miser *et al.* (Miser *et al.* 1987; Yaniv *et al.*, 1990) (Table 23.5). In relapsing or resistant forms, high dose melphalan and ABMT achieved good response rates in phase II studies. However, only short durations of response were experienced, with only a few

Table 23.5 Megatherapy for soft tissue sarcomas

Year	Author	Drug	Dose/day	−8	−7	−6	−5	−4	−3	−2	−1	0
1986	Pinkerton	L-PAM	200 mg/m²								X	
		CYC	300 mg/m²	X								
1985b	Philip	VCR	1.5 mg/m² bolus				X					
			0.5 mg/m² ctn				X	X	X	X	X	
		TBI	2×2 Gy				X	X	X			
		L-PAM	180 mg/m²								X	
1987	Williams	CYC	2.5 g/m²					X		X		X
		TT	1.8–7 mg/kg					X		X		X
1987	Hartmann	1st:VCR	1.5 mg/m²					X				
			0.5 mg/m²					X	X	X	X	X
		BCNU	200 mg/m²						X	X	X	
		L-PAM	180 mg/m²								X	
		2nd: PCB	400 mg/m²				X	X	X	X		
		VP16	300 mg/m²				X	X	X			
		CYC	3 g/m²								X	X
1989	Pinkerton	L-PAM	180 mg/m²									X
		CBDCA	250 mg/m²				X	X	X	X	X	
1990	EBMT-STR	L-PAM	180–220 mg/m²								X	
		L-PAM	60 mg/m²				X	X	X			
		TBI	2×2 Gy							X	X	X
1990	SIOP	CBDCA	adapted*				X	X	X	X	X	
	study	L-PAM	180 mg/m²								X	

L-PAM = melphalan; CYC = cyclophosphamide; CBCDA = carboplatin; TBI = total body irradiation, TT = thiotepa; ENSG = European Neuroblastoma Study Group; EBMT-STR = European Bone Marrow Transplantation – Solid Tumour Registry; 1st/2nd: refers to double graft programmes for first and second graft, CBCDA adapted * = [glomular filtration rate ml/min + (15 × body surface area)] × 20.

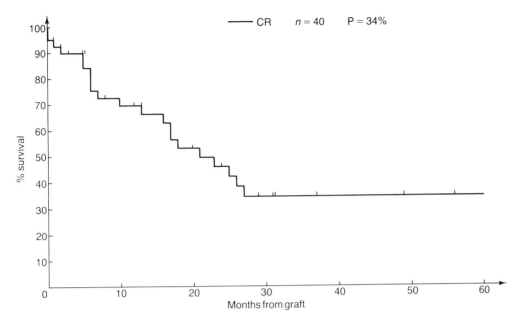

Fig. 23.3 EBMT 90 Soft tissue sarcoma: CR versus PR.

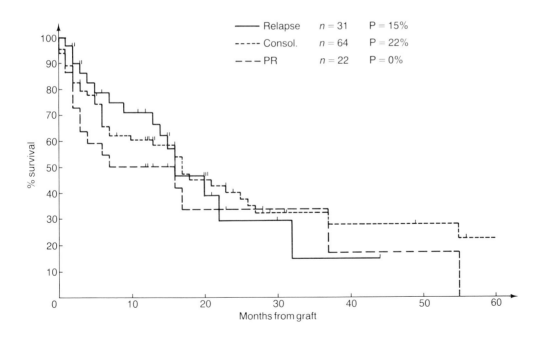

Fig. 23.4 EBMT 90 Soft tissue sarcoma: Relapse, versus consolidation in CR, versus PR.

long-term survivors. In Lyon, after adding TBI, disease-free survival has been observed in six out of nine children with metastatic disease at 20 months. The VACA/TBI regimen produced a response rate of 93%, leaving 45% survivors but observed at a rather short median follow-up of one year.

The last report from the European Solid Tumour registry included 95 patients receiving BMT either as consolidation treatment (as was the case in 64 patients) or after relapse had occurred (31 patients). Twenty-one patients received double grafts. Rhabdomyosarcoma was diagnosed in 46 cases; other soft tissue sarcomas were seen in a further 44. The overall survival rate was 30% at 30 months. As previously experienced in other solid tumours, sensitive relapses still had a second chance of a 20% survival versus none for resistant cases. Metastatic patients receiving BMT in complete remission achieved an overall survival rate of 34% at 40 months (EBMT database, Lyon) (Figs. 23.3 and 23.4).

23.3.2 CONCLUSION

The overall survival rate at three years may be superior in high risk soft tissue sarcoma patients using high dose chemotherapy regimens followed by bone marrow rescue than observed in patients treated only by conventional Stage 4 regimens. The issue of TBI remains controversial. Several studies are currently underway to try to establish the role of high dose chemotherapy in the treatment of this disease.

23.3.3 EWING'S SARCOMAS

Peripheral non-bulky Ewing's sarcoma have a good prognosis. However, in axial and large volume tumours, chemotherapy is usually only temporarily effective. Metastatic disease at diagnosis has a dismal outcome with only few survivors at two years (15%)

and no survivors at four years when conventional therapy is used.

Several reports have evaluated the role of megatherapy for metastatic Ewing's sarcoma. The efficacy of high dose melphalan as a single agent followed by marrow rescue was documented by Cornbleet *et al.* (1981) and Graham-Pole *et al.* (1984). This treatment concept resulted in a very high response rate of more than 75% but, unfortunately with mainly partial responses of short duration. Pilot studies reported by Miser *et al.* (1987) in patients with high risk Ewing's sarcoma suggested that TBI may be of benefit. The National Cancer Institute's experience is the largest single centre report using the VACA massive therapy regimen and TBI. With this regimen, 26 out of 57 selected very bad prognosis patients were at continuous remission at two years follow-up (Miser *et al.*, 1987). In another single centre report from the Institute Gustave-Roussy, Hartmann *et al.* (1990) reported the experience with 32 children treated for metastatic Ewing's sarcoma by high dose chemotherapy followed by autologous BMT. Fourteen patients entered phase II studies of high-dose alkylating agents, displaying a response rate of 61%. High-dose chemotherapy was involved as consolidation treatment in complete remission in 18 patients. Only a slight improvement in disease-free survival duration was achieved in comparison with conventional chemotherapy (Table 23.6).

The European BMT solid tumour registry contains 90 patients, half of them in the paediatric age group (Dini *et al.*, 1989b). Fifty-two patients received megatherapy as consolidation treatment, whereas 38 patients were grafted for relapse, 26 being sensitive and 18 resistant relapses. TBI was given in 40% of patients. At the median follow-up time of 38 months after graft, the overall survival for these 90 patients is 30%. Megatherapy as consolidation treatment resulted in a five-year survival of 46% for

Table 23.6 Megatherapy for Ewing's sarcoma

Year	Author	Drug	Dose/day	−8	−7	−6	−5	−4	−3	−2	−1	0
1985	Philip	VCR	1.5 mg/m² bolus		X							
			0.5 mg/m² ctn		X	X	X	X	X			
		TBI	2×2 Gy					X	X	X		
		L-PAM	180 mg/m²								X	
1987	Miser	VCR	2 mg/m²							X		
		CYC	1.2 g/m²							X	X	
		DXR	35 mg/m²							X	X	
		TBI	4 Gy					X	X			
1990	Hartmann	BCNU	300 mg/m²			X						
		PCB	400 mg/m²			X	X	X	X			
		L-PAM	180 mg/m²							X		
		BCNU	300 mg/m²					X				
		L-PAM	180 mg/m²							X		
		L-PAM	140 mg/m²	X								
		BU	4×1 mg/m²		X	X	X	X				
		CYC	60 mg/m²							X	X	
		BU	4×1 mg/m²				X	X	X	X		
		L-PAM	140 mg/m²								X	
		BU	4×1 mg/m²	X	X	X	X					
		CYC	50 mg/kg					X	X	X	X	
		TT	350 mg/m²						X	X	X	

BCNU = carmustine; PCB = procarbazine; L-PAM = melphalan; BU = busulfan; CYC = cyclosphosphamide; TT = thiotepa; VCR = vincristine; DXR = doxorubicin; ctn = continuous infusion.

patients in first complete remission but was only 13% for patients grafted in first partial remission. Patients grafted for relapse, sensitive or resistant, have all died of disease at the time of reevaluation (resistant relapses: 0% at 13 months; sensitive relapses: 0% at 40 months). The outcome of patients grafted in terms of disease progression was equally fatal (Figs. 23.5 and 23.6).

23.3.4 CONCLUSION

If one considers the results of aggressive conventional chemotherapy which is still the first choice therapy for these patients, the place of high dose chemotherapy and ABMT is still unclear (Hayes *et al.*, 1987; Miser *et al.*, 1987; Dini *et al.*, 1989b; Hartmann *et al.*, 1990; Pinkerton *et al.*, 1989). There is a clear need for randomized studies comparing conventional protocols to megatherapy to define the optimal approach for these patients.

23.4 WILMS' TUMOUR

In Wilms' tumour, an advance in paediatric oncology has been achieved. With conventional therapies, long-term survival in up to 80% patients is reported, so that nowadays more attention can be given to reduction of treatment toxicity and prevention of long-term sequelae. However, 20% are not curable by conventional methods. This population comprises patients with unfavourable histol-

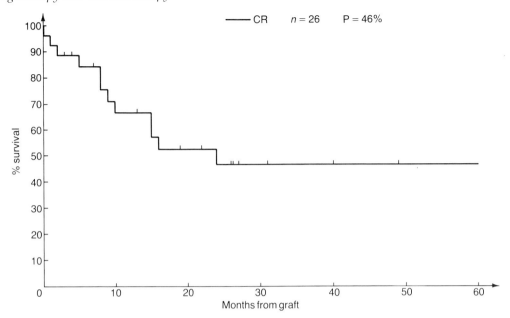

Fig. 23.5   EBMT 90 Ewing's sarcoma: CR.

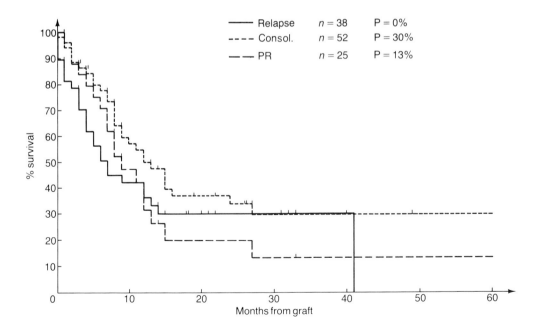

Fig. 23.6   EBMT 90 Ewing's sarcoma: Relapses versus consolidation in CR, versus PR.

Table 23.7 Different high-dose regimens reported to the EBMT-STR registry for Wilms' tumour

Drug	Dose/day	−6	−5	−4	−3	−2	−1	−0
L-PAM	180 mg/m²					X		
VCR	1.5 mg/m²	X						
	0.5 mg/m² ctn	X	X	X	X	X		
L-PAM	180 mg/m²					X		
VCR	1 mg/m²	X						
	0.5 mg/m² ctn	X	X	X	X			
BCNU	300 mg/m²	X						
BU	20 mg/kg	X	X	X	X			
CYC	120 mg/kg	X	X	X	X			
L-PAM	140 mg/m²						X	
IFO	2 g/m²	X	X	X	X	X		
VP16	200 mg/m²	X	X	X	X	X		
L-PAM	180 mg/m²						X	
CDDP	40 mg/m²	X	X	X	X	X		
VM26	200 mg/m²	X	X	X	X	X		
IFO	2 g/m²	X	X	X	X	X		
VP16	200 g/m²	X	X	X	X	X		
DXR	40 mg/m²	X	X					
L-PAM	180 mg/m²						X	
VP16	200 mg/m²	X	X	X	X	X		
CBCDA	350 mg/m²	X	X	X	X	X		
CYC	1.5 g/m²	X	X	X	X			
BCNU	300 mg/m²	X						
VP16	200–300 mg/m²	X	X	X				

Drug	Dose/day	−8	−7	−6	−5	−4	−3	−2	−1	0
BU	150 mg/m²	X	X	X	X					
CYC	2 g/m²							X	X	

L-PAM = melphalan; DXR = doxorubicin; VP16 = etoposide; VM26 = teniposide; CYC = cyclophosphamide; BU = busulfan; VCR = vincristine; BCNU = carmustine; CDDP = *cis*platinum; CBDCA = carboplatinum; IFO = ifosfamide; ctn = continuous infusion.

ogy, those with metastatic disease, and patients resistent to first line treatment.

High-dose melphalan produced complete remissions in six out of six patients with two long-term survivors (Pinkerton *et al.*, 1986). Adding cisplatin and etoposide plus whole lung irradiation or local radiotherapy, produced complete remissions in seven patients in another study (Lanino, 1987). The National Wilms' Tumour Study Group reported on 367 relapses treated by conventional regimens achieving an overall long-term survival of 30%. The following risk factors were described:

unfavourable histology and one of the following criteria:

477

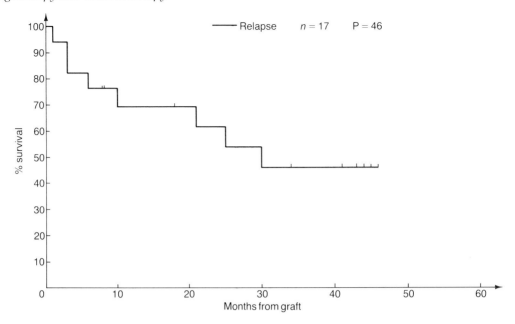

Fig. 23.7 EBMT 90 Wilms' tumour: Relapses.

1. + extrapulmonary relapse;
2. or/+ abdominal relapse after radiation;
3. or/+ > Stage I;
4. or/+ more than a two-drug regimen;
5. or/+ relapse within one year.

The last evaluation of the EBMT Solid Tumour Registry revealed a 34% EFS at 45 months for relapsed Wilms' tumour patients treated by different myeloablative regimens (Table 23.7). Renal and pulmonary complications were observed in many of these heavily pretreated patients, a factor that has to be given special attention in the design of alternative treatment approaches in the future. Nevertheless, a salvage attempt with megatherapy seems to be justified in poor prognosis recurrent Wilms' tumour (Garaventa *et al.*, 1989) (Fig. 23.7).

23.4.1 CONCLUSION

Pilot studies are promising and thus prospec-tive international studies are warranted in selected Wilms' tumour patients who relapse or progress while on conventional therapy.

23.5 BRAIN TUMOURS

Brain tumours constitute almost 25% of childhood cancers. Nearly half are low-grade astrocytic tumours but the majority still present as high-grade tumours with a poor outlook despite conventional therapeutic approaches including surgery and irradiation. The prognosis for children with high-grade astrocytomas, including anaplastic astrocytoma and glioblastoma multiforme, is hardly better than for their adult counterparts.

The Children's Cancer Study Group has reported a pilot study for children with recurrent brain tumours involving thiotepa and etoposide. Pharmacological data had previously indicated excellent penetration of thiotepa into cerebrospinal fluid and brain tissue. (Finlay *et al.*, 1989)

Table 23.8 Megatherapy regimens for paediatric brain tumours

Year	Author	Drug	Dose/Day	−8	−7	−6	−5	−4	−3	−2	−1	0
1987	Johnson	BCNU	350 mg/m²				X	X	X			
1989	Biron	BCNU	800 mg/m²				X					
1989	Finlay	TT	300 mg/m²				X	X	X			
		VP16	500 mg/m²				X	X	X			
1989	ongoing	BU	120 mg/m²	X	X	X	X					
	SFOP	TT	350 mg/m²					X	X	X		
	protocols											
		BCNU	200 mg/m²				X	X				
		CBCDA	250 mg/m²				X	X	X	X	X	
		L-PAM	180 mg/m²								X	
1990	Hartmann	BU	150 mg/m²	X	X	X	X					
		TT	300 mg/m²					X	X	X		

BCNU = carmustine; TT = thiotepa; VP16 = etoposide; BU = busulphan; L-PAM = melphalan; CBCDA = carboplatin; SFOP = Société Française d'Oncologie Pediatrique

Virtually all of the larger series of megatherapy for brain tumours have included high-dose BCNU, but results were still disappointing when used alone (Hildebrand *et al.*, 1980; Takvorian *et al.*, 1983; Phillips *et al.*, 1986; Mbidde *et al.*, 1988; Biron *et al.*, 1989).

The role of high-dose BCNU in combination with whole-brain radiotherapy can be summarized in the following way: short treatment duration; good quality of life but with the median survival still not dramatically changed. Recent approaches using BCNU at

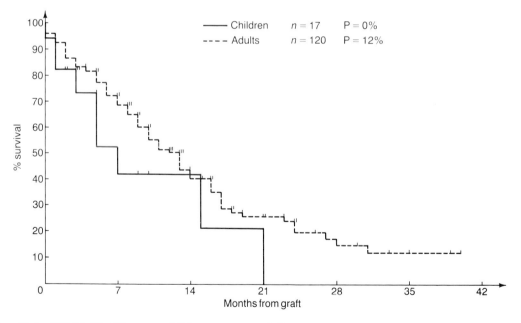

Fig. 23.8 EBMT 90 Gliomas: children versus adults.

high dose followed by ABMT, has so far enrolled only a few children. An improved survival for the whole patient group at 18 months has been observed, but was not apparent at 24 months (Biron *et al.*, 1989a). The EBMT registry was able to analyse 139 patients with gliomas with 17 patients being in the paediatric age group, demonstrating the still poor outcome in these patients (Fig. 23.8).

Approaches recently evaluated for children in ongoing SFOP studies involve etoposide and cyclophosphamide for recurrent medullo-blastoma, peripheral neuroectodermal tu-mours and ependymomas. Megatherapy has included BCNU, carboplatin and melphalan for patients in second complete remission. Other patients have entered a phase II study involving thiotepa and busulphan. Brain stem tumours are known for their almost invariably fatal prognosis. A further SFOP pilot study involves cisplatin and irra-diation followed by megatherapy with VP16 and thiotepa. High dose chemotherapy regimens are summarized in Table 23.8.

23.5.1 CONCLUSION

The outlook of patients is still poor and not dramatically changed by the high dose regi-mens reported. Results of ongoing studies are too preliminary at this time but are of interest since they reflect innovative ap-proaches for this poor prognosis patient group.

23.6 RETINOBLASTOMA

Local control and survival is achieved in 90% of patients by surgery and/or radiotherapy, and chemotherapy is reserved for cases with locally extensive disease, through the *lamina cribrosa* or along the optic nerve with the risk of meningeal involvement, a particular poor prognostic feature, or showing disseminated disease, which most commonly involves, as in neuroblastoma, bones, bone marrow and lymph nodes.

The response rates achieved with conven-tional chemotherapy (White, 1983; Zucker *et al.*, 1982; Pratt *et al.*, 1985; Grabowski, 1987) are the basis for using megatherapy in high risk retinoblastoma following dose escalation theories. Ekert *et al.*, reported as early as 1982 on the possible role of ABMT for retinoblast-oma. Recent treatment guidelines of the SFOP for megatherapy recommend the use of 'CEC' (carboplatin, etoposide and cyclo-phosphamide) (Table 23.9) as treatment regi-men for children with distant metastases in 1st complete remission and for local or dis-tant relapses achieving a 2nd complete or local good partial remission.

23.7 GERM CELL TUMOURS

The prognosis of metastatic non-seminom-atous germ cell tumours (NSGT) has been considerably improved since the introduction of multidrug chemotherapy involving cis-platin, bleomycin, and either etoposide or vinblastine followed by surgery. However,

Table 23.9 Megatherapy proposed for retinoblastoma

Year	Author	Drug	Dose/day	−7	−6	−5	−4	−3	−2	−1	0
1989	Zucker	CYC	1.6 g/m^2	X	X	X	X	X			
	(SFOP protocol)	VP16	350 mg/m^2	X	X	X	X	X			
		CBCDA	250 mg/m^2	X	X	X	X	X			

CYC = cyclophosphamide; CBCDA = carboplatin; VP16 − etoposide

Table 23.10 Megatherapy regimens reported for germ cell tumours

Year	Author	Drugs	Dose/day	−7	−6	−5	−4	−3	−2	−1	0
1989	Pico	CDDP	40 mg/m²	X	X	X	X	X			
		VP16	350 mg/m²	X	X	X	X	X			
		CYC	1600 mg/m²		X	X	X	X			
1989b	Biron	CDDP	40 mg/m²	X	X	X	X	X			
		VP16	200 mg/m²	X	X	X	X	X			
		IFO	3 g/m²		X	X	X	X			
1989	Jansen	CBCDA	500 mg/m²	X		X		X			
		VP16	400 mg/m²	X		X		X			

CDDP = cisplatin; CBCDA = carboplatin; VP16 = etoposide; CYC = cyclophosphamide; IFO = ifosfamide.

relapsing patients failing to achieve a second complete remission on conventional regimens have a dismal prognosis, and need more aggressive treatment potentially involving marrow rescue. Several agents, carboplatin, ifosphamide, cyclophosphamide and etoposide, are known to induce a steep dose-response curve, achieving remissions in patients who are pretreated and refractory to conventional doses of these drugs. To date, the experience with high dose chemotherapy for relapsed NSGCT is still limited to only a few patients in the paediatric age group. Reports on high dose regimens are detailed on Table 23.10. As previously found in lymphomas, only sensitive relapses gained benefit from intensification treatments although most patients (60%) will reach a complete remission. In adults, even in the presence of poor prognostic factors such as large tumour load, elevated beta-HCG and elevated number of metastatic sites, results are encouraging since more than 50% are still alive after 1.5 years in a recent French study (Biron *et al.*, 1989b).

23.7.1 CONCLUSION

The concept of high dose therapy is still based on the Goldie-Coldman hypothesis. In the field of modern paediatric oncology two conclusions are clear:

(a) The concept of consolidation at the time of minimal residual disease is still appropriate. However, we are not able yet to overcome drug resistance in most cases.
(b) The concept of alternating non cross resistant regimens may have been counterproductive in the field of high dose therapy. In multidrug regimens the dose for each effective drug is often reduced and frequently more than two drug regimens are no better than one drug. Future directions will involve either double graft programmes with a regimen using each effective drug at maximum dosage or single agent high dose regimens with or without ABMT. The concept of maximum tolerated dose of each single agent should be emphasized in new strategies.

Autologous bone marrow transplantation has been used up to now as a rescue for haematological toxicities. Immunological effects against tumour cells have been demonstrated in leukaemia and lymphoma (Santos, 1990; Jones, 1990) and should still be studied in solid tumours. Preliminary results of our group and of the Memorial Sloan Kettering group for neuroblastoma suggest ways to try to transform rescue to therapy. This is probably the future for ABMT. Growth factors will not replace ABMT in all cases but may decrease toxicity and the cost of ABMT allowing new directions and innovative therapies to be developed.

23.8 THE ROLE OF IMMUNOTHERAPY

23.8.1 INTRODUCTION

Cytokines are biological proteins which permit the transmission of signals from one cell to another. These proteins are secreted by groups of specialized cells and are fixed on specific receptors on the surface of responding cells. However, since receptors may be widely distributed, and since the activation of cells usually permits the release of other cytokines and a succession of reactions, cytokines have pleiotropic effects. Cloning of the genes encoding for these cytokines and their large scale production by genetic recombination techniques have allowed a better understanding of their biological characteristics and their use in therapy (Favrot *et al.*, 1990c).

23.8.2 DEVELOPMENT OF CONCEPTS

The immune system plays a role in proliferation and differentiation events in various tissues. Any disregulation of the latter may allow the emergence of a cancer. On the other hand, immune modulation can be stimulated and regulated using the cytokines as therapeutic tools.

Basic insights into the possible role of immunological phenomena have been gained by clinical observations. Allogenic bone marrow transplantation has been able to cure patients who would otherwise have had no chance and there are three major aspects that contribute to this advance:

(1) myeloablative chemotherapy (Armitage and Gale, 1989; Cheson *et al.*, 1989; Santos, 1990);
(2) the graft versus leukaemia (or tumour) effect (Butturini *et al.*, 1987; Jones, 1990);

(3) the transfer of donor effector mechanisms into the tumour-bearing recipient (Slavin *et al.*, 1988).

The most convincing observation advocating immunotherapy was the result in allogeneic BMT for AML in first remission, demonstrating a 18% failure rate for matched siblings versus a relatively poor outcome for identical twins with 59% relapse rate (Champlin and Gale, 1987; Gale *et al.*, 1989). The role of GVHD is well known and it has been demonstrated that the incidence of leukaemia relapses is inversely correlated to GVHD (Butturini *et al.*, 1987). Several studies have been carried out by Slavin and co-workers trying to simulate graft versus leukaemia effect without occurrence of GVHD, first by a series of mouse models, and then transferring the work into clinical phase II studies. It does not seem important to eliminate the last tumour cell, which is virtually impossible, but rather to activate host immune defence mechanisms to control minimal residual disease (Slavin *et al.*, 1988). A next step from the Jerusalem group was to question the possible role of T-cells within this network. Again, a clinical observation was helpful. The incidence of relapse in CML with T-cell depleted bone marrow is higher than in non T-cell depleted allogeneic BMT without occurrence of GVHD, giving rise to the conclusion that T-cell depletion impairs GVL-like effects (Goldman *et al.*, 1988). Further studies from animal models to clinical phase II trials went on to ask the question if T-donor cells can be given safely without causing severe GVHD. Finally, T donor lymphocytes following T-depleted BMT were given to the hosts successfully (Slavin *et al.*, 1988). First preliminary results and observations seem to support the concept that immunotherapy by allogeneic cells is an approach that really can cure patients (Slavin, 1990, personal communication). A further major task is to ask if such anti-leukaemic effects can be stimulated in the autologous or syngeneic situation. Basically it appears that GVL does not rely directly on an allogeneic mediated mechanism and that it may be an effect mediated by NK or IL-2 activated cells. Therefore the most compelling goals of recent phase I and II trials are to learn how to administer IL-2 tolerably and to give it at a time where it can work with maximum efficacy (Favrot *et al.*, 1988; 1990a–d).

For the moment, the following conclusions can be drawn:

(1) one should administer IL-2 (alone or in combinations with other regulators of the cytokine network) at the time of minimal residual disease;
(2) elimination of the last tumour cell is neither feasible nor necessary;
(3) minimal residual disease can be controlled by active immune mechanisms;
(4) tumour cell 'dormancy' will finally lead to tumour cell death.

23.8.3 CLINICAL STUDIES IN NEUROBLASTOMA

Spontaneous remissions of neuroblastoma in children below one year of age as well as the better prognosis of infants with advanced metastatic disease, the regression of neuroblast 'embryonal rests' in the newborn and the spontaneous maturation in some Stage II patients, suggested an important role for the immune system. In the past, despite *in vitro* evidence (Sidell, 1982; Thiele, 1985), attempts to achieve tumour maturation (such as with vitamin B_{12} or retinoic acid) have been singularly unsuccessful. A double-blind study is being conducted by the ENSG evaluating the role of retinoic acid for children who achieved complete or good partial remission after intensive therapy (Lie, 1990).

The potential beneficial effect of stimulation of the antitumour defence, therefore, was the rationale for immunotherapy trials in neuroblastoma. To date, very little is known

about the possible role of immunotherapy in other solid tumours in childhood (Nasr, 1989).

23.8.4 INTERLEUKIN

One therapeutic approach is the generation of cytotoxic effector cells, capable of lysing a wide variety of tumour cells, by culturing human peripheral blood mononuclear cells (PBMC) with recombinant interleukin-2 (IL-2) (Favrot *et al.*, 1990c; Lotzova, 1987). The induction of these potent effector cells by IL-2 has been termed the lymphokine activated killer cell (LAK) phenomenon. Since cells mediating LAK activity possess a broad range of cytotoxic activity against malignant but not normal cells, the therapeutic potential for these activated killer cells has evoked considerable enthusiasm (Rosenberg *et al.*, 1985; 1987; Lotze *et al.*, 1985). For example, IL-2 has been shown to induce partial or complete response in end stage disease, in particular in metastatic renal cell carcinoma (Sosman *et al.*, 1988; Philip *et al.*, 1989) or melanoma (Rosenberg *et al.*, 1987) resistant to conventional therapy. The lack of major or non reversible toxicity of this therapy and its potential value for eradication of residual neuroblastoma cells has led to prospective studies. These models of phase II studies were the rationale to start the evaluation of the efficacy of continuous infusion of IL-2 with LAK cells in advanced Stage IV neuroblastoma in Lyon (Favrot *et al.*, 1989d; 1990b; 1990c). Fourteen out of 14 patients progressed. This result was explained by the inability of end stage neuroblastoma to produce NK cells under IL-2 stimulation and also because of the excess of T8 suppressor cell proliferation. Further experimental results suggested that the optimal timing for IL-2 immunotherapy could be during the first months following high-dose chemotherapy and BMT (Favrot *et al.*, 1989e; 1990d). Patients have profound T-cell defects with undetectable IL-2 secretion (Favrot *et al.*,

1988) during the first months after BMT. Nevertheless, these T-cells respond to exogenous IL-2 *in vitro* suggesting that at this time there may be functional natural killer (NK) cells with potential LAK activity after IL-2 stimulation (Favrot *et al.*, 1990e). These observations have been the basis for the introduction of IL-2 immunotherapy in children with advanced neuroblastoma after autologous BMT. Thus, a second pilot study was set up in Lyon to enter patients two months after autologous ABMT. This demonstrated that, in contrast to the former patient group, there was an excess of NK cells at this time as well as a deficit in T8 suppressor cells. Two out of the four initial patients did respond to IL-2 therapy and their NK cells were shown to produce regression of neuroblastoma. A new prospective study post autologous marrow transplantation is currently under evaluation in the LMCE group in France (Michon *et al.*, 1990).

23.8.5 ANTI GD$_2$

Monoclonal antibodies have the ability to target selectively to occult metastases. The availability of radioisotopes and the development of conjugation chemistry has greatly expanded the potentials of these antibodies. The ganglioside GD$_2$ is an antigen expressed in many human tumours and also detectable in the serum of neuroblastoma patients. It has been demonstrated to be an ideal tumour antigen to target neuroblastoma. The murine IgG3 antibody 3F8 to ganglioside GD2 was selected for *in vivo* studies to evaluate both its diagnostic and therapeutic potentials. Firstly, using a radio-labelled antibody as transport vehicle for targeted radiotherapy (Cheung *et al.*, 1988) or secondly, as a direct cytotoxin in the absence of a radioisotope, the mechanism of action being dependant on complement activation properties and antibody-dependent cell-mediated tumour cytotoxicity (ADCC).

In a phase I study, the antibody 3F8 was administered intravenously to 17 patients with metastatic GD$_2$ positive neuroblastoma or malignant melanoma with dose escalations up to 100 mg/m^2 (Cheung *et al.*, 1987). Observed toxicities included pain, hypertension, urticaria and complement depletion but were controllable with symptomatic therapy. Anti tumour responses ranging from complete clinical remissions to mixed responses have been reported (Cheung *et al.*, 1987). Equivalent pilot studies are now carried out in Lyon in heavily pretreated, relapsed neuroblastoma patients. The results on six patients tested so far are preliminary, but do not seem to further support this treatment approach. Further studies are underway in other European and French units.

23.8.6 CONCLUSION

Two major approaches to increase the chance of cure have been reviewed in this chapter. Firstly, the use of dose intensity with megatherapy regimens, which are still the best understood concept in overcoming resistant neoplastic disease. Secondly, enrolling the host's immune system in the fight against the residual tumour. Much is still unknown about the normal structure and function of immunological control mechanisms such as self-recognition, tolerance (Nossal, 1989; Coutinho and Bandiera, 1989; Gopas *et al.*, 1989) and concomitant immunity as well as the relationship between the (non) expression of MHC-I antigens by cancer cells and the host response (Cayeux *et al.*, 1989a; 1989b; Favrot *et al.*, 1988; 1989d; 1990a; Gilewski and Colomb, 1990; Blaise *et al.*, 1990; Gottlieb *et al.*, 1989; Coutinho, 1989; Fidler and Radinsky, 1990). Several studies have been initiated in this field. It is our opinion that these two different approaches will, in the future, more frequently be used in conjunction with or without bone marrow transplantation and will provide further innovative therapies in paediatric oncology.

REFERENCES

Appelbaum, F.R. and Buckner, C.D. (1986) Overview of the clinical relevance of autologous bone marrow transplantation. *Clin. Haematol.*, **1**, 1–10.

Armitage, J.O. and Gale, R.P. (1989) Bone marrow autotransplantation. *Am. J. Med.*, **86**, 203–6.

Armitage, J.O. (1989) Bone marrow transplantation in the treatment of patients with lymphoma. *Blood*, **73**, 1749–58.

Armitage, J.O. and Bierman, P.J. (1989) Is there an optimum conditioning regimen for patients with lymphoma undergoing autologous bone marrow transplantation? in ABMT. Proceedings of the 4th international symposium (eds K.A. Dicke, G. Spitzer, S. Jagannath, M.J. Evinger-Hodges) Houston, pp. 299–303.

Athanasou, N.A., Quinn, J., Brenner, M.K. *et al.* (1990) Origin of marrow stromal cells and haemopoietic chimaerism following bone marrow transplantation determined by *in situ* hybridisation. *Br. J. Cancer*, **61**, 385–9.

Atkins, M.B. (1986) Phase I evaluation of recombinant IL-2 in patients with advanced malignant disease. *J. Clin. Oncol.*, **4**, 1380–91.

August, C.S., Serota, F.T., Kich, P.A. *et al.* (1984) Treatment of advanced neuroblastoma with supralethal chemotherapy, radiation and allogenic or autologous marrow reconstitution. *J. Clin. Oncol.*, **2**, 609–16.

August, C.S. and Auble, B. (1989) Autologous bone marrow transplantation for advanced neuroblastoma at the Children's Hospital of Philadelphia: an update, in ABMT. Proceedings of the fourth international symposium (eds K.A. Dicke, G. Spitzer, S. Jagannath, M.J. Evinger-Hodges) Houston, pp. 567–73.

Bast, R.C., De Fabrities, P., Lipton, J. *et al.* (1985) Elimination of malignant clonogenic cells from human bone marrow using multiple monoclonal antibodies and complement. *Cancer Res.*, **45**, 499–502.

Beck, D., Maritaz, O., Gross, N. *et al.* (1988) Immunocytochemical detection of neuroblastoma cells infiltrating clinical bone marrow samples. *Eur. J. Pediatr.*, **147**, 609–12.

Berenson, R.J., Bensinger, W.I., Kalamasz, D. *et al.* (1986) Elimination of daudi lymphoblasts from human bone marrow using avidin-biotin immunoadsorption. *Blood*, **67**, 509–11.

Biron, P., Mornex, F., Colombat, P. *et al.* (1989a) High dose BCNU and ABMT, surgery and radiotherapy in gliomas. in ABMT. Proceedings of the 4th international symposium on autologous bone marrow transplantation. (eds K.A. Dicke, G. Spitzer, S. Jagannath, M.J. Evinger-Hodges) Houston, pp. 437–47.

Biron, P., Brunat-Mentigny, M., Bayle, J.Y. *et al.* (1989b) Centre Léon Bérard, experience of massive chemotherapy in non seminomatous germ cell tumors. Analysis of first regimens in progressive disease and VP16-IPM-CDDP (VIC) in sensitive patients, in ABMT. Proceedings of the 4th international symposium on autologous bone marrow transplantation. (eds K.A. Dicke, G. Spitzer, S. Jagannath, M.J. Evinger-Hodges) Houston, pp. 477–86.

Blaise, D., Olive, D., Stoppa, A.M. *et al.* (1990) Hematologic and immunologic effects of the systemic administration of recombinant interleukin-2 after autologous bone marrow transplantation. American Society of Hematology. *Blood*, **76**, 1092–7.

Borden, E.C. and Sondel, P.M. (1990) Lymphokines and cytokines as cancer treatment. Immunotherapy realized. *Cancer*, **65**, 800–14.

Bouffet, E., Philip, I., Chauvin, F. *et al.* (1990a) Analysis of parameters influencing recovery from aplasia following autologous bone marrow transplantation (ABMT). *Med. Ped. Oncol.*, **18**, 386.

Bouffet, E., Favrot, M., Biron, P. *et al.* (1990b) Place de la chimiothérapie massive dans le traitement des lymphomes malins non Hodgkiniens. *Bull. Cancer*, **77**, 159–67.

Bourhis, J., De Vatnaire, F., Wilson, G.D. *et al.* (1991) Combined analysis of DNA ploidy index and N-myc genomic content in neuroblastoma, *Cancer Res.*, **51**, 33–6.

Bowman, F., Chastagner, P., Palau, R. *et al.* (1990a) Histological and immunohistochemical detection of bone marrow involvement by neuroblastoma. *Med. Ped. Oncol.*, **18**, 23.

Bowman, L.C., Castelberry, R.P., Altshuler, G. *et al.* (1990b) Therapy based on DNA index (DI) for infants with unresectable and disseminated neuroblastoma (NB): preliminary results of the pediatric oncology group 'better risk' study *Med. Ped. Oncol.*, **18**, 364.

Brodeur, G.M., Hayes, F.A., Green, A.A. *et al.* (1987) Consistent N-*Myc* copy number in simultaneous or consecutive neuroblastoma samples from sixty individual patients. *Cancer Res.*, **47**, 4248–53.

Brodeur, G.M., Seeger, R.C., Barret, A. *et al.* (1988) International criteria for diagnosis, staging and response to treatment in patients with neuroblastoma. *J. Clin. Oncol.*, **6**, 1874–81.

Brodeur, G.M. and Fong, C.T. (1989) Molecular biology and genetics of human neuroblastoma. *Cancer Genet. Cytogenet.*, **41**, 153–74.

Butturini, A., Bortin, M.M., Gale, R.P. *et al.* (1987) Graft-vs-leukaemia following bone marrow transplantation. *Bone Marrow Transplantation*, **2**, 233–42.

Butturini, A. and Gale, R.P. (1989) How can we cure leukemia? *Br. J. Haematol.*, **72**, 479–85.

Cabanillas, F., Jagannath, S. and Philip, T. (1990) Management of recurrent or refractory disease. *Non Hodgkin's Lymphomas*, (ed. I. Magrath) Edward Arnold, London, pp. 359–71.

Canon, J.L., Humblet, Y., Symann, M. *et al.* (1990) Resistance to cisplatin: how to deal with the problem? *Eur. J. Cancer*, **26**, 1–3.

Carlsen, N.L.T., Christensen, I.J., Schroeder, H. *et al.* (1986) Prognostic factors in neuroblastomas treated in Denmark from 1943 to 1980. A statistical estimate of prognosis based on 253 cases. *Cancer*, **58**, 2726–35.

Cayeux, S., Meuer, S. Pezutto, A. *et al.* (1989a) Allogeneic mixed lymphocyte reactions during a second round of ontogeny, normal accessory cells did not restore defective Interleukin-2 (IL-2) synthesis in T cells but induced responsiveness to exogeneous IL-2. *Blood*, **74**, 2278–84.

Cayeux, S., Meuer, S., Pezutto, A. *et al.* (1989b) T cell oncogeny after autologous bone marrow transplantation: failure to synthesize interleukin-2 (IL-2) and lack of CD2- and CD3-mediated proliferation by both CD4+ and CD8+ cells even in the presence of exogeneous IL-2. *Blood*, **74**, 2270–7.

Chabner, B.A. and Fojo, A. (1989) Multidrug resistance, P-glycoprotein and its allies – the elusive focus. *J. Nat. Cancer Inst.*, **81**, 910–3.

Champlin, R.E. and Gale, R.P. (1987) Acute myelogenous leukemia: Recent advances. *Blood*, **69**, 1551–62.

Cheson, B.D., Lacernax, L., Leyland-Jones, B. *et al.* (1989) Autologous bone marrow transplantation. *Ann. Int. Med.*, **110**, 51–65.

Cheung, H.K.V., Lazarus, H., Miraldi, F.D. *et al.* (1987) Ganglioside GD2 specific monoclonal antibody 3F8: a phase I study in patients with neuroblastoma and malignant melanoma. *J. Clin. Oncol.*, **5**, 1430–40.

Cheung, N.K. and Miraldi, F.D. (1988) Iodine 131 labelled G_{D2} monoclonal antibody in the diagnosis and therapy of human neuroblastoma, in *Advances in Neuroblastoma Research.* 2nd edn pp. 595–604.

Christiansen, H. and Lampert, F. (1988) Tumour karyotype discriminates between good and bad prognostic outcome in neuroblastoma. *Br. J. Cancer*, **57**, 121–6.

Colombat, P., Biron, P., Binet, C. *et al.* (1989) High dose chemotherapy with autologous bone marrow transplantation in low grade non-Hodgkin's lymphomas, in ABMT. Proceedings of the fourth international symposium (eds K.A. Dicke, G. Spitzer, S. Jagannath, M.J. Evinger-Hodges) Houston, pp. 317–25.

Combaret, V., Favrot, M.C., Kremens, B. *et al.* (1987) Eliminating Burkitt's cells from bone marrow with an immunomagnetic purging procedure, in ABMT. 3rd International Conference on Autologous Bone Marrow Transplantation (eds K. Dicke, G. Spitzer and S. Jagannath) Houston, pp. 443–8.

Combaret, V., Favrot, M.C., Chauvin, F. *et al.* (1989a) Immunomagnetic depletion of malignant cells from autologous bone marrow graft: from experimental models to clinical trials. *J. Immunomagnetics*, **16**, 125–36.

Combaret, V., Favrot, M.C., Kremens, B. *et al.* (1989b) Immunological detection of neuroblastoma cells in bone marrow harvested for autologous transplantation. *Br. J. Cancer*, **59**, 844–7.

Combaret, V., Wang, Q., Favrot, M.C. *et al.* (1989c) Clinical value of n-*myc* oncogene amplification in 52 patients with neuroblastoma included in recent therapeutic protocols. *Eur. J. Cancer Clin. Oncol.*, **24**, 1607–12.

Combaret, V., Viehl, P., Bouffet, E. *et al.* (1990) Immunological detection of minimal residual disease in the bone marrow of neuroblastoma patients: interest and limit for therapeutic strategies. *Med. Ped. Oncol.*, **18**, 369.

Cornbleet, M., Corringham, R., Prentice H. *et al.* (1981) Treatment of Ewing sarcoma with high dose melphalan and autologous bone marrow transplantation. *Cancer Treat. Rep.*, **63**, 241–4.

Couanet, D. and Geoffray, A. (1988) Etude en imagerie par résonance magnétique (IRM) des métastases ostéomédullaires des neuroblastomes. *Bull. Cancer*, **75**, 91–6.

Coutinho, A. and Bandeira, A. (1989) Tolerize one, tolerize them all, tolerance is self-assertion. *Immunol. Today*, **10**, 264–6.

Coutinho, A. (1989) Beyond clonal selection and network. *Immunol. Rev.*, **110**, 63–87.

Daniel, C.P. and Dexter, T.M. (1989) The role of growth factors in haematopoietic development, clinical and biological implications. *Cancer and Metastasis Reviews*, **8**, 253–62.

De Kraker, J., Hartmann, O., Voûte, P.A. *et al.* (1982) The effect of high dose melphalan with autologous bone marrow transplantation in neuroblastoma patients with advanced disease. *Pediatr. Oncol.*, **570**, 165–70.

De Vita, V. (1986) Dose response is alive and well. *J. Clin. Oncol.*, **4**, 1157.

De Witte, T., Hoogenhout, J., de Pauw, B. *et al.* (1986) Depletion of donor lymphocytes by counterflow centrifugation successfully prevents acute graft-versus-host disease in matched allogeneic marrow transplantation. *Blood*, **67**, 1302–6.

Deacon, J.M., Wilson, P.A., Peckham, M.J. *et al.* (1985) The radiobiology of human neuroblastoma. *Radioth. Oncol.*, **3**, 201–9.

Dexter, T.M. and White, H. (1990) Growth without infiltration. *Nature*, **344**, 380–1.

Dini, G., Garaventa, A., Lanino, E. *et al.* (1990) Pattern of failure in patients receiving unpurged autologous bone marrow transplantation for neuroblastoma, in *Autologous Bone Marrow Transplantation, 5th International Conference* (eds. K. Dickie, J. Armitage and M.J. Dickie-Evinger), Omaha, pp. 611–20.

Dini, G., Philip, T., Hartmann, O. *et al.* (1989a) on behalf of the EBMT Group. Bone marrow transplantation for neuroblastoma: a review of 513 cases, in Bone Marrow Transplantation in children and adults. (eds C. Bernasconi and G.R. Burgio) Pavia, Italy, pp. 42–6.

Dini, G., Hartmann, O., Pinkerton, R. *et al.*

(1989b) Autologous bone marrow transplantation in Ewing's sarcoma: an analysis of phase II studies from the European Bone Marrow Transplantation Group, in ABMT. Proceedings of the fourth international symposium. (eds K.A. Dicke, G. Spitzer, S. Jagannath, M.J. Evinger-Hodges) Houston, pp. 593–9.

Ekert, H., Ellis, W.M., Waters, K.D. *et al.* (1982) Autologous bone marrow rescue in the treatment of advanced tumors of childhood. *Cancer*, **49**, 603.

Espevik, T., Waage, A., Faxvaag, A. *et al.* (1990) Regulation of interleukin-2 and interleukin-6 production from T-cells: involvement of interleukin-1 beta and transforming growth factor beta. *Cell Immunol.*, **126**, 47–56.

Evans, A.E., D'Angio, G.J., Propert, K. *et al.* (1987) Prognostic factors in neuroblastoma. *Cancer*, **59**, 1853–9.

Favrot, M.C., Philip, I., Philip, T. *et al.* (1986) Bone marrow purging procedure in Burkitt lymphoma with monoclonal antibodies and complement. Quantification by a liquid cell culture monitoring system. *Br. J. Cancer*, **64**, 161–4.

Favrot, M.C., Philip, I., Combaret, V. *et al.* (1987) Experimental evaluation of an immunomagnetic bone marrow purging procedure using a Burkitt lymphoma model. *Bone Marrow Transplantation*, **2**, 59–66.

Favrot, M.C., Philip, T., Biron, P. *et al.* (1988) *In vivo* therapy by CD8 monoclonal antibody for delays to hematological recovery after autologous bone marrow transplantation, in *Lymphocyte Activation and Differentiation*. Walter de Gruyter, Berlin, pp. 855–8.

Favrot, M.C. and Philip, T. (1989a) Bone marrow purging, in *New Directions in Cancer Treatment*, (ed. I. Magrath) UICC, Berlin, pp. 343–57.

Favrot, M.C., Philip, I. Pavone, E. *et al.* (1989b) *Ex vivo* BM purging is efficient in Burkitt Lymphoma but high dose chemotherapy is ineffective in patients with active disease in the bone marrow, in *Autologous Bone Marrow Transplantation* Proceedings of the 4th International Symposium (eds K.A. Dicke, G. Spitzer, S. Jagannath, M.J. Evinger-Hodges) Houston, pp. 331–8.

Favrot, M.C., Combaret, V., Coze, C. *et al.* (1989c) Is bone marrow purging efficient and necessary for ABMT in solid tumors? in *Bone Marrow*

Transplantation: Current Controversies, Alan R. Liss, New York, pp. 289–99.

Favrot, M.C., Floret, D., Michon, J. *et al.* (1989d) Phase II study of adoptive immunotherapy with continuous infusion of Interleukin 2 in children with advanced neuroblastoma. A report of 11 cases. *Cancer Treat. Rev.*, **16** (suppl. A), 129–42.

Favrot, M.C., Floret, D., Negrier, S. *et al.* (1989e) Systemic IL2 therapy in children with progressive neuroblastoma after high dose chemotherapy and bone marrow transplantation. *Bone Marrow Transplantation*, **4**, 499–503.

Favrot, M.C., Coze, C., Combaret, V. *et al.* (1990a) Lymphokine activated killer cell expansion for clinical trials of adoptive immunotherapy with IL2. Optimization of the culture technique. *Molecular Biotherapy*, **2**, 32–7.

Favrot, M.C., Michon, J., Bouffet, E. *et al.* (1990b) rIL2 immunotherapy for 19 children with advanced metastatic neuroblastoma, in *Cytokines in Hemopoiesis, Oncology and AIDS*, (eds. Freund *et al.*), Springer Verlag, Berlin, pp. 683–90.

Favrot, M.C., Combaret, V., Bouffet, E. *et al.* (1990c) Stimulation of the immune system for the therapy of advanced stage neuroblastoma, in *Experimental Hematology Today* (ed. N.C. Gorin), Springer Verlag, New York, pp. 88–92.

Favrot, M.C., Michon, J., Floret, D. *et al.* (1990d) IL 2 immunotherapy in children with neuroblastoma after high dose chemotherapy and autologous bone marrow transplantation. *Ped. Hemat. Oncol.*, **7**, 275–84.

Favrot, M.C., Philip, T., Combaret, V. *et al.* (1990e) Effect of CD8 *in vivo* therapy on delay to engraftment after an autologous bone marrow transplantation. *Bone Marrow Transplantation*, **5**, 33–8.

Fidler, I.J. and Radinsky, R. (1990) Genetic control of cancer metastasis. *J. Natl. Cancer Inst.*, **82**, 166–8.

Filipovich, A.H., Vallera, D.A., Voule, R.J. *et al.* (1984) *Ex vivo* treatment of donor bone marrow with anti-T cell immunotoxins for prevention of graft-versus-host disease. *Lancet*, **1**, 469–72.

Finlay, J., August, C., Packer, R. *et al.* (1989) High dose chemotherapy with autologous bone marrow rescue in children with recurrent brain tumors, in ABMT. Proceedings of the fourth international symposium (eds K.A. Dicke, G.

Spitzer, S. Jagannath, M.J. Evinger-Hodges) Houston, pp. 449–55.

Frei, E., Evinger-Hodges, M.J., Canellos, G.P. (1980) Dose: a critical factor in cancer chemotherapy. *Am. J. Med.*, **69**, 585–94.

Frei, E., Teicher, B.A., Holden, S.A. *et al.* (1988) Preclinical studies and clinical correlation of the effect of alkylating dose. *Cancer Res.*, **48**, 4717–23.

Gale, R.P., Horowitz, M.M., Biggs, J.C. *et al.* (1989) Transplant or chemotherapy in acute myelogenous leukemia. For the Advisory Committee of the International Bone Marrow Transplant Registry *Lancet*, **1**, 119–22.

Garaventa, A., Bernard, J.L., Badell, I. *et al.* (1989) High-dose chemotherapy with autologous bone marrow transplantation in Wilms' tumor: a survey of the European Bone Marrow Transplantation Group, in ABMT. Proceedings of the fourth international symposium. (eds K.A. Dicke, G. Spitzer, S. Jagannath, M.J. Evinger-Hodges) Houston, pp. 601–7.

Gehan, E. (1984) Dose response relationship in clinical oncology. *Cancer*, **54**, 1204–7.

Gilewski, T.A. and Colomb, H.M. (1990) Design of combination biotherapy studies: future goals and challenges. *Semin. Oncol.*, **17**, 3–10.

Goldie, J.H. and Coldman, A. (1979) A mathematical model for relating the drug sensitivity of tumors to their spontaneous mutation rate. *Cancer Treat. Rep.*, **63**, 1727–9.

Goldie, J.H. and Coldman, A. (1983) Quantitative model for multiple levels of drug resistance in clinical tumors *Cancer Treat. Rep.*, **67**, 923–31.

Goldie, J.H. and Coldman, A. (1985) Genetic instability in the development of drug resistance. *Semin. Oncol.*, **13**, 222–30.

Goldman, J.M., Gale, R.P., Horowitz, M.M. *et al.* (1988) Bone Marrow Transplantation for chronic myelogenous leukemia in chronic phase: Increased risk or relapse associated with T-cell depletion. *Ann. Intern. Med.*, **108**, 806–14.

Goldstein, L.J., Fojo, A.T., Veda, K. *et al.* (1990) Expression of the multidrug resistance, MDR1, gene in neuroblastomas. *J. Clin. Oncol.*, **8**, 128–36.

Gopas, J., Rager-Zisman, B.R., Bar-Eli, M. *et al.* (1989) The relationship between MHC antigen expression and metastasis. *Advances in Cancer Research*, **53**, 89–115.

Gorin, N.C., Douay, L., Laporte, J.P. *et al.* (1986)

Autologous bone marrow transplantation using marrow incubated with Asta-Z 7557 in adult acute leukemia. *Blood*, **67**, 1367–70.

Gottlieb, D.J., Prentice, H.G., Heslop, H.E. *et al.* (1989) Effects of recombinant Interleukin-2 administration on cytotoxic function following high-dose chemo-radiotherapy for hematological malignancy. *Blood*, **74**, 2335–42.

Grabowski, E.F. and Abramson, D.H. (1987) Intraocular and extraocular retinoblastoma. *Hematol. Oncol. Clin. N. Amer.*, **1**, 721–35.

Graham, G.J., Wright, E.J., Hewick, R. *et al.* (1990) Identification and characterisation of inhibitors of haemapoietic stem cell proliferation. *Nature*, **344**, 442–4.

Graham-Pole, J., Lazarus, H.M., Herzig, R.H. *et al.* (1984) High dose melphalan for the treatment of children with refractory neuroblastoma and Ewing's sarcoma. *Am. J. Pediatr. Hematol. Oncol.*, **6**, 17–26.

Graham-Pole, J., Gee, A.P., Gross, S. *et al.* (1988) Bone marrow transplantation (BMT) for advanced neuroblastoma (NBL). A multicenter POG pilot study, in *Advances in Neuroblastoma Research 2*, (eds A. Evans, G.L. D'Angio, R.C. Seeger), 215–33.

Graham-Pole, J. (1989) The role of marrow autografting in neuroblastoma, *Bone Marrow Transplantation*, **4**, 3–7.

Hann, H.L., Evans, A.E., Siegel, S.E. *et al.* (1985) Prognostic Importance of serum ferritin in patients with stages III and IV neuroblastoma: The Children's Cancer Study Group Experience. *Cancer Res.*, **45**, 2843–8.

Hartmann, O., Kalifa, C., Beaujean, F. *et al.* (1985) Treatment of advanced neuroblastoma with two consecutive high-dose chemotherapy regimens and ABMT, in *Advances in Neuroblastoma Research*, (eds A.E. Evans, G.L. D'Angio, R.C. Seeger), Alan R. Liss, New York, 565–8.

Hartmann, O., Benhamou, E., Beaujean, F. *et al.* (1986) High dose busulfan and cyclophosphamide with autologous bone marrow transplantation support in advanced malignancies in children: A phase II study. *J. Clin. Oncol.*, **4**, 1804–10.

Hartmann, O., Benhamou, E., Beaujean, F. *et al.* (1987) Repeated high-dose chemotherapy followed by purged autologous bone marrow transplantation as consolidation therapy in metastatic neuroblastoma. *J. Clin. Oncol.*, **5**, 1205–11.

Hartmann, O., Oberlin, O., Beaujean, F. *et al.* (1990) Place de la chimiothérapie à hautes doses suivie d'autogreffe médullaire dans le traitement des sarcomes d'Ewing métastatiques de l'enfant. *Bull. Cancer*, **77**, 181–7.

Hayashi, Y., Kanda, N., Inaba, T. *et al.* (1989) Cytogenetic findings and prognosis in neuroblastoma with emphasis on marker chromosome 1. *Cancer*, **63**, 126–32.

Hayes, F.A., Thompson, E.I., Parvey, L. *et al.* (1987) Metastatic Ewing's sarcoma: remission induction and survival. *J. Clin. Oncol.*, **5**, 1199–204.

Hervé, P., Cahn, J.Y., Plouvier, E. *et al.* (1984) Autologous bone marrow transplantation for acute leukemia using transplants chemopurified with metabolites of oxazaphosphorine (ASTA Z 7557, INN mafosfamide). First clinical results. *New Drugs*, **2**, 245–50.

Hildebrand, J., Badjou, R., Collard-Ronge, E. (1980) Treatment of brain gliomas with high dose of CCNU and autologous bone marrow transplantation. *Biomedicine*, **32**, 71–4.

Ho, A.D., Haas, R., Wulf, G. *et al.* (1990) Activation of lymphocytes induced by recombinant human granulocyte-macrophage-colony-stimulating factor in patients with malignant lymphoma. *Blood*, **75**, 203–12.

Imashuku, S., Yamanaka, H., Morioka, Y. *et al.* (1988) Serum ferritin in stage IV neuroblastoma. *Am. J. Pediatr. Hematol. Oncol.*, **10**, 39–41.

Ivy, S.P., Ozols, R.F., Cowan, K.H. *et al.* (1989) Drug resistance in cancer treatment, in *New Directions in Cancer Treatment*, (ed. I. Magrath) Springer-Verlag, Berlin, pp. 191–215.

Janossy, G., Campana, D., Galton, J. *et al.* (1987) Applications of monoclonal antibodies in bone marrow transplantation (BMT). 3rd Workshop in Leucocyte Differentiation Antigens, Oxford, p. 43.

Jansen, J., Nichols, C., Besien, K.V. *et al.* (1989) Phase I/II Study of high dose Carboplatin/VP 16 with marrow rescue in refractory germ cell cancer, in *ABMT 4th International Symposium* (eds K.A. Dicke, G. Spitzer, S. Jagannath, M.J. Evinger-Hodges), Houston, 487–91.

Johnson, D.B., Thompson, J.M., Corwin, J.A. *et al.* (1987) Prolongation of survival for high-grade malignant gliomas with adjuvant high-dose

BCNU and autologous bone marrow transplant-ation. *J. Clin. Oncol.*, **5**, 783–9.

Jones, R.J. (1990) The existence of a clinical graft-versus-lymphoma effect. *Experimental Hemato-logy*, **18**, abst 522.

Kaizer, H., Stuart, R.K., Brookmeyer, R. *et al.* (1985) Autologous bone marrow transplantation in acute leukemia: a phase I study of in vitro treatment of marrow with 4-hydroperoxycyclo-phosphamide to purge tumor cells. *Blood*, **65**, 1504–7.

Kemshead, J.T. (1988) Monoclonal antibodies to the small round cell tumours of childhood: an international workshop. Advances in Neuro-blastoma Research 2, Alan R. Liss, New York, pp. 535–46.

Kingston, J.E., Malpass, J.S., Stiller, C.A. *et al.* (1984) Autologous bone marrow transplantation contributes to haemopoietic recovery in children with solid tumors treated with high dose mel-phalan. *Br. J. Haematol.*, **58**, 589–95.

Kinsella, T.J., Glaubiger, D., Diesseroth, A. *et al.* (1983) Intensive combined modality therapy including low-dose TBI in high-risk Ewing's sar-coma patients. *J. Radiation Oncology Biol. Phys.*, **9**, 1955–60.

Kogner, P., Theodorsson, E., Bjôrk, O. (1990) Neuropeptide Y in the plasma; a tumor marker with prognostic significance in children with neural crest tumors. SIOP XXII Meeting Rome. *Med. Ped. Oncol.*, **18**, 373.

Korbling, M., Hess, A.D., Tutshka, P.J. *et al.* (1987) 4-hydroperoxycyclophosphamide: a model for eliminating residual human tumour cells and T-lymphocytes from the bone marrow graft. *Br. J. Haematol.*, **52**, 89–90.

Ladisch, S., Wu, E.L., Feig, S. *et al.* (1987) Shed-ding of GD$_2$ ganglioside by human neuroblast-oma. *Int. J. Cancer*, **39**, 73–6.

Lanino, E., Garaventa, A., Miniero, R. *et al.* (1987) High dose cisplatin plus VP16 ablative therapy and autologous bone marrow rescue in relapsed and resistant Wilm's tumour. In: *Bone Marrow Transplantation* **2** (Suppl 2), 221.

Le Tourneau, J.N., Bernard, J.L., Hendren, W.H. *et al.* (1985) Evaluation of the role of surgery in 130 patients with neuroblastoma. *J. Pediat. Surg.*, **3**, 244–7.

Lebein, T.W., Stepan, D.E., Bartholomew, R.H. *et al.* (1985) Utilization of a colony assay to assess the variables influencing elimination of leukemic cells from human bone marrow with monoclonal antibodies and complement. *Blood*, **65**, 945–9.

Lie, O.S. (1990) 13-*Cis* retinoic acid as continuation therapy in children with advanced neuroblast-oma in complete or good partial response. A toxicity study. *Med. Ped. Oncol.*, **18**, 384.

Ling, V., Juranka, P.F., Endicott, J.A. *et al.* (1988) Multidrug resistance and P-glycoprotein expression, in *Mechanisms of Drug Resistance in Neoplastic Cells*. Academic Press, London, pp. 197–209.

Lord, B.I., Bronchud, M.M., Owens, S. *et al.* (1989) The kinetics of human granulopoiesis following treatment with granulocyte stimulating factor *in vivo*. *Proc. Nat. Acad. Sci.*, **86**, 9499–503.

Lotze, M.T. *et al.* (1985) *In vivo* administration of purified human interleukin-2:II. Half life immunologic effects, and expansion of peripheral lymphoid cells *in vivo* with recom-binant IL-2. *J. Immunol.*, **135**, 2865–75.

Lotzova, E. (1987) Interleukin-2 generated killer cells: Their characterization and role in cancer therapy. *Bull. Cancer*, **39**, 30–8.

Mauch, P.L., Ferrara, J., Hellman, S. *et al.* (1989a) Stem cell self-renewal considerations in bone marrow transplantation. *Bone Marrow Transplant-ation*, **4**, 601–7.

Mauch, P.L. and Hellman, S. (1989b) Loss of hema-topoietic stem cell self-renewal after bone mar-row transplantation. *Blood*, **74**, 872–5.

Mbidde, E., Selby, P., Perren, T.J. *et al.* (1987) High dose BCNU with ABMT and full dose radiotherapy for grade IV astrocytoma. *Br. J. Cancer*, **58**, 779–82.

Michon, J., Phillip, T., Harmann, O. *et al.* (1989) A new protocol using an alternating non-cross resistant induction regimen and two different modalities of massive consolidation chemother-apy in treatment of metastatic neuroblastoma children, in ABMT (eds K.A. Dicke, G. Spitzer, S. Jagannath, M.J. Evinger-Hodges), Houston, pp. 529–41.

Michon, J., Favrot, M., Bouffet, E. *et al.* (1990) Toxicity and efficacy of IL2 with or without LAK cells in the treatment of metastatic neuroblast-oma. A report of 26 cases. *Med. Ped. Oncol.*, **18**, 394.

Migliaccio, A.R., Migliaccia, G., Johnson, G. *et al.* (1990) Comparative analysis of hematopoietic growth factors released by stromal cells from normal donors or transplanted patients. *Blood*, **75**, 305–12.

Miser, S., Kinsella, A.T., Triche, A. *et al.* (1987) Treatment of high risk sarcomas with an intensive consolidation followed by autologous bone marrow transplantation. Proceedings ASCO meeting, Abstract 859.

Moore, D. and Malcolm, A.S. (1990) Hematopoietic Growth Factors in Cancer. *Cancer*, **65**, 836–44.

Moyes, J., McCready, V.R. and Fullbrook, A. (1989) Neuroblastoma: *m*-IBG in its diagnosis and management, in *Neuroblastoma*, Springer-Verlag, Berlin p. 26.

Nakagawara, A., Ikeda, K., Tsuda, T. *et al.* (1987) N-*myc* oncogene amplification and prognostic factors of neuroblastoma in children. *J. Ped. Surg.*, **22**, 895–998.

Nakagawara, A., Ikeda, K., Tasaka, H. (1988) Dopaminergic neuroblastoma as a poor prognostic subgroup. *J. Pediat. Surg.*, **23**, 346–9.

Nasr, S., McKolanis, J., Pais, R. *et al.* (1989) A phase I study of interleukin-2 in children with cancer and evaluation of clinical and immunologic status during therapy. A pediatric oncology group study. *Cancer*, **64**, 783–8.

Negrier, S., Biron, P., Favrot, M. *et al.* (1990) Autologous bone marrow transplantation in pediatric solid tumor. *Ped. Hematology and Oncol.*, **7**, 35–46.

Norton, L. and Simon, R. (1977) Tumor size, sensitivity to therapy and design of treatment schedules. *Cancer Treat. Rep.*, **61**, 1307–9.

Norton, L. (1985) Implications of kinetic heterogeneity in clinical oncology. *Semin. Oncol.*, **12**, 232–6.

Nossal. G.J.V. (1989) Immunologic tolerance, collaboration between antigens and lymphokines. *Science*, **147**, 147–53.

Philip, I., Favrot, M.C., Philip, T. (1987) Use of a liquid cell culture assay to quantify the elimination of Burkitt lymphoma cells from the bone marrow. *J. Immun. Meth.*, **97**, 11–17.

Philip, T., Biron, P., Philip, I. *et al.* (1985a) Autologous bone marrow transplantation for very bad prognosis neuroblastoma, in *Advances in Neuroblastoma Research* (eds A. Evans, G.L. D'Angio and R.C. Seeger) Liss, New York, pp. 568–86.

Philip, T. (1985b) Chimiotherapie massive et autogreffe de moelle dans les tumeurs des parties molles (15 cas). *Bull. Cancer*, 72–62.

Philip, T., Armitage, J.O., Spitzer, G. *et al.* (1987a) High dose therapy and autologous bone marrow transplantation after failure of conventional chemotherapy in adults with intermediate grade or high grade non-Hodgkin's lymphoma. *N. Engl. J. Med.*, **316**, 1493–8.

Philip, T., Nelson, L., Bernard, J.L. *et al.* (1987b) Definition of response and remission in children over one year of age with advanced neuroblastoma. Proposition of a scoring system. *Ped. Hematol. and Oncol.*, **4**, 25–51.

Philip, T., Frappaz, D., Biron, P. *et al.* (1987c) A single institution's experience of autologous bone marrow transplantation for neuroblastoma, in 3rd International Conference on Autologous Bone Marrow Transplantation (eds K. Dicke, G. Spitzer and S. Jagannath). Houston, 419–23.

Philip, T., Bernard, J.L., Zucker, J.M. *et al.* (1987d) High dose chemotherapy with bone marrow transplantation as consolidation treatment in neuroblastoma: an unselected group of stage IV patients over one year of age. *J. Clin. Oncol.*, **5**, 266–71.

Philip, T. and Pinkerton, R. (1989a) Neuroblastoma, in *New Directions in Cancer Treatment* (ed. I. Magrath) UICC Springer-Verlag, Berlin, pp. 605–11.

Philip, T. and Pinkerton, R. (1989b) Very high dose therapy in lymphomas and solid tumors, in *New Directions in Cancer Treatment* (ed. I. Magrath), Springer-Verlag, Berlin, pp. 119–42.

Philip, T., Bouffet, E., Biron, P. *et al.* (1989a) Facteur dose/facteur temps en chimiothérapie. *Bull. Cancer*, **76**, 979–94.

Philip, T. Chauvin, F. Michon, J. *et al.* (1989b) A pilot study of double ABMT in advanced neuroblastoma. 4th International Conference on Autologous Bone Marrow Transplantation, (eds K. Dicke, G. Spitzer, S. Jagannath and M.J. Evinger-Hodges), Houston, 799–805.

Philip, T., Mercatello, A., Negrier, S. *et al.* (1989c) Interleukin-2 with and without LAK cells in metastatic renal cell carcinoma: the Lyon first-year experience in 20 patients. *Cancer Treatment Reviews*, Academic Press, suppl.A, 91–104.

Philip, T., Zucker, J.M., Bernard, J.L. *et al.* (1991)

High dose chemotherapy with BMT as consolidation treatment in neuroblastoma. The LMCE1 unselected group of patients revisited with a median follow up of 55 months after BMT, in *Advances in Neuroblastoma Research*, (eds A.E. Evans, G.J. D'Angio, A.G. Knudson Jnr and R.C. Seeger), Wiley-Liss, New York, pp. 517–25.

Phillips, G., Fay, J., Herzig, G. (1985) Autologous bone marrow transplantation in malignant glioma. *Int. J. Cell. Cloning*, **3**, 257–60.

Phillips, G. *et al.* (1989) Autologous bone marrow transplant conditioning regimens for non-Hodgkin's lymphoma, in ABMT 4th International Symposium (eds K.A. Dicke, G. Spitzer, S. Jagannath and M.J. Evinger-Hodges), Houston, 305–15.

Phillips, G.L., Wolf, S.N., Fay, J.W. *et al.* (1986) Intensive 1, 3-bis (2 chloroethyl) 1-nitrosourea (BCNU) monochemotherapy and autologous marrow transplantation for malignant gliomas. *J. Clin. Oncol.*, **4**, 639–43.

Pico, J.L., Droz, J.P., Ostronoff, M. *et al.* (1989) High dose chemotherapy with autologous bone marrow transplantation for poor prognosis non seminomatous germ cell tumors, in ABMT 3rd international symposium (eds K.A. Dicke, G. Spitzer, S. Jagannath, M.J. Evinger-Hodges), Houston, 469–76.

Pino, Y., Torres, J.L., Bross, D.S. *et al.* (1982) Risk factors in interstitial pneumonitis following allogeneic bone marrow transplantation. *Int. J. Radiat. Oncol. Biol. Phys.*, **8**, 1301–4.

Pinkerton, C.R., Philip, T., Bouffet, E. *et al.* (1986) Autologous bone marrow transplantation in pediatric solid tumors. *Clin. Haematol.*, **15**, 187–94.

Pinkerton, C.R., Phillip, T., Hartmann, O. *et al.* (1989) High-dose chemo-radiotherapy with autologous bone marrow rescue in pediatric soft tissue sarcomas, in ABMT. Proceedings of the fourth international symposium. (eds K.A. Dicke, G. Spitzer, S. Jagannath, M.J. Evinger-Hodges), Houston, 617–20.

Pinkerton, C.R. (1990) Where next with therapy in advanced neuroblastoma? *Br. J. Cancer*, **61**, 351–3.

Poynton, C.H. *et al.* (1983) Immunomagnetic removal of CALLA positive cells from human bone marrow. *Lancet*, **1**, 524–5.

Pratt, C.B., Crom, D.B., Howarth, C. (1985) The use of chemotherapy for extra ocular retinoblastoma. *Med. Ped. Oncol.*, **13**, 330–3.

Pritchard, J., McElwain, T.J., Graham-Pole, J. *et al.* (1982) High-dose melphalan with autologous marrow for treatment of advanced neuroblastoma. *Br. J. Cancer*, **45**, 86–94.

Pritchard, J., Germond, S., Jones, D. *et al.* (1986) Is high dose melphalan of value in treatment of advanced neuroblastoma? Preliminary results of a randomization trial by the European Neuroblastoma Study Group. Proc. ASCO, **5**, 205–8.

Reisner, Y., Kapoor, D., Kirkpatrick, D. *et al.* (1983) Transplantation for severe combined immunodeficiency with HLA-A, B, D, DR, incompatible parental marrow cells fractionated by soybean agglutinin and sheep red blood cells. *Blood*, **61**, 341–4.

Reynolds, C.P., Reynolds, D.A., Frenkel, E.P. *et al.* (1982) Selective toxicity of 6-hydroxydopamine and ascorbate for human neuroblastoma *in vitro*: a model for clearing marrow prior to autologous transplant. *Cancer Res.*, **42**, 1331–6.

Reynolds, C.P., Seeger, R.C., Vod, D. *et al.* (1986) Model system for removing neuroblastoma cells from bone marrow using monoclonal antibodies and magnetic immunobeads. *Cancer Res.*, **46**, 5882–4.

Reynolds, C.P., Moss, T.J., Stephen, A.F. *et al.* (1989) Treatment of poor prognosis neuroblastoma with intensive therapy and autologous bone marrow transplantation. In ABMT, (eds K.A. Dicke, G. Spitzer, S. Jagannath, M.J. Evinger-Hodges), Houston, 575–83.

Rodary, C., Flamant, F., Donaldson, S.S. *et al.* (1989) (for the SIOP-IRS Committee) An attempt to use a common staging system in rhabdomyosarcoma: a report of an international workshop initiated by the international society of pediatric oncology (SIOP). *Med. Ped. Oncol.*, **17**, 210–5.

Rosen, E.M., Cassady, J.R., Frantz, C.N. *et al.* (1984) Neuroblastoma, the joint center for radiation therapy/Dana-Farber Cancer Institute/Children's Hospital experience. *J. Clin. Oncol.*, **2**, 719–22.

Rosenberg, S.A., Lotze, M.T., Muul, L.M. *et al.* (1985) Observations on the systemic administration of autologous lymphokine activated killer cells and recombinant interleukin-2 to patients with metastatic cancer. *N. Engl. J. Med.*, **313**, 1485–8.

Rosenberg, S.A., Lotze, M.T., Muul, L.M. *et al.*

(1987) A progress report on the treatment of 157 patients with advanced cancer using lymphokine activated killer cells and interleukin-2 or high dose interleukin-2 alone. *N. Engl. J. Med.*, **316**, 889–97.

Rothenberg, M. and Ling, V. (1989) Multidrug resistance: molecular biology and clinical relevance. *J. Nat. Cancer Inst.*, **81**, 907–10.

Saarinenu, M., Coccia, P.F., Gerson, S.L. *et al.* (1985) Eradication of neuroblastoma cells in vitro by monoclonal antibody and human complement: method for purging autologous bone marrow. *Cancer Res.*, **45**, 5969–70.

Santos, G.W. (1990) Bone Marrow Transplantation in Hematologic Malignancies. *Cancer*, **65**, 786–91.

Scanlon, K.F., Kashani-Sabet, M., Miyachi, Y. *et al.* (1989) Molecular basis of cisplatin resistance in human carcinomas: model systems and patients. *Anticancer Res. Q.*, 1301–12.

Schwab, M. (1991) Is there a neuroblastoma anti-oncogene? In *Advances in Neuroblastoma Research 3*, Alan Liss, New York, 1–9.

Seeger, R.C., Brodeur, G.M., Sather, H. *et al.* (1985) Association of multiple copies of the n-*myc* oncogene with rapid progression of NBL's. *N. Engl. J. Med.*, **313**, 1111–16.

Shimada, H., Chatten, J., Newton, W.A.J. *et al.* (1984) Histopathologic prognostic factors in neuroblastic tumors: definition of subtypes of ganglioneuroblastoma and an age-linked classification of neuroblastoma. *J. Natl. Cancer Inst.*, **73**, 405–16.

Shimada, H., Aoyama, C., Chiba, T. *et al.* (1985) Prognostic subgroups for undifferentiated neuroblastoma: immunohistochemical study with anti-S-100 protein antibody. *Hum. Pathol.*, **16**, 471–6.

Sidell, N. (1982) Retinoic acid-induced growth inhibition and morphologic differentiation of human neuroblastoma cells *in vitro*. *J. Nat. Cancer Inst.*, **68**, 589–96.

Sieber, F., Spivak, J.L., Sutcliffe, A.M. *et al.* (1984) Selective killing of leukemic cells by merocyanine 540-mediated photosensitization. *Proc. Natl. Acad. Sci.*, **81**, 7584–6.

Skipper, H.E., Schabel, F.M. Jr, Wilcor, W.S. *et al.* (1964) Experimental evaluation of potential anti-cancer agents. On the criteria and kinetics associated with 'curability' of experimental leukemia. *Cancer Chemother. Rep.*, **35**, 1–111.

Slavin, S., Naparstek, E., Or, R. *et al.* (1988) Prevention of GVHD and induction of graft-versus-leukemia effects: will it be possible? *Bone Marrow Transplantation*, **3**, suppl 1, 208–9.

Sosman, J.A., Kohler, P.C., Hank, J.H. *et al.* (1988) Repetitive weekly cycles of recombinant human interleukin-2: Responses of renal carcinoma with acceptable toxicity. *J. Natl. Cancer Inst.*, **80**, 60–3.

Stepan, D.E., Bartholomew, R.M., Lebien, T.W. (1984) *In vitro* cytodestruction of human leukemic cells using murine monoclonal antibodies and human complement. *Blood*, **6**, 1120–4.

Stephenson, S.R., Cook, B.A., Merse, A.D. *et al.* (1986) The prognostic significance of age and pattern of metastases in stage IV-S neuroblastoma. *Cancer*, **58**, 372–5.

Takvorian, T., Parker, L.M., Hockberg, F.H. (1983) Autologous bone marrow transplantation: host effects of high dose BCNU. *J. Clin. Oncol.*, **1**, 610–14.

Thiele, C.J. (1985) Decreased expression of N-*myc* precedes retinoic acid-induced morphological differentiation of human neuroblastoma. *Nature*, **313**, 404–6.

Treleaven, J.G., Gibson, F.M., Ugelstad, J. *et al.* (1984) Removal of neuroblastoma cells from bone marrow with monoclonal antibodies conjugated to magnetic microspheres. *Lancet*, **14**, 70–3.

Tsuchida, Y., Honna, T., Iwanaka, T. *et al.* (1987) Serial determination of serum neurone-specific enolase in patients with neuroblastoma and other pediatric tumors. *J. Pediat. Surg.*, **22**, 419–24.

Tsuda, T., Obara, M., Hirand, H. *et al.* (1987) Analysis of n-*myc* amplification in relation to disease stage and histologic types in human neuroblastomas. *Cancer*, **60**, 820–6.

Vossen, J.M. (1990) Autologous bone marrow rescue as part of a curative approach for pediatric solid tumors: the case of neuroblastoma. *Pediatr. Hematol. Oncol.*, **7**, 3–7.

Waldman, H., Hale, G., Cividalli, G. *et al.* (1984) Elimination of graft-versus-host disease by *in vitro* depletion of alloreactive lymphocytes with a monoclonal rat anti-human lymphocyte antibody (Campath-1) *Lancet*, **2**, 483–6.

Waxman, S. (1988) The importance of the induction of gene expression and differentiation by cytotoxic chemotherapy. *Cancer Invest.*, **6**, 747–53.

Weichselbaum, R.R., Schmit, A., Little, J.B. (1982) Cellular repair factors influencing radiocurability of human malignant tumors. *Br. J. Cancer*, **45**, 10–6.

West, C.M.L., Sandhu, R.R., Stratford, J. (1984) The radiation response of V79 and human tumor multicellular spheroids-cells. Survival and growth delay studies. *Br. J. Cancer*, **50**, 143–51.

White, L. (1983) The role of chemotherapy in the treatment of retinoblastoma. *Retina*, **3**, 194–9.

Williams, G.T., Smith, C.A., Spooncer, E. *et al.* (1990) Haemopoietic colony stimulating factor promotes cell survival by suppressing apeptosis. *Nature*, **343**, 76–9.

Williams, S.F., Bitran, J.D., Kominer, L. *et al.* (1987) A phase 1–11 study of bialkylator chemotherapy, high-dose thiotepa, and clyclophosphamide with autologous bone marrow reinfusion in patients with advanced cancer. *J. Clin. Oncol.*, **5**, 260–5.

Yaniv, I., Bouffet, E., Irle, C. *et al.* (1990) Autologous bone marrow transplantation in pediatric solid tumors. *Ped. Hematol. Oncol.*, **7**, 35–46.

Yeager, A.M., Kaizer, J., Santos, G.W. *et al.* (1986) Autologous bone marrow transplantation in patients with acute non-lymphocytic leukemia, using *ex vivo* marrow treatment with 4-hydroperoxycyclophosphamide. *N. Engl. J. Med.*, **315**, 141–7.

Zeltzer, P.M., Marangos, P.J., Evans, A.E. *et al.* (1986) Serum neurone-specific enolase in children with neuroblastoma. Relationship to stage and disease course. *Cancer*, **57**, 1230–4.

Zucker, J.M., Lemercier, N., Schlienger, P. *et al.* (1982) Chemotherapeutic conservative management in 23 patients with locally extended bilateral retinoblastoma. *Eur. J. Cancer. Clin. Oncol.*, **10**, 1046.

Zucker, J.M., Quintana, E., Asselain, B. *et al.* (1990) Extra ocular retinoblastoma: effectiveness of a multiagent chemotherapy including adriamycin and CDDP (In press).

Chapter 24

An overview of the clinical potential of targeted therapy

J.T. KEMSHEAD and L. S. LASHFORD

24.1 INTRODUCTION

The idea of selectively targeting therapy to tumours is not new. Over 100 years ago Hericourt and Richet (1895) attempted to treat a patient with a sarcoma using serotherapy. Progress in the field has been slow, but in recent years a resurgence of interest has followed the development of monoclonal antibody technology. Many groups have raised monoclonal antibodies to a variety of cell surface antigens expressed on tumour cells. Without exception, no reagent has been developed to date that is truly tumour specific. It is often forgotten that antibodies are capable of binding to a range of epitopes with differing affinities and, therefore, the search for truly tumour-specific reagents is probably fallacious. In spite of this, many antibodies have been developed that have greater operational tumour specificity than is implied from their immunoreactivity with a variety of tissue sections. This chapter reviews the different approaches taken to using antibodies as carriers of 'cytotoxic' agents to tumour cells. In addition, we point out problems associated with this type of therapy and some of the new approaches being made to improve its effectiveness.

In addition to monoclonal antibodies, biochemical approaches to targeting 'therapy' to tumour cells have been made. These rely on the differential expression of various biochemical pathways in cells of different lineages. The best studied of these is the selective uptake of iodine into thyroid carcinoma cells. Of paediatric interest are the mechanisms involved in the uptake, storage and release of biogenic amines in cells of neuroectodermal origin. *Meta*-iodobenzylguanidine (*m*IBG) is a guanethidine analogue that is taken up into cells in a fashion similar to adrenaline and noradrenaline (Shapiro *et al.*, 1985). As its name implies, *m*IBG can be made using a variety of the isotopes of iodine and may be used as a radiopharmaceutical agent for either the imaging or treatment of malignancies such as pheochromocytoma and neuroblastoma. The use of *m*IBG for diagnosis and therapy of tumours will be reviewed along with recent data on its mode of storage within neuroblastoma cells. Rather like monoclonal antibodies, *m*IBG has enormous potential as a selective delivery agent, but a great deal of work is necessary before we understand fully how best to use both of these targeted forms of therapy.

24.2 IMMUNOLOGICAL TARGETING

24.2.1 BASIC BIOLOGICAL MODELS

Several approaches to studying the efficacy of targeted compounds have been made. These include both tissue culture systems and a variety of animal models using either syngeneic tumours or immuno-compromized animals where human tumours can be grafted into the host. None of these have proved reliable indicators of the efficacy of the targeted agents in the clinical situation (Jones *et al.*, 1987). However, pre-clinical assessment of compounds can supply useful information regarding the stability of the conjugate, the affinity/avidity of the antibody for its antigen, and whether the binding of the antibody to the cell membrane causes capping, shedding or internalization of the antigen-antibody complex. This point is critical for work with drugs and immunotoxins where internalization is important for therapeutic effect. Several groups have used soft agar cloning techniques to judge the efficacy of specific antibody conjugates as compared to non-specific antibodies carrying the same 'therapeutic agent' (Courtney and Mills, 1978). In addition, spheroid model systems have been employed to ascertain how different immuno-conjugates can penetrate and kill small tumour 'clumps' (Walker *et al.* 1990).

Animal model systems have been used to a much wider extent to judge the efficacy of therapy. Many groups have shown the potential of antibody targeted therapy in the nude mouse xenografted with a variety of different human tumours. In this model, established tumours of greater than 1 cm in diameter have been at least temporarily eradicated from the host (Jones *et al.* 1987). The model has again enabled researchers to judge the efficacy of targeted therapy as compared to similar agents with no specificity for tumour. It was through the encouraging data obtained from studies of this type that much of the enthusiasm for targeted therapy arose. In these studies, it was not unusual for between 5–15% of the injected dose of immunoconjugate to be targeted selectively to each gram of tumour xenografted into the animal. However, as will be discussed below, the animal model systems are poor predictors of what happens to immunoconjugates when they are administered to humans. The reasons behind this are unclear, but probably reflect both different rates of clearance from the vasculature of the mouse as compared to humans, and the blood supply of the xenograft in the animal. Whilst the nude mouse can act as a 'carrier' of human xenografts, the blood supply to that tumour is murine in nature. It would appear from many experimental studies that this vasculature is far more 'leaky' than its equivalent human counterpart.

24.3 TYPES OF TARGETING AGENTS

24.3.1 IMMUNOTOXINS

Toxins are natural products existing in plants and bacteria. Much of the work on immunotoxins was undertaken with ricin isolated from the castor bean *Ricinus communis*. More recently, a host of other toxins have been isolated and attached to immunoglobulins. These include diptheria toxin (Hertler *et al.*, 1990), saporin (Davis *et al.*, 1989), gelonin (Reimann *et al.*, 1989), abrin (Sallustio *et al.*, 1990), holoricin and momorcochin-S (Sallustio *et al.*, 1990; Marsh and Klinman, 1990). These reagents act on cells in a common manner by functioning as ribosomal inhibitor proteins. Molecules such as ricin are dimers consisting of two chains, A and B. The B chain of the molecule contains a galactose recognition site that allows the molecule to bind non-specifically to a variety of cell types. The A chain of the molecule is the one that blocks ribosomal activity once the toxin enters the cell. To confer specificity on to an immunotoxin the binding of the B chain has to be blocked. This can only be achieved by linking the A chain of the molecule to immunoglobulin, by chemically modifying the B chain so that it is no longer capable of binding carbohydrate molecules, or *in vitro* by using the immunotoxins in the presence of sufficiently high concentrations of galactose to block B chain binding (Thorpe *et al.*, 1988). The search for alternative toxins to ricin has revealed natural compounds, such as gelonin, which are single glycoproteins that are similar to the ricin A chain.

Problems that are related to the use of immunotoxins have been addressed in detail. In early studies, the stability of toxin/ antibody binding *in vivo* was a major problem, as was the immunogenicity of the conjugates. The question of antibody toxin stability has been mainly resolved through the use of heterobifunctional binding agents. Deglycosylation of the toxin prior to its conjugation to antibody has also markedly reduced its immunogenicity, but this problem has not been eliminated (Thorpe *et al.*, 1988). A further problem relating to the use of immunotoxins is that it is not easy to predict which antibody/toxin conjugate will be efficacious. It has been shown that two immunotoxins, consisting of the same antibody but differing toxins, can vary markedly in their effectiveness. The rationale behind this observation remains ill understood.

Irrespective of the above problems, immunotoxins have proved highly effective at killing tumour cells either *in vitro* or in animal model systems. This has led to a cautious appraisal of their activity in the clinic. As with other targeted agents, low levels of uptake and uneven penetration of the immunotoxin into solid tumour deposits have been identified as the major problem concerning their use (see below). Few, if any, detailed immunotoxin studies have been carried out in children. However, in adult patients with either metastatic colorectal carcinoma or B cell lymphoma phase I, toxicity studies have revealed side effects which manifest as a capillary leak syndrome (Byers *et al.*, 1990). Symptoms included a decrease in serum albumin, oedema, proteinurea, mild fever and flu-like characteristics. In the study of patients with carcinoma, changes in mental status were also noted, whilst in the lymphoma study, myalgia was observed. In both of these studies on systemic administration of immunotoxins, partial but not complete remissions were noted in an encouraging number of patients. Whilst the use of immunotoxins in body compartments has been explored in animals, no detailed clinical studies have been undertaken to date.

24.3.2 DRUGS

Several drugs have been conjugated to monoclonal antibodies in an attempt to increase their therapeutic index. Mitomycin-C (Liang *et al.*, 1989), platinum (Plotnikov *et al.*, 1989), several vinca alkaloids (Schneck *et al.*, 1990), cytorhodin-S (an anthracycline derivative) (Iwahashi *et al.*, 1989) and methotrexate (Kralovec *et al.*, 1989) have been coupled to monoclonal antibodies and their efficacy as immunoconjugates tested in a variety of systems. In general, drug antibody conjugates have proved less effective than immunotoxins. Many of the problems associated with the use of drug antibody conjugates also apply to toxins. Links between the cytotoxic drug and the antibody need to be sufficiently stable to allow the conjugate to be targeted to the tumour site without dissociation. Once the conjugate binds to the cell, it needs to be internalized and the drug released so that it can exert its cytotoxic effect. Perhaps the best studied exceptions to this mode of action are adriamycin (doxorubicin)/antibody conjugates. As well as the accepted mode of action of adriamycin

(DNA chelation, free radical formation, and metal chelation), the compound has been described as exerting a cytotoxic effect on cells via interaction with undefined components of the cell membrane (Priestman, 1989). This is thought to induce a cytotoxic effect on the cell by bringing about changes in membrane fluidity. Within this context, adriamycin antibody conjugates may have a direct cytotoxic effect by simple targeting to cell membrane antigens.

To increase the efficacy of drug conjugates, monoclonal antibodies have been modified so that they are capable of carrying greater amounts of drug. This has been achieved by linking pre-defined peptides to the antibody backbone (Baldwin and Byers, 1989). For example, polylysine has been linked to antibodies and this has served as a peptide core onto which daunomycin has been linked. This type of modification has been shown to effect the half-life of the conjugate in the blood, indicating that it is critical to select the appropriate linker technology for efficient drug targeting. A further approach to drug targeting has been through the use of bispecific antibodies (Stevenson, 1989). In this instance, hybrid antibodies are produced so that one arm of the molecule recognizes the target antigen on tumour cells and the other serves as a capture arm to bind to the cytotoxic agent.

24.3.3 ISOTOPES

Much of the early work on antibody/isotope conjugates was undertaken with isotopes of iodine. These studies added an extra element to those undertaken with either toxins or drugs, as isotope targeting also allows the imaging of metastatic disease. The linker technology involved in the coupling of iodine to antibodies is similar for both imaging and therapeutic applications of the conjugates. What differs is the choice of isotope used. Initial scintigraphic studies were undertaken with ^{131}I linked to antibodies using a simple oxidation, reduction procedure. These investigations were, in many ways, a compromise, as this isotope is far from ideal for scintigraphic imaging. Using the same technology, ^{123}I can be linked to antibodies. This has better properties as an isotope for imaging in nuclear medicine, but its use is restricted by having a short half-life, limited availability, and by its cost. Results with many iodine/antibody conjugates were encouraging, but they revealed that while new lesions were detected, some lesions that were detectable by other imaging modalities were missed.

The search for better scintigraphic agents has proceeded in two directions: the development of antibody fragments that may allow better penetration of the conjugates into tumour, and alternative technologies for linking different isotopes to antibodies (Kalofonos *et al.*, 1988). The former is relatively straightforward, but experience has shown that difficulties may be encountered in producing (Fab)$_2$ and Fab fragments from certain monoclonal antibodies. In addition, caution needs to be taken in the use of Fab fragments as these will bind less avidly to their target antigen than whole Ig and (Fab)$_2$ dimers.

^{111}In was the first alternative to iodine to be explored for immunoscintigraphy. This was linked to antibodies through diethylenetriamine pentaacetic acid (DTPA), which cross links to proteins and serves as a metal chelator. ^{111}In antibody conjugates have probably improved the sensitivity of immunoscintigraphy, but problems remain concerning the stability of the binding of isotope to the metal chelate (Pimm *et al.*, 1987). ^{111}In has been found in the liver of the majority of patients undergoing scintigraphy. This is thought to occur as transferrin and has a higher affinity for the DTPA chelate than ^{111}In and it therefore displaces the isotope. In addition to ^{111}In, a variety of other isotopes have been conjugated to DTPA. These include ^{99}m technetium (Tc) for conventional immunoscintigraphy and [67]gadolinium (Ga) for the enhancement of nuclear magnetic resonance imaging (Kornguth *et al.*, 1987). To improve the stability of metal chelate antibody complexes *in vivo* other approaches to labelling antibodies have been sought. These include the use of alternative metal chelating agents such as deferoxamine to bind ^{67}Ga to antibodies (Koizumi *et al.*, 1988) and the use of macrocycles. These can be thought of as molecules that can be linked to antibodies and hold 'radiometals' with high stability (Moi *et al.*, 1990). Examples of such molecules are 1,4,7,10-tetraazacyclododecane-N,N',N'',-N'''-tetraacetic acid (DOTA) that has been used to chelate both ^{111}In and [90]yttrium (Y) to monoclonal antibodies. In addition to these studies, alternative approaches to linking ^{99m}Tc and iodine to antibodies have been made. Mather and Ellison (1990) have developed an elegant alternative for incorporating ^{99m}Tc into antibodies. Sulphydryl groups within the antibody molecule are reduced using 2-mercaptoethanol so that two heavy/light chain fragments are generated. Labelling is performed via Sn^{++} reduction of pertechnetate in the presence of a low affinity chelating ligand. This methodology provides a very convenient way of labelling antibodies using an isotope provided by a conventional bone scanning kit.

Recently, Zalutsky *et al.* (1989) have also radiolabelled antibodies with iodine using N-succinimidyl 3-(tri-n-butylstannyl) benzoate. Animal studies indicate that this approach to conjugating iodine to antibodies results in significantly less dehalogenation *in vivo* as compared to conventional iodine labelling chemistry.

In parallel with scintigraphic studies ^{131}I was the first isotope to be conjugated to antibodies for targeted radiation therapy. In the paediatric field, two antibodies have been predominantly used, UJ13A which recognizes the neural cell adhesion molecule

(NCAM) (Patel *et al.*, 1990), and 3F8 which primarily binds to the ganglioside GD_2, but also may cross react with a carbohydrate moiety on NCAM (Patel *et al.*, 1989). In these studies (and others) myelosuppression has been the predominant side effect. This occurs particularly in children that have been heavily pretreated with combination chemotherapy. While responses to targeted radiation have unquestionably been observed, both scintigraphic studies and direct tumour biopsy indicates that little antibody penetrates a solid tumour deposit. In contrast to the 5–15% of the injected dose per gram of tumour seen in the human tumour xenograft/nude mouse model, approximately 0.001% gram finds its way into solid tumour deposits in patients. This universal finding has prompted three avenues of investigation:

1. to attempt to increase antibody penetration into tumours (see below);
2. to develop more toxic antibody-isotope conjugates;
3. to investigate tumours where access is inherently less of a problem.

[131]I emits both beta and gamma radiation. For the purposes of targeted radiation therapy it is the β component that is important, this having a mean particle range of approximately 1.0 mm. This implies that if penetration into solid tumour deposits is limited, tumour kill will only occur in the area directly adjacent to where antibodies bind. Thin layer autoradiography and studies on the penetration of antibodies into tumour spheroids in culture indicate that antibodies unevenly penetrate even small nodules of cells. Furthermore, ^{131}I is not an ideal isotope for killing individual tumour cells as the particle range of β radiation emitted is too long in comparison to the average diameter of a tumour cell (10 μm). For these reasons, alternative isotopes have been examined. [90]Y, a β emitter, has been attached to antibodies via the

DTPA chelate. The β emissions from this isotope have a mean particle range of 5 mm and ^{90}Y is therefore more applicable for the treatment of solid tumour deposits. In early studies with ^{90}Y, problems were encountered with the linkage of the isotope to antibody. This was because DTPA was used as a metal chelator. Recently, through the use of macrocycle linkers, more stable antibody conjugates of ^{90}Y have been produced.

Another β emitter that has been considered for targeted radiation therapy is ^{32}P which has been used for the treatment of polycythaemia rubra vera. The main problem with this radionuclide is associated with its conjugation to antibody. Foxwell *et al.* (1988) have described a method of linking ^{32}P to proteins via a synthetic heptapeptide. The peptide chosen is kemptide, which acts as a substrate for kinases. This can be phosphorylated using protein kinases and [^{32}P]-gamma-ATP. This procedure has only been used experimentally to date, but tumour responses in animals have been reported. The main toxicity observed with the conjugates was myelosuppression, thought to occur due to release of ^{32}P from the antibody conjugate.

Alpha emitters also have a role to play in targeted radiation therapy, and may be particularly appropriate for the elimination of single cell disease from the body. Alpha emissions from ^{211}astatine (At) have a mean range of 0.05 mm and in theory can be linked to antibodies via a similar chemistry to that used in iodine conjugation. Although preclinical work has been undertaken, no clinical studies with ^{211}At have been reported to date reflecting both its limited availability and problems associated with handling the isotope. The main physical drawback of ^{211}At is its very short half-life of seven hours.

In parallel with the new developments in preparing conjugates, attention has also focussed on the treatment of diffuse tumours where antibody permeability is not a limita-tion. Epenetos *et al.* (1987) were amongst the first groups to explore this area through their studies on the administration of ^{131}I labelled antibodies to patients with malignant ascites. Similar studies on both the systemic and intrathecal administration of radiolabelled antibodies to patients with leukaemia have been undertaken. In addition, encouraging responses have been noted following the instillation of ^{131}I labelled antibodies directly into the cerebrospinal fluid of patients suffering from malignant meningitis secondary to a number of different neoplasms (Moseley *et al.*, 1990). Further preclinical and clinical studies are necessary to establish the efficacy of the above conjugates. In addition, work is being undertaken on linking other isotopes to antibodies such as ^{10}boron (B) (Coderre *et al.*, 1988). After tumour is targeted with ^{10}B, the area is exposed to a beam of slow neutrons which cause the release of highly damaging short range emissions. Ideally these should kill the tumour cells and spare the surrounding tissue.

It is likely that no ideal isotope antibody combination will be found and in fact a combination of different antibodies and isotopes will almost certainly prove to be the most efficacious. Such combinations will both deal with the problem of antigen heterogeneity upon tumour cells and in addition be designed to optimize kill of both solid tumour deposits and micro-metastatic disease.

24.3.4 BIOLOGICAL RESPONSE MODIFIERS

One of the conceptual difficulties associated with targeting 'therapeutic' agents to tumours is to establish whether any observed effect is due to the targeted agent rather than the vector. It is clear that monoclonal antibodies can elicit cytotoxic effects either via antibody-dependent cell-mediated cytotoxity (ADCC) or complement-mediated cytotoxicity. These effects are mediated through antibodies of differing isotypes and it is therefore often possible to design conjugates which minimize the inherent cytotoxic nature of the antibody. A number of studies have observed late responses to targeted therapy which are difficult to explain solely on the basis of the delivery of the targeted agent to the tumour. An explanation for this is that human anti-idiotype is generated to the antigen binding site of the mouse antibody and this may be responsible for the cytotoxic effect (O'Connell *et al.*, 1990). Several studies specifically aimed at establishing anti-idiotype networks in patients have been set up and some responses noted. While some groups are examining the effects of anti-idiotype antibodies alone, others are attempting to enhance their efficacy via the introduction of other biological response modifiers such as alpha interferon (Brown *et al.*, 1990).

In addition to being used alone as biological response modifiers, antibodies have been used as carriers of proteins such as interferon. Furthermore, bispecific antibodies have been constructed to target lymphocyte activated killer (LAK) cells to tumours. Bispecific antibodies can be constructed through the chemical linkage of two different monoclonal antibodies *in vitro* or by the fusion of two hybridomas and the selection of a hybrid secreting the relevant combination of heavy and light chains (Ferrini *et al.*, 1989).

Nitta *et al.* (1990) have treated glioma patients with hybrid antibodies consisting of reagents with specificity for CD3 antigen and an antigen expressed on glial cells. These chemically modified bispecific reagents were targeted to LAK cells through the antibody to CD3. When injected into the cerebrospinal fluid the intention is that the anti-glial antibody targets the complex to tumour cells. While 4/10 tumours regressed as a result of this therapy, the time from treatment is relatively short. Moreover, the antibody used to target the cell antibody complexes to tumour cells has recently been shown to recognize NCAM. This antigen is found in large amounts on cells throughout the CNS. It is also present on LAK cells and consequently it is difficult to see just how effective LAK cell targeting was achieved. In spite of these problems, this approach to targeting is intriguing and may result in a far less toxic approach to LAK cell therapy.

24.4 FUTURE DIRECTIONS OF ANTIBODY-TARGETED THERAPY

As has been said, the major problem identified with any form of antibody targeting is the poor penetration of antibody into solid tumour deposits. For progress to be made in this field improvements are necessary. Reduction of the size of the antibody complex has been attempted through the use of Fab fragments. However, this approach has not resulted in substantial improvements in the degree of uptake; this suggests that fundamental changes in the size of the antibody 'conjugate' need to be made. This can only be achieved through a molecular approach where the actual antigen binding site of an immunoglobulin molecule can be synthetically engineered. Whether these antibody fragments will function well and dramatically improve 'antibody' access into tumours has still to be resolved. The problem of access may be difficult to address in well encapsulated tumours simply because of increased interstitial pressure within the neoplasm (Jain, 1990). If this is the case then ways of increasing the 'leakiness' of tumours will have to be investigated prior to antibody therapy.

It is now clear that the generation of an anti-mouse Ig response within an individual changes the pharmacokinetics of antibody handling. Briefly, antibodies are complexed, trapped in the reticuloendothelial system, and subsequently excreted. While it can be clearly demonstrated that anti-mouse Ig

501

responses are generated as a result of administering murine and rat monoclonal antibodies to patients, the number of injections that can be given prior to induction of the response is not clear. This depends on the dose of antibody given, whether it is aggregated, and the immune status of the individual (i.e. whether or not they have received extensive chemotherapy to suppress their immune system). The obvious approach to resolve this problem is to use human antibodies. This can be achieved by a molecular approach to humanize a monoclonal antibody (Winter, 1989). Alternatively, human monoclonal antibodies can be produced; however, this field has been fraught with problems of obtaining cells producing appropriate immunoglobulins for fusions, the stability of the hybrids and the low level of antibody production from the ensuing hybridomas (Wong *et al.*, 1989).

Humanization of antibodies may itself lead to a problem as this will increase the circulating time of the antibody conjugate in the bloodstream and almost certainly reduce its therapeutic index (dose to tumour as compared to normal tissue – i.e. whole body). This problem and the problem of rapidly clearing mouse Ig from the circulation of patients has been addressed by administering anti-mouse Ig to patients after the monoclonal has been allowed to circulate for a period of time (Stuart *et al.*, 1990). A similar idea to increase the therapeutic index of the targeted agent is to use bispecific antibodies. Molecules such as biotin can be linked to antibodies and allowed to target to tumour. The intention is that the antibody remains in tumour for a longer period of time than either in the circulation or non-specifically trapped in other organs. Once clearance from normal tissues occurs, streptavidin carrying a cytotoxic agent can be administered and this is captured by the biotin labelled antibody in the tumour (Paganelli *et al.*, 1990). In general biotin has a much higher affinity for streptavidin than monoclonal antibodies have for antigens.

Which of these options will ultimately enhance the efficacy of targeted therapy remains to be resolved. More work in the field is necessary to resolve where targeted therapy using antibodies will ultimately prove beneficial. Almost certainly this will not be through the use of antibodies alone but in combination either with other cytotoxic agents or external beam radiation.

24.5 *m*IBG AS A RADIOPHARMACEUTICAL AGENT

24.5.1 SCINTIGRAPHY

Meta-iodobenzylguanidine, a guanethidine analogue, was first developed as an imaging agent for pheochromocytoma (Shapiro *et al.*, 1985). In recent years it has found a wider application in both the diagnosis and therapy of tumours which possess the ability to take up biogenic amines. Several studies have now demonstrated that *m*IBG is an excellent imaging agent for neuroblastoma, particularly when used at diagnosis (Hoefnagel *et al.*, 1987). Results differ from centre to centre on the overall tumour detection rate and there is still debate as to whether it is more sensitive than conventional bone scanning for identifying tumour deposits in bone. Equally uncertain is its overall role in the detection of the metastatic spread of neuroblastoma to bone marrow. Questions about the overall efficacy of *m*IBG as a scintigraphic agent have undoubtedly arisen through the use of different amounts of *m*IBG, the time for which images are taken, and the actual isotope of iodine attached to the guanethidine analogue. Sufficient data has accrued on the use of [131]I *m*IBG to have shown that the sensitivity of imaging increases with the amount of the compound used. Furthermore, as discussed above, [123]I *m*BG is a better imaging agent than ^{131}I *m*BG simply due to the physical properties of the two isotopes of iodine. Unfortunately, the former isotope is relatively expensive and is currently available in limited quantities.

In addition to being highly effective as an imaging agent for pheochromocytoma and neuroblastoma, ^{131}I*m*IBG has been used as a scintigraphic agent for other tumours and disease states. It has been successfully used to image retinoblastoma (Bomanji *et al.*, 1989), medullary carcinoma of the thyroid (Sinzinger *et al.*, 1984), and insulomas (Geatti *et al.*, 1989). Less successful results have been obtained with melanoma and bronchial cell carcinoma (Osei-Bonsu *et al.*, 1989). Outside cancer medicine, ^{131}I*m*IBG has been used experimentally for the early detection of myocardial infarction (Fagret *et al.*, 1989). Care has to be taken in the use of *m*IBG to make sure that other medication does not interfere with its uptake into cells. Antagonists of adrenergic receptors and some calcium blockers can interfere with the uptake of *m*IBG.

24.5.2 THERAPY

Many groups have now attempted to treat relapsed neuroblastoma with ^{131}I *m*IBG. The results of these studies vary markedly from centre to centre, but in the majority of cases, responses have been noted. Voute *et al.* (1990) recently reported the results of a study of 47 relapsed neuroblastoma patients who received a total of 135 doses of *m*IBG. In the majority of cases, 7.4 GBq (200 mCi) was administered as the first doses, followed by subsequent doses of 3.7 GBq (100 mCi). Seven complete remissions were recorded lasting for periods of between 5–23 months. In addition, 22 partial remissions were obtained, ten patients showed no change in their disease status and eight progressed on therapy. The results underline one major difficulty in this type of therapy, this being how to determine response. If overall tumour

shrinkage/disappearance of disease is important, then one should not use *m*IBG scintigraphy to determine the efficacy of *m*IBG therapy. It is now clear that after one or several *m*IBG therapies, tumour may no longer take up the guanethidine analogue and even appear as 'filling defects' after *m*IBG scintigraphy. The alternative argument used by individuals assessing *m*IBG therapy in the above manner is that it is the biologically active disease that is important. If tumour does not take up *m*IBG then it is presumed inert and therefore not a therapeutic problem. It is not known which of these arguments is correct although cases have been reported where further shrinkage of tumour has been observed by CT scan after patients with 'non-imagable' *m*IBG tumour have received alternative chemotherapy. A further problem relating to *m*IBG therapy is the difficulty in obtaining accurate tumour dosimetry. This naturally depends upon accurate measurement of disease. Even CT and NMR cannot supply information about the uniformity of *m*IBG deposition within solid tumours and therefore accurate dosimetry is impossible. Despite these problems, Voute *et al.* (1990) have clearly demonstrated efficacy of *m*IBG in relapsed patients and, as a consequence, are currently treating patients with the material at diagnosis. Due to logistical reasons, they give patients one course of chemotherapy and then directly follow this with *m*IBG therapy.

An alternative to giving patients set doses of *m*IBG is to administer the material in such a way as to give patients a set total body dose of radiation. This approach has been explored by the UK Children's Cancer Study Group (UKCCSG) in a multi-centre study. Patients who failed induction chemotherapy with imagable disease were initially given an *m*IBG scan and the dose calculated to give a whole body dose between 1 and 2.5 Gy. Twenty-six treatments were undertaken in 24 children, indicating that individuals predominantly received only one injection of the guanethidine analogue. Patients were assessed for response based on conventional imaging. Seven of 22 fully accessible patients had a partial response, nine had stable disease, and six progressed through therapy. Toxicity noted in this study (and in several others including that of Voute) was primarily haemopoietic and clear responses to therapy were noted.

Despite inaccuracies in determining the dose of radiation targeted to tumours, most estimates indicate that it is insufficient to irradiate a solid tumour deposit. This conclusion is implied by the work of Moyes *et al.* (1989) who administered diagnostic amounts of radiolabelled *m*IBG prior to surgery. At tumour resection, values of between 0.0013% and 0.07% of the injected dose per gram of tumours were obtained. These results suggest *m*IBG needs to be used in combination with other therapeutic modalities to maximize its efficacy. One possibility is to use targeted radiation therapy to replace external beam total body irradiation as part of the high dose chemo-radiation regimens used with autologous bone marrow rescue. Another option is to replace a fraction of external beam radiation with targeted radiation as a way of increasing the therapeutic index. A final option is to attempt to replace the iodine with another halogen, namely [211]astatine, which is more cytotoxic (see below). Further work is necessary to discover which of these options, if any, will prove the most efficient for therapy.

24.5.3 BASIC STUDIES

Until recently, few human neuroblastoma cell lines have been available to study the uptake of *m*IBG. Extrapolation from pheochromocytoma cell line studies has been made and this suggests that uptake is via the type one mechanism involved in amine transport into cells. This mechanism is dependent on an energy-dependent sodium gradient and is specifically blocked by the tricyclic anti-depressant desipramine. Storage of *m*IBG in pheochromocytoma cells has been shown to occur in neurosecretory granules. Three neuroblastoma cell lines have now been identified and all take up *m*IBG in a similar manner to pheochromocytoma cells. However, all three lines store *m*IBG cytoplasmically rather than in neurosecretory granules. Whether this is simply due to a paucity of granules within these cells or to a fundamentally different biochemical pathway is not known. This information is critical to understanding the overall mechanism of *m*IBG toxicity particularly as Smets *et al.* (1989) have demonstrated that the guanethidine analogue can interfere with mono-ADP-ribosyl transferases. To extrapolate from this study, *m*IBG may have a direct cytotoxic effect upon cells. This has been reported at non-physiological levels but preliminary data from the study of the SK-N-BR(2c) cell line indicates that this may also occur with concentrations of drug similar to those found in the serum of patients receiving therapeutic amounts of *m*IBG. The biodistribution of *m*IBG is also critical in deciding on the isotope of iodine to be used for therapy. Some groups have suggested a role for [125]I *m*BG, particularly in killing neuroblasts in bone marrow. Cytotoxicity of ^{125}I depends on Auger electrons (Woo *et al.*, 1990) resulting in the deposition of energy within extremely limited ranges. For [125]I *m*IBG to be effective, it needs to be close to or within the nuclear membrane for it to exert its effect on DNA.

24.5.4 FUTURE DIRECTIONS FOR *m*IBG RESEARCH

Both *in vivo* and *in vitro* studies on the accumulation of *m*IBG into cells have profound implications for its further development. In particular, pharmacokinetic strategies may be found for increasing the retention of *m*IBG into tumour deposits. For example, nifedipine has been shown to improve the accumulation of *m*IBG into pheochromocytoma cells (Blake *et al.*, 1989). However, other studies have reported that some calcium antagonists can block *m*IBG uptake into cells. At least theoretically [211]As can be linked to *m*IBG via the same chemistry as iodine, both elements being members of the halogen family. Whether this is practically possible and whether *m*ABG will be taken up into cells in a similar manner to *m*IBG needs to be resolved. For the longer term, a search for an alternative compound to *m*IBG and ways to modify its uptake and release from cells could be a fruitful area of research. Whatever developments take place in the next few years it is clear that radiopharmaceuticals, like monoclonal antibodies, do not offer immediate solutions to specific cancer therapy. They will almost certainly find a role in future treatments but this is likely to be in combination with other modalities.

REFERENCES

Baldwin, R.W. and Byers, V.S. (1989) Monoclonal antibody immunoconjugates for cancer treatment. *Curr. Opin. Immunol.*, **1**(5), 891–4.

Blake, G.M., Lewington, V.J., Zivanovic, M.A. and Ackery, D.M. (1989) Glomerular filtration rate and the kinetics of [123]I *meta*-iodobenzylguanidine. *Eur. J. Nucl. Med.*, **15**(9), 618–23.

Bomanji, J., Hungerford, J.L., Kingston, J.E., *et al.* (1989) [123]I *meta*-iodobenzylguanidine (MIBG) scintigraphy of retinoblastoma: preliminary experience. *Br. J. Ophthalmol.*, **73**(2), 146–50.

Brown, S.L., Miller, R.A., Horning, S.J. *et al.* (1990) Treatment of B-cell lymphomas with anti-idiotype antibodies alone and in combination with alpha inferon. *Blood*, **73**(3), 651–61.

Byers, V.S., Rodvien, R., Grant, K. *et al.* (1990) Phase I study of monoclonal antibody-ricin A chain immunotoxin XomaZyme-791 in patients with metastatic colon cancer. *Cancer Res.*, **49**(21), 6153–60.

Coderre, J.A., Kalef-Ezra, J.A., Fairchild, R.G. *et al.* (1988) Boron neutron capture therapy of a murine melanoma. *Cancer Res.*, **48**(22), 6313–6.

Courtney, V.D. and Mills, J. (1978) An *in vitro* colony assay for human tumours growing in immune special mice treated *in vivo* with cytotoxic agents. *Br. J. Cancer*, **37**, 261–8.

Davis, T.L. and Wiley, R.G. (1989) Anti-Thy-1 immunotoxin, OX7-saporin, destroys cerebellar Purkinje cells after intraventricular injection in rats. *Brain Res.*, **504**(2), 216–22.

Epenetos, A.A., Courtenay-Luck, N. and Snook, S.J. (1987) Antibody guided irradiation of advanced ovarian carcinoma with intra-peritoneally administered radiolabelled monoclonal antibody. *J. Clin. Oncol.*, **12**, 1890–9.

Fagret, D., Wolf, J.E. and Comet, M. (1989) Myocardial uptake of *meta* (^{123}I) Iodo-benzylguanidine ([123]I *m*IBG) in patients with myocardial infarct. *Eur. J. Nucl. Med.*, **15**, 624–31.

Ferrini, S., Prigione, I., Mammoliti, S. *et al.* (1989) Re-targeting of human lymphocytes expressing the T-cell receptor gamma/delta to ovarian carcinoma cells by the use of bispecific monoclonal antibodies. *Int. J. Cancer*, **44**(2), 245–50.

Foxwell, B.M., Band, H.A., Long, J. *et al.* (1988) Conjugation of monoclonal antibodies to a synthetic peptide substrate for protein kinase: a method for labelling antibodies with [32]P. *Br. J. Cancer*, **57**(5), 489–93.

Geatti, O., Shapiro, B. and Barillari, B. (1989) Scintigraphic depiction of an insulinoma by [131]I *meta*-iodobenzylguanidine. *Clin. Nucl. Med.*, **14**(12), 903–5.

Hericourt, J. and Richet, C. (1895) Treatment of a case of sarcoma with chemotherapy. *Proc. Natl. Acad. Sci.*, **120** 984–50.

Hertler, A.A. and Frankel, A.E. (1990) Immunotoxins: a clinical review of their use in the treatment of malignancies. *J. Clin. Oncol.*, **7**(12), 1932–42.

Hoefnagel, C.A., Voute, P.A., De Kraker, J. and Marcuse, H.R. (1987) Radionuclide diagnosis and treatment of neural crest tumours using [131]I *meta*-iodobenzylguanidine. *J. Nucl. Med.*, **28** 308–14.

Iwahashi, T., Tone, Y., Usui, J. *et al.* (1989) Selective killing of carcinoembryonic antigen (CEA)-producing cells *in vitro* by the immunoconjugate cytorhodin-S and CEA-reactive cytorhodin-S antibody CA208. *Cancer Immunol. Immunother.*, **30**(4), 239–46.

Jain, R.K. (1990) Tumour physiology and antibody delivery, in *The Present and Future Role of Monoclonal Antibodies in the Management of Cancer.* (eds J.M. Vaeth and J.L. Meyer) Karger, Basle **24** 32–46.

Jones, D., Lashford, L.S., Dicks-Mireaux, C. and Kemshead, J.T. (1987) Therapeutic application of radiolabelled monoclonal antibody UJ13A in patients and animal models. *Nat. Cancer Inst. Monographs*, **3**, 125–30.

Kalofonos, H.P., Sivolapenko, G.B., Courtenay Luck, N.S. *et al.* (1988) Antibody guided targeting of non-small cell lung cancer using ^{111}In-labelled HMFG1 F(ab')$_2$ fragments. *Cancer Res.*, **48**, 1977–84.

Koizumi, M., Endo, K., Kunimatsu, M. *et al.* (1988) ^{67}Ga-labelled antibodies for immunoscintigraphy and evaluation of tumour targeting of drug-antibody conjugates in mice. *Cancer Res.*, **48**, 1189–94.

Kornguth, S.E., Turski, P.A., Perman, W.H. *et al.* (1987) Magnetic resonance imaging of gadolinium-labelled monoclonal antibody polymers directed at human T lymphocytes implanted in canine brain. *J. Neurosurg.*, **66**(6), 898–906.

Kralovec, J., Spencer, G., Blair, A.H. *et al.* (1989) Synthesis of methotrexate-antibody conjugates by regiospecific coupling and assessment of drug and antitumor activities. *J. Med. Chem.*, **32**(11), 2426–31.

Liang, Y.Y., Wang, N.Q., Li, N. *et al.* (1989) The selective cytotoxicity of monoclonal antibody conjugated with mitomycin C on human gastric cancer cells. *Yao Hsueh Hsueh Pao* (Acta Pharmaceutica Sinica [Peking]) **24** (11), 801–6.

Marsh, J.W. and Klinman, D.M. (1990) Development of a diphtheria toxin mutant conjugate directed against antigen-specific B cells expressing high affinity surface Ig. *J. Immunol.*, **144**(3), 1046–51.

Mather, S.J. and Ellison, D. (1990) Reduction mediated technetium-[99]m labelling of monoclonal antibodies. *J. Nucl. Med.*, **31**, 692–7.

Moi, M.K., DeNardo, S.J. and Meares, C.F. (1990) Stable bifunctional chelates of metals used in radiotherapy. *Cancer Res.*, **50**, 789s–793s.

Moseley, R.P., Davies, A.G., Richardson, R.B. *et*

al. (1990) Intrathecal administration of ^{131}I radiolabelled monoclonal antibody as a treatment for neoplastic meningitis *Br. J. Cancer.*, **62**, 637–47.

Moyes, J.S., Babich, J.W., Carter, R. *et al.* (1989) Quantitative study of radiodirected *meta*-iodobenzylguanadine uptake in children with neuroblastoma in correlation with tumour histopathology. *J. Nucl. Med.*, **30**, 474–80.

Nitta, T., Sato, K., Yagita, H. *et al.* (1990) Preliminary trial of specific targeting therapy against malignant glioma. *Lancet*, **i**, 368–71.

O'Connell, M.J., Chen, Z.J., Yang, H. *et al.* (1990) Active specific immunotherapy with anti-idiotypic antibodies in patients with solid tumours. *Semin. Surg. Oncol.*, **5**(6), 441–7.

Osei-Bonsu, A., Kokoschka, E.M., Ulrich, W. and Sinzinger, H. (1989) [131]I *meta*- iodobenzylguanidine (*m*IBG) for bronchial oat cell cancer and melanoma detection? *Eur. J. Nucl. Med.*, **15**, 629–31.

Paganelli, G., Magnani, P., Siccardi, A.G. and Fazio F. (1990) Radiolocalization of tumour pretargeted with biotinylated monoclonal antibody. *The 7th International Meeting on Advances in the Application of Monoclonal Antibodies in Clinical Oncology*, abstract. *Eur. J. Cancer*, **26**, (9), 1013

Patel, K., Rossell, R.J., Bourne, S. *et al.* (1990) Monoclonal antibody UJ13A recognizes the neural cell adhesion molecule (NCAM). *Int. J. Cancer*, **44** 1062–8.

Patel, K., Rossell, R.J., Pemberton, L.F. *et al.* (1989) Monoclonal antibody 3F8 recognises the neural cell adhesion molecule (NCAM) in addition to the ganglioside GD2. *Br. J. Cancer*, **60**, 861–6.

Pimm, M.V., Perkins, A.C. and Baldwin, R.W. (1987) Diverse characteristics of ^{111}In labelled anti-CEA monoclonal antibodies for tumour immunoscintigraphy: radiolabelling, biodistribution and imaging studies in mice with human tumour xenografts. *Eur. J. Nucl. Med.*, **12**(10), 515–21.

Plotnikov, V.M., Kazakov, S.A. and Merkulov, V.G. (1989) Immunobiological activity of platinum coordination compounds in a complex with immunoglobulin fragments *Biull. Eksp. Biol. Med.*, **108**(9), 313–5.

Priestman T.J. (1989) The Pharmacology of Cytotoxic Drugs in Cancer Chemotherapy: An Intro-

506

duction 3rd edn (ed T.J. Priestman) Chapter 3 Springer-Verlag, Berlin pp. 27–51.

Reimann, K.A., Turner, S., Lambert, J.M. *et al.* (1989) *In vivo* administration of lymphocyte-specific monoclonal antibodies in nonhuman primates. V. Evidence that humoral immune response to monoclonal antibodies and immunotoxin conjugates abrogates their cytotoxic activity. *Transplantation*, **48**(6), 906–12.

Sallustio, S. and Stanley, P. (1990) Isolation of Chinese hamster ovary ribosomal mutants differentially resistant to ricin, abrin, and modeccin.: *J. Biol. Chem.*, **265**(1), 582–8.

Schneck, D., Butler, F., Dugan, W. *et al.* (1990) Disposition of a murine monoclonal antibody vinca conjugate (KS1/4-DAVLB) in patients with adenocarcinomas *Clin. Pharmacol. Ther.*, **47**(1), 36–41.

Shapiro, B., Copp, J.E., Sisson, J.C. *et al.* (1985) [131]I *meta*-iodobenzylguanidine for the locating of suspected pheochromocytoma: experience with 400 cases (441 studies). *J. Nucl. Med.*, **26**, 576–85.

Stevenson, G.T. (1989) Attack on neoplastic cell membranes by therapeutic antibody. *Mol. Cell Biochem.*, **91**(1–2), 33–8.

Sinzinger, H., Renner, F. and Granegger, S. (1984) Unsuccessful [131]I *m*IBG imaging of carcinoid tumours and apudomas. *J. Nucl. Med.*, **25**, 1221–22.

Smets, L.A., Loesberg, C., Janssen, M. *et al.* (1989) Active uptake and extravesicular storage of *meta*-Iodobenzylguanidine in human neuroblastoma SK-N-SH cells. *Cancer Res.*, **49**, 2941–44.

Stuart, J.S., Sivolapenko, G.B., Hird, V. *et al.* (1990) Clearance of ^{131}I-labeled murine monoclonal antibody from patients' blood by intra-venous human anti-murine immunoglobulin antibody. *Cancer Res.*, **50**(3), 563–7.

Thorpe, P.E., Wallace, P.M., Knowles, P.P. *et al.* (1988) Improved antitumor effects of immunotoxins prepared with deglycosylated ricin A-chain and hindered disulfide linkages. *Cancer Res.*, **48**(22), 6396–403.

Voute, P.A., Hoefnagel, C.A., de Kraker, J. and Valdez Olmos, R. (1990) Results of treatment with [131]I *m*IBG in patients with neuroblastoma: Future Prospects. *Progress in Clinical and Biological Research Advances in Neuroblastoma Research 3,* (Eds) A.E. Evans, G.J. D'Angio, A.G. Knudson Jnr and R.C. Seeger. Fifth Symposium, Philadelphia, **366**, 439–45.

Walker, K.A., Mairs, R., Murray, T. *et al.* (1990) Tumour spheroid model for the biologically targeted radiotherapy of neuroblastoma micrometastases. *Cancer Res.*, **50** (3 Suppl), 1000s–1002s.

Winter, G.P. (1989) Antibody engineering. *Philos. Trans. R. Soc. Lond. Biol.* **324**(1224), 537–46.

Wong, J.H., Irie, R.F. and Morton, D.L. (1989) Human monoclonal antibodies: prospects for the therapy of cancer. *Semin. Surg. Oncol.*, **5**(6), 448–52.

Woo, D.V., Dervi, L., Brady, L.W. *et al.* (1990) Auger electron damage induced by radioiodinated ^{125}I monoclonal antibody, in *The Present and Future Role of Monoclonal Antibody in the Management of Cancer.* (eds J.M. Vaeth and J.L. Meyer) Karger, Basle 24: 32–46.

Zalutsky, M.R., Noska, M.A., Colapinto, E.V. *et al.* (1989) Enhanced tumour localization and *in vivo* stability of a monoclonal antibody radioiodinated using N-succinimidyl 3-(tri-n-butyl-stannyl) benzoate. *Cancer Res.*, **49**(20), 5543–9.

Chapter 25

Recent advances and future trends in cancer chemotherapy

D.R. NEWELL

25.1 INTRODUCTION

There can be little doubt that chemotherapy has had a major impact on the treatment of malignant neoplasms. This impact has perhaps been greatest in the setting of paediatric oncology where over 50% of patients can be expected to be alive five years after diagnosis (Craft and Pearson, 1989; Stiller and Bunch, 1990). This was certainly not the case 30 years ago and, although other modalities and early diagnosis have also played a role, the successful treatment of disseminated disease owes much to the use of cytotoxic chemotherapy. In adult oncology the success of chemotherapy is more limited and according to one estimate only 10% of adults with cancer can expect to be cured by drug treatment (Frei, 1985). Thus there is clearly still much to be achieved; this chapter will review recent advances in cancer chemotherapy and attempt to highlight certain areas which might lead to improved therapies in the future.

25.2 SUPPORTIVE CARE AND HIGH DOSE THERAPY

Over the last decade there have been major advances in the general area of supportive care in order to both reduce the impact of cytotoxic chemotherapy on patient quality of life and allow the more routine use of high dose chemotherapy. The first of these developments and, from the point of view of the patient, arguably the most significant, has been the advent of the 5-hydroxy-tryptamine receptor type 3 antagonists as anti-emetics (Merrifield and Chaffee, 1989). Compounds such as ondansetron, granisetron and ICS 205–930 are potent and selective anti-emetics and are devoid of many of the side effects of more conventional therapies, most notably sedation. The compounds are extremely effective in controlling cytotoxic-induced nausea and vomiting even when produced by such emetogens as cisplatin. Although they are not universally effective, particularly in the case of anticipatory vomiting, they are nonetheless a great advance and serve to illustrate well how effective drug therapy can be when the underlying target is defined.

The second significant development in supportive care is the management of haematological toxicity. Here, two advances have been made: the more frequent, although not routine, use of autologous bone marrow transplantation (Frei *et al.*, 1989), and the introduction of haematopoietic growth factors (Dexter, 1989; Devereux and Linch, 1989). In both cases, the major impetus for the bone marrow support has been the desire to administer higher doses of cytotoxic drugs in the expectation that, with higher doses, high response rates will be achieved. Although there are substantial data from retrospective studies that increased dose intensity leads to increased response rates (Hryniuk, 1988; Dodwell *et al.*, 1990), well controlled prospective clinical studies are harder to find. Furthermore, whilst improved response rates have been reported with greater dose intensity, the impact on patient survival has rarely been reported. In the absence of data to show improved survival it is hard to argue for high dose therapy which is often extremely toxic. With the advent of haematopoietic growth factors, prospective studies on the impact of dose intensity on survival should become more feasible. However, it should be noted that while growth factors to lessen leucopenia (G-CSF; GM-CSF) and anaemia (erythropoietin) are now widely available, this is not the case for thrombocytopenia. Furthermore, once haematological toxicity is overcome, a second dose limiting toxicity will be encountered and this is usually in an organ where amelioration is extremely difficult. For example, with alkylating agents, which are common candidates for high dose therapy, gastrointestinal, cardiac and neuronal toxicities (from melphalan, cyclophosphamide and busulphan respectively) become apparent at high doses (Newell and Gore, 1991). To what extent non-haematological toxicity can be overcome by the use of combinations of alkylating agents remains to be seen.

25.3 DEVELOPMENT OF NOVEL ANTICANCER DRUGS

The history of the development of cancer chemotherapy is a mixture of science, serendipity and random screening (Calvert, 1989). Although there is a tendency to belittle the contribution of early workers, the scientific intuition employed was often every bit as good as that achieved today, particularly in view of the limited equipment and resources available. Thus, for example, the observations concerning the effect of mustard gas on soldiers (Krumbhaar and Krumbhaar, 1919) led to the identification of nitrogen mustards as an extremely useful class of anticancer compounds. In this development there was good clinical observation (the identification of degeneration of lymphatic tissue), lateral thinking (the realization that the same effect might occur in tumours of lymphoid origin) and chemistry (the synthesis of the nitrogen mustards as less vesicant derivatives of sulphur mustard). Similarly, the original observation by Rosenberg (Rosenberg *et al.*, 1966) of elongation in bacteria subjected to electrical currents led to the development of cisplatin, another extremely useful drug. In this case the purely serendipitous observation was exploited when it was realized that elongation was due to growth inhibition and that this was not a result of the electrical current but a property of the platinum complexes released from the platinum electrodes used to supply the current. Again, careful reasoning led to the suggestion that tumour inhibition might also be achieved by the use of platinum complexes and, lastly, substantial clinical expertize was required in order to develop clinical schedules (hydration and diuresis) which allowed the routine use of cisplatin.

25.3.1 ANALOGUE DEVELOPMENT

Once a successful lead compound, such as nitrogen mustard or cisplatin, has been identified, analogue studies can be performed and this approach has been the single most successful area of new drug development in cancer chemotherapy. As shown in Table

509

Table 25.1 Analogue development in cancer chemotherapy

Drug class	Parent compound	Analogues
Alkylating agents	Mechlorethamine	Melphalan
		Chlorambucil
		Cyclophos-phamide
		Ifosfamide
	BCNU	CCNU
		MeCCNU
		Fotemustine
Platinum complexes	Cisplatin	Carboplatin
Antimetabolites	Aminopterin	Methotrexate
	Mercaptopurine	Thioguanine
	Fluorouracil	Fluorodeoxy-uridine
Anthracyclines	Daunorubicin	Doxorubicin
		Epirubicin
		Mitozantrone
Plant products	Vincristine/	Vindesine
	Vinblastine	Vinzolidine
	Podophyllotoxin	Etoposide
		Teniposide

25.1, most of the effective agents available today are in fact analogues of earlier compounds and in some cases the original lead compound now only finds occasional if any use.

In general, analogues are developed for the following four major reasons:

1. an analogue is required that has reduced toxicity in comparison to the parent compound, e.g. carboplatin versus cisplatin;
2. a compound is required with a broader spectrum of activity than that of the parent compound, e.g. doxorubicin versus daunorubicin;
3. a new drug is sought with superior pharmacokinetic properties in comparison to the parent, e.g. improved oral bioavailability, as with chlorambucil versus nitrogen mustard;
4. a derivative is needed with superior pharmaceutical properties, e.g. easier formula-

tion, as with etoposide phosphate versus etoposide.

The success of drug development in this area is undoubtedly due to the fact that the underlying problem is usually well defined, i.e. the target properties for the new drug are clear. However, by definition, this approach is dependent upon the identification of new lead compounds and this in turn requires studies on new targets or the use of antitumour screens which will identify compounds with targets different from those already discovered. With currently identified agents most of the obvious goals for analogue synthesis have been successfully achieved with the possible exceptions of a bleomycin analogue which does not produce lung damage and an anthracycline which produces no cardiac toxicity. Although it is appreciated that in the latter case close analogues (e.g. epirubicin) or distant analogues (e.g. mitozantrone) with reduced cardiac side effects are known, they have yet to replace doxorubicin.

25.3.2 NOVEL AGENTS DIRECTED AT THE CELL MEMBRANE AND GROWTH SIGNAL TRANSDUCTION PATHWAYS

Most, although not all, authors would accept that the majority of the currently available cytotoxic drugs act at the level of the nucleus by interrupting DNA replication. This action readily explains the antiproliferative nature of cytotoxic drugs and the relatively limited toxicity of these agents to non-proliferating tissues. In attempting to discover new targets for drug discovery a number of groups have turned away from the nucleus and have focussed their attention on the cell membrane and growth signal transduction pathways. This approach is not purely a reaction, as over the last decade there has been an explosion in our understanding of the biochemistry of cell proliferation and of the lesions that occur in the transformed cell. A central factor in this

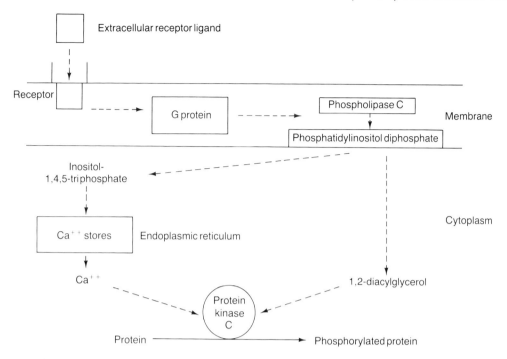

Fig. 25.1 Schematic representation of phospholipase C-G protein coupled signal transduction. (For clarity, protein kinase C and diacylglycerol are shown as being detached from the plasma membrane although they are both bound to the cell membrane *in vivo*.)

understanding was the realization that many viral oncogenes and their cellular counterparts code for components of growth signal transduction pathways thereby providing a mechanistic basis for transformation. An example is the *ras* oncogene family which code for GTP binding proteins which are involved in coupling cell surface receptors to intracellular signal cascades (Bourne *et al.*, 1990). In the transformed state, the aberrant *ras* gene products give rise to inappropriately sustained signals for growth. Similarly, a number of oncogenes code for growth factors or growth factor receptors which again, when inappropriately expressed, give rise to sustained signals for cell division. Figure 25.1 shows in schematic form some of the growth signal transduction pathways which have been identified and in the remainder of this section

some of the attempts made to exploit these as targets for drug design will be considered.

(a) Growth factor receptor targeted agents

The identification of growth factor receptors on the surface of the tumour cells has brought cancer chemotherapy closer than ever before to classical pharmacology. Thus tumour control by molecules which act as antagonists at the growth factor receptor can be seen as analogous to histamine receptor antagonists blocking acid secretion in the stomach. The problem is that while neurotransmitters and autocoids generally have molecular weights of less that 500, most, though not all, growth factors are relatively large polypeptides. Thus drug design in this area has to take on the challenge of working with peptide antagonists.

Of the growth factors implicated in human cancer, gastrin releasing peptide (GRP), the human equivalent of the amphibian peptide bombesin, is one of the smallest (27 amino acids). A seven amino acid segment is further implicated as being the critical moiety for the mitogenic effect of the peptide. GRP and related bombesins are mitogens in human small cell lung cancer lines and hence attempts have been made to block the binding of these growth factors to their receptors by the use of peptide antagonists. Most successful in the field has been Rozengurt and colleagues (Woll and Rozengurt, 1988). These workers have demonstrated that certain 11 amino acid peptides related to substance P can reduce GRP binding in Swiss 3T3 cells and mitogenic effects in small cell lung cancer cell lines. However, it has been shown recently that such peptides can directly interact with G-proteins and hence this effect may not be as specific as originally thought (Mousli *et al.*, 1990). An alternative method of blocking the GRP receptor on small cell lung cancer lines which has also received attention is the use of antibodies to the receptor. This approach has been shown by the group at the US National Cancer Institute to produce antitumour effects against human small cell lung tumours when grown in nude mice (Cuttitta *et al.*, 1985). However, since the antibody used was of murine origin, it suffers from the general clinical limitations inherent in the use of foreign antibodies (see below).

Although GRP has been useful as a model for the development of growth factor receptor antagonists, it suffers from the problem that it is not widely implicated as a growth factor in human cancer. This is not the case for tumour growth factor α (TGFα) which is found in a range of human tumours. TGFα is a close analogue of epidermal growth factor (EGF) and TGFα is thought to promote growth by binding to the EGF receptor (Wells, 1989). In certain tumours, for example, breast cancer, the expression of high levels of EGF receptors has been identified as a poor prognostic factor and hence the EGF receptor has been explored as a target for drug design. In the area of peptide analogues, the early claims by Todaro and coworkers (Nestor *et al.*, 1985) that a relatively small peptide acted as an antagonist have not been substantiated and a more detailed investigation produced only agonists or completely inactive peptides (Defeo-Jones *et al.*, 1988). This area is frustrated by the lack of a three dimensional structure for EGF or its receptor which makes the rational design of EGF receptor antagonists extremely difficult.

Another approach to the modulation of growth factor-receptor interactions involves the removal of extracellular growth factor so that it is not available for receptor binding and hence growth stimulation. This approach is best exemplified by the use of suramin, an acidic molecule which binds a number of polypeptides including TGFα and EGF. In tissue culture, suramin can antagonize the mitogenic effects of a number of growth factors and this observation stimulated clinical trials of the drug, in particular for the treatment of prostatic cancer (Stein *et al.*, 1989; Van Oosetrom *et al.*, 1990; Armand and Cvitkovic, 1990). In early trials, activity has been reported; so, however, has toxicity and it is clear that suramin can only be given with therapeutic drug monitoring if satisfactory levels are to be achieved without the risk of severe toxicity. In general, this is an interesting approach and the design of small molecules to bind to and inactivate growth factors would appear both a feasible and worthwhile goal.

In general terms, the modulation of growth factor receptor-growth factor interactions suffers from the theoretical constraint of being a cytostatic but not a cytotoxic modality. Thus tumour control will in theory only be maintained while there is continual exposure to the agent. In addition, the presence of the antagonist would presumably exert a significant selective pressure on the tumour cell population in favour of growth factor-independent proliferation and thus resistance to the growth factor antagonist might be anticipated. In this respect, growth factor receptor antagonists might well suffer from the problems of antimetabolite cytotoxic chemotherapy where resistance is commonplace. However, set against this is the long-term and highly successful clinical experience with antioestrogens which can be seen as antagonists of the breast tumour growth factor oestradiol (Lerner and Jordan, 1990). In this case the receptor is of course intracellular rather than membrane bound; however, the same general principles apply and, despite this, antioestrogens are extremely useful drugs with breast tumour control being obtained for many years in some patients. Thus there is every reason to hope that growth factor receptor antagonists will also turn out to be useful agents. Perhaps of greater concern is the widespread distribution of growth factor receptors on normal tissues – this may in the long-term limit the clinical utility of antagonists; however, until the antagonists are developed, this question cannot be fully addressed.

(b) Protein kinase C and tyrosine protein kinases

Intracellular protein phosphorylation, catalysed by protein kinases, is an important mechanism in signal transduction, and two kinase activities have been shown to be heavily involved in growth regulation, namely protein kinase C and growth factor receptor-associated tyrosine kinase activities. As shown in Figure 25.1, G-protein linked cell surface receptors activate phospholipase C and this in turn leads to the release of diacylglycerol and inositol 1,4,5-triphosphate (IP3) (see below) by catabolism of

membrane-bound phosphatidylinositol 4,5-diphosphate. The released diacylglycerol itself then activates protein kinase C which is known to be an important event in the regulation of cell division (Krauss *et al.*, 1990). Thus protein kinase C has become a clear target for the development of novel antitumour agents. Attempts to produce potent protein kinase C inhibitors are only now proving successful (Gescher and Dale, 1989) and in any case it is by no means clear that it is an inhibitor that is required. For example, the marine product bryostatin 1 is in fact a protein kinase C activator yet it has antitumour properties and will soon enter clinical trial (Smith *et al.*, 1985). In more general terms, a major concern with protein kinase C, as with most signal transduction pathways, is the ubiquitous nature of the enzyme with the result that antitumour selectivity may be difficult to achieve. As a counter to this concern, it is now known that there are various isoenzyme forms of protein kinase C and hence it may be possible to achieve tumour selectivity (Jaken and Leach, 1988). The area of protein kinase C modulation is clearly still evolving and with the massive industrial and academic activity in this area, active compounds for clinical trial will almost certainly be identified during the next few years.

The second group of kinases that have received extensive attention are the growth factor-associated tyrosine protein kinases. Certain growth factor receptors, for example, EGF and platelet-derived growth factor receptors, have the ability to phosphorylate proteins at tyrosine residues (Wells, 1989; Coughlin and Keating, 1989). This kinase activity is stimulated by binding of the growth factor to the extracellular receptor domain and hence tyrosine kinase activity is implicated in signal transduction. The protein substrates for phosphorylation are not well defined; however, in some cases they include the growth factor receptor itself.

Attempts to synthesize inhibitors of tyrosine kinase activity have met with some success. For example, compounds have now been described that inhibit EGF receptor kinase activity at low μM concentrations which also inhibit EGF stimulated cell growth in culture (Levitzki, 1990). However, as in the case of EGF receptor antagonists, the *in vivo* anti-tumour selectivity of such compounds is still to be defined.

(c) Inositol phosphate analogues to inhibit growth signal transduction

The second arm of the G-protein/ phospholipase C catalysed signal transduction pathway is the release of calcium from intracellular stores, primarily the endoplasmic reticulum. The released calcium acts in concert with diacylglycerol to stimulate protein kinase C (Fig. 25.1). The release of calcium is stimulated by IP3 and the involvement of this inositol phosphate brings into play the whole complex area of inositol phosphate synthesis and catabolism (Downes, 1989; Michell, 1989; Shears, 1989). Obviously, the synthesis of agents based on inositol phosphates has to contend with the problem of how to get the compounds into cells, given that they are likely to be carrying a net negative charge. However, it may be possible to approach this by using pro drug technology. The second area of concern in designing molecules to interact with inositol phosphate signalling is the sheer complexity of the pathway. New inositol phosphates, catabolic and anabolic enzymes are continually being discovered; despite this complexity, however, there is now evidence that it might be possible to develop agents which selectively modify these pathways (Nahorski and Potter, 1989). The use of such compounds in conjunction with our expanding understanding of the role of inositol phosphates should again lead to some interesting new agents. As encouragement in this area we should not forget that lithium, which is thought to act by inhibition of inositol phosphate catabolism, is a useful and safe therapeutic agent. Thus modulation of inositol phosphate metabolism is therapeutically feasible.

(d) Ion fluxes

The final area that has attracted attention in the intracellular transduction pathway of growth signals is that of ion fluxes. Thus, for example, mitogen stimulation in Swiss 3T3 cells leads to an early activation of the sodium/hydrogen antiport which in turn leads to cytoplasmic alkalinization (Rozengurt, 1989). Also, as indicated above, there is an increase in intracellular calcium as a result of IP3 release. These changes in ion fluxes have led to the suggestion that ion channel blockers could be used to produce antiproliferative effects and if this could be achieved selectively in tumour cells it would again be of interest.

Before leaving the area of growth factors and signal transduction pathway modifiers, it is worth pausing for a moment to consider how such agents might be tested in the laboratory and taken into clinical trial. As discussed above, these compounds may only be cytostatic and as such they will be unlikely to produce any effect if one uses traditional clinical criteria to define response. Thus, in clinical trials, an agent that produces no tumour regression, i.e. cytostasis or 'no change', is defined as being inactive. Preclinical pharmacologists are in general more generous with their response criteria scoring compounds which only produce growth inhibition as being active. In either case it is essential that preclinical and clinical scientists adopt the same language to avoid any misunderstanding as these exciting new agents come through into clinical trial.

(e) Novel DNA active agents

Although it is generally accepted that most of

the currently used antitumour agents have the cell nucleus as their target there is a school of thought that argues that we have only just began to exploit DNA as a target for anticancer drug design (Hurley, 1989). By definition, the transformed state is a heritable phenotype and as such the nucleus must contain the information which codes for those characteristics which constitute malignant neoplasia. Indeed, a large number of oncogenes, either mutated, rearranged, or over-expressed, have now been identified in human tumour samples. Thus DNA can be seen as the root cause of transformation in the cancer cell and hence it should perhaps be the prime target for curative cancer chemotherapy. The good antitumour activity of a wide range of DNA interactive agents is taken by many as support for the theory that the nucleus is where anticancer drugs should be directed and thus DNA remains a prime target.

Recent work on the development of agents which interact with DNA has followed two separate but convergent paths. The first concerns studies on the mechanism of action of established DNA interactive drugs. It has been recognized for some time that there is some base sequence preference within the DNA duplex for reaction with, for example, alkylating agents or binding by, for example, anthracyclines. With the application of modern biochemical methods it has been possible to define these in considerable detail. For example, it is now known that the alkylation of guanine at the N^7-position by nitrogen mustards displays some sequence specificity (Kohn *et al.*, 1987) and it is tempting to speculate that the antitumour selectivity of these agents is in some way related to the alkylation of specific sequences critical to survival in tumour cells. Interestingly, the favoured sequences for alkylation are found in the DNA sequence of the c-H-*ras* oncogene and again specific damage to the oncogene

might explain why these agents display antitumour selectivity.

On a more basic point, the development of DNA sequence-specific agents offers the potential for the synthesis of genuinely selective anticancer drugs for the first time. On statistical grounds, a consecutive sequence of 15–16 bases will be unique within the human genome, i.e. the same sequence will not be found anywhere else on the DNA polymer. Given that mutated oncogene sequences have now been described in a number of human cancers, e.g. *ras* oncogenes (Bos, 1989), the ability to uniquely target the mutated DNA sequence would offer the opportunity to selectivity target the DNA of the tumour cell and hence the tumour itself. Broadly speaking there are two reasons why one would want to target a mutated oncogene. Firstly, if expression of the mutated oncogene were essential to tumour cell survival, an agent which damages the gene should switch off its expression and hence kill the tumour cell. Secondly, the mutated oncogene sequence could be used to target generally toxic species to the tumour, for example, free radical generating agents. It is likely that the latter approach would be necessary for tumours where expression of the mutated gene was not vital for survival since it is extremely unlikely that damage to a single gene, i.e. at only one site in the DNA if there is only one gene copy, would itself be a lethal event for the cell.

In terms of the types of agent that have been looked at as models for DNA sequence-specific drugs, three broad types can be identified:

1. derivatives of known DNA reactive agents;
2. DNA sequence-specific oligopeptides;
3. oligodeoxynucleotides.

1. Derivatives of known DNA reactive agents

As discussed above, certain nitrogen mus-

515

tards have been shown to preferentially react, by N[7] alkylation, with guanine bases in particular sequences, GGG for example, in the case of nitrogen mustard, melphalan and chlorambucil (Kohn *et al.*, 1987). In contrast, uracil mustard was found to show equal reactivity towards GGG and 5'-GC-3' sequences. Furthermore, in the case of quinacrine mustard, the introduction of a DNA binding function led to an alteration in the pattern of DNA alkylation. These observations suggest that relatively small molecules can display some sequence-specificity; however, it is debateable as to whether this is of a sufficient level for true antitumour selectivity. Thus it is difficult to see how these agents could be made to recognize the 10–15 base sequences that would be required for complete tumour DNA targeting.

2. DNA sequence-specific oligopeptides

It is now thought that control of transcription is achieved primarily through the interaction of DNA binding proteins with the genome. For this to happen in a selective manner there must be specific protein–DNA interactions in a manner analogous to the adenine:thymine; cytosine.guanine interactions which dictate the interaction of the two strands of the DNA duplex. Although the rules for DNA–protein interactions have yet to be defined in any detail, certain oligopeptides have already been identified which display DNA sequence-specific binding ability. These sequence-specific peptides, most extensively studied by Lown and colleagues (Rao *et al.*, 1990), have been termed lexitropsins and in theory it should be possible to design compounds capable of recognising 10–15 base sequences in DNA. In addition, certain of these compounds possess inherent antitumour activity and this might be increased by the introduction of alkylating and/or free radical generating moieties. In this respect, other natural compounds already combine alkylating activity and sequence-specificity,

e.g. the anthramycins (Hurley, 1989), and again these agents are being used as models for the development of sequence-specific drugs. Although this field is still at an early stage of development, one series of compounds have already reached clinical trial. CC-1065 is a tri-pyrroloindole antibiotic which binds in the minor groove of DNA and reacts covalently with the N[3] of adenine (Hurley *et al.*, 1988). Clinical trials of an analogue of CC-1065 are currently underway and the results are eagerly awaited.

Finally one general point should be kept in mind with compounds of this class. Mechanistically, these agents all bind in the minor groove of DNA and as such the number of recognition points between the drug and DNA are limited. In contrast, DNA binding proteins occupy the major groove which offers far more sites for sequence recognition; thus it is not clear at the moment whether the minor groove will offer sufficient potential for high fidelity sequence-specificity.

3. Oligodeoxynucleotides

In addition to the use of oligonucleotides to suppress translation, i.e. antisense nucleotides, direct interaction of oligonucleotides with DNA to form a triplex has been reported (review by Helene, 1989). In this case, binding is in the major groove and again DNA damage can be induced in a sequence-specific manner if a free radical generating system is included in the molecule, for example, as in EDTA-Fe. One general problem with the use of natural oligonucleotides is that of degradation by nucleases, and, as is described below, phosphate ester modification has been investigated in an attempt to overcome this.

From the discussion in the previous sections it will be clear that the area of DNA sequence-specific agents is still very much in its infancy. Despite that, the potential of genuine tumour selectivity is already clear. Recent methodological advances, e.g. in x-ray crystallography, high field NMR and molecular biology, make rational drug development in this area a reality; however, the time scale for the evolution of clinically useful drugs in this field should be thought of in terms of decades rather than years.

(f) Antisense oligonucleotides

The use of antisense oligodeoxynucleotides is somewhat analogous to the last approach discussed except that it is RNA rather than DNA that is the target. An antisense oligodeoxynucleotide is one with a sequence that is opposite to that of the normal mRNA for a given gene such that a duplex forms between the mRNA and the antisense DNA (Stein and Cohen, 1988). Formation of the duplex will be reversible unless a reactive moiety is attached to the antisense molecule. However, even when a reactive group is not present there may be irreversible damage due to the action of RNase H on the ribonucleotide/deoxyribonucleotide duplex (Helene, 1989). Depletion of the levels of mRNA for the target gene leads to a cessation of translation and, if the gene is required for cell growth, cytostasis will be produced. Using antisense oligodeoxynucleotides, inhibition of gene expression (e.g. *myc*) has been shown *in vitro* and this resulted in an inhibition of cell growth. As an indication of the specificity that can be achieved, in one study N-*myc* expression was inhibited but c-*myc* was not (Rosolen *et al.*, 1990). Again, the *in vivo* application of antisense oligodeoxynucleotides raises a large number of problems and approaches to these are under investigation. Thus, in order to improve nuclease stability, oligomethylphosphonate, oligophosphorothioate and oligo-(α)-deoxynucleosides are being investigated. In addition, to improve cell uptake and mRNA binding, intercalator-oligonucleotide conjugates have been synthesised (Helen, 1989). Although this is another extremely difficult area the potential rewards are high

with ultra specific antitumour agents being a real possibility.

25.4 MODULATION OF DRUG RESISTANCE

Since the earliest days of cytotoxic chemotherapy, the phenomenon of drug resistance has been recognized as a significant clinical problem. Thus early responses to the antifolate aminopterin were short-lived and on retreatment the patients were clearly resistant to the effects of the drug. This problem is still with us today; however, over the last decade, remarkable advances have been made in our understanding of the mechanisms which underlie drug resistance. In uncovering these mechanisms it becomes possible to design strategies for overcoming resistance with the result that it may be possible to prolong response duration or even achieve cures in diseases which hitherto have been classed as chemosensitive but incurable. Clinically, the most impressive example of drug resistance must be small cell lung cancer where initial response rates are high yet recurrence is the rule and second line therapy of any kind is essentially ineffective. Large numbers of mechanisms for resistance are now known and certain of these are summarized in Table 25.2. In the remainder of this section, specific mechanisms will be covered in more detail, along with clinical manoeuvres aimed at their modulation.

25.4.1 P-GLYCOPROTEIN MEDIATED MULTIDRUG RESISTANCE

The 170 000 MW membrane bound P-glycoprotein is found at high levels in a number of tumour cell lines selected for their resistance to natural product cytotoxic drugs. A common feature of this phenotype is that, in addition to the agent used for the selection of the resistant cells, resistance to other

Table 25.2 Examples of cellular mechanisms of resistance to cytotoxic drugs

Mechanism of resistance	Effect	Drugs*
Elevated P-glycoprotein	Increased drug efflux	Doxorubicin Vinca alkaloids Etoposide
Elevated GSH levels	Increased drug detoxication	Melphalan Platinum complexes

Altered target enzyme:
Dihydrofolate reductase
  Topoisomerase II
  Topoisomerase I
	Inadequate enzyme inhibition	Methotrexate
		Etoposide
		Camptothecin

Elevated aldehyde dehydrogenase levels	Increased drug detoxication	Cyclophosphamide Ifosfamide

Elevated O^6-alkylguanine
  alkyltransferase levels
	Repair of drug-induced DNA
	  damage
		Nitrosoureas
		Dacarbazine
		Procarbazine

* For references, see those given in the text.

natural products is also seen. For example, cells made resistant to doxorubicin will often also be insensitive to vincristine and etoposide. This phenotype is described as multidrug resistance. Another common feature of the phenotype is reduced drug accumulation and this has led to the hypothesis that the P-glycoprotein acts as a drug efflux pump thereby reducing intracellular levels. This hypothesis is now generally accepted and there are also now data from a range of human tumour samples which suggests that elevated P-glycoprotein levels underlies certain types of clinical drug resistance (reviews Kaye, 1988; Gerlach, 1989; Fojo, 1989).

Two strategies are being studied to overcome multidrug resistance, namely the co-administration of agents which block the P-glycoprotein pump and the development of novel cytotoxic agents which are not substrates for the P-glycoprotein. In the first strategy, a large number of *in vitro* studies have shown that resistance can be overcome or reduced by the co-administration of agents

such as verapamil, quinidine and cyclosporin. Preclinical *in vivo* demonstrations of reversal of resistance are much harder to find, yet, despite this, a number of clinical trials have been performed. By and large these clinical studies have been unimpressive – for example, studies with verapamil rapidly identified the fact that the cardiac effects of the drug were extreme at the doses needed to achieve the levels required to overcome multidrug resistance *in vitro* (Ozols *et al.*, 1987a). Although other agents might be less toxic and are currently undergoing evaluation (Larson and Fischer, 1989), it is still hard to see why clear evidence for reversal in animal models is not obtained prior to clinical trials. Furthermore, such *in vivo* studies would address the question of antitumour selectivity of P-glycoprotein blockade since potentiation of cytotoxic drug retention in normal tissues cannot be excluded.

The second approach to the circumvention of multidrug resistance has been the development of agents which are not substrates for the P-glycoprotein pump. Thus, for example, the 9-alkylanthracyclines appear to be equipotent against wild-type and multidrug resistant cells whilst 4'-deoxy-4'-iododoxo-rubicin is also active against such cells (Coley *et al.*, 1990; Gianni *et al.*, 1990). This is another area of intense research activity and new agents or drug combinations will be coming to clinical trial in increasing numbers in the near future.

25.4.2 GLUTATHIONE AND GLUTATHIONE-S-TRANSFERASES

A number of antitumour agents are either electrophilic (e.g. alkylating agents) or can give rise to electrophilic species within the cell (e.g. aquated platinum drugs). The sul-phydryl group is amongst the most nucleo-philic species found in the cell and hence sulphydryl groups represent a prime site for reaction with electrophilic antitumour agents or electrophilic species derived from cytotoxic drugs (Hinson and Kadlubar, 1988). Of the non-protein-bound thiols in the cell, gluta-thione (GSH) is the most concentrated, being present at concentrations of 5-10mM in most mammalian cells. Since reaction with GSH is not itself a toxic event, this reaction consti-tutes an inactivation pathway for electro-philic cytotoxic drugs. The reaction of electrophilic drugs with GSH can occur spon-taneously or it may require enzymatic cataly-sis by the family of enzymes known as the glutathione-S-transferases (GSTs) which are widely distributed and can constitute up to 5% of the total cellular protein content.

As reaction with GSH constitutes inactiva-tion, a number of studies have investigated the link between GSH levels, GST levels and sensitivity to electrophilic cytotoxic drugs (Waxman, 1990). In view of the importance of platinum complexes in cancer treatment, a number of the studies have focused on plati-num resistance. A number of cell lines have been described where resistance to platinum

drugs and elevations in cellular GSH are associated (Hamilton *et al.*, 1989). This has also been the case for some cell lines resistant to the alkylating agent melphalan. Given that elevated GSH protects the cell from electro-philic cytotoxic drugs it is logical that deple-tion of cellular GSH should sensitize the tumour cell. GSH depletion can readily be achieved *in vitro* by the use of buthionine sulfoximine (BSO), an irreversible inhibitor of glutamyl-cysteine synthase, an enzyme in the biosynthetic pathway for GSH. In mice, BSO selectively reduced GSH levels in tumours as opposed to bone marrow and this led to a potentiation of the antitumour activ-ity of melphalan (Ozols *et al.*, 1987b). On the basis of these results, BSO is currently under-going clinical evaluation as a modulator of alkylating agent and platinum drug resist-ance.

The role of GSTs in GSH-mediated drug resistance is less well defined (Tew, 1988; Waxman, 1990). Although slightly elevated GST levels have been described in a number of cell lines, it is by no means clear that the elevation of the GST level is the cause of resistance. Furthermore, experiments involv-ing transfection of GST genes have produced conflicting results as to the chemosensitivity of the transfected cells and thus the role of GST elevations in drug resistance remains open. However, if GSTs are found to be important their inhibition could be achieved by the use of inhibitors such as ethacrynic acid and again this offers the potential for clinical studies.

25.4.3 O⁶-ALKYLGUANINE ALKYLTRANSFERASE

For monofunctional alkylating agents (e.g. dacarbazine, procarbazine) or agents which initially form mono adducts (e.g. chloroethyl-nitrosoureas) reaction with guanine at the O⁶ position is an important mechanism of cyto-toxicity. This is despite the fact the reaction at the N^7 position of guanine is quantitatively more important. The role of O^6 alkylation is implied by the observation that cell lines with high levels of the DNA repair enzyme O^6-alkylguanine alkyltransferase (AT), are resistant to the cytotoxicity of this type of agent (D'Incalci *et al.*, 1988; Pegg, 1990). Thus inhibition of the activity of this repair enzyme should lead to a potentiation of the activity of monofunctional alkylating drugs. Mechanistically, AT acts as a suicide protein, i.e. reaction with its substrate leads to irreversible inactivation of the protein, and hence it may even be incorrect to call the AT protein an enzyme since it is not catalytic in the normal sense. It is known that simple O^6-alkyl and aryl guanines can act as substrates for, and hence depletors of, AT. Thus agents such as O^6-methyl and O^6-benzyl guanine can potentiate the activity of monofunctional alkylating drugs *in vitro*. Clinical trials of O^6-methylguanine are currently being considered in the USA although this agent is not particularly potent and it is likely that the successful application of AT inhibitors must await the development of more potent molecules such as O^6-benzylguanine. The importance of attempting to develop AT inhibitors is shown by the fact that whilst chloroethylnitrosoureas, e.g. BCNU, CCNU and methyl-CCNU, are extremely effective in treating rodent tumours, this class of compound is very unimpressive in patients. The only consistent difference between rodent and human tumours which might explain this is the presence of much higher levels of AT in human cancers. If the combined clinical use of AT inhibitors and nitrosoureas led to the antitumour activity seen in mice with nitrosoureas alone this approach would indeed be a major clinical advance.

The above examples of the enzymes and proteins involved in drug resistance serve to illustrate the substantial improvements in our level of understanding of drug resistance in the last decade. These and certain other enzyme systems implicated are outlined in Table 25.2. It is likely that further examples are still to be revealed and in so doing new targets for the modulation of drug resistance will be exposed.

25.5 ANTIBODY TARGETED THERAPY

With the advent of monoclonal antibody technology the production of antibodies of sufficient quality and quantity for widespread pharmaceutical use has become possible for the first time. Cancer therapists have not been slow to exploit this and five general approaches to the therapeutic use of antibodies are now being studied:

1. direct antibody therapy;
2. antibody directed radiotherapy, i.e. the use of antibodies labelled with therapeutic isotopes;
3. antibody targeting of conventional cytotoxic drugs (Baldwin and Byers, 1989);
4. antibody targeting of potent toxins (Blakey *et al.*, 1988; Hertler and Frankel, 1989);
5. antibody directed enzyme pro drug therapy (ADEPT) (Bagshawe, 1989).

The first two of these approaches should more accurately be regarded as immunotherapy and immunoradiotherapy, rather than chemotherapy, and hence will not be discussed here. The other approaches have received substantial attention over the last decade with clinical trials underway for some agents. For all these approaches the foremost problem is the identification of tumour-associated antigens against which antibodies can be raised. It is interesting that the term 'tumour associated' has tended to replace that of 'tumour specific' as it has become clear that tumour-associated antigens are invariably also present on some normal tissues at some developmental stage. A recent clinical example of this problem was the use of the 'breast cancer specific' 260F9 monoclonal antibody recombinant ricin A chain immunotoxin (Gould *et al.*, 1989). Although preclinical studies failed to detect significant normal tissue binding, clinical studies soon identified serious neurotoxicity and it was subsequently found that the target antigen was expressed on Schwann cells. These types of observation are extremely worrying and pose major questions as to the type of preclinical toxicology that is relevant to the development of antibody targeted drugs.

A second general problem in the development of antibody targeted drugs is the development of host antibodies to the antibody administered. The majority of therapeutic antibodies studied to date have been of murine origin and hence, predictably, they produce human anti mouse antibodies (the HAMA response) when given to patients. This dictates that with murine antibodies the total amount of antibody that can be administered is limited and as such the agent should ideally be extremely effective, that is potentially curative on a single or short course administration schedule. This concern is one of the reasons for the study on antibody toxin conjugates or immunotoxins (ITs) which are highly potent *in vitro* – ITs, for example, are often toxic to cells bearing the target antigen in the region of 10^{-10}M.

Other problems faced by antibody targeted drugs include heterogeneity of antigen expression in the tumour, i.e. not all tumour cells will express the target antigen, and access of these large molecules (usually MW >150,000) to all viable cells within the tumour. As an approach to these latter two problems, Bagshawe *et al.* (1989) have developed the ADEPT philosophy in which the antibody is used to target an enzyme and not a drug or toxin. The enzyme is chosen so as to be able to activate a low molecular weight pro drug which is given once the antibody-enzyme conjugate has been cleared from the normal tissues and the circulation. As the pro drug is converted to the active cytotoxic in

the extracellular fluid is has the potential to damage both antigen positive and negative cells. Furthermore, the low molecular weight of the cytotoxic agent generated should allow good tumour penetration.

25.5.1 ANTIBODY TARGETING OF CONVENTIONAL CYTOTOXIC DRUGS

The central hypothesis in this approach is that cytotoxic drugs, albeit for reasons poorly understood, often possess considerable antitumour selectivity. If this selectivity can be enhanced by antibody targeting then improved clinical results might be expected. The advantage of this approach is that clinicians are already expert in dealing with the side effects of cytotoxic drugs and hence antibody-cytotoxic drug conjugates might prove relatively easy to handle. However, the disadvantage is that large numbers of cytotoxic drug molecules are usually required to kill a single tumour cell. By linking the drug directly to the antibody it may not be possible to achieved satisfactory intracellular levels, i.e. there may be insufficient target cell surface antigens. Since high levels of cytotoxic drug molecules linked directly to the antibody leads to poor antigen recognition, the solution has been to use a carrier, albumin, for example, onto which the cytotoxic drug is loaded. The albumin-drug conjugate is then linked to the antibody for targeting. Foremost in this field has been the Cancer Research Campaign group at Nottingham, (Baldwin and Byers, 1989) which has studied a number of cytotoxic drugs including methotrexate and the vinca alkaloids. In general, the choice of cytotoxic is limited to the more potent agents since, as discussed above, the number of drug molecules that can be delivered to the cell is limited. Although, in experimental systems, *in vivo* data have been produced to support this approach, most workers in the field are of the opinion that the limited potency of these reagents and the ability of cells to develop resistance to conventional cytotoxic drugs limit its overall utility.

25.5.2 IMMUNOTOXINS

The solution to the potency problem identified in the previous section is to link the antibody to extremely potent molecules such as the plant ribosome inactivating proteins (RIPs). These RIPs include ricin, abrin and gelonin which, once internalized, are thought to be able to kill cells at a level of only one molecule per cell. This effect is achieved by catalytically inactivating ribosomes and, in the case of ricin the most widely used toxin, this is performed by the A chain of the toxin. In the intact native toxin, internalization of the A chain is achieved by the B chain of the molecule which is jointed to the A chain by a single disulphide bond. In ITs the B chain is replaced by the antibody which is conjugated to the A chain by a short chain chemical linker and a disulphide bond.

A number of ITs have already been the subject of clinical investigations although to date the results have not been impressive (Spitler *et al.*, 1987; Gould *et al.*, 1989; Byers *et al.*, 1989). Problems observed include binding and toxicity to normal tissues expressing the target antigen (Gould *et al.*, 1989), rapid IT degradation and blood clearance, and the development of the HAMA response. In addition, IT administration is associated with a non-specific vascular leak syndrome, the aetiology of which is not well understood. In general, more specific, stable and potent ITs are needed to overcome these problems and with regard to stability and blood clearance significant advances have been made. Thus it is known that the use of deglycosylated or recombinant ricin A chain produces ITs which persist for longer *in vivo*. Reduced IT clearance in this case is due to the lack of carbohydrate residues on the A chain which aid recognition by the reticuloendothelial sys-

tem. Also, chemical linkers have been developed with hindered disulphide bonds that reduce systemic A chain-antibody cleavage and hence again improve IT persistence. Other current developments include the use of antibody fragments to reduce the molecular weight of ITs and to improve their tumour penetration, and the development of humanized antibodies to reduce the immunogenicity of ITs (Reichmann *et al.*, 1988). It is still too early to comment on the viability of IT therapy in general, in particular the latter approaches; however, this is a field that continues to stimulate a large volume of research and novel agents for clinical trial are likely to be produced in some numbers for the foreseeable future.

25.5.3 ANTIBODY DIRECTED ENZYME PRO DRUG THERAPY (ADEPT)

Although the pro drug concept has been active in cancer chemotherapy for many years it has recently been given a new lease of life with the advent of the ADEPT approach. The major problem with the conventional pro drug approach was the identification of tumour-specific enzymes which could be exploited to selectively catalyse pro drug activation. However, in the ADEPT approach this is no longer a problem as the enzyme can be supplied exogenously and targeted to the tumour by the antibody. Examples of enzymes that have been used for linking to antibodies include carboxypeptidase G2 (Bagshawe, 1989) and alkaline phosphatase (Senter, 1988). In the case of the former, the pro drug is the glutamic acid derivative of benzoic acid mustard; in the latter, phosphates of both etoposide and mitomycin have been used. *In vivo* data with xenografts have shown the feasibility of the ADEPT approach and clinical trials with one pro drug, benzoic acid mustard glutamate, are ongoing in order to define a safe dose of the pro drug for subsequent use with the antibody enzyme conjugate (Bagshawe, 1989). Finally, as a subtle addition to the ADEPT approach, recent work has shown that the use of a second antibody to the enzyme-antibody conjugate can help to remove non-tumour bound enzyme prior to the administration of the pro drug, a manoeuvre which may help to reduce host toxicity due to non-specific release of active drug (Bagshawe, 1989).

In conclusion, antibody targeted therapies clearly have enormous potential in terms of antitumour selectivity. However, as yet, this potential has not been realized in the clinical setting. Since the human being is the only relevant species for toxicological studies, the true value of antibody targeted therapy will only become apparent after extended clinical trials. Although this may take some time, antibody targeted therapy offers the first real chance of achieving Erhlich's goal of the 'magic bullet' and even if there are a few hurdles to jump on the way we should not be discouraged.

25.6 RECENT INITIATIVES IN ANTICANCER DRUG SCREENING

Despite the enormous recent advances in our understanding of the molecular biology of cancer we are still some considerable distance from a full and satisfactory understanding of exactly why cells become and remain transformed, particularly in the clinical setting. Thus, although we may have a number of new targets against which to direct novel drugs, we still need model tumour systems in which to evaluate the likely clinical utility of new agents. In addition to this there remains a need to screen novel chemicals, primarily natural products, in the hope that we might by chance discover useful new drugs. A number of effective agents are either natural products or semi synthetic derivatives thereof – anthracyclines, bleomycins, vinca alkaloids and epipodophyllotox-

ins for example – and as yet only a small fraction of the potential natural products have been examined. Given the depressing rate at which the human race is destroying the ecosystem of our planet, there is a very real possibility that we are losing plants and animals that may yield useful anticancer agents before we have even identified them. Thus there is a very real need for a screening system which can function rapidly and one that is capable of evaluating compounds in large numbers. Such a system should be seen as stop-gap for use while we overhaul rational drug design; given that the latter is still some way off, every attempt should be made to make the screen as predictive as possible.

Historically, the major (quantitatively) drug screening programme has been that carried out at the National Cancer Institute (NCI) in Washington (Goldin *et al.*, 1981). Up until the mid 1980s, the major focus was on *in vivo* activity against mouse tumours with a few agents going through to testing against human tumour xenografts. In various guises this *in vivo* screen has been used to evaluate over half a million compounds since 1955 but since only 40 or so useful drugs were developed during that time, it was deemed to be ineffective. In reviewing the screen, three major weaknesses were identified. Firstly, the majority of the studies were against rodent not human tumours. Secondly, the initial tumours studied in the old *in vivo* rodent screen in order to select out potentially active agents were leukaemic/ lymphoma in origin. Finally, only small numbers of tumours of any one histological type were examined hence the screen was not representative of the heterogeneity of human cancer. Taken together it was felt that these limitations were likely to explain why the only compounds with activity that were selected were active in leukaemia and lymphoma whilst essentially all agents were inactive against common solid adult tumours.

As an alternative to the *in vivo* rodent screen Boyd (1989) proposed the use of panels of immortal human tumour cell lines grown *in vitro* as the primary screen. The major histological types of human cancer were selected for the panel with at least 5–6 different cell lines in each disease category. In practice, it proved difficult to develop sufficient breast cancer cell lines but in the other major disease types sufficient cell lines have been established, i.e. lung, colon, melanoma, renal, CNS and ovary. Obviously, a number of criticisms can be levelled against such an *in vitro* screen. Firstly, the screen will not differentiate between selective anti-tumour agents and general poisons. Secondly, compounds which require host metabolic activation will not be identified. Thirdly, agents which act via complex host-tumour interactions will not be selected. As a response to first criticism, the NCI have stated that it is activity against selected tumour histologies that is being sought and this will exclude general cell poisons. With regard to the second point, it could be argued that metabolic activation by the host as a prerequisite for activity is best avoided. Furthermore, even if mice are used there is no guarantee that they will metabolize compounds in the same way as humans. Finally, where complex host-tumour mechanisms are operative, it is probably best to attempt to understand the mechanism rather than hope that any *in vivo* rodent system will model it satisfactorily.

Thus the new NCI screening initiative certainly deserves a chance to prove itself. The screen is now established and is being used to screen compounds in large numbers. It is probably unreasonable to judge the screen in a period of less than 10 years and in any case given the current, and completely justified, moves away from large scale animal experimentation it is rather difficult to see what could be put in its place. Purists might argue that all the funding should be put into basic research as the more cost effective way of identifying new therapies, but that is not an easy stance to defend on the basis of past success.

Regardless of the mechanism by which a new agent is selected for clinical trial, the advent of human tumour xenografts has provided a method of evaluating likely clinical utility with far more certainly than has hitherto been feasible. Studies by a number of groups, with a number of drugs and in a number of diseases, have shown that the response to human tumours, when grown as xenografts in immune incompetent mice, closely mirrors the response of the tumour in the patient. This is the case for both individual tumour response and the response of disease types in general. Thus pseudo phase II data can be obtained before the new drug has even entered clinical trials (Boven *et al.*, 1988) and clinicians involved in new drug development now expect to see xenograft data included in the preclinical profile of novel agents.

25.7 PHARMACOLOGICALLY GUIDED CYTOTOXIC DRUG ADMINISTRATION

Of all areas of therapeutics, cancer chemotherapy is the one with the smallest therapeutic index. The vast majority of anticancer treatments only show activity, and then to an often limited degree, at toxic doses. In the light of this it seems amazing that for so long cytotoxic drug administration has depended almost exclusively on doses calculated on the basis of surface area alone. The original reasons for doing so are logical and well defined, i.e. a number of parameters vary more closely with surface area than with body weight – metabolic rate, renal function, volumes of blood and extracellular fluid, for example (Pinkel, 1958). However, drug concentrations in the plasma and hence in extracellular fluid, are determined by factors other than these alone and thus surface

Table 25.3 Examples of pharmacokinetic determinants of the activity and toxicity of cytotoxic drugs

Pharmacokinetic parameter	Drug and effect[1]
Poor and/or variable oral bio-availability	MTX – relapse in leukaemia
Peak plasma level	Cisplatin – nephrotoxicity Doxorubicin – cardiotoxicity
Duration of exposure	Etoposide – response in small cell lung cancer MTX – myelosuppression
Plasma AUC/clearance, steady state plasma level	5FU – myelosuppression/gastrointestinal toxicity Busulphan – neurotoxicity[2] Carboplatin – thrombocytopenia Etoposide – response in solid tumours[3] MTX – response in ALL Teniposide – activity in leukaemia/solid tumours Vinblastine – leucopenia Vincristine – neurotoxicity
Toxic metabolite formation	Cyclophosphamide/ifosfamide – urotoxicity Ifosfamide – neurotoxicity
Active metabolite level	AraC – response in leukaemia 6MP – neutropenia

1. References as given in the text.
2. Vassal *et al.*, 1990
3. Desoize *et al.*, 1990

area will not account for all the inter individual variation seen. For example, inter individual variation may be genetic in origin, i.e. pharmacogenetic, or result from specific organ abnormalities due to prior treatment or disease. Taken together, these variables are best dealt with by therapeutic drug monitoring (TDM) which is already commonplace in other areas of therapy, as for example phenytoin and cardiac glycoside chemotherapy.

The evidence for host drug handling, i.e. pharmacokinetics, as a major determinant of the activity and toxicity of cytotoxic drugs, is now overwhelming (Newell, 1989; Evans and Relling, 1989) and specific examples are summarized in Table 25.3. Attempts are already being made to prospectively validate phar-macokinetically guided dosing. In the field of paediatric oncology, the treatment of acute lymphocytic leukaemia by TDM is underway at the St Jude Hospital in Memphis and the results from this trial are eagerly awaited. This initiative is built on the earlier observation that for both methotrexate and teniposide pharmacokinetics are a major independent determinant of response (Evans and Relling, 1989). Clearly, if the ongoing TDM studies prove to be positive and response rates and/or duration of remission are improved by the application of TDM, the resource implications will be significant. However, analytical techniques continue to improve and there is no fundamental reason why assays for the more commonly used agents cannot be fully automated.

Another area of clinical oncology where pharmacokinetically guided dosing is making a major impact is in the field of new drug trials. This is an area fraught with ethical problems as patients offered experimental chemotherapy are often in a psychologically compromised position. Thus extra care is needed to ensure that therapy stands a chance of offering what the patient expects, activity, without risking what the clinician fears, life threatening toxicity. These problems are particularly acute at the initiation of a new drug trial when there are absolutely no human data on which to base the dose to be given. Retrospective data from a very large number of studies have shown that for conventional cytotoxic drugs 1/10th the dose which gives 10% lethality in mice (the LD10) is a safe phase I starting dose when expressed in terms of mg/m^2 (Greishaber and Marsoni, 1986). However, similar retrospective studies also show that the safe dose for therapeutic studies in humans, usually just below the maximum tolerated dose (MTD), can lie anywhere between 1 and 100 times the phase I starting dose. In the mid 1980s, Collins and co-workers at the NCI made a major contribution to experimental cancer chemotherapy when they identified pharmacokinetic variability as a major reason for the discrepancy between the LD10 dose in mice and the MTD in patients (Collins *et al.*, 1986). In Table 25.4, the ratios of the MTD in patients to the LD10 in mice, and the ratios of the areas under the plasma drug concentration versus time curves (AUCs) at these doses, are given for a number of drugs. As can be seen, for most compounds, the ratios of the AUC values are much closer to unity that the ratios of the doses, which implies that much of the dose variation can be explained by pharmacokinetics. The AUC is used in these comparisons as a single measure of whole body exposure to the drug, that is, it reflects both the level of the drug and its persistence. AUC is a valid measure of drug exposure for agents which interact with their target either by tight binding (e.g. DNA binding drugs), or covalent reaction (e.g. alkylating agents). For enzyme inhibitors, duration of exposure at or above a given plasma level is more likely to relate to cytotoxic activity and this may explain why AUC related no better to toxicity than did dose for antimetabolites.

The realization that AUC values may relate

Table 25.4 Comparison of doses and areas under plasma concentration versus times curves (AUCs) in mice (LD10 dose) and patients (MTD)[1]

Drug	MTD/LD10 Dose ratio	MTD/LD10 AUC ratio
Alkylating agents/ platinum complexes		
Carboplatin	1.1	1.0
Cisplatin	2.2	1.3
Diaziquone	1.0	1.0
Teroxirone	4.3	0.8
Thio-TEPA	0.4	1.0
Antimetabolites		
5-Azacytidine	6.0	1.1
Dihydroazacytidine	1.2	0.3
Fludarabine	0.1	0.1
PALA	2.8	3.3
Pentostatin/DCF	0.7	1.1
Tiazofurin	0.7	0.9
DNA binding drugs		
Amsacrine	0.8	1.3
CI941[2]	0.9	1.1
Doxorubicin	5.0	0.8
Iododoxorubicin[3]	4.4	0.7
Piroxantrone[4]	2.1	1.0
Miscellaneous		
Indicine-N-oxide	0.9	0.6
Trimelamol[5]	4.8	1.3

1. References as given in the text.
2. Graham *et al.*, 1989 and unpublished
3. Gianni *et al.*, 1990
4. Hantel *et al.*, 1990; Ames *et al.*, 1990
5. Judson *et al.*, 1989

more closely to toxicity than dose led Collins and co-workers to propose that AUC values be used in dose escalation strategies during phase I clinical trials. The intention in so doing is to allow more aggressive dose escalation at non-toxic doses and to control dose increments more carefully at or near the MTD. A number of schemes have been proposed as to how this might be done (Collins *et al.*, 1986, EORTC Pharmacokinetics and Metabolism Group, 1987) and prospective clinical data are now becoming available. Although it is still too early to comment on the overall value of the approach, it is already clear that the inclusion of more basic science in early clinical trials is improving their quality. In addition, it is easy to see how early clinical trials could be improved even further by the inclusion of basic mechanistic investigations. Thus drug-target interactions can now be studied in the clinical setting with such techniques as NMR, flow cytometry, and antibody detection of drug induced damage. Failure to include detailed pharmacokinetic and mechanistic studies in early clinical trials might almost be considered unethical, given the substantial commitment made by the patient in accepting experimental therapy. As such, early clinical trials should only be attempted in specialist centres that can offer good laboratory backup.

In summary, although the clinical pharmacology of antitumour agents has been under study for over three decades, it is only now that the benefits are being reaped. The improved use of existing and novel antitumour agents, through an improved understanding of their clinical pharmacology, will almost certainly make a major impact on response rates and, it is hoped, on survival in chemosensitive diseases.

25.8 CONCLUSIONS

There is every reason to be extremely optimistic about the future prospects for cancer chemotherapy. Improved antitumour selectivity, shown as both reduced toxicity and greater activity, can be anticipated in a number of diseases and with a number of agents. Furthermore, there is no evidence of any shortage of targets for the development of new drugs. Every angle of the molecular biology of cancer that is opened up offers new loci at which antitumour agents can be directed. In developing these agents, the experimental chemotherapist can call upon the powerful methods of computer-assisted drug design and biotechnology, thereby both improving the efficiency of drug development and the spectrum of agents that can be contemplated. Once detailed pharmacology, preclinical and clinical, is added to this recipe for new drug development, substantial improvements in cancer therapy must follow.

REFERENCES

Ames, M.M., Loprinzi, C.L., Collins, J.M. *et al.* (1990) Phase I and clinical evaluation of piroxantrone hydrochloride (oxantrazole). *Cancer Res.*, **59**, 3905–9.

Armand, J.P. and Cvitkovic, E. (1990) Suramin: A new therapeutic concept. *Europ. J. Cancer*, **26**, 417–9.

Bagshawe, K.D. (1989) Towards generating cytotoxic agents at cancer sites. *Br. J. Cancer*, **60**, 275–81.

Baldwin, R.W. and Byers, V.S. (1989) Monoclonal antibody immunoconjugates for cancer treatment. *Curr. Opin. Immunol.*, **1**, 891–4.

Blakey, D.C., Wawrzynczak, E.L., Wallace, P.M. *et al.* (1988) Antibody-toxin conjugates: a perspective, in *Monoclonal Antibody Therapy*, (ed. H. Waldmann), Karger, Basel, pp. 50–90.

Bos, J.L. (1989) *ras* Oncogenes in human cancer: A review. *Cancer Res.*, **49**, 4682–9.

Bourne, H.R., Sanders, D.A. and McCormick, F. (1990) The GTPase superfamily: a conserved switch for diverse cell functions. *Nature*, **348**, 125–32.

Boven, E., Winograd, B., Fodstad, O. *et al.* (1988) Preclinical phase II studies in human tumour lines: a European multicenter study. *Europ. J. Cancer Clin. Oncol.*, **24**, 567–73.

Boyd, M.R. (1989) Status of the NCI preclinical antitumor drug discovery screen. *Principles and Practice of Oncology Updates*, **3**, 1–12.

Byers, V.S., Rodvien, R., Grant, K. *et al.* (1989) Phase I study of monoclonal antibody-ricin A chain immunotoxin Xomazyme-791 in patients with metastatic colon cancer. *Cancer Res.*, **49**, 6153–60.

Calvert, A.H. (1989) Introduction: A history to the progress of anticancer chemotherapy. *Cancer Surveys*, **8**, 493–509.

Coley, H.M., Twentyman, P.R. and Workman, P. (1990) 9-Alkyl, morpholinyl anthracyclines in the circumvention of multidrug resistance. *Europ. J. Cancer*, **26**, 665–7.

Collins, J.M., Zaharko, D.S., Dedrick, R.L. *et al.* (1986) Potential roles for preclinical pharmacology in phase I clinical trials. *Cancer Treat. Rep.*, **65**, 89–95.

Coughlin, S.R. and Keating, M.T. (1989) The platelet-derived growth factor system. *Cancer Treat. Res.*, **47**, 169–76.

Craft, A.W. and Pearson, A.D.J. (1989) Three decades of chemotherapy for childhood cancer: from cure 'at any cost' to 'cure at least cost'. *Cancer Surveys*, **8**, 605–29.

Cuttitta, F., Carney, D.N., Mulshine, J. *et al.* (1985) Bombesin-like peptides can function as autocrine growth factors in small-cell lung cancer. *Nature*, **316**, 823–6.

Defeo-Jones, D., Tai, J.Y., Wegrzyn, R.J. *et al.* (1988) Structure-function analysis of synthetic and recombinant derivatives of transforming growth factor alpha. *Mol. Cell Biol.*, **8**, 2999–3007.

Desoize, B., Marechal, F. and Cattan, A. (1990) Clinical pharmacokinetics of etoposide during 120 hours continuous infusions in solid tumours. *Br. J. Cancer*, **62**, 840–1.

Devereux, S. and Linch, D.C. (1989) Clinical significance of the haematopoietic growth factors. *Br. J. Cancer*, **59**, 2–5.

Dexter, T.M. (1989) Haematopoietic growth factors. *Br. Med. Bull.*, **45**, 337–49.

D'Incalci, M., Citti, L., Taverna, P. *et al.* (1988) The importance of the DNA repair enzyme O^6-alkyl guanine alkyltransferase (AT) in cancer chemotherapy. *Cancer Treat. Rev.*, **15**, 279–92.

Dodwell, D.J., Gurney, H. and Thatcher, N. (1990). Dose intensity in cancer chemotherapy. *Br. J. Cancer*, **61**, 789–94.

Downes, C.P. (1989) The cellular functions of *myo*-inositol. *Biochem. Soc. Trans.*, **17**, 259–68.

EORTC Pharmacokinetics and Metabolism Group (1987). Pharmacokinetically guided dose escalation in Phase I trials. Commentary and proposed guidelines. *Eur. J. Cancer Clin. Oncol.*, **23**, 1083–7.

Evans, W.E. and Relling, M.V. (1989) Clinical pharmacokinetics-pharmacodynamics of anticancer drugs. *Clin. Pharmacokinetics*, **16**, 327–36.

Fojo, A.T. (1989) Multidrug resistance in human tumours. *Cancer Treat. Res.*, **48**, 27–36.

Frei, E. III. (1985) Curative cancer chemotherapy. *Cancer Res.*, **45**, 6523–37.

Frei, E. III., Antman, K., Teicher, B. *et al.* (1989) Bone marrow autotransplantation for solid tumours – prospects. *J. Clin. Oncol.*, **7**, 515–26.

Gerlach, J.H. (1989) Structure and function of P-glycoprotein. *Cancer Treat. Res.*, **48**, 37–53.

Gescher, A. and Dale, I.L. (1989) Protein kinase C – a novel target for rational anticancer drug design? *Anticancer Drug Des.*, **4**, 93–105.

Gianni, L., Vigano, L. and Surbone, A. (1990) Pharmacology and clinical toxicity of 4'-iodo-4'deoxydoxorubicin: An example of successful application of pharmacokinetics to dose escalation in phase I trials. *J. Natl. Cancer Inst.*, **82**, 469–77.

Goldin, A., Venditti, J.M., MacDonald, J.S. *et al.* (1981) Current results of the screening program at the Division of Cancer Treatment, National Cancer Institute. *Eur. J. Cancer*, **17**, 129–42.

Gould, B.J., Borowitz, M.J., Groves, E.S. *et al.* (1989) Phase I study of an anti-breast cancer immunotoxin by continuous infusion: Report of a targeted toxic effect not predicted by animal studies. *J. Natl. Cancer Inst.*, **81**, 755–81.

Graham, M.A., Newell, D.R., Foster, B.J. *et al.* (1989) The pharmacokinetics and toxicity of the anthrapyrazole anti-cancer drug CI-941 in the mouse: a guide for rational dose escalation in patients. *Cancer Chemother. Pharmacol.*, **23**, 8–14.

Greishaber, C.K. and Marsoni, S. (1986) Relation of preclinical toxicology to findings in early clinical trials. *Cancer Treat. Rep.*, **70**, 65–72.

Hamilton, T.C., Lai, G.M., Rothenberg, M.L. *et al.*

(1989) Mechanisms of resistance to cisplatin and alkylating agents. *Cancer Treat. Res.*, **48**, 151–69.

Hantel, A., Donehower, R.C., Rowinsky, E.K. *et al.* (1990) Phase I study and pharmacodynamics of piroxantrone (NSC 349174), a new anthra-pyrazole. *Cancer Res.*, **50**, 3284–8.

Helene, C. (1989) Artificial control of gene expression by oligodeoxynucleotides covalently linked to intercalating agents. *Br. J. Cancer*, **60**, 157–60.

Hertler, A.A. and Frankel, A.E. (1989) Immuno-toxins: a clinical review of their use in the treatment of malignancies. *J. Clin. Oncol.*, **7**, 1932–42.

Hinson, J.A. and Kadlubar, F.F. (1988) Gluta-thione and glutathione transferases in the de-toxification of drug and carcinogen metabolites, in *Glutathione Conjugation* (eds H. Sies and B. Ketterer). Academic Press, New York, pp. 235–280.

Hryniuk, W.M. (1988) The importance of dose intensity in the outcome of chemotherapy, in *Important Advances in Oncology 1988* (eds V.T. De Vita, S.M. Hellman and S.A. Rosenburg). J.B. Lippincott, Philadelphia, pp. 121–41.

Hurley, L.H., Lee, C.S., McGovern, J.P. *et al.* (1988) Molecular basis for sequence-specific DNA alkylation by CC-1065. *Biochemistry*, **27**, 3886–92.

Hurley, L.H. (1989) DNA and associated targets for drug design. *J. Med. Chem.*, **32**, 2027–33.

Jaken, S. and Leach, K.L. (1988) Isozymes of protein kinase C. *Ann. Rep. Med. Chem.*, **23**, 243–51.

Judson, I.R., Calvert, A.H., Rutty, C.J. *et al.* (1989) Phase I trial and pharmacokinetics of trimelamol (N^2,N^4,N^6-trihydroxymethyl-N^2,N^4,N^6-trim-ethylmelamine). *Cancer Res.*, **49**, 5475–9.

Kaye, S.B. (1988) The multidrug resistance pheno-type. *Br. J. Cancer*, **58**, 691–4.

Kohn, K.W., Hartley, J.A. and Mattes, W.B. (1987) Mechanism of DNA sequence alkylation of guanine-N7 positions by nitrogen mustards. *Nucleic Acids Res.*, **24**, 10531–49.

Krauss, R.S., Housey, G.M., Hsiao, W.L. *et al.* (1990) The role of protein kinase C in signal transduction and cellular transformation. *Prog. Clin. Biol. Res.*, **340D**, 175–82.

Krumbhaar and Krumbhaar (1919) The blood and bone marrow in yellow cross gas (mustard gas) poisoning: changes produced in the bone marrow of fatal cases. *J. Med. Res.*, **40**, 497–507.

Larson, E.R. and Fischer, P.H. (1989) New approaches to antitumour therapy. *Ann. Rep. Med. Chem.*, **24**, 121–8.

Lerner, L.J. and Jordan, V.C. (1990) Development of antiestrogens and their use in breast cancer: Eighth Cain Memorial award lecture. *Cancer Res.*, **50**, 4177–89.

Levitzki, A. (1990) Tryphostins – potential antipro-liferative agents and novel molecular tools. *Biochem. Pharmacol.*, **40**, 913–8.

Merrifield, K.R. and Chaffee, B.J. (1989) Recent advances in the management of nausea and vomiting caused by antineoplastic drugs. *Clin. Pharmacy*, **8**, 187–99.

Michell, R.H. (1989) Phosphoinositides and inosi-tol phosphates. *Biochem. Soc. Trans.*, **17**, 1–3.

Mousli, M., Bueb, J.-L., Bronner, C. *et al.* (1990) G protein activation: a receptor-independent mode of action for cationic amphiphilic neuro-peptides and venom peptides. *Trends in Pharm. Sci.*, **11**, 358–62.

Nahorski, S.R. and Potter, B.V.L. (1989) Molecular recognition of inositol polyphosphates by intra-cellular receptors and metabolic enzymes. *Trends in Pharm. Sci.*, **10**, 139–44.

Nestor, J.J., Newman, S.R., DeLustro, B. *et al.* (1985) A synthetic fragment of rat transforming growth factor alpha with receptor binding and antigenic properties. *Biochem. Biophys. Res. Commun.*, **129**, 226–32.

Newell, D.R. (1989) Pharmacokinetic determinants of the activity and toxicity of antitumour agents. *Cancer Surveys*, **8**, 557–603.

Newell, D.R. and Gore, M.E. (1991) The toxicity of alkylating agents – clinical characteristics and pharmacokinetic determinants, in *The Toxicity of Anticancer Drugs*, (eds G. Powis and M. Hacker), Pergamon Press, New York, pp. 44–62.

Ozols, R.F., Cunnion, R.E., Klecker, R.W. *et al.* (1987a) Verapamil and adriamycin in the treat-ment of drug-resistant ovarian cancer patients. *J. Clin. Oncol.*, **5**, 641–7.

Ozols, R.F., Louie, K.G., Plowman, J. *et al.* (1987b) Enhanced melphalan cytotoxicity in human ovarian cancer *in vitro* and in tumour-bearing nude mice by buthionine sulphoximine deple-tion of glutathione. *Biochem. Pharmacol.*, **36**, 147–53.

Pegg, A.E. (1990) Mammalian O^6-alkylguanine-DNA alkyltransferase: Regulation and importance in response to alkylating carcinogens and therapeutic agents. *Cancer Res.*, **50**, 6119–29.

Pinkel, D. (1958) The use of body surface area as a criterion of drug dosage in cancer chemotherapy. *Cancer Res.*, **18**, 853–6.

Rao, K.E., Shea, R.G., Yadagiri, B. *et al.*, (1990). Molecular recognition between oligopeptides and nucleic acids: DNA sequence specificity and binding properties of thiazole-lexitropsins incorporating the concepts of base site acceptance and avoidance. *Anticancer Drug Des.*, **5**, 3–20.

Reichmann, L., Clark, M., Waldmann, H. *et al.* (1988) Reshaping antibodies for therapy. *Nature*, **332**, 323–7.

Rosolen, A., Whitesell, L., Ikegaki, N. *et al.* (1990) Antisense inhibition of single copy N-*myc* expression results in decreased cell growth without reduction of c-*myc* protein in a neuroepithelioma cell line. *Cancer Res.*, **50**, 6316–22.

Rosenberg, B., Van Camp, L., Grimley, E.B. *et al.* (1966) The inhibition of growth or cell division in *E. coli* by different ionic species of platinum complexes. *Nature*, **242**, 1347–52.

Rozengurt, E. (1989) Signal transduction pathways in mitogenesis. *Br. Med. Bull.*, **45**, 515–28.

Senter, P.D., Schreiber, G.J., Hirschberg, D.L. *et al.* (1988) Enhancement of the *in vitro* and *in vivo* antitumour activities of phosphorylated mitomycin and etoposide by monoclonal antibody-alkaline phosphatase conjugates. *Cancer Res.*, **49**, 5789–92.

Shears, S.B. (1989) Metabolism of inositol phosphates produced upon receptor activation. *Biochem. J.*, **260**, 313–24.

Smith, J.B., Smith, L. and Petit, G.R. (1985) Bryostatins: potent, new mitogens that mimic phorbol ester promoters. *Biochem. Biophys. Res. Comm.*, **132**, 939–45.

Spitler, L.E., de Rio, M., Khentigan, A. *et al.* (1987) Therapy of patients with malignant melanoma using a monoclonal antimelanoma antibody-ricin A chain immunotoxin. *Cancer Res.*, **47**, 1717–23.

Stein, C.A. and Cohen, J.S. (1988) Oligodeoxynucleotides as inhibitors of gene expression: a review. *Cancer Res.*, **48**, 2659–68.

Stein, C.A., LaRocca, R.V., Thomas, R. *et al.* (1989) Suramin: An anticancer drug with a unique mechanism of action. *J. Clin. Oncol.*, **7**, 499–508.

Stiller, C.A. and Bunch, K.J. (1990) Trends in survival for childhood cancer in Britain diagnosed 1971–85. *Br. J. Cancer*, **62**, 806–15.

Tew, K.D. (1988) Enzyme changes linked to anticancer drug resistance. *Ann. Rep. Med. Chem.*, **23**, 265–74.

Van Oosterom, A.T., De Smedt, E.A., Denis, L.J. *et al.* (1990) Suramin for prostatic cancer: A phase I/II study in advanced extensively pretreated disease. *Eur. J. Cancer*, **26**, 422.

Vassal, G., Deroussent, A., Hartmann, O. *et al.* (1990) Dose-dependent neurotoxicity of high dose busulphan in children: A clinical and pharmacological study. *Cancer Res.*, **50**, 6203–7.

Waxman, D.J. (1990) Glutathione S-transferases: Role in alkylating agent resistance and possible target for modulation chemotherapy – a review. *Cancer Res.*, **50**, 6449–54.

Wells, A. (1989) The epidermal growth factor receptor and its ligands. *Cancer Treat. Res.*, **47**, 143–68.

Woll, P.J. and Rozengurt, E. (1988) Bombesin and bombesin antagonists: Studies in Swiss 3T3 cells and human small cell lung cancer. *Br. J. Cancer*, **57**, 579–86.

Chapter 26

Growth and endocrine function following treatment of childhood malignant disease

W.H.B. WALLACE and S.M. SHALET

26.1 INTRODUCTION

The overall cure rate for childhood cancer in the UK is now over 60%, and for some tumours it is over 90%. It has been estimated that by the year 2000 at least one in 1000 young adults will have been cured of childhood cancer. This improved survival has stimulated great interest in the adverse effects of radiotherapy and cytotoxic chemotherapy on growth and the endocrine system following treatment.

Radiation therapy may directly impair hypothalamic, pituitary, thyroid, and gonadal function or, alternatively, it may induce the development of hyperparathyroidism and thyroid adenomas or carcinomas. Cytotoxic chemotherapy may damage the gonad, and both irradiation and cytotoxic chemotherapy may interfere with the normal growth of bone.

A variety of clinical presentations may result from these complications of treatment, including short stature, failure to undergo normal pubertal development, precocious puberty, hyperparathyroidism (Rao *et al.*, 1980), hypothyroidism, tumour of the thyroid, gynaecomastia, infertility, and varying degrees of hypopituitarism (Littley *et al.*, 1990).

26.2 GROWTH IMPAIRMENT

There are a number of factors which may adversely affect growth in children treated for the common malignant diseases of childhood. These include direct radiation damage to the hypothalamic-pituitary axis (Littley *et al.*, 1990), the long bones (Gonzales and Van Dyjk, 1983), and the spine (Probert *et al.*, 1973). Additionally important factors include cytotoxic drugs (Clayton *et al.*, 1988c), malnutrition, steroid therapy, and the presence of residual tumour.

26.2.1 BRAIN TUMOURS

Short stature is a common complication after the treatment of brain tumours in childhood. These include gliomas, ependymomas and medulloblastomas, all lesions that do not directly affect the hypothalamic-pituitary axis (Onoyama *et al.*, 1975; Bamford *et al.*, 1976). The treatment of these tumours may include neurosurgery, cranial or craniospinal irradiation, and chemotherapy. The final height achieved by the patients may be adversely influenced by a number of factors including radiation-induced growth hormone deficiency, impaired spinal growth, precocious puberty, chemotherapy, malnutrition and occult tumour. The impact of malnutrition and residual tumour on growth has not yet been studied in these children and there are few studies that have examined cytotoxic chemotherapy and growth retardation.

(a) Growth hormone deficiency

Irradiation of the hypothalamic-pituitary axis may produce a range of pituitary hormone deficiencies – from isolated growth hormone deficiency to panhypopituitarism (Shalet *et al.*, 1988). Of the six anterior pituitary hormones, the first to be affected by radiation damage is always GH, followed by gonadotrophin and ACTH secretion. The degree of pituitary hormonal deficit is related to the radiation dose received by the hypothalamic-pituitary axis. Thus, after lower radiation doses, isolated GH deficiency ensues, whilst higher doses may produce panhypopituitarism. The speed with which individual pituitary hormone deficiencies occur is also dose-dependent. The greater the radiation dose, the earlier GH deficiency will develop after treatment. Thus, between two and five years after irradiation, 100% of children receiving >30 Gy to the hypothalamic-pituitary axis show subnormal GH responses to an insulin tolerance test while 35% of those receiving <30 GY show a normal GH response (Shalet and Clayton, 1990).

While both the hypothalamus and pituitary may be directly damaged by irradiation, evidence has accumulated that the hypothalamus is more radiosensitive than the pituitary (Shalet *et al.*, 1988). The primary pathophysiological defect in these children, therefore, is likely to be subnormal endogenous secretion of growth hormone releasing hormone rather than inadequate growth hormone production from pituitary somatotrophs. Thus an ideal treatment for children with radiation-induced GH deficiency may prove to be an intranasal or a suitable depot preparation of a growth hormone releasing hormone analogue if this becomes available.

(b) Spinal irradiation and growth

Children treated for medulloblastomas, ependymomas and certain other brain tumours, receive spinal as well as cranial irradiation. After a dose of spinal irradiation of 27 to 35 Gy over 22 to 27 days spinal growth may be appreciably impaired (Shalet *et al.*, 1987). The younger the child at the time of irradiation, the greater the loss in growth potential. It has been estimated that the loss in height is at least 9 cm if the child is irradiated at one year and 5.5 cm if irradiation is given at ten years of age. It is likely that these estimates of eventual loss in height are conservative. Furthermore, in centres where the dose of irradiation to the spine is greater than that used in the above study, even more potential growth may be lost. It is during puberty when most of the impairment in spinal growth occurs, irrespective of the age at irradiation. Consequently, the prognosis for spinal growth in an irradiated child who is still prepubertal should not be too optimistic.

(c) Precocious puberty

Puberty that is early (Winter and Green, 1985) or precocious (Brauner *et al.*, 1984) has been reported in some children who have received cranial irradiation as part of their treatment for a brain tumour. The onset of puberty in children with radiation-induced GH deficiency is at significantly earlier chronological and bone ages than in children with isolated idiopathic GH deficiency and may affect both sexes (Shalet *et al.*, 1988). In a group of irradiated children aged one to 13 years, we have shown that the age of pubertal onset is positively correlated to the age at irradiation (Fig. 26.1). It is therefore the children who are youngest at irradiation who are likely to have the most profound disturbances in the timing of puberty. The mean age at puberty of these children with radiation-induced GH deficiency is similar to that of normal children, unlike isolated idiopathic GH deficiency, which is normally associated with delay in the onset of puberty.

The clinical implication for the treatment of children with radiation-induced GH deficiency and early puberty is to forshorten the time available for treatment with growth hormone. The effect of arresting pubertal maturation using a gonadotrophin-releasing hormone (GnRH) analogue in combination with GH therapy is currently under investigation.

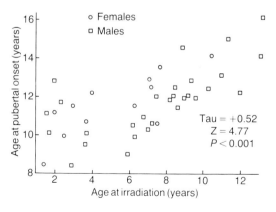

Fig. 26.1 Relationship between age at irradiation and age at pubertal onset in 41 children who received cranial/craniospinal irradiation for a brain tumour or irradiation for ALL.

(d) Treatment with growth hormone

Final height data in children with radiation-induced growth hormone deficiency following the treatment of brain tumours (Clayton *et al.*, 1988a and b) indicate that their growth in response to GH treatment is less impressive than that seen in children with isolated idiopathic growth hormone deficiency. It is apparent that there are additional factors, such as spinal irradiation and early puberty, which combine to attenuate the response to GH treatment in children with radiation-induced GH deficiency. The impairment of spinal growth following spinal irradiation means that it is inappropriate to compare the growth responses of children who have received cranial irradiation with those receiving craniospinal irradiation. Thus these two groups must be considered separately.

In our centre, the growth response to GH therapy has been studied in 12 children with GH deficiency following cranial irradiation and in 14 children with idiopathic GH deficiency (Clayton *et al.*, 1988a). Before treatment, the cranially irradiated patients had higher standard deviation scores (SDS) for standing height, sitting height, and subischial leg length, and less bone age retardation. Both groups started GH treatment at a similar age (11–12 years) with a similar pretreatment height velocity and peak GH response to standard provocative tests. GH therapy administered in a schedule of four units intramuscularly three times per week produced a significant and similar increase in height velocity over the first two years of treatment in both groups. At completion of growth, however, cranially irradiated children ($n = 7$) showed no change in height SDS with GH therapy, compared to marked catch-up growth in the idiopathic GH-deficient children ($n = 14$) (Fig. 26.2 and 26.3). Nonetheless, GH has enabled cranially irradiated patients to maintain their percentile position and to achieve a more acceptable

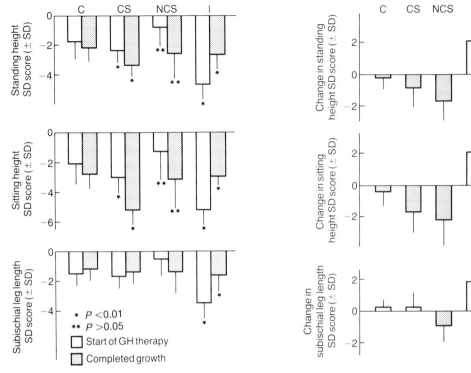

Fig. 26.2 Mean standing height, sitting height and leg length standard deviation (SD) scores at the start of GH therapy/clinic review, and at completed growth, in GH-treated cranially irradiated (C), craniospinal irradiated (CS), and idiopathic GH-deficient children (I) and in an untreated group of craniospinal irradiated children (NCS).

Fig. 26.3 Mean change in standard deviation (SD) scores for standing height, sitting height and leg length over the period of GH therapy/clinic review in GH-treated cranial irradiated (C), craniospinal irradiated (CS) and idiopathic GH-deficient children (I) and in an untreated group of craniospinal irradiated children (NCS).

final height than if they had remained untreated.

For the children with radiation-induced GH deficiency who had received craniospinal irradiation, those who had received GH therapy were compared with those who remained untreated (Clayton *et al.*, 1988b). The mean age at diagnosis was 11 years in both groups and the duration of GH therapy or clinic review in the treated and untreated groups, respectively, was four years. GH therapy produced a significant increase in

height velocity over the first three years in the treated group, with a mean first year increment of three centimetres. Patients treated to completion of growth ($n = 8$) showed a significant increase in leg length SD ($+0.2$) compared to that (-0.9) of the untreated group (-0.9; $n = 7$). Sitting height SDS decreased equally in both groups (by -1.7 for the treated and -2.2 for the untreated), indicating that GH therapy had not ameliorated the impairment of spinal growth caused by spinal irradiation (Fig. 26.2 and

534

26.3). At completion of GH therapy there was a mean decrease in standing height SDS of 0.9 in the treated group, but a decrease of 1.7 SD in those not treated with GH. Thus, although GH therapy failed to induce 'catch up' growth in craniospinally irradiated patients, it did restrict further loss to adult stature, with a mean final height SDS of −3.4 in treated patients (Clayton *et al.*, 1988b).

These studies indicated that GH therapy is of benefit in children with radiation-induced GH deficiency; however, the height gained or rather the 'height loss' prevented was disappointingly small and much less than that seen in GH-treated children with idiopathic GH deficiency.

A further important adverse factor in the height prognosis of these children was the time interval between irradiation and the initiation of treatment with GH which averaged between 5.5 and 6.7 years (Clayton *et al.*, 1988a and b). There is little doubt that better results would have been achieved if treatment with GH had been started earlier. Until recently there has been a tendency to wait until the child exhibits a poor growth rate before instituting GH therapy. This should not now be considered a prerequisite before GH therapy is commenced as the natural history of radiation-induced GH deficiency is well documented and height lost cannot be recaptured.

For many years the standard GH schedule for the treatment of GH-deficient children in the UK was four units administered three times per week irrespective of the patient's size or pubertal status. It has now become clear that the frequency of administration and the dose of GH are critical factors which influence the growth response. The children reported by Clayton *et al.* (1988a and b) received a mean total weekly GH dose of 0.4 units per kg in three injections per week. Our current GH schedule is 0.5 units per kg per week administered by daily injection. The growth velocity of our GH-deficient children

was 7.4 cm per year in the cranial irradiated and 6.2 cm per year in the craniospinal irradiated during the first year of GH therapy. Recently, Lannering and Albertsson-Wikland (1989) reported a mean growth velocity during the first year of GH therapy of 8.2 cm per year in a group of 15 Swedish children with radiation-induced GH deficiency, four of whom had received craniospinal irradiation. The mean pretreatment growth velocity of the Swedish children was similar to that of the children studied by Clayton *et al.* (1988a and b), but the Swedish children received 0.7 units GH per kg per week, administered by daily injection. Their improved growth velocity results were maintained during the second year of GH therapy. What, if any, tests of growth hormone secretion should be carried out? Lannering and Albertsson-Wiklund (1987) suggested that spontaneous 24-hour GH profiles provide the most useful information. However, after the higher doses of cranial irradiation used in the treatment of brain tumours, discordancy between physiological GH secretion and the GH response to pharmacological stimuli is uncommon. The majority of such children will therefore show a subnormal GH response to an insulin tolerance test as well as blunted physiological GH secretion. A 24-hour GH profile, with its heavy demands on clinical and laboratory staff, is likely to remain a research investigation rather than become a routine method of investigation in paediatric endocrinology. If tests of GH secretion are carried out, the insulin tolerance test remains a particularly useful investigation in the child who has received cranial irradiation (Ahmed *et al.*, 1986).

A persistent cause of concern in children treated with GH therapy for radiation-induced GH deficiency is the possibility of a relapse of the original malignancy. The chances of recurrence of a brain tumour are greatest within two years of the primary treatment of the tumour. Late relapse rates are similar for children treated for medullo-blastoma, those who received GH therapy (two out of 11) and those who did not receive GH therapy (three out of 17). Similarly, in children treated for glioma, the prognosis was unaltered by GH therapy (Clayton *et al.*, 1987). Consequently, there is no evidence that treatment with GH increases the risk of recurrence of a brain tumour in children with radiation-induced GH deficiency.

A reasonable policy would be to treat all the children with a brain tumour who are treated by standard radiation schedules, including a dose to the hypothalamic-pituitary axis in excess of 30 Gy, with GH two years after their primary treatment. By this time the chance of tumour recurrence is low, the children would no longer be receiving cytotoxic chemotherapy, and it is already established that the majority will be GH deficient. This policy would not require routine tests of GH secretion to be performed. One drawback, however, is that a minority of the children would receive GH at a time when they have not yet become GH deficient.

Many of the children irradiated for a brain tumour who have received a dose of 25 to 30 Gy will be GH deficient by two years after primary treatment. These children should undergo standard provocative tests of GH release at two years and if the results are abnormal receive GH therapy. If GH secretion appears normal and the growth rate is appropriate for bone age and pubertal status, then growth should be observed and the GH stimulation tests repeated annually. However, if the growth rate is subnormal in the presence of normal GH responses to pharma-cological stimuli, a combination which is very unusual in our experience, then radiation-induced neurosecretory dysfunction may be a possible explanation. The alternative approaches would be either an appraisal of physiological GH secretion, such as a 24-hour profile, or an empirical trial of GH therapy. Whatever policy an individual centre prac-

tices, the principle of administering GH therapy earlier in this group of children is central to their ultimate height prognosis.

26.2.2 ACUTE LYMPHOBLASTIC LEUKAEMIA (ALL)

(a) Growth abnormalities

Much controversy has been generated over the growth patterns and growth hormone requirements of the child with ALL treated with cranial irradiation and combination cytotoxic chemotherapy for several years. Children irradiated for ALL, rather than for a brain tumour, tend to receive a lower radia-tion dose to the hypothalamic pituitary axis. Most of the growth studies have been carried out in children who received a total cranial radiation dose of 24 to 25 Gy. The prevalence of GH deficiency in such children will depend on the number of fractions, fraction size, and duration of the radiation schedule (Shalet *et al.*, 1979).

The influence of cytotoxic chemotherapy on growth has received little attention to date. The most detailed *in vitro* experimental studies were performed by Morris (1981) using the isolated perfused rat liver for soma-tomedin production and a porcine costal car-tilage bioassay to study the uptake of (^{35}S)-sulphate and (^{3}H)-thymidine in response to stimulation by somatomedins. The effects of seven different anti-leukaemic drugs on these two systems were investigated. In the carti-lage bioassay, 6-mercaptopurine, metho-trexate and cyclophosphamide had no inhibi-tory effects at all; prednisolone, sodium sul-phate and doxorubicin hydrochloride in-hibited (^{35}S)-sulphate and (^{3}H)-thymidine uptake; vincristine sulphate inhibited only (^{35}S)-sulphate uptake whilst cytosine arabi-noside inhibited only (^{3}H)-thymidine uptake.

In the liver perfusion system, methotrexate and low concentrations of doxorubicin hydro-chloride and prednisolone sodium sulphate had no effect on somatomedin production in response to GH; 6-mercaptopurine and vincristine sulphate rapidly showed a significant inhibition of somatomedin production, whilst cyclophosphamide and cytosine arabinoside showed less inhibition. More recently, interest has shifted towards somatomedin production by the chondrocyte rather than the hepatocyte. These experimental studies indicate that cytotoxic chemotherapy may have a profound effect on the GH-cartilage growth plate.

In the child treated for ALL, the duration and nature of the combination cytotoxic chemotherapy will influence the growth prognosis. A few children with ALL who have received chemotherapy alone have grown normally (Sunderman and Pearson, 1969; Wells *et al.*, 1983). However, in a study of 82 children treated for ALL with combination chemotherapy and cranial irradiation in Manchester (Clayton *et al.*, 1988c), there is unequivocal evidence to indicate that chemotherapy has an effect on growth. In these children, who received two years of chemotherapy, catch-up growth was seen in the third year after diagnosis, irrespective of the radiation schedule; when chemotherapy was maintained for a further year, this phenomenon was delayed by a year.

In a study of 77 children, Kirk *et al.* (1987) reported significant growth retardation after treatment for ALL with cranial irradiation (24 Gy) and combination chemotherapy. At four years from diagnosis, 32% of 60 survivors had shown a decrease in standing height by more than one standard deviation from the population mean. At six years from diagnosis this had risen to 71% of 38 children, and seven children were more than two standard deviations below the population mean. After standard GH provocation tests, 30 out of 46 patients had partial or complete GH deficiency and the mean pulsatile GH secretion was low in the 34 patients assessed. Radiation-induced GH deficiency was implicated as the main aetiological agent in this growth retardation, and treatment with exogenous GH was instituted in a high proportion of these children.

The findings of the Manchester study (Clayton *et al.*, 1988c) did not support the conclusions of Kirk *et al.* (1987). Six years after diagnosis, the Manchester children had shown a mean standing height standard deviation score (SDS) of −0.44 compared with −1.5 in the Australian study. Furthermore, the Manchester children were less growth retarded after ten years (mean height SDS −0.84) than were the Australian children after six years (mean SDS −1.5). While systematic studies of GH secretion were not performed in the Manchester children, comparison of the radiation doses and fractionation schedules in the two studies indicates that an equal or even greater frequency of abnormalities in GH secretion would be expected in our children. If GH deficiency is the main cause of the growth failure, then the extent of growth restriction should have been equal or greater in our patients, which was not the case. Thus the different degree of growth retardation in these two studies cannot be explained by a variation in the frequency of GH deficiency. However, there were significant differences in the chemotherapy protocols employed by the two groups.

In the Manchester series, all the children received vincristine, prednisolone, L-asparaginase, 6-mercaptopurine and methotrexate. Early protocols also included cytosine arabinoside, doxorubicin and cyclophosphamide. Drugs administered intrathecally included methotrexate and in some children cytosine arabinoside. The treatment schedule UKALL VIII, introduced in 1980 and associated with a significant improvement in survival, differed from preceding protocols in that asparaginase was used early in treatment, 6-mercaptopurine was given at full dose through the latter part of the remission induction period, and maximum drug dosages were sustained throughout remission mainte-

537

nance. At two years, all patients were randomly allocated to discontinue treatment or receive a further year of maintenance therapy.

The ALL children studied by Kirk *et al.* (1987) were treated with a modified LSA_2L_2 protocol (Wollner *et al.*, 1980) which included cyclophosphamide, vincristine, prednisolone, methotrexate, daunorubicin, cytosine arabinoside, thioguanine, L-asparaginase, lomustine, and hydroxyurea in an induction, consolidation and maintenance regimen. Six doses of intrathecal methotrexate 12 mg/m^2 were given during the radiotherapy and two doses (6.25 mg/m^2) were given every ten weeks during maintenance therapy. In 1980, the intrathecal methotrexate dose was changed to a standard 12 mg for patients aged three years and older, 10 mg for those aged two to three years, and 8 mg for those under two years. Six doses were given as early CNS directed therapy with one dose every ten weeks during continuing therapy. The duration of therapy was three to four years (mean 3.5 years).

There is no doubt that the protocol received by the Australian children is more 'intense', both in content and duration, than the UK schedule. We believe that this is the major reason for the dissimilar growth patterns seen in the two studies. This has important implications; all UK and most European centres will have used the same or a very similar protocol to UKALL VIII, and therefore the long-term growth data of their ALL children should be similar to the findings in the Manchester children. Furthermore, the likely site of chemotherapy damage in the ALL children studied by the Australian group is the epiphyseal growth plate (Cowell *et al.*, 1988). This may mean that the dose of GH required to improve the growth prognosis of these children is greater than is necessary to achieve a similar effect in children with isolated GH deficiency. Both the experimental and clinical studies suggest

that there is a need for much more research into the mechanism of action of cytotoxic treatment on growth.

(b) Precocious puberty

Early and precocious puberty have been described in girls after treatment for ALL (Leiper *et al.*, 1987). The onset of puberty, defined as the attainment of Tanner breast stage 2 in the girls and 4 ml testicular volumes in the boys, occurred at more than 2 SD from the mean in 24 girls (20%) and 4 boys (3%). The early onset of puberty is significantly in excess of that expected from the normal distribution in the girls but not in the boys. Early puberty combined with GH deficiency will lead to severe growth impairment, particularly as an attenuated pubertal growth spurt may be misinterpreted as a normal growth velocity. In conjunction with the data of Clayton *et al.* (1988e), it would appear that although irradiation may cause precocious puberty in either sex, the female is more vulnerable at lower radiation doses.

(c) Treatment with growth hormone

For a number of reasons, the demand for treatment with GH is more difficult to predict after treatment for ALL than after a brain tumour. In the children with severe growth retardation (Kirk *et al.*, 1987) even though cytotoxic chemotherapy is a serious adverse factor, radiation-induced GH deficiency is common. It is appropriate therefore that most of these children are offered treatment with GH – in Manchester we have only treated a minority (Clayton *et al.*, 1988c).

Moell *et al.* (1987) have studied the growth patterns of children with ALL during different phases of childhood. In this group, the girls treated for ALL lost very little standing height SD score during prepubertal life but showed an attenuated pubertal growth spurt. Physiological GH secretion was blunted in the prepubertal girls and there was no increase in GH secretion associated with puberty (Moell *et al.*, 1989). Since 1980, the total dose in early cranial irradiation for ALL has been reduced to 18 Gy. A pilot study of 24-hour GH secretion in 19 ALL children who received 18 Gy cranial irradiation and 17 normal children has been completed recently (Crowne *et al.*, 1990). The mean area under the GH curve (AUC) in the prepubertal ALL children was not significantly different from that of the normal prepubertal children. However, there was a significant increase in the GH AUC between the prepubertal and pubertal normal children but not in those who had received 18 Gy. These preliminary results would suggest that after low dose cranial irradiation, prepubertal GH secretion is normal in the majority but GH secretion during puberty may be attenuated in a significant proportion of children. Thus after 18 Gy cranial irradiation, GH therapy needs to be considered around the onset of puberty in those children whose height lies below the 10th percentile. In the original long-term study following 24–25 Gy (Clayton *et al.*, 1988c), the mean loss in standing height over a period of ten years was 0.84 SD score. For an adult male this represents 5.6 cm and for a female 5 cm. We do not consider that the mean loss in final height of our children is sufficient to justify long-term GH therapy in the majority. Our own practice is to offer a therapeutic trial of GH treatment to those children with GH deficiency who are below the 10th percentile for standing height, or whose growth rate is persistently poor after completion of cytotoxic treatment.

26.2.3 BONE MARROW TRANSPLANTATION

High dose therapy and bone marrow transplantation has become a life saving procedure for an increasing number of children and young adults with either non-malignant or malignant haemotological disorders, in particular leukaemia. High dose regimens are designed to suppress the immune system and to eradicate the underlying haematological disorder or malignancy. The agents commonly used include high dose cyclophosphamide or busulphan given alone or in combination with total body irradiation (TBI). Follow-up studies evaluating growth and development have shown that the delayed effects are related to the regimen used before bone marrow transplantation.

TBI has been given in single dose exposures of 7.5 to 10 Gy, and more recently in fractionated exposures of total doses ranging from 12 to 15.75 Gy given over three to seven days. Severe growth impairment is common and may be due to various aetiological factors including GH deficiency, thyroid dysfunction, radiation-induced skeletal dysplasia, or graft versus host disease and its treatment.

In a study by Sanders *et al.* (1986), after TBI and bone marrow transplantation for leukaemia, 27 out of 43 patients (63%) had subnormal GH levels following L-dopa or insulin stimulation. Of the 27 patients with GH deficiency, 21 had received cranial irradiation before their transplant. However, Borgstrom and Bolme (1988) have described GH deficiency occurring after TBI in children who had not previously received cranial irradiation. Their children received TBI at a mean dose rate of <0.05 Gy per minute to a total dose of 10 Gy, given in one session of about four hours. At three years after their TBI, ten out of 18 children tested had subnormal GH responses, and seven of nine children had reduced GH secretion when assessed by a 24-hour GH profile.

Following TBI in adults (ten to 13.2 Gy in five to six fractions over three days), the GH response to an insulin tolerance test was normal, suggesting intact GH secretion (Shalet *et al.*, 1990). It remains unclear whether the GH deficiency described by

Borgstrom and Bolme (1988) reflects greater radiosensitivity of the hypothalamus in childhood compared to adults, or, perhaps more likely, is due to the different TBI fractionation schedules employed by the different groups.

There remains a pressing need for more information on the impact of single and fractionated courses of TBI on the incidence of GH deficiency, GH neurosecretory dysfunction, speed of onset of GH deficiency, and cartilage growth. Without such information, the growth problems of this group of patients remain among the most difficult encountered in clinical practice. In a child with growth failure after TBI, once hypothyroidism and graft versus host disease have been excluded, standard provocative tests of GH secretion should be performed. If the GH responses are subnormal then GH therapy should be offered. If the GH responses are normal, however, then it is possible that the growth failure is due either to GH neurosecretory dysfunction, or radiation-induced impairment of cartilage growth. The former may be investigated by a 24-hour GH profile; alternatively, the child may be offered an empirical trial of GH therapy. If GH therapy is to be instituted, the optimum schedule in the likely presence of GH deficiency and radiation-induced skeletal dysplasia remains unknown.

26.2.4 ABDOMINAL TUMOURS

In 1952, Neuhauser *et al.* described 34 children who had received irradiation that included the spine within the field, and concluded that the severity of the irradiation effects on the vertebrae which were detected radiologically, were directly related to dosage and inversely related to age at treatment. A large study by Riseborough *et al.* (1976) of 81 patients treated with radiotherapy for a Wilms' tumour, reported spinal deformity occurring in 70%. They found significant correlations between the dose of irradiation

and the age at irradiation with the severity of the spinal deformity. In a recent study of 30 long-term male survivors who received abdominal irradiation as part of their treatment for a Wilms' tumour (Wallace *et al.*, 1990), we have found a modest reduction in final standing height SDS (−1.15) accompanied by a marked reduction in final sitting height SDS (−2.41) with no apparent effect on subischial leg length SDS (0.04) (Fig. 26.4). During puberty there is a significant fall in sitting height SDS after both whole abdominal and

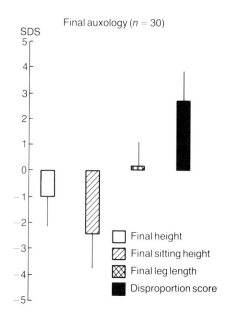

Fig. 26.4 Disproportionate short stature after abdominal irradiation as part of the treatment for a Wilms' tumour in 30 long-term male survivors. There is a modest reduction in final standing height standard deviation score (SDS, −1.15) accompanied by a marked reduction in final sitting height SDS (−2.41) with no apparent effect on sub-ischial leg length SDS (0.04) The disproportion score, which represents the sub-ischial leg length SDS minus the sitting height SDS, is strongly positive reflecting the post-irradiation spinal shortening in these patients.

flank irradiation; this is reflected in a significant increase in disproportion. The younger the patient is at treatment the more severe is the restriction on spinal growth and the shorter and more disproportionate they become as an adult. The estimated eventual loss in potential height from abdominal irradiation at the age of one is 10 cm and at five years is 7 cm. As flank irradiation remains an important adjunct to the treatment of Wilms' tumours in a significant minority of children, we recommend that the measurement of sitting height, in addition to standing height, is necessary to document the full effects of irradiation on the growing spine.

26.3 THYROID DISEASE

26.3.1 THYROID CANCER

Along with hypothyroidism, thyroid tumours are one of the most serious complications of radiation to the thyroid gland. In 1950, Duffy and Fitzgerald reported that nine of a series of 28 children with thyroid carcinoma had previously received irradiation for thymic enlargement and suggested the possibility that irradiation was an aetiological factor in the development of thyroid tumours. Subsequently, a number of large-scale surveys were undertaken, which confirmed unequivocally a causal relationship between external irradiation to the neck in childhood and thyroid cancer. Important determinants of cancer risk are radiation dose, age at exposure, and length of time since exposure. Thus, after neck irradiation, young children are more vulnerable to the subsequent development of thyroid cancer than older children and all children are much more at risk than adults.

The risk of carcinogenesis is present over an extremely wide range of radiation dose and that risk extends over a period of at least 50 years. An estimated dose of 0.09 Gy was linked to a fourfold increase of malignant thyroid tumours in children irradiated for *tinea capitis* (Ron *et al.*, 1989), and by 1986 a total of 21 patients with thyroid cancer following irradiation for Hodgkin's disease had been reported (Moroff and Fuks, 1986). Of the Hodgkin's disease patients, 74% had received a radiation dose equal to or exceeding 20 Gy, and the latent period between radiation and the presentation with a thyroid cancer spanned from six to 48 years.

Histologically, the large majority of radiation-induced thyroid cancers are well-differentiated papillary carcinomas but follicular tumours also occur. An important factor in the prognosis for spontaneously occurring thyroid cancer is the size of the lesion at diagnosis: those less than 1.5 cm in diameter when detected have little or no effect on life span. Many radiation-induced tumours are small but approximately half are greater than 1.5 cm in diameter and there is an increased incidence of multicentric disease, local invasion and distant metastases compared with tumours occurring in nonirradiated patients.

26.3.2 BENIGN NODULES

Abnormalities of thyroid morphology, other than cancer, are frequently found in patients exposed to radiation. These include focal hyperplasia, single or multiple adenomas, chronic lymphocytic thyroiditis, colloid nodules, and fibrosis. Certain studies suggest that palpable thyroid abnormalities occur in about 20–30% of an irradiated population as compared to a 1–5% prevalence of palpable nodular thyroid disease within the general population. Benign thyroid nodularity occurs much more frequently in an irradiated population than thyroid cancer but the exact incidence is less precisely documented. After surgical removal, radiation-induced benign thyroid nodules have a high recurrence rate which may be decreased by treatment with thyroxine to suppress TSH secretion.

26.3.3 THYROID DYSFUNCTION

The degree of thyroid dysfunction after thyroid irradiation may range from frank hypothyroidism with an increased TSH concentration and low thyroxine concentration, to subtle disturbance with increased TSH and normal thyroxine concentrations. Most accumulated data about radiation-induced hypothyroidism are derived from studies performed in patients treated for lymphoma (Schimpff *et al.*, 1980) or head and neck cancer. These individuals have generally received doses of irradiation in the range of 30–50 Gy given in multiple fractions over several weeks. Following a radiation dose to the neck of between 40–50 Gy over 4–5 weeks, approximately 25% of patients showed an elevated TSH and low thyroxine concentration whilst in a further 41% there was a raised TSH concentration in the presence of a normal thyroxine concentration (Schimpff *et al.*, 1980). The time interval between thyroid irradiation and the peak incidence of thyroid dysfunction is unknown. Schimpff *et al.* (1980) noted thyroid dysfunction in 14% of patients during the first year after irradiation with the cumulative incidence rising to a maximum of 66% six years post-irradiation. Recovery of normal thyroid function, several years after radiation-induced thyroid dysfunction has been documented, may occur occasionally.

Apart from patients receiving neck irradiation for a lymphoma or head and neck cancer, there are other groups of patients who are vulnerable to radiation-induced thyroid dysfunction or thyroid tumours. Direct irradiation is received by the thyroid gland during the spinal component of craniospinal irradiation used to treat some childhood brain tumours. Similarly at risk are children who receive total body irradiation before bone marrow transplantation.

In a series of 116 children who were transplanted for malignancy after treatment with high dose cyclophosphamide and total body irradiation (Sanders *et al.*, 1986), 18% developed compensated thyroid dysfunction (raised TSH and normal thyroxine levels) and 11% developed asymptomatic hypothyroidism. In this series, two children developed secondary thyroid malignancies at four and eight years after administration of total body irradiation.

A recent study of thyroid dysfunction after radiotherapy and chemotherapy for brain tumours (Livesey and Brook, 1989), investigated thyroid function in 119 survivors. They described raised concentrations of TSH in 11 of 47 children who had spinal irradiation but no chemotherapy. Chemotherapy further increased the risk of thyroid dysfunction such that two out of four patients who had cranial irradiation and chemotherapy and 20 out of 29 patients who had spinal irradiation and chemotherapy had increased TSH concentrations. In their study, six patients had frank hypothyroidism and four had secondary hypothyroidism. The precise influence of chemotherapy on radiation-induced thyroid dysfunction needs to be substantiated.

In children with obvious biochemical hypothyroidism, thyroxine replacement therapy is indicated. In those patients with compensated thyroid dysfunction who have been irradiated, we believe treatment with thyroxine is indicated for several reasons. Firstly, there is strong circumstantial evidence that an increased concentration of TSH may increase the risk of thyroid tumour developing in an irradiated thyroid gland. Secondly, in a child in whom growth may be compromised for a number of reasons, it is important to maximize the remaining growth potential by ensuring that the child is euthyroid. In those children and young adults who are at risk from developing radiation-induced thyroid disease we would recommend annual palpation of the neck and assessment of the basal TSH and thyroxine concentrations.

26.4 GONADAL DYSFUNCTION

Testicular damage from cytotoxic drugs was
first described by Spitz in 1948. At autopsy,
the absence of spermatogenesis and the presence of tubules lined only by Sertoli cells
was noted in 27 out of 30 men who had
been treated with nitrogen mustard. Subsequently Louis *et al.* (1956) reported amenorrhoea in women treated with busulphan for
chronic myeloid leukaemia.

The impact of combination cytotoxic chemotherapy on gonadal function is dependent on
the nature and dosage of the drugs received
by the child. Drugs that have been shown to
cause gonadal damage include the alkylating
agents such as cyclophosphamide, chlorambucil, and the nitrosoureas, in addition to
procarbazine, vinblastine, cytosine arabinoside and *cis*-platinum.

It is known that the normal adult testis is
extremely sensitive to the effects of external
irradiation (Rowley *et al.*, 1974). However,
neither the threshold dose of irradiation
required to damage the germinal epithelium
in childhood, nor the dose above which irreversible damage occurs, are known. In irradiated women, the response of the ovary
involves a fixed pool of oocytes which once
destroyed cannot be replaced. The LD_{50} for
the human oocyte has recently been estimated not to exceed 4 Gy (Wallace *et al.*,
1989c).

26.4.1 ACUTE LYMPHOBLASTIC
LEUKAEMIA (ALL)

(a) Combination chemotherapy and the testis

Lendon *et al.* (1978) studied testicular histology in 44 boys treated with combination
chemotherapy for ALL. At the time of testicular biopsy, 21 boys were still receiving cytotoxic drugs and 23 had completed their chemo-

therapy some time earlier. Evidence of
leukaemic infiltration was seen in five (11%),
interstitial fibrosis in 24 (55%) and basement

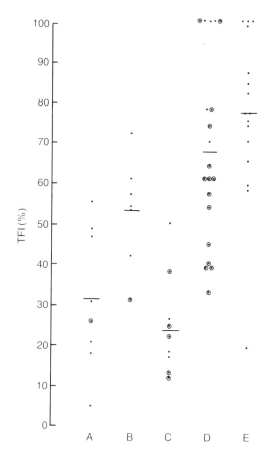

Fig. 26.5 Tubular fertility index (TFI) in boys
with acute lymphoblastic leukaemia. Group A received cyclophosphamide but not cytosine arabinoside (total dose: >1 g/m²); group B received cytosine arabinoside (total dose: >1 g/m²); group C
received both cyclophosphamide and cytosine arabinoside (total dose >1 g/m²); group D received
neither cyclophosphamide nor cytosine arabinoside; group E received very little or no chemotherapy. Horizontal bars indicate mean TFI in each
group and circles indicate subjects still receiving
treatment.

543

membrane thickening in six (14%). Based on a count of at least 100 cross-sections of tubules per biopsy, the tubular fertility index (TFI) was calculated as the percentage of seminiferous tubules containing identifiable spermatogonia. The mean TFI in the 44 biopsies was 50% of that in age-matched controls and 18 of the biopsies had a severely depressed TFI of 40% or less. Three variables had a highly significant effect on the TFI. Previous chemotherapy with cyclophosphamide or cytosine arabinoside (total dose >1 g/m^2) depressed the TFI whereas with increasing time after completion of chemotherapy the TFI improved (Fig. 26.5). These conclusions were supported by the findings of Uderzo *et al*. (1984).

In a prospective study of 14 boys with ALL (Blatt *et al*., 1981) who were treated with a combination of vincristine, prednisolone, methotrexate and 6-mercaptopurine, normal testicular function was documented through puberty as determined by normal testicular maturation and appropriate gonadotrophin and serum testosterone levels. Semen analysis was normal in the six boys studied. Not surprisingly perhaps, they concluded that testicular damage did not occur if the chemotherapy did not include drugs known to cause testicular damage.

Shalet *et al*., (1981) studied testicular function in the 44 boys whose testicular biopsies were reported by Lendon *et al*. (1978). They reported normal Leydig cell function as assessed by the testosterone response to human chorionic gonadotrophin, but described abnormalities of FSH secretion, consistent with germ cell damage, in the pubertal boys. In this study, all the patients achieved normal adult secondary sexual characteristics and had a serum testosterone within the normal adult range consistent with normal Leydig cell function.

In a recent study of testicular function in 25 boys treated with a modified LSA$_2$L$_2$ protocol (Quigley *et al*., 1989), that consisted of ten

cytotoxic agents including cyclophosphamide and cytosine arabinoside, given for three or four years, severe testicular damage was reported. In 24 testicular biopsies assessed at the time of completion of chemotherapy, there was an absence of germ cells in 13 and in the remaining 11 the germ cells were markedly depleted. Elevation of the basal FSH and an exaggerated FSH response to an acute bolus of GnRH were reported in the majority of boys who were pubertal at assessment. Furthermore, all 13 pubertal boys had pathologically small testes below the mean testicular size for their pubertal stage. Inhibin, which is a product of both the Sertoli and Leydig cells, was undetectable in five of 18 prepubertal and one of seven pubertal boys, providing further evidence of testicular damage.

To assess the reversibility of documented germ cell damage after chemotherapy for ALL in childhood, our group (Wallace *et al*., 1991) have studied testicular function in 37 male long-term survivors. This study was conducted at two separate time points; initially a wedge testicular biopsy was performed at or near completion of chemotherapy to assess the incidence of occult testicular relapse. The TFI was calculated as described earlier (Lendon *et al*., 1978), and subsequently, at a median time of 10.7 years after stopping chemotherapy; the patients were reassessed by clinical examination, measurement of gonadotrophins and testosterone levels and, in 19, by semen analysis. The median TFI for all 37 biopsies was 74% and at reassessment six men had evidence of severe damage to the germinal epithelium. Five of these men had azoospermia and one, who did not provide semen for analysis, had a reduced mean testicular volume and a raised basal FSH consistent with severe germ cell damage.

Of 11 males who had a TFI $<50\%$ at testicular biopsy, five recovered normal germ cell function at a median of 10.1 years after completing chemotherapy. Twenty-three of the 26 males who had a TFI >50%, showed completely normal testicular function when reassessed subsequently, and in the remaining three men the results were inconclusive. Clearly, with increasing time after completion of treatment, germ cell function can improve so that normal fertility may be a possibility for some patients who have sustained damage to the germinal epithelium. Nonetheless, the long-term prognosis for fertility may remain poor for at least ten years in those most severely affected.

(b) Combination chemotherapy and the ovary

Ovarian damage following combination chemotherapy for ALL has been reported only rarely. Siris *et al.* (1976) studied the pubertal development of 35 girls and women with ALL treated with the standard drugs: prednisolone, vincristine, methotrexate and 6-mercaptopurine and also, in nine, cyclophosphamide and, in one, busulphan. Seventeen were treated when prepubertal, 11 during puberty, and seven when postmenarchial. The median follow up time was 74 months and 15 were still on therapy at the time of the study. Only one among the prepubertal and pubertal groups had primary ovarian failure with maturational arrest of the primordial follicles. That patient had received busulphan. Three developed low gonadotrophin and oestradiol levels. Among the postmenarchial females, two had experienced prolonged but reversible amenorrhoea. The remainder had progressed through puberty, achieved menarche, or continued to menstruate normally. In contrast, morphological studies have shown that the ovaries from girls treated for ALL between one and 12 years of age and studied one week to four years after diagnosis, demonstrated inhibition of follicular development

(Himmelstein-Braw *et al.*, 1978). The girls who had received chemotherapy for only a short period of time had normal ovaries with ample follicular growth and many small non-growing follicles. This implied that cytotoxic drugs rather than the disease itself had disrupted ovarian morphology.

In a study by Pasqualini *et al.* (1987), twenty-four girls, fourteen prepubertal and ten pubertal, were studied following long-term treatment for ALL. Five of the fourteen prepubertal girls underwent pubertal development and were reevaluated. Ten of the total fifteen pubertal girls achieved menarche during the study, and in three of the original ten pubertal girls, FSH concentrations were transiently elevated. Only one pubertal patient had oligomenorrhoea, and of five patients who had a luteal phase progesterone measured, three showed evidence of adequate luteal function. To evaluate ovarian function and pregnancy outcome after treatment of ALL, Green *et al.* (1989) reported 27 pregnancies in 12 out of 39 women who had been treated for ALL during childhood or adolescence. There were four spontaneous abortions, one stillbirth, and 22 liveborn infants. Two of the liveborn infants had congenital anomalies (one heart murmur; one epidermal naevus) and none of the children (ages one month to ten years) had developed childhood cancer.

In a more recent study, however, Quigley *et al.* (1989) described a high incidence of ovarian damage in 20 girls treated with a modified LSA_2L_2 protocol. Basal and peak FSH levels after administration of GnRH were significantly higher in both the prepubertal and pubertal girls than in the comparable control groups. Further evidence of ovarian damage was the undetectable serum inhibin, a granulosa cell product, in a high proportion of the girls. Despite clear evidence of primary ovarian damage, none of the girls had a delay in reaching puberty and oestradiol levels were normal.

(c) Testicular irradiation

Brauner *et al.* (1983) studied 12 boys with ALL who had received direct testicular irradiation (24 Gy in 12 fractions over 18 days) between ten months and 8.5 years earlier for a testicular relapse (in nine) and as testicular phrophylaxis (in three). Leydig cell dysfunction, manifested by a low testosterone response to human chorionic gonadotrophin (hCG), or an increased basal level of plasma LH or both, was present in ten of the 12 boys. Similar findings were reported by Leiper *et al.* (1983) who studied 11 prepubertal boys who had received 24 Gy in 10–12 fractions over 14–16 days.

In a study of 11 boys between one and five years after testicular irradiation (24 to 25 Gy in 12 to 16 fractions over 16 to 22 days) for a testicular relapse of ALL, Shalet *et al.* (1985) investigated both the time of onset of radiation-induced Leydig cell damage and the question of reversibility. Six of the seven boys irradiated during prepubertal life had no response to human chorionic gonadotrophin (hCG) stimulation. Four of these seven prepubertal boys had a normal testosterone response to an hCG test performed before irradiation. Two of the four boys irradiated during puberty had an appropriate basal testosterone level, but the testosterone response to hCG was subnormal in three of the four. All five boys studied within one year of irradiation showed Leydig cell dysfunction and, in four, a completely absent testosterone response to hCG stimulation. Brauner *et al.* (1983) had suggested that Leydig cell failure may not occur for a number of years after irradiation. However, the evidence from the study by Shalet *et al.* (1985), showed that severe Leydig cell damage was present fairly soon after irradiation. There was no evidence of Leydig cell recovery up to five years after irradiation.

A recent study by Castillo *et al.* (1990) has examined the effect of 'intermediate' doses of testicular irradiation on Leydig cell function in boys treated for ALL. Fifteen boys were studied, twelve received 12 Gy 'prophylactic' testicular irradiation in six 2 Gy fractions over eight days, and the other three were treated for overt testicular relapse with 24 Gy (in two patients) and 15 Gy (in one patient). The seven patients old enough to provide semen for analysis were azoospermic. Eleven of the 12 patients who received 12 Gy, as well as the patient who had received 15 Gy, had normal pubertal development for their age, with an appropriate basal testosterone level and response to hCG. Elevated basal, or post GnRH stimulation, LH levels in the pubertal boys suggests that subclinical Leydig cell damage is common. The problem of whether or not a lower dose, such as 12 to 15 Gy testicular irradiation, combined with aggressive multiagent chemotherapy, will be curative in boys with isolated testicular relapse remains to be evaluated.

All boys who have received direct testicular irradiation for ALL will require a biochemical assessment of testicular function. In the presence of results that indicate Leydig cell failure, if there are no signs of puberty by 12 to 13 years of age, or if there is failure to progress through puberty, then androgen replacement therapy should be initiated.

26.4.2 BRAIN TUMOURS

Both the adjuvant cytotoxic chemotherapy and the spinal fields of irradiation may damage the gonads in children treated for brain tumours. In 1982, Rappaport *et al.* described three girls with primary ovarian failure after treatment for medulloblastoma in childhood. The ovarian failure was attributed to radiation-induced ovarian damage associated with spinal irradiation. However, all three girls received adjuvant chemotherapy, the details of which were not disclosed. Subsequently, Ahmed *et al.* (1983) studied gonadal function in children previously treated for medulloblastoma with surgery, followed by postoperative craniospinal irradiation. The nine children in the group that received adjuvant chemotherapy with nitrosoureas (BCNU or CCNU) plus procarbazine (in three patients), showed clinical and biochemical evidence of gonadal damage with elevated FSH concentrations and, in the boys, small testes for their stage of pubertal development. There was no evidence of gonadal damage in the group that did not receive chemotherapy, all eight children completed pubertal development normally; the boys had adult size testes and the girls regular menses. Ahmed *et al.* (1983) concluded that nitrosoureas were responsible for the gonadal damage, with procarbazine contributing to the damage in the three children who received this drug.

Subsequently, long-term follow-up in 21 girls and 29 boys who had received a nitrosourea (carmustine [BCNU] or lomustine [CCNU]) with or without procarbazine has shown that there is a high prevalence of primary gonadal dysfunction (Clayton *et al.*, 1988d and 1989). Both sexes progressed through puberty normally, with consistently raised basal concentrations of FSH and, occasionally, increased concentrations of LH. The girls achieved menarche at an appropriate age. As adults, most of the boys had inappropriately small testicular volumes, which are likely to be associated with severe oligospermia or azoospermia, and infertility. A sex difference in the reversibility of damage was observed. The boys showed no evidence of recovery of germinal epithelial function and no deterioration in Leydig cell function in a follow-up extended to 11 years. In contrast, several girls who had previously been shown to have ovarian damage, have continued with regular menses and normal FSH and oestradiol concentrations. Although it was not known whether these cycles were ovulatory, it is likely that these girls had recovered

from the ovarian damage. The prospects of fertility among such girls are good in the early child-bearing years; however, a premature menopause remains a possibility. Many of these children also received spinal irradiation, which results in a scattered irradiation dose to the gonad. In the boys, this results in a small dose to the testis estimated at 0.46 to 1.2 Gy (following a fractionated course of radiotherapy delivering a total dose of 35 Gy to the whole spine in the Manchester centre). This small radiation dose is likely to contribute to the observed testicular damage. At other centres, individual boys who were treated with craniospinal irradiation but no chemotherapy have developed testicular dysfunction (Brown *et al.*, 1983); however, the scattered testicular irradiation dose is unknown.

In girls, the dose of irradiation received by the ovary may show greater variation. In the Manchester centre, a total dose in the range 0.9 to 10 Gy has been estimated to reach the ovaries. The position of the ovaries in relation to the spinal field, and therefore the radiation dose received, can be difficult to estimate as the ovaries are mobile and their position may vary throughout the course of treatment. Nonetheless, the radiation dose received may contribute appreciably to ovarian dysfunction and this may be irreversible.

The scattered dose to the ovary will differ among treatment centres depending on the radiotherapy technique. In a large study of gonadal dysfunction following treatment of intracranial tumours (Livesey and Brook, 1988), 18 of 42 girls (43%) showed evidence of primary ovarian dysfunction. Seven out of 11 girls who received craniospinal irradiation but no chemotherapy, and nine out of 14 who had both craniospinal radiotherapy and adjuvant chemotherapy, had ovarian dysfunction. The authors concluded that spinal irradiation was the dominant gonadotoxic treatment. Hence the individual contributions of spinal irradiation and cytotoxic chemotherapy to ovarian damage following the treatment of intracranial tumours will vary depending on the radiotherapy techniques used and the nature of the adjuvant chemotherapy.

26.4.3 ABDOMINAL TUMOURS

(a) Radiation damage to the ovary

There have been few studies of ovarian function following ovarian irradiation, uncomplicated by the effects of other cytotoxic agents, in humans. Shalet *et al.*, (1976) studied ovarian function in 18 females treated for abdominal tumours in childhood. Treatment consisted of abdominal irradiation in each case (20–30 Gy over 25–44 days) and chemotherapy in seven cases. Only one girl received a cytotoxic drug known to damage the ovary (cyclophosphamide). All 18 showed elevated FSH levels and low oestradiol levels typical of primary ovarian failure. The clinical manifestations of ovarian failure in these young women included amenorrhoea or oligomenorrhoea and poor or absent breast development. Sex steroid replacement therapy was required to induce breast development and prevent the subsequent development of osteoporosis.

Ovarian morphology following whole abdominal radiation (20–30 Gy) has been studied by Himmelstein-Braw *et al.*, (1977) in seven girls who died from malignant disease. They found that follicle growth was inhibited and, in the majority, the number of oocytes was markedly reduced.

We have recently studied the natural history of ovarian function (Wallace *et al.*, 1989b) in 53 patients treated in childhood for an abdominal malignancy by surgery and radiotherapy. Of 38 patients who received whole abdominal irradiation (20–30 Gy), 27 failed to undergo or complete pubertal development (pubertal failure) and a prema-

ture menopause (median age 23.5 years) occurred in a further ten. Of 15 girls who received flank irradiation (20–30 Gy), ovarian function was normal in all but one in whom pubertal failure occurred. The median age at last assessment of this latter group is only 15 years. In only one patient, who developed pubertal failure after whole abdominal irradiation and required sex steroid replacement therapy to achieve normal secondary sex characteristics, has there been evidence of reversibility of ovarian function with a documented conception at the age of 22.7 years. Five patients who developed pubertal failure required bilateral augmentation mammoplasties despite sex steroid replacement therapy. Four patients in our series have had six conceptions; all received whole abdominal irradiation and subsequently developed a premature menopause. There were no live births with all miscarriages occurring in the second trimester. There have as yet been no conceptions or live births from the group who received flank irradiation.

It is clear that the outlook for normal ovarian function following whole abdominal irradiation is poor. Flank irradiation, which was introduced intermittently from 1972, has resulted in less pubertal failure but the possibility of a premature menopause still exists. By further study of the 18 of these girls who received megavoltage whole abdominal radiotherapy (30 Gy), and developed pubertal failure (Wallace *et al.*, 1989c), we have been able to estimate that the LD_{50} for the human oocyte does not exceed 4 Gy. Knowledge of the radiosensitivity of the human oocyte provides a more factual basis on which to provide fertility counselling for such patients. The dose of irradiation received by an ovary is dependent on the position in relation to the radiation field; this can be determined by pelvic ultrasound examination. If the dose received by the ovary furthest from the radiation field is calculated, then the surviving fraction of oocytes can be estimated and the predicted age at ovarian failure determined assuming an average complement of oocytes for age at the time of irradiation.

The influence of abdominal radiotherapy on reproductive outcome is not restricted to radiation-induced ovarian failure. Li *et al.* (1987) reported the outcome of pregnancy in 99 patients or wives of patients who were cured of childhood Wilms' tumour at seven paediatric centres between 1931 and 1979. These patients carried or sired 191 singleton pregnancies of at least 20 weeks' duration. Among the 114 pregnancies in women who had received abdominal radiotherapy for Wilms' tumour, an adverse outcome occurred in 34 (30%). There were 17 perinatal deaths (five in premature infants of low birth weight) and 17 other infants were of low birth weight. Compared with White women in the United States, the irradiated women had an increased perinatal mortality rate (relative risk 7.9) and an excess of infants of low birth weight (relative risk 4.0). In contrast, an adverse outcome was found in two (3%) of the 77 pregnancies in non-irradiated female patients with Wilms' tumour and wives of male patients.

There are a number of reasons why abdominal irradiation might result in an adverse pregnancy outcome. Radiation damage may affect uterine distensibility through the presence of fibrosis following a direct action on connective tissue; this may explain our own findings of a high incidence of mid-trimester miscarriage and the observed excess risk of preterm delivery and low birth weight. Uterine vascular insufficiency in pregnancy may be another factor, although the expected outcome would be intrauterine growth retardation rather than prematurity.

(b) Radiation damage to the testis

There remain very few studies of testicular function following relatively low dose irradiation to the testes in childhood. Shalet *et al.* (1978) studied testicular function in ten men aged between 17 and 36 years who had received irradiation for a Wilms' tumour in childhood. The dose of scattered irradiation to the testes ranged from 2.7–9.8 Gy (20 fractions over four weeks). Eight men had either oligo- or azoospermia (sperm count 0 to 5.6 million/ml) and seven of these had an elevated FSH level. All patients progressed through puberty spontaneously.

The relationship between Leydig cell function and pubertal status at irradiation has been further explored by Shalet *et al.* (1989). They studied testicular function in three groups of patients previously treated for malignant disease. Group one consisted of 16 men (median age 28 years) who had previously undergone a unilateral orchidectomy for a testicular teratoma at a median of 1.25 years earlier. Group two consisted of 49 men (median age 36 years), who had previously been treated for a testicular seminoma by unilateral orchidectomy and post-operative radiotherapy to the remaining testis at a median of 2.5 years earlier. The radiation dose was 30 Gy administered in 20 fractions over 27–28 days. In group three there were five subjects studied between the ages of 12 and 34 years, all of whom had been treated for testicular or pelvic tumours by unilateral orchidectomy and postoperative radiotherapy (22.5–30 Gy in 20–28 fractions) between the ages of one and five years. The control group consisted of 41 men with a median age of 28 years.

In group one the median basal FSH and LH concentrations were significantly greater than in age-matched controls. Circulating beta-hCG was undetectable in all 16 men whilst the median basal testosterone was not significantly different from normal. In group two the median basal FSH and LH concentrations were significantly higher and median basal testosterone levels significantly lower than in group one. All five patients in group three showed grossly elevated FSH and LH levels (>32 IU-l) with a median basal testosterone level (0.7 nmol/l) significantly lower than in groups two and three. None of the five, irradiated during childhood, showed a testosterone response to an hCG stimulation test or underwent puberty spontaneously.

The normal testosterone and mildly elevated gonadotrophin levels in group one

reflect a resetting of the pituitary-testicular axis following unilateral orchidectomy in adult life. In group two the lowered testosterone and greatly elevated gonadotrophins, compared to group one, reflect the capacity of irradiation in adult life to damage both the germinal epithelium and Leydig cells. The severe reduction in testosterone levels in group three (Fig. 26.6), compared to group two, despite the similar radiation doses received, suggests a much greater vulnerability to radiation-induced Leydig cell damage in the prepubertal boy than in the adult male.

In a series of studies using the rat model, Delic *et al.* (1985; 1986a, and b) provided supporting evidence that the pubertal status modified the testicular response to radiation injury. The threshold dose for induction of Leydig cell dysfunction in prepubertal, pubertal and adult rats was about 5 Gy; however, the younger animals appeared to be more vulnerable to persistent Leydig cell damage.

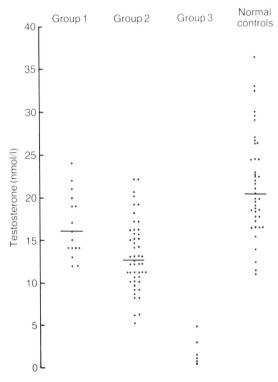

Fig. 26.6 Patients in group one (*n* = 16) underwent an orchidectomy in adult life, whilst those in group two (*n* = 49) and three (*n* = 5) received high-dose irradiation to the remaining testis after orchidectomy; however, patients in group two were treated as adults and those in group three during prepubertal life. The control group consisted of 41 men (age range: 20 to 50 years). The dots represent the basal serum testosterone concentrations and the horizontal lines indicate the median values.

26.4.4 BONE MARROW TRANSPLANTATION

(a) The testis

Sklar *et al.* (1984) examined eight males aged between ten and 17 years at the time of transplant who were followed up for between 13 and 77 months after the bone marrow transplant. Therapy before bone marrow transplant consisted of high dose cyclophosphamide alone (two patients), high dose cyclophosphamide plus total lymphoid irradiation (one patient); the remaining five patients received total body irradiation and either high dose cyclophosphamide or a combination of BCNU, cyclophosphamide and cytosine arabinoside. Total lymphoid irradiation was given as a single dose of 7.5 Gy; the calculated dose of irradiation to the testis is 0.35 to 0.99 Gy. Total body irradiation was also delivered as a single dose of 7.5 Gy. The basal serum FSH was elevated in six patients and small testes were noted in four. Of the six with abnormal FSH levels, four, who were followed serially, showed a return of the basal FSH level to the normal range. Semen analysis, performed in one patient, revealed oligospermia despite normal basal gonado-trophins. Leydig cell function was less impaired in that seven of the eight patients had normal adult male levels of testosterone and all eight progressed through puberty normally.

The largest study to date of growth and development following bone marrow trans-plantation in childhood is from the Seattle group (Sanders *et al.*, 1986). They studied 142 patients, aged between one and 17 years at the time of transplantation, who have sur-vived disease-free for more than one year after marrow transplantation for haemato-logical malignancies. Before transplant all children received multi-agent chemotherapy and 55 also received central nervous system irradiation. Marrow transplant preparation included high dose chemotherapy and total body irradiation given as a single dose of 9.2 to 10 Gy (79 patients) or as fractionated doses of 2 to 2.25 Gy/day for six to seven days (63 patients).

Sixty-three boys between the ages of one and 13 years were prepubertal at transplant. At study, 31 of these boys were between 13 and 22 years of age and 21 showed delayed development of secondary sexual character-istics. Biochemical investigations in 25 of the 31 boys who had entered puberty revealed isolated elevation of FSH concentration in seven boys and both FSH and LH levels raised in 10 of the remainder, four of whom had an undetectable testosterone level. All ten showed delayed development.

Biochemical investigations in 25 of 27 boys who were postpubertal at the time of trans-plant revealed raised FSH levels in 23, raised LH in ten, and a normal testosterone level in

all. Semen analysis in four boys revealed azoospermia thereby confirming the severe damage to the testicular germinal epithelium.

These results are in agreement with earlier conclusions on radiation-induced testicular damage. The Leydig cells of the prepubertal testis appear more vulnerable than those of the postpubertal testis to damage induced by total body irradiation. Severe damage to the germinal epithelium after total body irradia-tion is inevitable and the chances of reversi-bility remain to be quantified.

(b) The ovary

In view of the radiosensitivity of the human oocyte (LD$_{50}$, < 4 Gy: Wallace *et al.*, 1989c) it is not surprising that a high prevalence of prim-ary ovarian failure is found after total body irradiation. In the large study by Sanders *et al.* (1986), 35 girls were prepubertal at trans-plant (aged two to 12 years), and 16 of the 35 were progressing through puberty at the time of the study. Six girls achieved menarche at an appropriate age (four of these six had received fractionated total body irradiation) but the remaining ten girls showed delayed development of secondary sexual character-istics. Gonadotrophin and oestradiol levels in 11 of the 16 girls over the age of 12 years showed very high FSH and LH levels and an oestradiol level in the prepubertal range in seven, with transiently abnormal results in two of the remaining four girls.

Of the 17 girls who were postpubertal at the time of transplant, all had amenorrhoea with elevated FSH and LH levels and low oestradiol levels for the first two years post transplant. Among 14 girls followed up between three and 14 years after transplant, four have shown recovery of ovarian function between three and five years after transplant. In conclusion, the majority of girls who have received high dose chemotherapy and total body irradiation before bone marrow trans-plantation are likely to develop irreversible ovarian failure. Appropriate sex steroid replacement therapy may be necessary to induce secondary sexual characteristics, alleviate symptoms of oestrogen deficiency, prevent osteoporosis, and decrease the risk of ischaemic heart disease in these patients.

26.4.5 HODGKIN'S DISEASE

Combination chemotherapy has greatly improved the prognosis for patients treated for Hodgkin's disease. This has resulted in the survival of an increasing number of young patients, cured of this cancer, but at risk from the late effects of the treatment.

(a) Combination chemotherapy and the testis

Sherins *et al.* (1978) were the first to report chemotherapy-induced testicular damage in patients treated for Hodgkin's disease in childhood. They studied 19 Ugandan boys who had been treated for Hodgkin's disease with nitrogen mustard, vincristine, procarbazine and prednisone (MOPP) and were at least two years out from treatment. Eight out of nine pubertal boys had a raised basal FSH level, and in all six boys biopsied, testicular histology revealed germinal aplasia. They also studied six boys who received the same treatment but who were still prepubertal at the time of the study and found that serum FSH, LH, and testosterone concentrations were appropriate for their age. In this study, nine of the 13 pubertal boys had moderate to severe gynaecomastia associated with a mild elevation of LH and low serum testosterone levels. The authors suggested that the gynaecomastia was an accentuation of the transient breast enlargement observed normally in early puberty but enhanced by the relative decrease in serum testosterone. Alternatively, the marked prevalence of gynaecomastia may have reflected the improved nutritional status of the Ugandan

boys once they came under medical supervision. Whitehead *et al.* (1982a) also found evidence of severe damage to the germinal epithelium in patients who received MOPP in childhood. Six patients, two of whom had also received a small dose of testicular irradiation, provided semen for analysis between 2.4 and eight years after completion of chemotherapy and were found to be azoospermic. Four boys studied whilst still prepubertal showed normal basal gonadotrophin levels

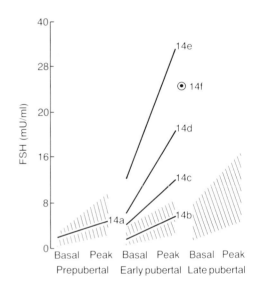

Fig. 26.7 Basal and peak FSH concentrations after GnRH in a boy treated with multiple courses of MOPP for Hodgkin's disease between the ages of six and nine years. The GnRH tests were performed at: (a) one year; (b) 1.5 years; (c) 1.7 years; (d) 2 years, and (e) 3 years after completion of treatment; (f) is the basal FSH level 5 years post-treatment. Normal ranges of values for each pubertal stage are shown (shaded areas). Note that basal and stimulated FSH levels remain normal until 1.7 years after completion of chemotherapy despite the fact that the testicular damage will have occurred at the time chemotherapy was administered. This illustrates the unreliability of FSH estimations in predicting testicular damage in prepubertal and peripubertal boys.

and gonadotrophin responses to GnRH. However, several subjects treated when pre-pubertal showed normal serum gonado-trophin levels in prepubertal life but an evolving pattern of abnormally elevated gonadotrophin levels in early puberrtly, despite the increasing length of time since completion of chemotherapy (Fig. 26.7).

Green *et al.* (1981) described five males who had received combination chemotherapy for Hodgkin's disease without pelvic irradiation; all had an elevated FSH when evaluated postpubertally. Three of the patients who were prepubertal at the time of treatment developed elevated serum FSH levels with the onset of pubertal development. It is clear from these studies that gonadotrophin esti-mations are unreliable markers of testicular damage in prepubertal life. In the study of Whitehead *et al.* (1982a) the marked preva-lence of gynaecomastia in the Ugandan boys described by Sherins *et al.* (1978) was not substantiated. They described gynaecomastia occurring in one out of 12 pubertal boys similar to the incidence reported in adult men (seven out of 74) treated with MVPP (mus-tine, vinblastine, procarbazine, predniso-lone) for Hodgkin's disease (Whitehead *et al.*, 1982b). Furthermore, although three pre-pubertal boys showed subnormal testoster-one response after stimulation with human chorionic gonadotrophin, all nine late puber-tal or adult males who had received MOPP earlier in childhood had normal testosterone levels and had progressed through puberty normally.

There is no doubt that the cytotoxic drugs which damage the testis predominantly affect the germinal epithelium. However, subtle impairment of Leydig cell function has been suggested in men treated with MVPP for Hodgkin's disease. While the circulating tes-tosterone concentration and response to hCG are normal, the basal LH concentration is frequently elevated and the LH response to a GnRH test exaggerated. The bioactive to immunoactive LH ratio is normal and there is no disturbance of LH pulse frequency; however, the amplitude of the LH pulses is significantly elevated. Due to this compensa-tory process, androgen replacement therapy is rarely indicated following chemotherapy-induced testicular damage (Tsatsoulis *et al.*, 1987).

(b) Combination chemotherapy and the ovary

There are very few reports of ovarian func-tion in girls treated for Hodgkin's disease with combination chemotherapy alone. Whitehead *et al.* (1982a) commented on two such girls treated between the ages of 11 and 12 years. Menarche had already occurred in one patient aged 11 years. Her periods were regular even while receiving chemotherapy. The second patient was aged 14 years when menarche subsequently occurred. Her men-strual cycle was regular and ovulatory, as indicated by a plasma progesterone level of 25 nmol/l on the 21st day of her cycle.

In adulthood, the age of a woman is an important factor in determining if ovarian failure is likely to follow MOPP or MVPP for Hodgkin's disease. As the number of oocytes decreases steadily with increasing age, it is likely that ovarian function in prepubertal and pubertal girls may be less susceptible to cytotoxic-induced damage than in adult life.

26.5 CONCLUSIONS

In this chapter we have reviewed the growth and endocrine consequences of the treatment of the more common childhood malignan-cies. Irrespective of the primary malignancy, it can be said that damage is caused if the radiation field includes an endocrine gland, or if a cytotoxic chemotherapy regi-men contains gonadotoxic drugs. As an example, if a child is growing slowly after irradiation for a rhabdomyosarcoma of the orbit, consider the possibility that an appreciable amount of irradiation reached the hypothalamic-pituitary axis and caused GH deficiency. Alternatively, if a boy has received combination cytotoxic chemotherapy for a bone tumour and has pathologically small testes, consider the possibility that the alkylating agent or cisplatin (Wallace *et al.*, 1989a) used in the cytotoxic chemotherapy regimen has caused severe damage to the germinal epithelium. The first boy may require treatment with GH, while, at the appropriate time, the second will need some advice and counselling about his potential infertility.

All children attending an oncology centre should have their standing height, weight and pubertal stage noted at each visit. The measurements should be recorded on standard Tanner growth charts. If all or part of the child's spine has been irradiated then the sitting height should be measured regularly. Standard charts are available for recording growth in leg length and sitting height. The oncologist can also screen for abnormalities of thyroid function and morphology, and some oncologists will feel competent to titrate the replacement dose of thyroxine against the clinical state, and the TSH and thyroxine concentrations of the child. Growth disturbance and the hormonal management of pubertal development are more complicated and require expertise in endocrinology.

The numbers of patients recovering from cancer in childhood are growing, and for optimum management, every major paediatric oncology centre should offer a combined clinic service to which both the paediatric oncologist and the paediatric endocrinologist contribute.

REFERENCES

Ahmed, S.R., Shalet, S.M., Campbell, R.H.A. and Deakin, D.P. (1983) Primary gonadal damage following treatment of brain tumours in childhood. *J. Pediatr.*, **103**, 562–5.

Ahmed, S.R., Shalet, S.M. and Beardwell, C.G. (1986) The effects of cranial irradiation on growth hormone secretion. *Acta. Paediatr. Scand.*, **75**, 255–260.

Bamford, F.N., Morris-Jones, P.H., Pearson, D. *et al.* (1976) Residual disabilities in children treated for intracranial space-occupying lesions. *Cancer*, **37**, 1149–51.

Blatt, J., Poplack, D.G. and Sherins, R.J. (1981) Testicular function in boys after chemotherapy for acute lymphoblastic leukaemia. *N. Engl. J. Med.*, **304**, 1121–4.

Borgstrom, B. and Bolme, P. (1988) Growth and growth hormone in children after bone marrow transplantation. *Horm. Res.*, **30**, 98–100.

Brauner, R., Czernichow, P., Cramer, P. *et al.* (1983) Leydig cell function in children after direct testicular irradiation for acute lymphoblastic leukaemia. *N. Engl. J. Med.*, **309**, 25–8.

Brauner, R., Czernichow, P. and Rappaport, R. (1984) Precocious puberty after hypthalamic and pituitary irradiation in young children. *N. Engl. J. Med.*, **311**, 920.

Brown, I.H., Lee, T.J. Eden O.B. *et al.* (1983) Growth and endocrine function after treatment for medulloblastoma. *Arch. Dis. Child.*, **58**, 722–7.

Castillo, L.A., Craft, A.W., Kernahan, J. *et al.* (1990) Gonadal function after 12-Gy testicular irradiation in childhood acute lymphoblastic leukaemia. *Med. Pediatr. Oncol.*, **18**, 185–9.

Clayton, P.E., Shalet, S.M., Gattamaneni, H.R. and Price, D.A. (1987) Does growth hormone cause relapse of brain tumours? *Lancet* i, 711–3.

Clayton, P.E., Shalet, S.M. and Price, D.A. (1988a) Growth response to growth hormone therapy following cranial irradiation. *Eur. J. Pediatr.*, **147**, 593–6.

Clayton, P.E., Shalet, S.M. and Price, D.A. (1988b) Growth response to growth hormone therapy following craniospinal irradiation. *Eur. J. Pediatr.*, **147**, 597–601.

Clayton, P.E., Shalet, S.M., Morris-Jones, P.H. and Price, D.A. (1988c) Growth in children treated for acute lymphoblastic leukaemia. *Lancet*, i, 460–2.

Clayton, P.E., Shalet, S.M., Price, D.A. and Campbell, R.H.A. (1988d) Testicular damage after chemotherapy for childhood brain tumors. *J. Pediatr.*, **112**, 922–6.

Clayton, P.E., Shalet, S.M., Price, D.A. and Gattamaneni, H.R. (1988e) Does cranial irradiation cause early puberty? *J. Endocrinol.*, **117**, 56A.

Clayton, P.E., Shalet, S.M., Price, D.A. and Morris-Jones, P.H. (1989) Ovarian function following chemotherapy for childhood brain tumours. *Med. Ped. Onc.*, **17**, 92–6.

Cowell, C.T., Quigley, C.A., Moore, B. *et al.* (1988) Growth and growth hormone therapy of children treated for leukaemia. *Acta. Paediatr. Scand.* (suppl) **343**, 152–61.

Crowne, E.C., Wallace, W.H.B., Moore, C. *et al.* (1990) Pubertal rise in spontaneous growth hormone (GH) secretion is attenuated by low dose irradiation. *Horm. Res.*, **33** (suppl 3), 140.

Delic, J.I., Hendry, J.H., Morris, I.D. and Shalet, D.M. (1985) Dose and time related responses of the irradiated prepubertal rat testis: 1. Leydig cell function. *Int. J. Androl.*, **8**, 459–71.

Delic, J.I., Hendry, J.H., Morris, I.D. and Shalet, S.M. (1986a) Leydig cell function in the pubertal rat following local testicular irradiation. *Radiother. Oncol.*, **5**, 29–37.

Delic, J.I., Hendry, J.H., Morris, I.D. and Shalet, S.M. (1986b) Dose and time relationships in the endocrine response of the irradiated adult rat testis. *J. Androl.*, **7**, 32–41.

Duffy, B.J. and Fitzgerald, P.J. (1950) Thyroid cancer in childhood and adolescence. *Cancer*, **3**, 1018–32.

Gonzales, D.G. and Van Dijk, J.D.P. (1983) Experimental studies on the responses of growing bones to X-ray and neutron irradiation. *Int. J. Rad. Onc. Biol. Phys.*, **9**, 671–7.

Green, D.M., Brecher, M.L., Lindsay, A.N. *et al.* (1981) Gonadal function in paediatric patients following treatment for Hodgkin's disease. *Med. Pediatr. Oncol.*, **9**, 235–44.

Green, D.M., Hall, B. and Zevon, A. (1989) Pregnancy outcome after treatment for acute lymphoblastic leukaemia during childhood or adolescence. *Cancer*, **64**, 2335–9.

Himmelstein-Braw, R., Peters, H. and Faber, M. (1977) Influence of irradiation and chemotherapy on the ovaries of children with abdominal tumours. *Br. J. Cancer*, **36**, 269–75.

Himmelstein-Braw, R., Peters, H. and Faber, M.

(1978) Morphological study of the ovaries of leukaemic children. *Br. J. Cancer*, **38**, 82–7.

Kirk, J.A., Raghupathy, P., Stevens, M.M. *et al.* (1987) Growth failure and growth hormone deficiency after treatment for acute lymphoblastic leukaemia. *Lancet*, **i**, 190–3.

Lannering, B. and Albertsson-Wiklund, K. (1987) Growth hormone release in children after cranial irradiation. *Horm. Res.*, **27**, 13–22.

Lannering, B. and Albertsson-Wiklund, K. (1989) Improved growth response to GH treatment in irradiated children. *Acta. Paed. Scand.*, **78**, 562–7.

Leiper, A.D., Grant, D.B. and Chessells, J.M. (1983) The effect of testicular irradiation on Leydig cell function in prepubertal boys with acute lymphoblastic leukaemia. *Arch. Dis. Child.*, **58**, 906–10.

Leiper, A.D., Stanhope, R., Kitching, P. and Chessells, J.M. (1987) Precocious and premature puberty associated with the treatment of acute lymphoblastic leukaemia. *Arch. Dis. Child.*, **62**, 1107–12.

Lendon, M., Hann, I.M., Palmer, M.K. *et al.* (1978) Testicular histology after combination chemotherapy in childhood for acute lymphoblastic leukaemia. *Lancet*, **ii**, 439–41.

Li, F.P., Gimbrere, K., Gelber, R.D. *et al.* (1987) Outcome of pregnancy in survivors of Wilms' tumour. *JAMA*, **257**, 216–9.

Littley, M.D., Shalet, S.M. and Beardwell, C.G. (1990) Radiation and hypthalamic-pituitary function. *Clin. Endocrinol. Metab.*, **4**, 147–75.

Livesey, E.A. and Brook, C.G.D. (1988) Gonadal dysfunction after treatment of intracranial tumours. *Arch. Dis. Child.*, **63**, 495–500.

Livesey, E.A. and Brook, C.G. (1989) Thyroid dysfunction after radiotherapy and chemotherapy of brain tumours. *Arch. Dis. Child.*, **64**, 593–5.

Louis, J., Limarzi, L.R. and Best, W. (1956) Treatment of chronic granulocytic leukaemia with myleran. *Arch. Intern. Med.*, **97**, 299–308.

Moell, C., Garwicz, S., Westgren, V. and Wiebe, T. (1987) Disturbed pubertal growth in girls treated for acute lymphoblastic leukaemia. *Ped. Hem. Onc.*, **4**, 1–5.

Moell, C., Garwicz, S., Westgren, U. *et al.* (1989) Suppressed spontaneous secretion of growth hormone in girls after treatment for acute lymphoblastic leukaemia. *Arch. Dis. Child.*, **64**, 252–8.

Moroff, S.V. and Fuks, J.Z. (1986) Thyroid cancer following radiotherapy for Hodgkin's disease: A case report and review of the literature. *Med. Ped. Oncol.*, **14**, 216–20.

Morris, M.J. (1981) *In vitro* effects of anti-leukaemic drugs on cartilage metabolism and their effects on somatomedin production by the liver. Manchester University, 1981, PhD thesis.

Neuhauser, E.B.D., Wittenborg, M.H., Bereman, C.Z. and Cohen, J. (1952) Irradiation effects of roentgen therapy on the growing spine. *Radiology*, **59**, 637–50.

Onoyama, Y., Abe, M., Takahashi, M. *et al.* (1975) Radiation therapy of brain tumours in children. *Radiology*, **115**, 687–93.

Pasqualini, T., Escobar, M.E., Domene, H. *et al.* (1987) Evaluation of gonadal function following long-term treatment for acute lymphoblastic leukaemia in girls. *Am. J. Pediatr. Haematol. Oncol.*, **9**, 15–22.

Probert, J.C., Parker, B.R. and Kaplan, H.K. (1973) Growth retardation in children after megavoltage irradiation of the spine. *Cancer*, **32**, 634–9.

Quigley, C., Cowell, C., Jimenez, M. *et al.* (1989) Normal or early development of puberty despite gonadal damage in children treated for acute lymphoblastic leukaemia. *N. Engl. J. Med.*, **321**, 143–51.

Rao, S.D., Frame, B., Miller, M.J. *et al.* (1980) Hyperparathyroidism following head and neck irradiation. *Arch. Int. Med.*, **140**, 205–7.

Rappaport, R., Brauner, R., Czernichow, P. *et al.* (1982) Effect of hypothalamic and pituitary irradiation on pubertal development in children with cranial tumors. *J. Clin. Endocrinol. Metab.*, **54**, 1164–8.

Riseborough, E.J., Grabias, S.L., Burton, R.I. and Jaffe, N. (1976) Skeletal alterations following irradiation for Wilms' tumour. *J. Bone Joint Surgery*, (Am) **58**(4), 526–36.

Ron, E., Modan, B., Preston, D. *et al.* (1989) Thyroid neoplasia following low-dose radiation in childhood. *Radiat. Res.*, **120**, 516–31.

Rowley, M.K., Leach, D.R., Warner, G.A. and Heller, C.G. (1974) Effect of graded doses of ionising radiation on the human testis. *Radiat. Res.*, **59**, 665–78.

Sanders, J.E., Pritchard, S., Mahoney, P. *et al.* (1986) Growth and development following marrow transplantation for leukaemia. *Blood*, **68**, 1129–35.

Schimpff, S.C., Diggs, C.H., Wiswell, J.G. *et al.* (1980) Radiation-related thyroid dysfunction: Implications for the treatment of Hodgkin's disease. *Ann. Int. Med.*, **92**, 91–8.

Shalet, S.M., Beardwell, C.G., Morris-Jones, P.H. *et al.* (1976) Ovarian failure following abdominal irradiation in childhood. *Br. J. Cancer*, **33**, 655–8.

Shalet, S.M., Beardwell, C.G., Jacobs, H.S. and Pearson, D. (1978) Testicular function following irradiation of the human prepubertal testis. *Clin. Endocrinol.*, **9**, 483–90.

Shalet, S.M., Price, D.A., Beardwell, C.G. *et al.* (1979) Normal growth despite abnormalities of growth hormone secretion in children treated for acute leukaemia. *J. Pediatr.*, **94**, 719–22.

Shalet, S.M., Hann, I.M., Lendon, M. *et al.* (1981) Testicular function after combination chemotherapy in childhood for acute lymphoblastic leukaemia. *Arch. Dis. Child.*, **56**, 275–8.

Shalet, S.M., Horner, A., Ahmed, S.R. and Morris-Jones, P.H. (1985) Leydig cell damage after testicular irradiation for lymphoblastic leukaemia. *Med. Pediatr. Oncol.*, **13**, 65–8.

Shalet, S.M., Gibson, B., Swindell, R. and Pearson, D. (1987) Effect of spinal irradiation on growth. *Arch. Dis. Child.*, **62**, 461–4.

Shalet, S.M., Clayton, P.E. and Price, D.A. (1988) Growth and pituitary function in children treated for brain tumours or acute lymphoblastic leukaemia. *Horm. Res.*, **30**, 53–61.

Shalet, S.M., Tsatsoulis, A., Whitehead, E. and Read, G. (1989) Vulnerability of the human Leydig cell to radiation damage is dependent upon age. *J. Endocrinol.*, **120**, 161–5.

Shalet, S.M. and Clayton, P.E. (1990) Factors influencing the development of irradiation-induced growth hormone deficiency. *Horm. Res.*, **33** (suppl 3), 99.

Shalet, S.M., Littley, M.D., Morgenstern, D.P. and Deakin, D.P. (1990) Endocrine dysfunction following total body irradiation in adult life. *J. Endocrinol.*, **124**, 165A.

Sherins, R.J., Olweny, C.L.M. and Ziegler J.L. (1978) Gynacomastia and gonadal dysfunction in adolescent boys treated with combination chemotherapy for Hodgkin's disease. *N. Engl. J. Med.*, **299**, 12–16.

556

Siris, E.S., Leventhal, B.G. and Vaitukaitis, J.L. (1976) Effects of childhood leukaemia and chemotherapy on puberty and reproductive function in girls. *N. Engl. J. Med.*, **294**, 1143–6.

Sklar, C.A., Kim, T.H. and Ramsay, K.C. (1984) Testicular function following bone marrow transplantation performed during or after puberty. *Cancer*, **53**, 1498–501.

Spitz, S. (1948) The histological effects of nitrogen mustard on human tumours and tissues. *Cancer*, **1**, 383–98.

Sunderman, C.R. and Pearson, H.A. (1969) Growth effects of longterm anti-leukaemic therapy. *J. Pediatr.*, **75**, 1058–62.

Tsatsoulis, A.T., Whitehead, E., St. John, J. *et al.* (1987) The pituitary-Leydig cell axis in men with severe damage to the germinal epithelium. *Clin. Endocinrol.*, **27**, 683–9.

Uderzo, C., Locasciulli, A., Marzorati, R. *et al.* (1984) Correlation of gonadal function with histology of testicular biopsies at treatment discontinuation in childhood acute leukaemia. *Med. Pediatr. Oncol.*, **12**, 97–100.

Wallace, W.H.B., Shalet, S.M., Crowne, E.C. *et al.* (1989a) Gonadal dysfunction due to *Cis*-platinum. *Med. Pediatr. Oncol.*, **17**, 409–13.

Wallace, W.H.B., Shalet, S.M., Crowne, E.C. *et al.* (1989b) Ovarian failure following abdominal irradiation in childhood: Natural history and prognosis. *Clin. Oncol.*, **1**, 75–9.

Wallace, W.H.B., Shalet, S.M., Hendry, J.H. *et al.* (1989c) Ovarian failure following abdominal irradiation in childhood: the radiosensitivity of the human oocyte. *Br. J. Radiol.*, **62**, 995–8.

Wallace, W.H.B., Shalet, S.M., Lendon, M. and Morris-Jones, P.H. (1991) Male fertility in long-term survivors of acute lymphoblastic leukaemia in childhood. *Int. J. Androl.* (in press).

Wallace, W.H.B., Shalet, S.M., Morris-Jones, P.H. *et al.* (1990) Effect of abdominal irradiation on growth in boys treated for a Wilms' tumour. *Med. Pediatr. Oncol.*, **18**, 441–6.

Wells, R.J., Foster, M.B., D'Ercole, J. and McMillan, C.W. (1983) The impact of cranial irradiation on the growth of children with acute lymphocytic leukaemia. *Am. J. Dis. Child.*, **137**, 37–9.

Whitehead, E., Shalet, S.M., Morris-Jones, P.H. *et al.* (1982a) Gonadal function after combination chemotherapy for Hodgkin's disease in childhood. *Arch. Dis. Child.*, **57**, 287–91.

Whitehead, E., Shalet, S.M., Blackledge, G. *et al.* (1982b) The effects of Hodgkin's disease and combination chemotherapy on gonadal function in the adult male. *Cancer*, **49**, 418–22.

Winter, R.J. and Green, O.C. (1985) Irradiation-induced growth hormone deficiency, blunted growth response and accelerated skeletal maturation to growth hormone therapy. *J. Pediatr.*, **106**, 609–12.

Wollner, N., Wachtel, A.E., Exelby, P.R. and Centore, D. (1980) Improved prognosis in children with intra-abdominal non-Hodgkin's lymphoma following LSA_2L_2 protocol chemotherapy. *Cancer*, **45**, 3034–9.

Chapter 27

Non endocrine late effects of treatment

P. MORRIS JONES

27.1 INTRODUCTION

The increasing numbers of survivors of childhood cancers provide exciting evidence of the remarkable advances which have been made in paediatric oncology. These individuals are, however, not without therapy-associated problems. The first described long-term unwanted effects of treatment were those associated with radiation damage to growing bone; these were followed by evidence of radiation damage to other tissues. In the 1950s the enhancing effects of chemotherapeutic agents on radiation became obvious when there was augmentation of radiation damage and late recall of latent effects weeks and months after the radiation therapy was complete. Chemotherapy itself is not without late consequences either, particularly manifest in specific organ damage.

27.2 CARDIAC DAMAGE

The anthracyclines are the most frequent cause of cardiac damage and endomyocardial changes can be demonstrated microscopically after a single dose of doxorubicin. Many studies have now been carried out which demonstrate the use of echocardiography in detecting subclinical changes in cardiac func-

tion (Hutter *et al.*, 1981; Hausdorf *et al.*, 1988). As early as 1980, Henderson and Frei reported on the limited usefulness of serial non-invasive techniques in decreasing the incidence of doxorubicin-induced cardiotoxicity. The longer term follow-up of patients with doxorubicin-induced chronic heart failure shows that some can recover. Neither those who die nor those who recover can be predicted by clinical or laboratory parameters, however, and those who do recover can fail again under stress (Moreb and Oblon, 1988). The most worrying of these latter situations is the stress of pregnancy and labour (Steinherz *et al.*, 1987).

Cardiac damage is also caused by radiation to the mediastinum and early death due to coronary artery disease at ages when atherosclerosis is rare has been reported (Joensuu, 1989; J. Kingston, personal communication). When chemotherapy and irradiation are combined the risks are increased, and both mitozantrone and cyclophosphamide (alone and in combination with cytosine arabinoside) have been implicated. Care must be taken when planning chemotherapy protocols to consider the possibility of mediastinal radiation being necessary at a late stage and if so to limit the dose of potentially cardiotoxic drugs.

27.3 PULMONARY TOXICITY

Most reported pulmonary toxicity has been caused by irradiation and consists of fibrosis and a restrictive pattern due to limited thoracic cage size (Makiperbaa *et al.*, 1989). More recent studies of children who have received both chemotherapy and radiation – usually for Hodgkin's disease – show abnormality both of forced vital capacity and total lung capacity (Miller *et al.*, 1986); similar changes are shown even in children cured of acute lymphoblastic leukaemia, and are probably due to impairment of lung growth and the toxicity of methotrexate (Shaw *et al.*, 1989).

The pulmonary toxicity of carmustine (BCNU) has been documented for many years (Bailey *et al.*, 1978). This drug is now used very rarely for treatment of children but there are cohorts of patients in whom it was previously used (with devastating results) especially for adjuvant treatment of malignant brain tumours (O'Driscoll *et al.*, 1990). The toxicity of 1-(2-choroethyl)-3-cyclohexyl-l-nitrosourea (CCNU) is undoubtedly less but nevertheless detailed assessment of lung function in patients given this drug for treatment of brain tumours does show evidence of damage. CCNU has also been incorporated into some protocols for treatment of non-Hodgkin's lymphoma and so these patients may well also be at risk. The pulmonary toxicity of bleomycin is well documented and probably has the greatest effect in childhood (Eigen and Wyszomierski, 1985).

27.4 GASTROINTESTINAL SEQUELAE

27.4.1 HEPATOTOXICITY

Most liver toxicity during therapy is of an acute nature and includes hepatitis B infection drug-induced toxicity and veno occlusive disease. Any of these can proceed to chronic hepatitis or hepatitis may appear *de novo* and be associated with the use of 6-mercapto-purine, or busulphan. Severe portal hypertension and oesophageal varices may also ensue and the possibility of late hepatocellular carcinoma cannot be excluded.

27.4.2 ALIMENTARY TRACT

Oesophageal stenosis can follow infection and ulceration. The former is usually due to candidiasis while ulceration may follow anthracycline or methotrexate administration and thus can progress to fibrosis. Stenosis in the small or large bowel may follow the severe ulceration seen with typhilitis or following radiation. Children receiving x-ray therapy to the pelvis are at particular risk of developing stenosis and fibrotic changes in the rectum, often leading to faecal incontinence and the occasional need for colostomy. Patients who have undergone laparotomy either prior to or following radiation therapy to the abdomen are at increased risk of developing intestinal obstruction secondary to adhesions. This problem may become recurrent.

27.5 GENITOURINARY DAMAGE

27.5.1 RENAL DAMAGE

Renal dysfunction may be the result of surgery, radiation or chemotherapy. The most frequent reason for nephrectomy is Wilms' tumour and although current practice is to restrict radiation therapy to patients with residual intra-abdominal disease and to shield the remaining kidney, there are increasing numbers of reports of patients developing renal failure following long-term hyperfusion of that kidney (Welch and McAdams, 1986). Many of these older patients will have received some radiation to the kidney as well as chemotherapy; standard regimens do not now include any known nephrotoxic drugs. Hypertension is also a known complication, probably due to the effects of radiation on the vascular supply. It is therefore very important that all patients undergoing nephrectomy should have blood pressure and renal function regularly monitored. Children with resectable supra-renal neuroblastoma may also require nephrectomy in order to achieve complete removal of malignant tissue and should be similarly followed. This group of patients are also highly likely to have received cisplatin which has been one of the mainstays of treatment for this tumour. Cisplatin is also used to treat germ cell tumours and, in some protocols, for therapy of osteogenic sarcoma (Womer *et al.*, 1985). Glomerular damage is seen frequently – few children escape a fall in their glomerular filtration rate. While this does not usually deteriorate further on cessation of therapy, significant recovery has not been documented. Ifosfamide, which has also been used in the treatment of many childhood tumours, produces tubular dysfunction and glomerular damage (Skinner *et al.*, 1989; Patterson and Khojasteh, 1989). Renal toxicity can be exacerbated by the previous use of cisplatin and the concomitant aminoglycoside antibiotics, some of the most commonly used antibiotics to treat infection in immunosuppressed patients (Goren *et al.*, 1987).

27.5.2 BLADDER TOXICITY

Haemorrhagic cystitis is caused both by cyclophosphamide and ifosfamide. Sodium 2-mercapto-ethanesulphonate (MESNA) will to a large extent protect against this complication but cannot prevent it entirely. The consequent long-term fibrosis can cause very reduced bladder capacity and the potential for secondary malignant change (Brugières *et al.*, 1989). Radiation damage can also be incurred by the bladder when the field involves the pelvis. In young boys the fields used for radiation of the testes may include the bladder leading to fibrosis.

27.6 MUSCULO SKELETAL DAMAGE

Avascular necrosis of bone has long been known to be a complication of corticosteroid therapy. It is surprising therefore that more reports have not occurred of this complication in children treated for leukaemia and the lymphoreticular disorders and it is likely that the condition is under-diagnosed (Murphy and Greenberg, 1990). It may be that the symptoms have been mistaken for relapse or infection (Blauensteiner *et al.*, 1987).

Slipped epiphyses are a common complication of radiation therapy, occurring especially, but not exclusively, in weight-bearing bones such as the femur (Ederken *et al.*, 1982). Treatment of this problem is difficult in the young patient as pinning of the epiphysis can lead to early fusion and limb length discrepancy. Every effort should be made, without jeopardizing treatment, to exclude epiphyses from radiation fields.

Even low doses of radiation will impair bone growth and the radiation fields commonly used to treat nephroblastoma and neuroblastoma will cause significant loss of height due to reduced growth of the vertebrae. Whole spinal irradiation for treatment of medulloblastomas and as part of some leukaemia protocols in the 1970s cause even greater impairment of sitting height. This, with no loss in leg length, leads to disproportionate loss in ultimate height and if coupled with growth hormone deficiency is particularly worrying to the patient. The combination of bone biopsy, with cytotoxic chemotherapy and/or radiotherapy increases the risk of pathological fracture (Rosenstock *et al.*, 1978).

Severe craniofacial asymmetry occurs when radiation is given to the orbit or cheek of the young child and this problem is worsened by the concurrent use of chemotherapy (Fig. 27.1). Skin and soft tissue changes are less common since megavoltage irradiation became the treatment of choice for

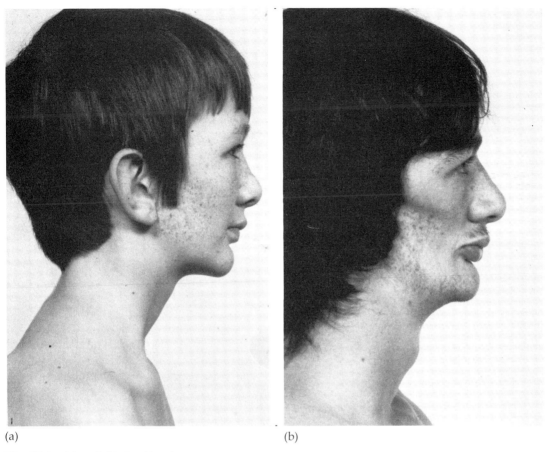

(a)   (b)

Fig. 27.1   (a) and (b) Profile of a patient seven and thirteen years after radiation and actinomycin D for a rhabdomyosarcoma of the cheek showing progressive deformity due to impaired bone growth.

paediatric patients but orthovoltage therapy is associated with significant thinning of the skin and the formation of telangiectases. Basal cell carcinomas have also been reported and soft tissue and muscle are reduced in bulk. These changes are particularly obvious in young patients receiving mantle irradiation for Hodgkin's disease (Fig. 27.2).

There have been recent reports of the increased incidence of melanocytic naevi in children who have received multi-agent chemotherapy (Hughes *et al.*, 1989; deWit *et al.*, 1990). The exact aetiology of these is unknown but they should be monitored with care as the possibility of subsequent develop-ment of malignant melanoma cannot be ruled out.

27.7 HAEMATOLOGICAL SEQUELAE

The majority of cytotoxic agents and radiation therapy have temporary or permanent effects on bone marrow elements and these can lead to the development of myelo-dysplastic syndrome (Levine and Bloomfield, 1986). The drugs most commonly implicated are the alkylating agents, particularly procar-bazine. Many patients show changes in chromosomes 5 and 7. Long-term changes can be demonstrated in the bone marrow

561

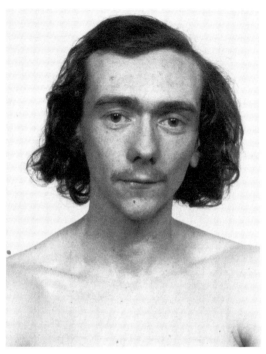

Fig. 27.2 Small jaw, thin neck and prominent clavicles following mantle irradiation for Hodgkin's disease.

following both treatment of acute lymphoblastic and acute myeloid leukaemias (Testa *et al.*, 1988; Bhavnani *et al.*, 1989).

27.8 NEUROLOGICAL SEQUELAE

The major neurological toxicity is that occurring secondarily to radiation of the brain, either for intracranial tumours or in acute leukaemia. The higher doses of radiation necessary to achieve cure in the former are associated with intellectual deterioration, leukoencephalopathy, and second primary neoplasms. Computerized tomography (CT) and magnetic resonance imaging (MRI) studies demonstrate atrophy and calcification. While the former may be due to the direct effects of the tumour causing pressure changes and disturbance of cerebrospinal

fluid (CSF) flow, the latter are shown to occur in areas distant from the tumour and are usually subcortical – at the grey/white matter junction – and can be demonstrated to progress with time (Davis *et al.*, 1986). Both conditions are worse in younger children especially those less than three years of age. White matter changes are much better demonstrated on MRI and these are well correlated with focal neurological changes and with mineralizing microangiopathy and demyelination found at postmortem (Atlas *et al.*, 1987). The true pathogenesis of these changes, however, is both incompletely explained and understood. It is likely to be due to direct effects on intra-cranial-endothelial cells, brain white matter, and damage of small blood vessels (Robain *et al.*, 1984).

All these complications are likely to increase in frequency with the introduction of chemotherapy of a more intensive nature both pre and post radiation. It has been suggested that pre radiation chemotherapy is less likely to be associated with late damage but nevertheless significant problems have been documented (Packer *et al.*, 1985). Radiation myelopathy most often presents as a transient acute problem but can present as a chronic progressive myelitis. Size of radiation dose fraction, total dose and length of cord irradiated have all been implicated but combined radiation and chemotherapy may increase the risk.

27.9 COGNITIVE SEQUELAE

Reports of impairment of cognitive function following therapy for malignant disease have been described in children with brain tumours and children treated for leukaemia. Radiation has been the most frequently implicated modality but deficits tend to be worse when intrathecal chemotherapy and radiotherapy are combined, especially in children receiving treatment before the age of five. Clear conclusions are difficult in children with brain tumours as treatment-associated damage cannot be separated from damage due to the tumour and its direct effect on cognitive function (Ellenberg *et al.*, 1987).

In patients treated for leukaemia most studies indicate that radiation is the major cause of problems (Copeland *et al.*, 1988). Other studies have demonstrated the importance of parental social class, age at diagnosis and dose of radiation (Trautmann *et al.*, 1988; Moore *et al.*, 1986; Bowman, 1987). A recent study from Canada has demonstrated a correlation between decline in head growth and cognitive function in survivors of leukaemia (Appleton *et al.*, 1990). The study demonstrated greater decline in growth (associated, in addition, with worse cognitive function) following 2400 cGy than 1800 cGy. In children under three years of age even the lower dose of radiation had a deleterious effect. Impaired visual motor skills, difficulties with mathematics, and fine motor control problems have all been documented along with poor attention/concentration, memory, and comprehension. Most studies demonstrate specific learning difficulties rather than global retardation. There is some evidence that remedial help and individualized instruction associated with parental support may go some way to minimize defects (Peckham *et al.*, 1988) and prospective intervention is recommended. There is also a need for better communication between hospital and school to minimize the tendency to set low standards of attainment and to correct the common belief that prognosis for life in these children is so poor that scholastic achievement is irrelevant (Larcombe *et al.*, 1990).

27.10 OTHER ORGAN DYSFUNCTION

27.10.1 DENTAL

Radiation has deleterious effects both on erupted teeth and developing dentition. Children who have received radiation to the jaw can be shown to have increased caries and may have malocclusion problems. When the salivary glands are included in the field, salivary secretion falls and this leads to difficulty in maintaining good dental hygiene leading to gingivitis.

Failure of tooth development, crown hypoplasia, and poor root development have all been demonstrated (Purdell Lewis *et al.*, 1988; Maguire *et al.*, 1987). Chemotherapy can lead to worsening of the effects of radiation by causing oral ulceration and hence poor hygiene and also by causing direct damage to microtubular function in the ondontoblasts (Macleod *et al.*, 1987) and impairment of enamel formation (Pajori *et al.*, 1988).

27.10.2 OPHTHALMIC

Cataracts described in children treated for leukaemia are posterior subcapsular in position and may be due either to steroids or radiation therapy (Elliot *et al.*, 1985). Children receiving radiation to the orbit for tumours such as rhabdomyosarcoma will also develop cataracts. They do not always impair vision but if they do, they can be successfully treated by cataract surgery (Heyn *et al.*, 1986).

27.10.3 OTOLOGICAL

High frequency hearing loss is well documented as a complication of platinum chemotherapy and the majority of patients thus treated can be shown to have damage. Carboplatin is less toxic then cisplatin but the former does cause significant morbidity. When cisplatin is given concomitantly with or following radiation in the area of the eighth nerve, the damage is increased and will lead to the use of hearing aids (Brock *et al.*, 1987; Schell *et al.*, 1989).

27.10.4 SECOND PRIMARY NEOPLASMS

The development of a second primary neoplasm is probably the most devastating late complication which can occur for a patient and their family and the one which they fear most. The earlier descriptions of this problem were largely confined to groups of patients with good prognosis, that is, malignancies which have been successfully treated in significant numbers for some years. However, increasingly, reports are now appearing for patients with leukaemia, non-Hodgkin's lymphoma and brain tumours. Most second primaries described prior to 1970 were due to late radiation effects and the majority arose within the radiation field or at its edge (Hawkins *et al.*, 1987; Miké *et al.*, 1982; Li *et al.*, 1983a). The commonest forms of second tumour are those of osteogenic sarcoma, soft tissue sarcoma, carcinoma of thyroid, breast and gastro-intestinal tract, and tumour of the central nervous system (CNS). It is well established that children with the familial form of retinoblastoma are at increased risk of second tumours – most often osteogenic sarcoma. In this case the cause is genetic as the tumour can arise in patients who have had no treatment other than surgery; the risk, however, is enhanced by radiation and chemotherapy. Children with Ewing's tumour have also been shown to be at significant increased risk of osteogenic sarcoma, probably due to previous radiotherapy, alkylating agent chemotherapy and disordered bone proliferation following pathological fracture.

Other genetic disorders associated with increased risk include Von Recklinhausen's disease and other phacomatoses, and Gorlin's syndrome. Patients with a history of malignancy within the family, especially with the pattern of the Li-Fraumeni syndrome, are also vulnerable (Birch *et al.*, 1984).

Thyroid carcinomas occur following irradiation to the neck and are most often seen following treatment for Hodgkin's disease but have also been reported following CNS tumours and soft tissue sarcomas of the head and neck.

Pulmonary irradiation is implicated in the development of carcinoma of the breast (Li *et al.*, 1983b). The use of chemotherapy in addition to radiation in patients with Hodgkin's disease may increase this risk.

The alkylating agents have been extensively investigated with reference to the development of second tumours and evidence is strong for their induction of malignancy, particularly in the case of acute myeloid leukaemia (Tucker *et al.*, 1987). Thus, patients with Hodgkin's disease are the most frequently reported with acute myeloid leukaemia (AML) or non-Hodgkin's lymphoma (NHL) following MOPP or COPP chemotherapy and it is of importance to note that no such risk has been shown for ABVD (Santoro *et al.*, 1987; Jenkin *et al.*, 1990).

Since there is a well established familial association between leukaemia and CNS tumours, the increasing use of alkylating agents, particularly procarbazine, in protocols for childhood CNS tumours, requires very careful follow-up of this cohort for any evidence of increased incidence of leukaemia. Conversely, children receiving high alkylating agents dose prior to bone marrow transplantation for haemopoetic malignancies may be at risk of CNS tumours.

Many attempts have been made to provide a figure for the overall increased risk of second malignancies following successful treatment of the first tumour. Clearly risks vary according to the type of first tumour, genetic factors, and treatment. Estimates from single and multi-institution studies carry a bias but nevertheless provide important pointers (Mike *et al.*, 1982). The population based study of Hawkins *et al.* (1987) probably provides the most accurate estimate at present available but the indications from their study of changing pattern and earlier onset gives considerable cause for concern.

27.11 PSYCHOSOCIAL DYSFUNCTION

During the earlier years of successful treatment of childhood tumours little attention was paid to the impact of the disease on the child, the family and the immediate community. Success was uncommon and in most instances the parents were warned of the high risk of death and the emotional impact of awaiting the event was not addressed in an open manner. This clearly led to many difficulties both for those who were ultimately bereaved and those who managed to avoid the sword of Damocles, some of whom, having cheated death themselves, felt ashamed to be alive and became resented by their families for having caused so much distress – the 'Lazarus syndrome'. Although nowadays severe problems of this kind are less common, they do occur.

The success of modern day treatment has led to its own problems, not least of which is the prolonged period of uncertainty which patient and family have to cope with before cure can be certain and this is then followed by the possibility of problems discussed in this chapter.

From the moment of diagnosis, the child and family have to face the problem of altered lifestyle and often also a change in ambitions. While both of these changes are to some extent inevitable, they can be minimized and professional support is essential to help families retain as much normality as possible and to encourage a continuation of setting of goals. It is natural for parents to become overprotective but this leads to regression in the child and separation anxiety in the parent; this can make medical intervention more difficult. In the very young child this can lead to failure of socialization and peer group interaction which can persist throughout school and adult life.

School absenteeism and school phobia are major problems amongst children with cancer and persist long after the completion of treatment (Lansky *et al.*, 1983; Mancini *et al.*, 1989). The intensive chemotherapy programmes used today make some loss of schooling inevitable but continuation of an ordered pattern of learning should be encouraged, persisting with teaching in hospital and by the short-term provision of home tuition. The latter however, should be seen as a temporary measure and early return to school and extra curricular activities encouraged (Larcombe *et al.*, 1990). The problems of cross infection tend to be exaggerated and must be put into perspective. School teachers need support in order to have a child with cancer in class and accurate information must be provided by the hospital staff (Charlton *et al.*, 1986). Even though treatment of the condition is free in this country families inevitably incur expenses, especially with regard to transportation. In other families, a mother will find it necessary to give up work or father may lose his job because of frequent absences. Carers should make strong efforts to prevent unnecessary expenditure, for example, on extra or special foods and clothing, expensive toys and inappropriate compensatory measures. Mothers should be encouraged to remain in work – not only for the monetary advantages but as a means of retaining social and supportive contacts. Intervention by hospital medical or social work staff may well achieve a sympathetic response from the father's employer who will adjust working hours or change the nature of the job for a limited period.

A more recently highlighted problem which has been previously neglected is the impact of cancer on siblings. This group of individuals has not only been forgotten by the doctor but also by the family. Their needs become of secondary importance and they tend to be pushed from pillar to post, farmed out to relatives, and their psychological problems given scant attention. Active efforts should be made to integrate them into the new family structure and function, and they should be fully informed of the seriousness of their sibling's illness and the possible outcome.

Young adult survivors of childhood cancer have problems with employment, life insurance and obtaining mortgages. The armed forces still refuse to employ these individuals and the problem is also considerable in some large multinational companies. The insistence on discharge from hospital follow-up before considering them for a job indicates ignorance on the part of medical assessors of the need for long-term surveillance. The larger insurance companies will now accept these young people for life insurance without loaded premiums when they have been disease-free and off treatment for ten years and similar arrangements are being introduced by building societies and other providers of mortgages. Education of the public remains inadequate and can lead to ostracization and discrimination but not all the changes must come from the community. Young cancer survivors should be encouraged to demonstrate their ability to compete on equal terms with their peer group and to feel confident in accepting the challenges of normal life. Their experiences during their illness in childhood should have equipped them well to cope with the problems inherent in modern day adult life.

27.12 CONCLUSIONS

Long-term effects of treatment of childhood cancer are many and varied as well as far reaching. They will continue to be present throughout the individual's life and new ones will develop both due to as yet undescribed toxicity and evolution of tissue damage. Minimization can be achieved by vigilant observation and a willingness on the part of clinicians to accept necessary modification of treatment, early intervention and prevention, and the co-operation of all disciplines involved in care. Every new treatment proto-

col should have a section built into it which makes provision for baseline assessment of organ function and psychological status and well designed prospective evaluation of treatment effects should be mandatory. Those in charge of the development of treatment for children with cancer must not bury their heads in the sand with regard to the now well established late effects, nor assume that toxicity will decline.

REFERENCES

Appleton, R.E., Farrell, K., Zaide, J. and Rogers, P. (1990) Decline in head growth and cognitive impairment in survivors of acute lymphoblastic leukaemia. *Arch. Dis. Child.*, **65**(5), 530–4.

Atlas, S.W., Grossman, R.I., Packer, R.J. *et al.* (1987) Magnetic resonance imaging diagnosis of disseminated necrotising leukoencephalopathy. *J. Comput. Tomogr.*, **11**(1), 39–43.

Bailey, C.C., Marsden, H.B., Jones, P.H. (1978) Fatal pulmonary fibrosis following 1,3-bis(2 chloro-ethyl)-1-nitrosourea (BCNU) therapy. *Cancer*, **43**(1), 74–76.

Bhavnani, M., Morris Jones, P.H. and Testa, N.G. (1989) Children in long term remission after treatment for acute lymphoblastic leukaemia showing persisting haematopoetic injury in clonal and long term cultures. *Br. J. Haematol.*, **71**(1), 37–41.

Birch, J.M., Hartley, A.L., Marsden, H.B. *et al.* (1984) Excess risk of breast cancer in mothers of children with soft tissue sarcomas. *Br. J. Cancer*, **49**, 325–9.

Blauensteiner, W., Gadner, H., Buch, J. and Grabno, A. (1987) Aseptic bone necrosis in leukaemia patients in childhood and adolescence. *Paediatr. Pathol.*, **22**(3), 251–8.

Bowman, J.D. (1987) Long-term sequelae of cranial irradiation of neuropsychological functioning of children treated for acute lymphoblastic leukaemia. *Diss. Abstr. Int.* (Sci.), **48**(3), 663.

Brock, P., Yeoman, L., Bellman, S. and Pritchard, J. (1987) Ototoxicity in children treated with *cis* platinum for germ cell and other tumours. *Med. Paed. Oncol.*, **15**(6), 138.

Brugières, L., Hartmann, O., Travagli, J.P. *et al.* (1989) Haemorrhagic cystitis following high dose chemotherapy and bone marrow transplantation in children with malignancies. Incidence, clinical course and outcome. *J. Clin. Oncol.*, **7**(2) 194–9.

Charlton, A., Pearson, D. and Morris Jones, P.H. (1986) Children's return to school after treatment for solid tumours. *Soc. Sci. Med.*, **22**(12), 1337–46.

Copeland, D.R., Dowell, R.E., Fletcher, J.B., *et al.* (1988) Neuropsychological effects of childhood cancer treatment. *J. Child. Neurol.*, **3**(1), 53–62.

Davis, P.C., Hoffman, J.C., Pearl, G.S. and Braun, I.F., (1986) CT Evaluation of effects of cranial radiation therapy in childhood. *Amer. J. Roentgenology*, **147**(3), 587–92.

de Wit, P.E.J., de Vaan, G.A.M., de Booth, M. *et al.* (1990) Prevalence of naevocytic naevi after chemotherapy for childhood cancer. *Med. Paed. Oncol.*, **18**(4), 336–8.

Ederken, B.S., Libshitz, H.I. and Cohen, M.A. (1982) Slipped proximal humeral epiphysis: a complication of radiotherapy to the shoulder in children. *Skeletal Radiol.*, **9**(1), 123–5.

Eigen, H. and Wyszomierski, D. (1985) Bleomycin lung injury in children. Pathophysiology and guidelines for management. *Am. J. Pediatr. Hematol. Oncol.*, **7**(1), 71–8.

Ellenberg, L., McComb, J.G. Siegel, S.E. and Stowe, S. (1987) Factors affecting intellectual outcome in paediatric brain tumour patients. *Neurosurgery*, **21**(5), 638–44.

Elliot, A.J., Oakhill, A. and Goodman, S. (1985) Cataracts in childhood leukaemia. *Br. J. Ophthalmol.*, **69**(6), 459–61.

Goren, M.P., Wright, R.K., Pratt, C.B., *et al.* (1987) The potentiation of ifosfamide neurotoxicity, hematotoxicity and tubular neurotoxicity by prior *cis*-diamminedichloroplatinum(II) therapy. *Cancer Res.*, **47**(5), 1457–60.

Hausdorf, G., Morf, G., Beron, G., *et al.* (1988) Long-term doxorubicin cardiotoxicity in childhood: non-invasive evaluation of the contractile state and diastolic filling. *Br. Heart J.*, **60**(4), 309–15.

Hawkins, M.M., Draper, G.J. and Kingston, J.E. (1987) Incidence of second primary tumours among childhood cancer survivors. *Br. J. Cancer*, **56**, 339–47.

Henderson, I.C. and Frei, E. (1980) Adriamycin cardiotoxicity. *Am. Heart J.*, **99**(5), 671–4.

Heyn, R., Ragab, A., Raney, R.B. *et al.* (1986) Late effects of therapy in orbital rhabdomyosarcoma in children: A report from the inter group rhabdomyosarcoma study. *Cancer*, **57**(9), 1738–43.

Hughes, B.R., Cunliffe, W.J. and Bailey, C.C. (1989) Excess benign melanocytic naevi after chemotherapy for malignancy in childhood. *Br. Med. J.*, **299**(1), 88–91.

Hutter, J.J., Sahn, D.J., Woolfenden, J.M. and Carnahan, Y. (1981) Evaluation of the cardiac effects of doxorubicin by serial echocardiography. *Am. J. Dis. Child.*, **135**(7), 653–7.

Jenkin, D., Doyle, J., Berry, M. *et al.* (1990) Hodgkin's disease in children: Treatment with MOPP and low-dose extended field irradiation without laparotomy; late results and toxicity. *Med. Ped. Oncol.*, **18**, 265–72.

Joensuu, H. (1989) Acute myocardial infarction after heart irradiation in young patients with Hodgkin's disease. *Chest*, **95**(2), 388–90.

Lansky, S.B., Zwartges, W. and Cairns, N.U. (1983) School attendance among children with cancer. *J. Psychosoc. Oncol.*, **2**, 75–82.

Larcombe, I.J., Walker, J., Charlton, A. *et al.* (1990) Impact of childhood cancer on return to normal schooling. *Br. Med. J.*, **301**, 169–71.

Levine, E.G. and Bloomfield, C.D. (1986) Secondary myelodysplastic syndromes and leukaemia. *Clin. Haematol.*, **15**(4), 1037–80.

Li, F.B., Yan, J.C., Sallan, S., *et al.* (1983a) Second neoplasms after Wilms' tumour in childhood. *J. Natl. Cancer Inst.*, **71**(6), 1205–9.

Li, F.P., Corkery, J., Wawter, G. *et al.* (1983b) Breast carcinoma after cancer therapy in childhood. *Cancer*, **51**, 521–3.

Macleod, R.I., Welbury, R.R., and Soames, J.V. (1987) Effects of cytotoxic chemotherapy on dental development. *J. R. Soc. Med.*, **80**(4), 207–9.

Maguire, A., Craft, A.W., Evans, R.G. *et al.* (1987) The long-term effects of treatment on the dental condition of children surviving malignant disease. *Cancer*, **60**(10), 2570–5.

Makiperbaa, A., Heino, M., Laitinen, L.A. and Siimes, M.A. (1989) Lung function following treatment of malignant tumours with surgery, radiotherapy or cyclophosphamide in childhood. A follow up study after 11 to 27 years. *Cancer*, **63**(4), 625–30.

Mancini, A.F., Rosita, P., Canino, R. *et al.* (1989)

School related behaviour in children with cancer. *Paed. Haem. Oncol.*, **6**, 145–54.

Miké, V., Meadows, A.T. and D'Angio, G.J. (1982) Incidence of second primary neoplasms in children: Results of an international study. *Lancet*, **ii**, 1326–31.

Miller, R.W., Fusner, J.E., Fink, R.J. *et al.* (1986) Pulmonary function abnormalities in long-term survivors of childhood cancer. *Med. Pediatr. Oncol.*, **14**(4), 202–7.

Moore, I.M., Kramer, J. and Ablin, A. (1986) Late effects of CNS prophylactic leukaemia therapy on cognitive functioning. *Oncol. Nurs. Forum.*, **13**(4), 45–51.

Moreb, J. and Oblon, D. (1988) The natural history of anthracycline induced cardiomyopathy. *Proc. Annu. Meet. Am. Soc. Clin. Oncol.*, **7**, A296.

Murphy, R.G. and Greenberg, M.L. (1990) Osteonecrosis in paediatric patients with acute lymphoblastic leukaemia. *Cancer*, **65**(8), 1717–9.

O'Driscoll, B.R., Hasleton, P.S., Taylor, P.M. *et al.* (1990) Active lung fibrosis up to 17 years after chemotherapy with Carmustine (BCNU) in childhood. *N. Eng. J. Med.*, **323**(6), 378–82.

Packer, R.J., Grossman, R.I., Rorke, L.B. *et al.* (1985) Brain stem necrosis after pre radiation high dose methotrexate. *Childs. Nerv. Syst.*, **1**(6), 355–8.

Pajori, U., Lanning, M. and Larmas, M. (1988) Prevalance and location of enamel opacities in children after anti neoplastic therapy. *Community Dent. Oral Epidemiol.*, **16**(4), 222–6.

Patterson, W.P. and Khojasteh, A. (1989) Ifosfamide induced renal tubular defects. *Cancer*, **63**(4), 649–51.

Peckham, V.C., Meadows, A.T., Bartel, N. and Marrero, C. (1988) Educational late effects in long term survivors of acute lymphoblastic leukaemia. *Paediatrics*, **81**(1), 127–33.

Purdell Lewis, D.J., Stalman, M.S. *et al.* (1988) Long-term results of chemotherapy on the developing dentition caries risk and development aspects. *Community Dent. Oral Epidemiol.*, **16**(2), 68–71.

Robain, O., Dulac, O., Dommergues, J.P. *et al.* (1984) Necrotising leukoencephalopathy complicating treatment of childhood leukaemia. *J. Neurol. Neurosurg. Psychiatr.*, **47**(1), 65–72.

Rosenstock, J.G., Jones, P.M., Pearson, D. and Palmer, M.K. (1978) Ewings' sarcoma adjuvant chemotherapy and pathological fracture. *Eur. J. Cancer*, **14**(6), 799–803.

Santoro, A., Bonadonna, G., Valagussa, P. *et al.* (1987) Long-term results of combined chemotherapy-radiotherapy approach in Hodgkin's disease: Superiority of ABVD plus radiotherapy versus MOPP plus radiotherapy. *J. Clin. Oncol.*, **5**(1), 27–37.

Schell, M., McHaney, V., Green, A.A. *et al.* (1989) Hearing loss in children and young adults receiving Cis platinum with or without prior cranial irradiation. *J. Clin. Oncol.*, **7**, 75.

Shaw, N.J., Tweeddale, P.M. and Eden, O.B. (1989) Pumonary function in childhood leukaemia survivors. *Med. Paediatr. Oncol.*, **17**(2), 149–54.

Skinner, R., Pearson, A.D.J., Price, L. *et al.* (1989) Hypophosphatemic rickets after ifosfamide treatment in children. *Br. Med. J.*, **29**, 1560–61.

Steinherz, L.H., Steinherz, P. and Tan, C. (1987) Cardiac failure more than six years post-anthracyclines. *Med. Ped. Oncol.*, **15**, 127.

Testa, N.G., Bhavnani, M., Will, A. and Morris Jones, P.H. (1988) Long-term bone marrow damage following treatment for acute lymphoblastic leukaemia. *Haematology*, (8) 279–87.

Trautmann, P.D., Erickson, C., Shaffer, D. *et al.* (1988) Prediction of intellectual deficits in children with acute lymphoblastic leukaemia. *J. Dev. Behav. Paediatr.*, **9**(3), 122–8.

Tucker, M.A., Meadows, A.T., Boice, J.D. *et al.* (1987) Leukaemia after alkylating agent therapy for childhood cancer. *J. Natl. Cancer Inst.*, **78**(3), 459–464.

Welch, T.R. and McAdams, A.J. (1986) Focal glomerulo-sclerosis as a late sequelae of Wilms' tumour. *J. Paediatr.*, **108**(1), 105–9.

Womer, R.B., Pritchard, J. and Barrett, M. (1985) Renal toxicity of cisplatinum in children. *J. Paediatr.*, **106**(3), 659–83.

Chapter 28

The management of morbidity from chemotherapy

A. OAKHILL

28.1 INTRODUCTION

The use of combination chemotherapy in the treatment of childhood cancer has led to a dramatic improvement in survival. The penalties for this improvement are the morbidity and mortality associated with therapy. Table 28.1 outlines the incidence and severity of toxicity in the most commonly used drugs in paediatric oncological practice. The management of both early and late effects provide the paediatric oncologist with a considerable number of taxing clinical problems. It is not possible to deal with all the early problems within this chapter but nausea and vomiting and the prevention and treatment of infection will be addressed. Late effects of treatment are reviewed in Chapters 26 and 27.

28.2 NAUSEA AND VOMITING

The nausea and vomiting associated with the administration of chemotherapy can be life threatening. Older children and adolescents may consider the suffering to be worse than the consequences of stopping treatment early and risking relapse. Chemotherapy-induced emesis should therefore be treated aggressively prior to the first course of treatment.

Morbidity from nausea and vomiting is both physical and psychological. Haematemesis from oesophageal tears, metabolic disturbance and dehydration may occur in poorly controlled emesis. The fear of receiving chemotherapy may be uppermost in a child's mind throughout treatment, leading to anxiety, depression, poor compliance and, in some patients, anticipatory nausea and vomiting.

Increasingly emetic combinations of drugs have been used to improve survival rates. cisplatin, the anthracyclines and ifosfamide, all potent anticancer agents, are vital constituents of protocols in the treatment of poorer prognosis tumours; they also have the highest emetic potential. Until recently, advances in antiemetic treatment have lagged far behind advances in treatment.

28.3 THE PHYSIOLOGY OF VOMITING

There are three phases in the process of vomiting:

Table 28.1 Commonly used drugs and the incidence and severity of toxicity

Toxicity \ Drug	Actinomycin D	Amsacrine	Asparaginase	Bleomycin	Busulphan	Carboplatin	Chlorambucil	Cisplatin	Cyclophosphamide	Cytosine	Daunorubicin	Doxorubicin	Epirubicin	Etoposide	Ifosfamide	Melphalan	6-Mercaptopurine	Methotrexate	Mitozantrone	Procarbazine	Teniposide	Thioguanine	Vinblastine	Vincristine
Nausea and vomiting	3	1	1	1	1	2	1	3	3	2	2	3	2	1	2	2	1	1	2	1/2	1	1	1	1
Haematological	3	3	1	1	2	3	3	3	3	3	3	3	3	2	3	3	2	3	2	3	2	2	1/2	1
Alopecia	2	1	1	2	1	1	1	1	2	2	2	3	2	2	2	2	1	2	1	1	1	1	2	2
'Gut'	2	1	2	1	1	1	1	1	1	2	2	2	2	1	1	1	1	2	1	1	1	1	2	2
Neurological	1	1	2	1	1	1	1	2	1	1/2	1	1	1	1	2	1	1	1/2	1	2	1	1	2	3
Cardiac	1	1	1	1	1	1	1	1	2	1	3	3	2	1	1	1	1	1	2	1	1	1	1	1
Respiratory	1	1	1	3	2	1	1	1	1	1	1	1	1	1	1	1	1	1	1	1	1	1	1	1
Nephrotoxicity	1	1	1	1	1	2	1	3	2	1	1	1	1	1	2/3	1	1	1	1	1	1	1	1	1
Hepatotoxicity	2	2	2	1	1	1	1	1	1	1	2	2	1	1	1	1	2	2	1	1	1	1	1	1
Ototoxicity	1	1	1	1	1	1	1	3	1	1	1	1	1	1	1	1	1	1	1	1	1	1	1	1

1. Little or no toxicity
2. Moderate toxicity
3. Severe toxicity

1. nausea, which is the sensation that vomiting may ensue. There is a concurrent autonomic reaction with bradycardia, sweating, pupillary dilatation and gastric stasis;
2. retching, which is the synchronized contraction of the muscles of respiration. This leads to a negative intrathoracic pressure and allows the static stomach contents to enter the oesophagus;
3. vomiting, where the contraction of the abdominal musculature leads to positive intrathoracic pressure and evacuation of the stomach contents through the mouth.

This complex sequence is probably controlled through the vomiting centre which lies in the lateral reticular formation of the medulla. Emetic agents (physical as well as chemical) do not act directly on the vomiting centre, but through the chemoreceptor trigger zone (CTZ), vagal afferents from the viscera and vestibular and cortical afferents.

In chemotherapy-induced nausea and vomiting, the gastrointestinal tract (through vagal and spinal visceral sympathetic nerves), the cerebral cortex (as seen in anticipatory vomiting), and the CTZ are believed to be the main sites of stimulation prior to input into the medullary vomiting centre. The CTZ is probably the most important element in this process. It is situated on the floor of the fourth ventricle and receptors within it are stimulated by emetic substances in the blood. Messages are then relayed to the vomiting centre.

The neurochemical properties of the CTZ are poorly understood. There is an abundance of histamine, dopamine and probably 5-hydroxytryptamine ($5HT_3$) receptors present and most antiemetic drugs act by blocking one or more of these receptors. Improved knowledge of the neurochemistry of the CTZ will surely lead to a better and more rational use of the drugs we use to prevent vomiting.

28.4 EMETIC POTENTIAL OF CHEMOTHERAPY

There are considerable differences in the emetic potential of chemotherapeutic agents and differences also in the emetic potential on individual patients. In particular, age is an important factor; the younger child is usually far more tolerant of chemotherapy than the adolescent and adult.

The measurement of emetic potential is extremely difficult. Whereas the number of vomits, quantity of vomitus and period of retching can be quantified, it is much more difficult to assess nausea, particularly in younger children. Table 28.2 lists the emetic potential of commonly used drugs in childhood cancer.

Table 28.2   The emetogenic potential of cytotoxics

High incidence
Cisplatin
Actinomycin D
Dacarbazine
Cyclophosphamide
Ifosfamide

Moderate incidence
CCNU
BCNU
Procarbazine
Adriamycin
Daunomycin
High dose cytosine arabinoside
Carboplatin
Epirubicin

Low incidence
Etoposide
6-Mercaptopurine
Methotrexate
Bleomycin
Hydroxyurea
Thioguanine
Vinblastine
Vincristine

28.5 THE PRINCIPLES OF TREATMENT OF CYTOTOXIC DRUG-INDUCED NAUSEA AND VOMITING

Great emphasis should be put on the preventative aspects of cytotoxic drug-induced vomiting. Perhaps the only half truth given to patients about their malignancy and its treatment should be to understate the unpleasantness of nausea and vomiting related to cancer therapy. High expectations of sickness will assuredly lead to cortical impulses into the vomiting centre.

The location where chemotherapy is administered is also important. A quiet and calm atmosphere may be more acceptable to adolescents, whilst younger children may benefit from a ward area with more distractions. Another important external stimulus is smell. Many children report hospital smells as inducing anticipatory nausea. In particular, alcohol wipes may upset them – and how necessary are they anyway?

There are a range of antiemetics available. Very few satisfactory trials however, have been performed on children. There are obvious reasons for this; it would, for example, be unethical to use a placebo on a newly diagnosed patient undergoing a first course of chemotherapy. Kearsley (1985) proposed that clinical trials of antiemetics should take place on patients with identical diagnoses treated on the same drug protocols and not having received prior chemotherapy. In addition to this, patients age could be similar. As can be seen, a randomized, double-blind, crossover trial would be very difficult to perform in paediatric practice. Most studies have relied on comparing the accepted 'in-house' combination to the new agent under investigation.

Various classes of antiemetics are used. Their site of action may be on the vomiting centre, CTZ, cerebral cortex, or peripheral nervous system. In some, the site of action is unknown and in others it is felt that they have more than one means of blocking neurotransmission. It is logical therefore that a combination of drugs may have greater efficacy than a single agent.

The most commonly used agents are dopamine antagonists acting primarily on the CTZ but in some instances having an additional peripheral effect. Perhaps the most interesting class of drugs, however, are the serotonin or $5HT_3$ antagonists.

28.6 ANTIEMETICS

28.6.1 SUBSTITUTED BENZAMIDES

Metoclopramide is a dopamine antagonist acting directly on the CTZ (Terrin *et al.*, 1984). It also has a peripheral antiemetic action, possibly associated with the acceleration of gastric emptying. Initially used in low dosage, it then fell out of favour, but the search for an effective antiemetic to match the emetic potential of cisplatin meant that it was reconsidered and employed at much higher dose.

28.6.2 PHENOTHIAZINES

This class of drugs appears to block dopamine receptors in the CTZ. Extrapyramidal reactions are again an undesired side effect, although patients are far more likely to complain of sedation and the sense of loss of control.

Prochlorperazine and chlorpromazine are the two most widely used antiemetics in paediatric practice. Unfortunately, they not only have undesirable toxicity but are poorly effective when the most emetic cytotoxic agents are given. Employed in combination with other agents such as promethazine or dexamethasone, they may be more efficacious.

28.6.3 CANNABINOIDS

The observation that patients who were regular users of cannabis and who smoked or ate it prior to chemotherapy had less severe vomiting, led to its investigation as an antiemetic. The major psychologically active substance is tetrahydrocannabinol (THC) and this agent was used in early investigations until the development of synthetic substances, the most commonly used of which is nabilone.

THC has been shown in several studies to be more effective than oral prochlorperazine and oral metoclopramide although these drugs hardly constitute a 'gold-standard' (Ekert *et al.*, 1979; Dalzell *et al.*, 1986). Nabilone also has the disadvantage of oral administration and has similar side effects including agitation, dysphoria, euphoria and a dry mouth. The use of these drugs is therefore limited unless they can be shown to have a role in pre-treatment of nausea and vomiting.

28.6.4 BENZODIAZEPINES

The main use for these drugs is in combination with antiemetics as they have little or no antiemetic activity on their own. Lorazepam is the most commonly used example (Anon., 1986). It has the benefits of mild sedation and amnesia and would therefore help patients who suffer from anticipatory nausea and vomiting.

28.6.5 CORTICOSTEROIDS

Ample evidence exists that dexamethasone and methylprednisolone are effective antiemetics. How they act is, however, unclear. They have been used to best effect in combination with other classes of antiemetic (Mehta *et al.*, 1986). Few side effects have been reported but euphoria and insomnia may be seen if they are used as a single agent.

28.6.6 DOMPERIDONE

This benzimidazole derivative acts, similarly

to metoclopramide, on the dopamine receptors in the CTZ and on gut motility. There was considerable interest in its use initially (Craft, 1983), but it appeared necessary to use higher doses than those recommended by the manufacturers and it then fell out of favour, with reports of cardiac toxicity in elderly patients.

28.6.7 5HT₃ ANTAGONISTS

This new class of agents is generating great interest as initial clinical trials show inhibition of emesis with few side effects. Ondansetron is a highly selective $5HT_3$ receptor antagonist acting both centrally in the CTZ and possibly on vagal afferent fibres in the upper gastrointestinal tract. Its effectiveness has shown that not only cholinergic, dopaminergic and histaminergic receptors are important in the CTZ (Peroutka and Snyder, 1982), but also serotonergic receptors (Kilpatrick *et al.*, 1987). Dose ranging phase 1 studies from single and multiple institutions have now been reported on groups of adult patients receiving both non-cisplatin and cisplatin-containing chemotherapy (Hesketh *et al.*, 1989). They appear not only to be highly effective but also to have minimal toxicity with headache and mild sedation being reported on occasion.

Marty *et al.* (1990) looked at the efficacy of ondansetron compared to high dose metoclopramide in a randomized, double-blind, crossover study and found it markedly superior in controlling acute emesis and nausea. This was true both for chemotherapy given over one day and over four to five days.

The role of ondansetron in the management of nausea and vomiting in the paediatric age group awaits results from a multicentre study presently taking place although results from single institutions suggest that the experience will be similar to that in the adult group.

In a study by Pinkerton *et al.* (1990), 30 children with cancer who received emetic combinations of chemotherapy were treated with ondansetron using an initial loading dose of 5 mg/m^2 intravenously, followed by an oral dose eight hourly for five days. The length of treatment was warranted because of the delayed vomiting seen with drugs such as ifosfamide.

The study emphasized the lack of toxicity with this drug although transient rises in liver enzymes were seen. Almost complete control of emesis was seen in patients receiving rapid VAC (vincristine, adriamycin, cyclophosphamide) but the results for patients receiving cisplatin and ifosfamide were disappointing. There appeared to be good control in the first twenty-four hours but late emesis was then seen. This may be due to the dose regimen or the route of administration and emphasizes the need to look at various regimens and the addition of other drugs such as dexamethasone (Cunningham *et al.*, 1989; Smith *et al.*, 1991)

Ondansetron has been highly effective in the control of nausea and vomiting in children undergoing conditioning for bone marrow transplants with cyclophosphamide and total body irradiation (Hewitt *et al.*, 1991).

28.6.8 CONCLUSION

In most areas of paediatric oncology, supportive care has kept abreast of developments in chemotherapy. This has sadly not been the case in the field of nausea and vomiting induced by chemotherapy. Physicians have been in the main blind to the distress caused by this toxicity. The most frequently used antiemetics have failed singly and in combination to combat the problem. The advent of the 5HT$_3$ antagonists offer hope for the future, but it is imperative to look rationally at their use and to design combination regimens which will be highly effective and without side effects.

28.7 HAEMATOLOGICAL TOXICITY

The treatment of infection and provision of adequate transfusion support are two cornerstones of successful supportive care for children treated for cancer. The need for transfusion support is usually predictable and, by and large, there are few contentious issues involved, the management of disseminated intravascular coagulation and the use of granulocyte transfusions being the exceptions.

Infection remains one of the major obstacles to the cure of children with malignant disease. Recent developments in prevention of infection may have a dramatic impact on the incidence of infective morbidity and mortality. Meanwhile, the debate over which empirical antibiotics to use in febrile neutropenic patients continues.

28.8 PRINCIPLES OF INFECTION CONTROL

(a) Prophylaxis

Of bacterial infections found in neutropenic patients, 80% are caused by endogenous flora, the majority from the gastrointestinal tract. At least half of these are acquired in hospital (Schiuff *et al.*, 1972). Attempts have therefore been made to look at the efficacy of protected environments and on gut decontamination. The different approaches all have considerable problems, particularly those related to cost and patient acceptance. Fortunately, the most effective measure is cheap, simple, and acceptable to patients as long as it is performed using warm water – hand washing. (Nauseef and Maki, 1981).

The total protective environment offers no survival advantages to patients undergoing treatment for cancer. The exception, however, is in bone marrow transplantation where bacteria and fungi in the environment need to be reduced to protect patients with prolonged neutropenia, severe cellular and humoral immunodeficiency, and deficiencies or breaks in the body's integument.

Prophylaxis against bacterial, fungal and viral infections have largely proved unhelpful. Exceptions are the administration of trimethoprim-sulphamethoxazole to prevent *Pneumocystis carinii* infection (Hughes *et al.*, 1987) and the use of acyclovir and possibly gancyclovir post bone marrow transplantation to prevent herpes or CMV infections (Schmidt *et al.*, 1991).

The use of gut and selective gut decontamination has been poorly investigated. There are serious doubts about efficacy and compliance and the emergence of resistant strains of bacteria is worrying. Simlarly, antifungal prophylaxis has few benefits, with the exception of the prevention of candidiasis in children at great risk (for example, during remission induction of leukaemia). It is important to review the needs of each unit individually, however. If there is a high incidence of Aspergillosis, for example, attempts to control this such as the use of nebulized amphotericin B (Conneally *et al.*, 1990), may be necessary.

(b) Immunization

Passive immunization using specific and non-specific immunoglobulins is currently under investigation. The case has been proved for varicella-zoster immune globulin, which reduces the incidence of pneumonitis and mortality in immuno-suppressed patients at risk of developing infection. Pooled immunoglobulin preparations are also beneficial in children unfortunate enough not to be immunized against measles and then to have had an infectious contact. The use of CMV globulin as prophylaxis post allogeneic bone marrow transplantation and pooled immunoglobulin to prevent Gram-negative septicaemia, are under investigation.

Active immunization using live attenuated viruses should not normally be considered in immuno-compromized children. The seriousness of infection with varicella-zoster (VZ) has, however, led to clinical trials with attenuated varicella vaccine. The first clinical trial in healthy children took place in Japan using the OKA strain (Takahashi *et al.*, 1974). This was followed by trials in Japan and the USA in the latter part of the 1970s on children with leukaemia. By and large, these were successful with only minor adverse effects seen; VZ vaccine, however, is still not in general use. The probable reason for this is that some batches of vaccine contained a less attenuated form of the live virus leading to quite severe infection in some children.

The Varicella Vaccine Collaborative Study Group (VVCSG) has published several important papers on the use of vaccine in the immuno-suppressed child (Gershan and Sternberg, 1989). They have shown that it is feasible to acquire an 87% seroconversion with one dose of vaccine, but also that by revaccination after three months, seroconversion was as high as 98%. The reason for the second immunization was that some children appeared to lose their antibody as treatment for leukaemia continued. (This factor was not seen in healthy controls.)

The vaccine appeared to be highly effective in the 437 children who were immunized over a 10-year period; only 36 patients developed mild chickenpox, despite a high percentage of children having close contact with infection. The safety of the vaccine has also improved. Although 40% of 372 patients treated in the VVCSG study developed a rash, only four had severe infection. It is imperative, however, to review the safety of the vaccine before it is accepted for more general use. That such a vaccine is necessary is obvious as chickenpox contact and infection in the immuno-suppressed patient, apart from being life threatening, will lead to interruption of treatment (increasing the risk of relapse), loss of time from school, and the continued use of painful, intramuscular injections of zoster immune globulin (ZIG).

(c) Management of infection

The management of febrile neutropenia is the most controversial area of supportive care of the child with cancer. This area of debate may be made obsolete, however, by the prevention of neutropenia by the use of cytokines. Clinical trials using the colony-stimulating factors (CSFs) have now passed through phase I, II, and III studies. The two most interesting CSFs are granulocyte CSF (G-CSF) and granulocyte macrophage CSF (GM-CSF). It is likely that the normal role of these two CSFs is to increase production and function of myeloid cells, particularly during infection. It is not known whether they have any role in basal haematopoiesis. The immediate effect of both GCSF and GMCSF is to cause a fall in circulating neutrophils, eosinophils and monocytes (Morstyn *et al.*, 1989; Weschke *et al.*, 1989). Several hours later there is a rise in leucocyte numbers (sooner with GCSF than GMCSF). With continued administration of GMCSF there are two peaks in neutrophil levels at four days and seven to eight days. GCSF provides a more prolonged plateau.

The best route of administration is the subject of investigation. For GMCSF it would certainly appear that subcutaneous injection causes a higher leucocyte count than continuous intravenous or bolus intravenous administration (Lieschike *et al.*, 1989). These studies have been performed in adults in whom subcutaneous injection may be more acceptable than in children. Even so the actual mechanics of administering G and GMCSF on an out-patient or domicillary basis still needs to be addressed.

Most published studies of the use of G and GMCSF have examined their use in the prevention of chemotherapy-related neutropenia. Results from phase III randomized placebo-controlled trials are not yet available and very few studies involving children have been performed. Early phase I and II clinical trials have been published and have shown reduction of the period of neutropenia, the nadir of neutrophil count, and the avoidance of decreasing doses of chemotherapy. Several studies have shown a reduction in the number of days of pyrexia and the numbers of documented infections. (Antman *et al.*, 1988; Bronchud *et al.*, 1989; Hermann *et al.*, 1989).

CSFs have been used in both autologous and allogeneic bone marrow transplantation and Sheridan *et al.* (1989) and Nemunaitis *et al.* (1991) found a shortened period of neutropenia, less antibiotic and intravenous nutrition usage, and a shorter period in isolation.

The problems of use of the CSFs are those of determining the most effective dose and route of administration and the logistics of treatment in patients who would ordinarily be out-patients. There appears to be little toxicity from their use, apart from occasional bone pain and fever in normal volunteers. Fever may, however, be confused as a sign of infection and promote the use of empirical antibiotics. The cost of treatment with CSFs will have to be studied and compared to the cost of admission and management of febrile neutropenia. It would appear that G and GMCSF have little effect on anaemia and thrombocytopenia and so there will still be dose-limiting toxicities. Nor will they have any effect on decreasing morbidity and mortality from serious viral infections.

A further important issue is whether the CSFs can stimulate the proliferation of leukaemia and solid tumours. There is some evidence in the laboratory that this may be the case, with proliferation of breast cancer and osteosarcoma cell lines, although high concentrations of CSF were used (Dedhar *et al.*, 1988). Clinical studies in the future will need to carefully assess tumour or leukaemia response and leukaemia relapse. No evidence for an increased relapsed rate has so far been documented. Despite these reservations it is likely that the CSFs will have an important role when used judiciously in selected patients at risk of severe infection.

In the early years of chemotherapy the morbidity and mortality from infection was extremely high. Gram-negative septicaemia had a mortality as high as 70%. The use of empirical antibiotics, although contrary to the philosophy of the use of antimicrobials in other clinical settings, became the most important element in the care of immunocompromized neutropenic patients. Since this discovery, the argument has raged over which antibiotics are the most appropriate and whether they should be used singly or in combination. Before reviewing this argument, it is important to state that the experiences of the individual oncology unit and the range of pathogens and their sensitivities within that unit are of the greatest significance.

The EORTC International Antimicrobial Project Group organized some of the earliest trials on empirical antibiotic regimens. There are advantages and disadvantages associated with multinational, multi-centre trials: on the positive side, the large numbers of patients that can be accrued, and on the negative side, the wide variation in organisms and their sensitivities seen between different units.

The first reported trial (EORTC, 1978) compared gentamicin with carbenicillin to gentamicin, carbenicillin and cephalothin. The first combination offered both the best cure rate and the least nephrotoxicity.

The development of semisynthetic penicillins (e.g. azlocillin; piperacillin) and third generation cephalosporins (e.g. ceftazidime; moxalactam) led to the exploration of their use both as single agents and in combination. The third EORTC trial (Gaya, 1984) compared gentamicin with the addition of azlocillin, ticarcillin and cefotaxime. The latter had poor antipseudomonal activity and therefore was found to be the least appropriate.

Throughout these early trials, Gram-negative organisms were the most common and important isolates from infected patients. *S. aureus* infections, so common during the 1960s, had fallen in incidence to about 10% due to better hygiene and effective anti-staphylococcal antibiotics. During the 1980s, however, a new pattern of infection has emerged with gram-positive isolates now as common as Gram-negative. Coagulase-negative staphylococci have increased in importance and are now the commonest organisms implicated in infection of neutropenic patients. Central venous catheters are the major reason for this change. *S. epidermidis*, a common skin organism, easily colonizes these devices. It should be remembered, however, that coagulase-negative infections can arise from other sites in the body such as the gut and respiratory tract.

Currently, a combination of antibiotics as empirical treatment probably has the largest number of advocates. The use of an aminoglycoside with either a cephalosporin or an extended spectrum penicillin offers considerable cover and no combination has been shown to be superior to this. These combinations are, however, more expensive and more toxic (e.g. oto- and nephrotoxicity is seen with the aminoglycosides) and have led many investigators to seek a single antibiotic for empirical treatment. The National Cancer Institute, as reported in an important paper by Pizzo *et al.*, (1986), compared ceftazidime (a third generation cephalosporin) with combination therapy using cephalothin, carbenicillin and gentamicin in 550 episodes of febrile neutropenia. There was no significant difference in terms of success after randomization to either of the arms. The difficulty arises however when the number of modifications to antibiotic therapy are reviewed. Those patients receiving ceftazidime required significantly more changes to treatment when definitive microbiological isolates were available; when the initial clinical assessment was made, more patients were shown to have gingivitis or perirectal infection. In terms of overall outcome, however, Pizzo *et al.* (1986) found monotherapy with cefatzidime to be as effective as combination therapy.

Recently other broad spectrum antibiotics have claimed attention for their use as monotherapy. These include other third generation cephalosporins (e.g. cefoperazone) and carbapenims. These provide excellent Gram-negative cover but are much less active against common Gram-positive organisms. Pizzo argues that Gram-positive infections are not usually associated with severe morbidity or mortality and there was no danger in withholding the appropriate antibiotic, vancomycin, until the isolate and its sensitivities were known. Vancomycin it should also be remembered has considerable oto- and nephrotoxicity as well as being responsible for the 'Red-man' syndrome. Recently however, Morrison *et al.* (1990) have advocated the inclusion of vancomycin in empirical antibiotic treatment in all patients with a central venous catheter. They argue that delayed treatment of Gram-positive septicaemia may lead to metastatic infection and a longer period of hospitalization. This argument had previously been employed by Shenep *et al.* (1988) at the St. Jude Children's Hospital in Memphis, who showed a much higher incidence of treatment failure and breakthrough bacteraemia in patients receiving ticarcillin clavulanate and amikacin than in the combination of those two drugs plus vancomycin.

In summary, each oncology unit needs to take note of its in-house organisms and their sensitivities and decide on an empirical antibiotic therapy. Should this be monotherapy with a third generation cephalosporin or carbapenim? Should it be combination therapy with a cephalosporin or extended spectrum penicillin and aminoglycoside? Should vancomycin be included in the combination?

Whichever decision is made over empirical

therapy, two additional major problems have to be faced: when to add antifungal therapy, and when to stop antibiotic treatment. Pizzo *et al.* (1979; 1982) advocate the continuation of antibiotics until a recovering neutrophil count reaches $500/mm^3$ for patients considered to be at low risk (i.e. when the neutropenia is likely to last less than one week). The management of patients facing a prolonged neutropenia (for example, during the induction of remission and treatment of acute myeloid leukaemia) is more problematic. Pizzo and co-workers have again performed valuable studies looking at this group of patients and they have divided them into two groups – those in whom the fever resolved after starting treatment with antibiotics, and those who remained feverish.

In the first group, antibiotics were continued for seven days and then stopped despite patients still being neutropenic. Unfortunately, 41% of this group again developed pyrexia and antibiotics had to be reinstituted. If antibiotics were stopped after seven days in the second group, then over 60% developed a septicaemia. It is important to emphasize therefore that should patients in the second, non-responding, high risk group stop antibiotics, then a second septicaemia is highly likely and the patients should be kept under close observation. It would seem more appropriate to continue antibiotics for at least a 14-day course or until the neutropenia has resolved. Further studies need to be performed to answer the question of when to stop antibiotics in prolonged neutropenia (see also 9.4).

The difficulty with continuing antibiotics is the risk of developing invasive fungal disease and this may be as high as 30%. A second problem is the increased likelihood of resistant organisms, although this problem is theoretical. Patients facing prolonged neutropenia who remain febrile on antibiotics must be considered to have fungal infection. The optimal time to institute empirical antifungal therapy has not yet been addressed in a clinical trial. Stein *et al.* (1982) and Pizzo *et al.* (1982) suggest that seven days of fever on antibiotics warrants empirical treatment. Four days may be more appropriate, however, considering there is such a high risk of developing infection with marked morbidity and mortality should fungus continue to invade.

There has always been resistance to starting antifungal therapy because of the toxicity associated with the use of amphotericin B. Fever and rigors are commonly seen (and undesirable in a thrombocytopenic patient) and on more prolonged use, nephrotoxicity with hypokalaemia and hypomagnesaemia occurs. Investigations for the future will need to proceed along two lines: firstly, the more accurate and speedy diagnosis of fungal infections, and secondly, the evaluation of newer antifungal therapies in comparison with amphotericin B.

Serological tests for *Candida albicans* are difficult to interpret as false positivity is common. Methods for detection of *C. albicans* antigen have been devised and proven useful (Hopwood and Warnock, 1986). The detection of *Aspergillus fumigatus* and *flavus* antigen in the blood has been more problematic as it appears that the host (i.e. the patient) rapidly metabolizes fungal galactomannan. It is the policy of our BMT Unit to take blood from patients three times a week to try to detect fungal antigen.

Alternative antifungal therapy is now being investigated using liposomal amphotericin B and the newer imidazoles itraconazole and miconazole (Hopes-Berestein, 1987). The results of these trials are eagerly awaited but until their worth has been proven there remains no alternative to the use of amphotericin B.

28.9 CONCLUSION

The supportive care of the child with cancer remains a major part of the work of an oncology unit. Encouragingly, several advances appear to be on the horizon which may prevent or improve early morbidity from chemotherapy. Some of the areas of controversy regarding infection prophylaxis are considered in Chapter 29.

REFERENCES

Anonymous (1986) Corticosteroids and lorazepam as antiemetics in cancer chemotherapy. *Drug. Ther. Bull.*, **24**, 46–8.

Antman, K.S., Griffin, J.D., Elias, A. *et al.* (1988) Effect of recombinant human GM-CSF on chemotherapy induced myelosuppression. *New. Engl. J. Med.*, **319**, 593–8.

Bronchud, M.H., Howell, A., Crowther, D. *et al.* (1989) The use of GCSF to increase the intensity of treatment with doxorubicin in patients with advanced breast and ovarian cancer. *Br. J. Cancer*, **60**, 121–5.

Conneally, E., Cafferhey, M.T., Daly, P.A. *et al.* (1990) Nebulised amphotericin B as prophylaxis against invasive aspergillosis in granulocytopenic patients. *Bone Marrow Transplant.*, **5**, 403–6.

Craft, A.W. (1983) Clinical experience with domperidone in paediatric oncology patients. *Clin. Res. Rev.*, **3**, 45–8.

Cunningham, D., Turner, A., Hawthorn, J. *et al.* (1989) Ondansetron with and without dexamethasone to treat chemotherapy-induced emesis. *Lancet*, **i**, 1323.

Dalzell, A.M., Bartlett, H. and Lilleyman, J.S. (1986) Nabilone: an alternative antiemetic for cancer chemotherapy. *Arch. Dis. Child.*, **61**, 502–5.

Dedhar, S., Grabourg, L., Galloway, P. *et al.* (1988) Human GM-CSF is a growth factor active on a variety of cell types of non-haemopoietic origin. *Proc. Natl. Acad. Sci.*, **85**, 9253–7.

Ekert, H., Waters, K.D., Jurk, I.H. *et al.* (1979). Amelioration of cancer chemotherapy induced nausea and vomiting by delta-9-tetrahydrocannabinol. *Med. J. Aust.*, **2**, 657–9.

EORTC Antimicrobial Therapy Project Group (1978) Three antibiotic regimens in the treatment of infection in febrile granulocytopenic patients with cancer. *J. Infect. Dis.*, **137**, 14–20.

Gaya, H. (1984) Rational basis for the choice of regimens for empirical therapy of sepsis in granulocytopenic patients. *Clin. Haematol.*, **13**, 573–80.

Gershan, A.A. and Sternberg, S.P. (1989) Persistence of immunity in varicella in children with leukaemia immunised with live attenuated varicella vaccine. *N. Engl. J. Med.*, **320**, 892–7.

Hermann, F., Schulz, G., Lindemann, A. *et al.* (1989) Haematopoietic responses in patients with advanced malignancy treated with recombinant human GM-CSF. *J. Clin. Oncol.*, **7**, 159–67.

Hesketh, P.J., Murphy, W.K., Lister, E.P. *et al.* (1989) GR38032F: a novel compound effective in the prevention of acute cisplatin-induced emesis. *J. Clin. Oncol.*, **7**, 700–5.

Hewitt, M., Cornish, J., Pamphilon, D. *et al.* (1991) Effective emetic control during conditioning of children for bone marrow transplantation using ondansetron, a 5-HT$_3$ antagonist. *Bone Marrow Transplantation*, **7**, 431–5.

Hopes-Berestein, G. (1987) Treatment of hepatosplenic candidiasis with liposomal amphotericin B. *J. Clin. Oncol.*, **5**, 310–17.

Hopwood, V. and Warnock, D.W. (1986) New developments in the diagnosis of deep fungal infection. *Eur. J. Clin. Microbiol.*, **5**, 379–88.

Hughes, W.T., Riveira, G.K., Schell, M.J. *et al.* (1987) Successful intermittent chemoprophylaxis for *Pneumocystis pneumonitis*. *N. Engl. J. Med.*, **316**, 1627–32.

Kearsley, J.H. and Tattersall, H.N. (1985). Recent advances in the prevention or reduction of cytotoxic induced emesis. *Med. J. Aust.*, **143**, 4–6.

Kilpatrick, G.J., Jones, B.J. and Tyers, M.B. (1987) Identification and distribution of 5HT$_3$ receptors in rat brain using radioligand binding. *Nature*, **330**, 746–8.

Lieschike, G.S., Maher, D., O'Connor, M. *et al.* (1989) Phase 1 study of intravenously administered GM-CSF and comparison with subcutaneous administration. *Cancer Res.*, **50**, 606–14.

Marty, M., Pouillart, P., Scholl, S. *et al.* (1990) Comparison of the 5HT$_3$ antagonist ondansetron with high dose metoclopramide in the con-

trol of cisplatin-induced emesis. *N. Engl. J. Med.*, **322**, 816–8.

Mehta, P., Gross, S., Graham-Pole, J. *et al.* (1986) Methyl-prednisolone for chemotherapy induced emesis. *J. Pediatr.*, **108**, 774–6.

Morrison, V.A., Peterson, B.A. and Bloomfield, C.D. (1990) Nosocomial septicaemia in the cancer patient. The influence of central venous access devices, neutropenia and type of malignancy. *Med. Ped. Oncol.*, **18**, 209–16.

Morstyn, G., Lieschke, G., Sheridan, W. *et al.* (1989) Clinical experience with recombinant human G-CSF and GM-CSF. *Sem. Haematol.*, **26**, (Suppl. 2) 9–13.

Nemunaitis, J., Buckner, C.D., Appelbaum, F.R. *et al.* (1991) Phase I/II trial of recombinant human granulocyte-macrophage colony-stimulating factor following allogeneic bone marrow transplantation. *Blood*, **77**, 2065–71.

Neuseef, W.M. and Maki, D.G. (1981) A study of the value of simple protective isolation in patients with granulocytopenia. *N. Engl. J. Med.*, **304**, 448–53.

Peroutka, S.J. and Snyder, S.H. (1982) Antiemetics: neuro-transmitter receptor binding predicts therapeutic actions. *Lancet*, **1**, 658–9.

Pinkerton, C.R., Williams, D., Wootton, C. *et al.* (1990) 5HT$_3$ antagonist ondansetron – an effective out-patient antiemetic in cancer treatment. *Arch. Dis. Child.*, **65**, 822–5.

Pizzo, P.A., Robichaud, K.J., Gill, F.A. *et al.* (1979) Duration of empiric antibiotic therapy in granulocytopenic cancer patients. *Am. Med. J.*, **67**, 194–200.

Pizzo, P.A., Robichaud, K.J., Gill, F.A. *et al.* (1982) Empiric antibiotic and antifungal therapy for cancer patients with prolonged fever and granulocytopenia. *Am. Med. J.*, **72**, 101–11.

Pizzo, P.A., Hathorn, J.W., Hiemeniz, J.W. *et al.* (1986) A randomised trial comparing ceftazidime alone with combination antibiotic therapy in cancer patients with fever and neutropenia. *N. Engl. J. Med.*, **315**, 552–8.

Schiuff, S.C., Young, V.M., Greene, W.H. *et al.* (1972) Origin of infection in acute non-lymphocytic leukaemia. *Ann. Intern. Med.*, **77**, 707.

Schmidt, G.M., Horah, D.A., Niland, J.C., *et al.* (1991) A randomised controlled trial of prophylactic ganciclovir for CMV pulmonary infection in recipients of allogeneic bone marrow transplants. *N. Engl. J. Med.*, **324**, 1005–11.

Shenep, J.L., Hughes, W.T., Roberson, P.K. *et al.* (1988) Vancomycin, ticarcillin and amikacin compared with ticarcillin clavulonate and amikacin in the empirical treatment of febrile, neutropenic children with cancer. *N. Engl. J. Med.*, **319**, 1053–8.

Sheridan, W.P., Morstyn, G., Wolf, M. *et al.* (1989) Effects of GCSF following high dose chemotherapy and autologous bone marrow transplantation. *Lancet*, **ii**, 891–5.

Smith, D.B., Newlands, E.S., Rustin, G.J.S. *et al.* (1991) Comparison of ondansetron and ondansetron plus dexamethasone as anti-emetic prophylaxis during cisplatin-containing chemotherapy. *Lancet*, **338**, 487–90.

Stein, R.S., Kayser, J. and Flexner, J. (1982) Clinical value of empirical amphotericin B in patients with acute myelogenous leukaemia. *Cancer*, **50**, 2247–51.

Takahashi, M., Ofsuko, T., Okuno, Y. *et al.* (1974). Live vaccine used to prevent the spread of varicella in children in hospital. *Lancet*, **ii**, 1288–90.

Terrin, B.N., McWilliams, N.B. and Maurer, H.M. (1984). Side effects of metoclopramide as an antiemetic in childhood cancer. *J. Pediatr.*, **104**, 138–40.

Weschke, G.J., Maher, D., Cebon, J. *et al.* (1989) Effects of sub-cutaneously administered recombinant human GM-CSF in patients with advanced malignancy. *Ann. Int. Med.*, **110**, 357–64.

Chapter 29

Prophylaxis against infection during cancer treatment

I. VAN LOO

29.1 INTRODUCTION

Prolonged and severe neutropenia is a common sequel to many chemotherapy regimens and the possibly fatal risk of infection during granulocytopenic episodes is a major problem. Treatment-related and patient-related factors predisposing to infection and the major pathogens are listed in Tables 29.1 and

29.2 respectively. There is a strong correlation between the number of circulating neutrophils and the presence and severity of bacterial and fungal infections. (Bodey *et al.*, 1966). Susceptibility to infection is determined not only by the absolute neutrophil count, but also by the rate of decline and duration of neutropenia (Hathorn and Pizzo, 1988)

Table 29.1 Predisposing factors to infection during cytotoxic chemotherapy

I.	Treatment-related factors
	(a) Degree of leucopenia (particularly granulocyte counts below 500/mm^3)
	(b) Duration of leucopenia
	(c) Concomitant high dose corticosteroid therapy
	(d) Indwelling central venous cannulae
II.	Patient-related factors
	(a) Lesions in mucosa, skin, epithelium
	(b) Pre-existing foci of infection:
	* symptomatic: boil; periodontal sepsis
	* asymptomatic: cytomegalovirus or herpes carrier
	(c) Poor general hygiene
	(d) Immunodeficiency associated with the disease itself
III.	Hospital/environment-related factors
	(a) Poor hospital facilities
	(b) Poor aseptic techniques
	(c) 'Hospital' organisms (with differing 'adherence', colonization and antibiotic sensitivity profiles)

Table 29.2 Common pathogens in paediatric oncology

Bacteria
Gram positive: Staphylococci
Streptococci
Corynebacteria
Listeria
Gram negative: Enterobacilli
(particularly noteworthy are multiple drug resistant coliforms)
Anaerobes: *Clostridia*, e.g. *C. perfringens* and *C. septicum*, but also noteworthy is the antibiotic-associated
enterocolitis due to *C. difficile*)

Fungi
Candida sp.
Aspergillus sp.
Cryptococcus
Phycomycetes (e.g. *mucor, rhizopus*)

Viruses
Herpes (simplex, zoster)
CMV, EB, RSV, adenovirus, influenza, rotavirus, HIV

Other opportunist agents
Pneumocystis carinii
Toxoplasma
Strongyloides stercoralis
Cryptosporidia

The quality of neutrophil function may also be altered due to the underlying disease or secondary to chemotherapy/radiotherapy (Pickering *et al.*, 1978). Cell-mediated immunity, with predisposition to viral and other opportunistic infections, is similarly depressed.

In a historical series of 494 adult patients with acute leukaemia treated in Houston between 1966 and 1972, Bodey (1986) found that there were 1216 febrile episodes (2.4 febrile episodes per patient). Disseminated infections accounted for 35% of infection episodes, pneumonia for 34%, cellulitis for 11%, and urinary tract infections for 7%. The causative agent was identified in 73% of cases, and Gram-negative bacilli were the most common pathogens (*E. coli, Klebsiella* and *Pseudomonas* accounting for over three quarters of all cultured bacteria). Gram-positive organisms (predominantly *Staphylo-

coccus aureus*) were responsible for only 6% of infections, and fungi (predominantly *Candida*) for 8%. The overall fatality from established bacterial septicaemia during the studied period was up to 85%.

Since that time, the immediate initiation of (empirical) intravenous antibiotics when neutropenic patients become febrile has greatly reduced fatalities, despite the ever-increasing aggressiveness of modern (myelo-suppressive) chemotherapy regimens. The rate of fatal infections in relation to paediatric solid tumour chemotherapy regimens is below 5%; it only rises above 15% in cases of acute myeloblastic leukaemia (see Chapter 9).

Several other important changes have also occurred since that series was evaluated. Repeated peripheral venous cannulations, as well as the current routine placement of long-lasting in-dwelling venous cannulae, have increased the risk of *Staphylococcus epidermidis* bacteraemias. Furthermore, the introduction of effective intravenous antibiotics against Gram-negative bacilli, and bowel decontamination regimes during neutropenia, have led to a substantial shift towards organisms other than Gram-negative bacilli as the cause of infections.

29.2 PRINCIPLES OF PROPHYLAXIS

A list, albeit oversimplified, of prophylactic measures that may be taken to prevent infection in the child receiving aggressive chemotherapy is given in Table 29.3.

In many clinical studies that have investigated preventive measures against infection, the most important measure has been the basic practice of hygiene by the medical staff (hand washing; use of gowns or plastic aprons; a stethoscope reserved for individual patient use, etc.).

(a) Isolation

In order to ensure a so-called protected

Table 29.3 Possible prophylactic measures against infection during cytotoxic chemotherapy

I.	Environment
	(a) Hygiene-handwashing
	(b) Protected environment
II.	Host
	(a) Chemoprophylaxis
	* Bowel decontamination
	* Prevention of colonization of indwelling venous cannulae
	* Antivirals
	* Antifungals
	* Antiparasitics
	(b) Avoidance of CMV-positive blood products
	(c) Active immunization
	(d) Passive immunization
	(e) Acceleration of granulocyte recovery
	(f) Oral hygiene

environment, the technique of 'reverse isolation of the patient' was introduced; this involves single rooms for the patients, air filtration, and barrier nursing. Interestingly, there is no sound evidence that such measures reduce the mortality from infection in these patients compared with patients who are managed by medical staff observing the basic practice of hygiene, and where patients receive prompt intravenous antibiotics upon the development of a febrile intravenous episode (Ribas-Mundo *et al.*, 1981; Armstrong, 1984).

The 'totally protected environment' (TPE) is a more pan-sterile regimen. The patient's room has a constant positive-pressure air flow of filtered air, and an aggressive programme of sterilization of all objects entering the room (including a low microbial or gamma-irradiated diet). In addition, the patient is given skin and bowel decontaminating antibiotics.

The TPE may confer survival advantages in patients who are profoundly neutropenic for many weeks (typically, bone marrow transplant patients), but is not otherwise considered routinely advantageous. Nevertheless, in hospitals where *Aspergillus* is a problem, the use of air filtration/laminar air flow rooms is judicious. The avoidance of foods which are naturally heavily contaminated with bacteria (such as some fresh fruits and vegetables), and water purification, may all be sensible measures to be included under the 'basic hygiene' label.

(b) Selective bowel decontamination

The reason that protected environments have not been more successful is that, in most studies, 80–85% of organisms responsible for infections in cancer patients are derived from their own endogenous flora (this changes to 50% where these are hospital-based germs). Oral and gastrointestinal flora are found to be the most common cause of endogenous infection, accounting for the high incidence of Gram-negative bacilli in the Houston study (see above). Initial studies used oral prophylaxis, with non-absorbable antibiotics, with the intention of sterilizing the bowel. The antibiotics employed included neomycin, gentamycin, polymyxin, framycetin, colistin and vancomycin. However, those regimens were unpalatable, and compliance was poor.

Furthermore, infections by antibiotic-resistant strains (particularly aminoglycoside-resistant strains) nullified any gains, and *Clostridium difficile* enterocolitis was a threat. Subsequently, there has been great interest in 'selective bowel decontamination' (SBD), using antibiotics that preserve the normal anaerobic flora of the gut while greatly reducing the aerobic Gram-negative bacilli. The rationale for this is that the preserved natural anaerobic flora will colonize and provide resistance against new colonization by opportunistic organisms (aerobes and fungi) (Van der Waaij *et al.*, 1971; van der Waaij and Berghuis de Vries, 1974).

At the Emmakinderziekenhuis in Amsterdam, the impact of SBD on febrile neutropenic episodes has been studied in three serial cohorts of patients: 1979 (no SBD), 1982–1983 and 1989; the latter two patient groups having been treated with SBD comprising polymyxin, cotrimoxazole and nystatin.

In the 1982–1983 cohort (Ramaekers, 1986), it was concluded that the introduction of SBD had led to a considerable reduction in the number of infections, septicaemias and deaths (the latter by a factor of seven-fold), when compared to the historical control group.

The same SBD regimen, reported recently, was used in the 1989 group (van Loo, 1990). A febrile episode occurred in 64% of neutropenias (defined as neutrophil count less than $500/mm^3$ for more than seven days). An organism was identified in only 58% of these presumed infective episodes. Of the proven

organisms, 35% were still Gram-negative bacilli, but 55% were Gram-positive cocci (with a surprisingly high incidence of alpha-haemolytic streptococci); 3% were *Candida albicans*.

The conclusion from this Amsterdam study has been that, with good compliance, SBD will reduce the infection rate from Gram-negative rods in particular. However, with poor compliance (which remains a problem), and an emergence of Gram-positive infections, especially alpha-haemolytic streptococci, the advantages of SBD are less clear-cut than was concluded by this study. The emergence of resistant organisms also remains a problem.

Oral cotrimoxazole has been explored as an antibacterial/bowel decontamination prophylactic agent. It also has the advantage of being active against *Pneumocystis carinii*. However, many of the disadvantages listed above apply, and there is the additional problem that the agent delays the recovery time of the granulocyte count – a factor that is not fully circumvented by a regimen of administration of three times per week. If bone marrow transplantation and high risk acute leukaemias (where controversy remains) are excluded, there is at present no evidence that SBD has a routine place in management.

(c) Other techniques

As has been mentioned above, the adoption of tunnelled central venous catheters has led to a proportionately greater incidence of Gram-positive coccal septicaemias and bacteraemias due to other skin commensals. In a recent study, Schwartz and colleagues (1990) have shown that catheter flushes with vancomycin-containing solutions significantly reduce this high rate of bacteraemia. The authors did not encounter vancomycin-resistant strains, but their conclusions have yet to be routinely accepted.

The presence of skin or peridontal sepsis or

(1974) Selective elimination of *Enterobacteriae* species from the digestive tract in mice and monkeys. *J. Hyg. (Camb.)*, **72**, 205–11.

Waaij van der, D., Berghuis de Vries, J.N., Lekkerkerk van der Wees, J.E.C. *et al.* (1971) Colonization of the digestive tract in conventional and antibiotic treated mice. *J. Hyg. (Lond.)*, **69**, 405–11.

Ziegler, E.J., McCutchon, J.A., Fierer, J.A. *et al.* (1982) Treatment of Gram-negative bacteraemia and shock with human antiserum to mutant Escherichia coli. *N. Engl. J. Med.*, **307**, 1254–60.

Chapter 30

Minimization and management of morbidity from radiotherapy

D.M. TAIT

30.1 RADIATION MORBIDITY IN CHILDREN

Children treated with radiotherapy are at risk of developing a number of late radiation effects; these roughly divide into three categories: abnormal growth and development of tissue; abnormal functioning of organs; and the induction of second malignancies. The third is obviously a catastrophic event, but fortunately it is rare. Unfortunately, the other two can also result in physiological, cosmetic and psychological consequences which may have an enormous effect on the quality of life of children surviving from cancer. This issue is now an important part of the management of paediatric malignancies: not only in the treatment of late effects as they become apparent in the increasing number of surviving children, but also as a constant consideration in the design of new treatments.

The incidence and severity of late radiation effects is very variable, but there are certain parameters that are known to influence outcome. One of the major determinants is the dose of radiation and the way in which it is given. In general, the higher the total dose, the greater the chance of damage. Both the individual fraction size and the total time taken to complete the course of treatment can modify this considerably. This means both that the use of small-sized fractions, i.e. <2 Gy, is likely to be less toxic and that the incidence and severity of complications will rise as fraction size increases.

These principles hold true both for adults and children, but children appear to be more sensitive to radiation damage, at least in terms of late effects. In general, the most severe radiation effects are seen in children who were irradiated at a very early age, and this relationship is particularly obvious in the central nervous system and musculo-skeletal tissues. In the central nervous system, the first two to three years of life are a time of intense activity, and during this period the process of myelination is completed. This probably accounts for the susceptibility to damage during this period; after the age of five, on the other hand, tolerance is very similar to that seen in adults. For other tissues, increased radiosensitivity is presumed to relate to tissue kinetics and to the growth and development that occurs in childhood.

30.2 RISK-BENEFIT ANALYSIS

Although the tissues of children are more radiosensitive than those of adults, and therefore more likely to suffer radiation damage, most paediatric tumours are also more radiosensitive than their adult counterparts. This means that radiotherapy can provide an effective form of treatment and can achieve good results using lower doses than are commonly employed in adult practice. Unfortunately, most children with paediatric tumours have a systemic malignancy and local treatment alone can only offer cure to a minority. Before the introduction of effective chemotherapy, this was the only chance of cure and very severe morbidity was therefore accepted as the necessary price to pay for any chance of survival.

The availability of effective chemotherapy has transformed the management of paediatric malignancy, with two major consequences: successful eradication of micrometastases has improved survival, and adequate chemoreduction of primary tumours has altered the requirement for local treatment. This means that in many situations, traditional radiotherapy doses and volumes can either be avoided altogether, modified, or minimized, and much better survival rates can be achieved with a coincidental decrease in morbidity.

30.3 THE AVOIDANCE OF RADIATION MORBIDITY

30.3.1 AVOIDING RADIOTHERAPY

Avoiding radiotherapy completely is the only certain way of avoiding radiation morbidity. However, this policy can only ethically be pursued in situations where it has been clearly established that omitting radiation will not adversely affect the outcome. This requires successive, well-designed clinical trials, each addressing a simple treatment question so that the appropriate management policy can progressively be defined. This is a laborious process, and all the more difficult in rare tumours where multi-centre cooperation offers the only possibility of success. However, it has been done. The National Wilms' Tumour Study (NWTS) group, for example, has carried out a series of clinical trials investigating the indications for, and the required intensity of, radiotherapy while maintaining the same overall survival rate. As a result, children with a good prognosis disease, as defined by early stage and favourable histology, are now treated by surgery and chemotherapy alone without any compromise in survival. These children are therefore spared the risk of musculo-skeletal deformity (Riseborough *et al.*, 1976; Vaeth *et al.*, 1962) or damage to other abdominal organs such as bowel and liver (Tefft, 1977).

Similarly, randomized trials in rhabdomyosarcoma have established that radiotherapy is unnecessary in certain categories of disease. IRS-I looked at the need for radiotherapy following wide local excision of localized tumours with negative excision margins and found that the addition of radiotherapy made no difference in terms of disease-free or overall survival (Maurer *et al.*, 1988). The question of whether or not radiotherapy can improve outcome where there is more extensive disease at the start of chemotherapy, i.e. in Group 3 patients, was also addressed in a randomized SIOP trial. Again, no difference was found between the two arms of the trial in terms of control of local disease (Flamant *et al.*, 1985).

In acute lymphoblastic leukaemia, effective CNS directed treatment has already reduced the rate of central nervous system recurrence from more than 60% to around 5%. Initially, this was achieved with craniospinal irradiation, but the associated radiation morbidity led to a search for less toxic, but equally effective, alternatives. Successive clinical trials have confirmed the approximate equivalence of cranial irradiation combined with intrathecal methotrexate; first at a dose of 24 Gy, and subsequently at the reduced dose of 18 Gy (Bleyer and Poplack, 1985; Rivera *et al.*, 1986). The possibility of replacing radiotherapy altogether has also been investigated, and the current MRC leukaemia study (UKALL XI) includes a randomization of high risk patients to either cranial irradiation or high dose intravenous methotrexate, both in combination with intrathecal methotrexate. Obviously, if CNS treatment can be as effectively achieved without cranial irradiation, then this ought to be achievable with a consequent reduction in toxicity, mainly in terms of intellectual function, endocrine status, and cataract formation. However, it is critical that alternative treatments are also strictly appraised with regard to toxicity to ensure that there is a true therapeutic benefit.

The possibility of avoiding radiotherapy does not, as yet, apply to all paediatric tumours. For brain tumours in particular, where chemotherapy has so far not been able to achieve the enormous impact on survival seen with other childhood tumours, radiotherapy remains an important component of treatment. However, for infants where the results of radiotherapy in terms of survival are poor, and where radiation damage is particularly pronounced, intensive chemotherapy regimens are being investigated to see whether radiotherapy can be avoided or at least delayed until the central nervous system is more fully developed (Baram *et al.*, 1986; Duffner *et al.*, 1986; Jacobs *et al.*, 1989).

30.3.2 MODIFYING RADIATION DOSE AND TARGET VOLUME

As both dose and volume are important determinants of normal tissue damage, a reduction in either or both will decrease the probability of late effects occurring. Cytoreduction of primary tumours by chemotherapy has made such modifications possible in most situations where radiotherapy is employed for local control. Again, the best way to prove the adequacy of a modified radiotherapy treatment is to test it in a randomized clinical trial. The NWTS has done this in order to determine whether it is necessary to irradiate the entire abdominal cavity, as was standard practice for Wilms' tumour, or whether radiotherapy can be confined to the tumour bed. The results show that the entire abdomen need only be encompassed in children with pre-operative or intra-operative tumour rupture, diffuse peritoneal seeding, or massive abdominal disease. Other children requiring radiotherapy need only have the tumour bed irradiated.

As a result of NWTS studies which have addressed the question of radiation dose, it has been possible to successfully modify treatment with regard to this parameter also. Traditionally, doses in the region of 24–30 Gy were used in Wilms', but it is now clear that, depending on the chemotherapy combination employed, doses as low as 10 Gy may be equally effective (Thomas *et al.*, 1988).

Dose can also effectively be modified by altering the fractionation schedule. Fraction size is a critical determinant of late normal tissue damage, but for most malignancies it seems to have little effect on tumour cell kill. Theoretically, therefore, a radiation schedule using multiple small fractions should be able to achieve the same level of tumour cell kill while decreasing the probability of late damage. Hyperfractionated schedules of this type are, however, generally used at the moment as a means of increasing the effective tumour dose while keeping normal tissue toxicity at the level that is seen with conventional fractionation. In paediatric oncology, this approach has been tried in those tumours in which dose escalation might be beneficial, such as large pelvic Ewing's and brain stem glioma (Edwards *et al.*, 1989).

30.3.3 EXCLUSION OF NORMAL TISSUES

In the process of external beam radiotherapy planning, consideration is always given to the position of normal tissue structures and the radiation dose that they will receive with any given beam arrangement. Every attempt is made to avoid, or at least to minimize, the dose to critical tissues whilst ensuring that the tumour area is uniformly irradiated to the prescribed dose. The treatment plan which offers the best therapeutic gain in terms of these factors can then be implemented.

In a few situations, it may be possible to surgically reposition critical organs in order to ensure that they are excluded from the high dose volume. For example, a procedure to 'hitch' the ovaries out of the area of pelvic irradiation has been performed in Hodgkin's disease (Le Floch *et al.*, 1976). In addition, several mechanisms have been devised for holding normal bowel out of the radiation field and these could have particular application in paediatric oncology in pelvic Ewing's, where it is necessary to get a high radiation dose into the tumour. However, this sort of approach is limited to a very few situations, and a common alternative is to use lead shielding within the radiotherapy beam to protect critical underlying structures. Because of divergence of the treatment beam, and the partial transmission of radiation through lead, this can never totally protect the underlying organ. In addition, care has to be taken to ensure that there is no coincidental protection of tumour. A simple example of this type of normal tissue protection is the use of lead blocks to protect the optic lenses and to reduce the likelihood of cataractogenesis when irradiating the brain or head/neck region. Even so, despite this measure, it is not uncommon to find some degree of catar-

act formation, thus indicating the inadequacy of the system. In addition, care must be taken not to provide protection to potential sites of disease such as the cribriform plate.

The precision of placement of protective lead blocks has been greatly aided by the application of computer technology to radiotherapy planning. Using serial CT or MRI images, it is now possible to reconstruct a three-dimensional image of the tumour volume and of the adjacent normal tissues. Three-dimensional planning from this information allows for the high dose volume to conform as closely as possible to the tumour volume with maximum exclusion of normal tissues. Therapy of this type is becoming more commonplace in radiotherapy practice and offers a possibility not only of excluding normal tissues and thus decreasing the probability of radiation damage, but also of being able to escalate dose within the tumour area.

Another approach for altering the dose distribution in normal tissues is stereotactic radiotherapy which is currently being developed and evaluated for treatment of brain tumours. The aim of this technique, using a multiple beam arc, is to achieve a higher dose in a very limited area of brain while reducing the dose to the surrounding normal tissues. Generally, this means that more of the brain receives radiation than with conventional external beam treatment, but to a lower dose. It remains to be determined whether or not this will prove to be a useful therapeutic approach.

Brachytherapy is a form of radiotherapy in which the direct application of radioactive materials to accessible tumours provides a localized, high dose treatment volume with relatively good sparing of adjacent normal structures (Plowman *et al.*, 1988; Thomson *et al.*, 1988). This can be achieved by inserting radioactive sources into body cavities (intracavitary), directly into tissue (interstitial), or by applying sources directly to body surfaces (mould application). Because the dose distribution in brachytherapy is largely governed by the inverse square law, a high dose can be delivered near the sources, but this rapidly falls off at a short distance from the radioactive source. Sometimes it is appropriate to deliver the entire radiation dose using a brachytherapy technique. In other situations it is used in addition to external beam to boost the dose to the most 'at risk' area while sparing most of the adjacent normal tissues from further irradiation. In paediatric oncology, this is a technique which has been widely used for retinoblastoma, where plaques of ^{137}Cs or ^{192}Ir are directly applied to focal areas of retinal involvement (Bedford *et al.*, 1971; Bleyer *et al.*, 1985).

Brachytherapy has also been used in rhabdomyosarcoma and other soft tissue sarcomas where both intracavitary and interstitial applications may provide a useful means of increasing the tumour dose while sparing normal tissues (Goffinet *et al.*, 1983).

30.3.4 AVOIDANCE OF COMBINED TOXICITY

In general, a combined modality approach in the management of paediatric tumours has had a beneficial effect with regard to reducing late radiation effects and surgical morbidity. However, this is not necessarily always the case and it is important to bear in mind that chemotherapy can enhance both the acute toxicity of radiation, as can be seen in the mucositis associated with treatment of head and neck tumours, and certain late effects such as cardiac and pulmonary dysfunction. It is therefore essential that when a treatment schedule involves both chemotherapy and radiation, there is careful selection of drugs so as to avoid overlapping toxicity of this type. It is also important to consider sequencing of the two modalities as this can sometimes significantly influence the likelihood and severity of acute and late side effects (Berry, 1980).

30.4 TREATMENT OF THE PHYSIOLOGICAL SEQUELAE OF RADIATION MORBIDITY

As radiation damage can affect any organ or tissue, the discussion of its management is an enormous topic and beyond the scope of this chapter. Some of the commoner sequelae have therefore been selected, with particular emphasis on those in which effective 'treatment' is available.

30.4.1 THE DETECTION OF LATE EFFECTS

Although radiation damage *per se* is irreversible, many late effects can be treated or overcome. This means that organized, relevant follow-up is essential to ensure that late effects are considered and investigated, and that treatment measures are instituted as and when appropriate. Early intervention may be important, as in the detection of growth hormone deficiency following cranial irradiation when, to maximize growth potential, replacement therapy should be started as soon as a fall in growth velocity occurs. In other situations, such as cosmetic correction of facial deformity, the best time to implement corrective measures may be after many years, but this can best be assessed by early awareness of the problem and regular observation.

The detection of late effects is obviously important for individual children, but is also critical in terms of appreciating the toxicity associated with a particular treatment policy. Many centres now run late effects clinics in which the relevant organs and their function are systematically examined. This is likely to be much more sensitive, in terms of detecting late effects, than the somewhat random assessment of patients coming through general oncology clinics.

30.4.2 MUSCULO-SKELETAL DEFORMITY

Virtually any external beam radiotherapy

treatment will involve irradiation of normal musculo-skeletal tissues. The effect that this will have in the long term will depend upon the age of the child at the time of irradiation, the volume of normal tissue included, the dose-fractionation schedule employed, and whether or not chemotherapy was used concurrently. For many children the final effect may seem trivial, but for others it will have serious implications and, for some, it will be catastrophic.

The two most important measures of outcome are cosmetic result and function. Serious cosmetic sequelae are most common when areas in the head and neck region have been irradiated, and these carry obvious psychological implications. However abnormal development of any body site may significantly affect body image and severely influence quality of life. Because of these consequences, it is essential that the long-term side effects are discussed fully at the outset with the parents (and the child, depending on age), and to handle the late effects as sympathetically and effectively as possible, if and when they occur. From the point of view of function, musculo-skeletal deformity of any site or severity will affect the usual perfect symmetry of the system, thereby inducing abnormal strains and tending to produce premature arthritis, etc. However, deformity of musculo-skeletal tissue may have secondary effects on other organs and tissues, as, for example, when impairment of pulmonary function accompanies gross deformity of the bony thorax.

Many of these deformities can now be corrected, at least in part, by modern surgical techniques, and the head and neck region is an area where this has been enthusiastically pursued. Because of the likelihood of developing facial deformity and asymmetry, irradiation of the face is avoided or moderated, along the lines already discussed, whenever possible. However, this is not always possible and, in addition, there are many children attending oncology clinics now who were treated at a time when more reliance had to be placed on radiotherapy. For these children, plastic surgery techniques should be considered since even a minor objective improvement may carry an enormous benefit to the patient.

As facial bone growth is closely allied with the development of the dentition, a process completed by the eruption of wisdom teeth in early adulthood, radiation might be expected to have some effect on facial development up to late puberty (Jaffe *et al.*, 1984). However, naturally, the effects are likely to be much greater the younger the child is at the time of treatment. The mandible is the major impetus to facial growth, a process which occurs in spurts, the first being at around the age of five to seven years and the second being associated with puberty. The mandibular condyle is the major growth centre for mandible, and therefore radiation of this area is likely to have the most profound effect.

For children irradiated at an early age, the best way of applying corrective surgery is usually by a process of repeated operations. Often this involves a first operation around the age of six to eight years, a further one around puberty, and a final adjustment in early adult life. For this reason, these children are best managed by early consideration of surgical procedures and careful anticipation of the likely final outcome if there is no intervention.

In addition to abnormal bone development following radiotherapy, there may be an associated hypoplasia of all soft tissue elements, including muscle and skin. Well-established techniques for correcting bone deformity, such as transfer of growing bone and onlay of bone grafts, need therefore to be accompanied by some means of creating tissue expansion. This is a comparatively modern approach and usually involves the insertion of a balloon-like bag beneath the skin which is slowly inflated, thereby increasing the surface area of the overlying skin. This procedure generally takes many weeks, but can be performed on an out-patient basis. The resultant increased area of skin can then comfortably accommodate the bone graft. Alternatively, by microvascular tissue transfer, a cutaneous or muscle flap can be used to provide bulk for deficient tissues. For example, a de-epithelialized groin flap can be used to restore the bulk of the cheek.

Unfortunately, there is a price to pay for corrective surgery, and that is scarring. The more surgery that is undertaken, the greater the number of skin incisions required and the more gross the deformity from scarring. Paradoxically, scarring in young children often tends to be more marked, with a greater tendency to hyptertrophy and stretching. Thus, although a facial feature may be quite successfully reconstructed it may be accompanied by the production of a number of unsightly scars at other body sites.

Facial surgery is not undertaken entirely for the cosmetic outcome. Radiation sequelae may also result in poor function, the most common problem at this site being dental malocclusion. Lack of orbital bone growth, however, accompanied by relative absence of periorbital fat and lack of growth of the eyelids, will affect the normal functioning of the eye. Similarly, hypoplasia of the nose can interfere with upper airway function. Both the orbit and nose are difficult areas to correct cosmetically and it should be reiterated that there is always a price to pay both at the area corrected and at the donor site when tissue transfer is attempted.

30.4.3 ENDOCRINE DEFICIENCIES

Failure of endocrine function following radiotherapy is now well documented and it seems that at least some endocrine tissues are relatively radio-sensitive. For example, the threshold dose capable of damaging the region of the hypothalamic-pituitary axis

responsible for growth hormone secretion appears to be only in the range of 20–30 Gy (Blatt *et al.*, 1988; Kirk *et al.*, 1987), subject to the fractionation schedule employed. Likewise, traditionally fractionated doses of less than 26 Gy can induce thyroid abnormalities although the incidence rises sharply with doses above this level (Constine *et al.*, 1984). However, abnormal function following low dose radiotherapy may not produce obvious clinical deficiencies and is more commonly detected by biochemical measurement of hormone levels. In other words, the endpoints available for detecting this form of radiation damage are relatively sensitive compared with those employed for many other tissues. In addition, there is the advantage that the functional status of the irradiated organ can be assessed relatively non-invasively and with minimal time and effort on the patient's part. This contrasts sharply with the sort of studies necessary to pick up minor degrees of malfunction in, for example, heart, lung and bowel.

Documenting subtle endocrine dysfunction is, however, not merely an academic pursuit. The ubiquitous effect of hormone imbalance on the normal growth and development of children, together with the availability of effective treatment, makes this a worthwhile area of effort.

The commonest radiation-induced endocrine abnormalities are those in which the hypothalamic-pituitary axis, thyroid or gonads have been included in, or lie adjacent to, the high dose treatment volume. At-risk children are therefore easily defined and require regular long-term follow-up to ensure that all deficiencies are detected and corrected appopriately.

Although the majority of endocrine deficiencies become apparent within the first few years after treatment (Duffner *et al.*, 1985; Constine *et al.*, 1984), in some children it may be as long as five years before they are detectable (Constine *et al.*, 1989).

As children with acute lymphoblastic leukaemia and brain tumours form the bulk of paediatric oncology practice, irradiation of the hypothalamic-pituitary axis within the cranial treatment volume is the commonest source of post-treatment endocrine abnormality. However, there seems to be a big variation in radiosensitivity between the process responsible for the production of growth hormones and the mechanisms responsible for other hypothalamic-pituitary products. As a result, abnormalities of growth hormone secretion are the commonest type of radiation-induced abnormality.

(a) Growth hormone insufficiency

Discrepancies in the reported prevalence of growth hormone insufficiency following radiotherapy are probably principally due to differences in sensitivity of the diagnostic tests employed. For example, in a study of 17 children given 25 Gy cranial irradiation, 14 (82%) had an abnormal growth hormone response on insulin tolerance testing but were normal with respect to growth velocity, serum somatomedin activity, and bone age (Shalet *et al.*, 1976b). Recently, attention has been given to the pulsatile nature of normal growth hormone secretion, the effects that radiotherapy has on this pattern, and its subsequent correlation with growth failure. Using alteration in the profile of growth hormone secretion as a measure of radiation damage, it seems that children treated with 18 Gy are less affected than those given 24 Gy (Blatt *et al.*, 1988).

Many children who develop growth hormone insufficiency following cranial radiation will also have had radiotherapy to the spine as part of their primary management. Because of this, the magnitude of response that can be expected from growth hormone replacement therapy will be reduced, and measurement of growth in body segments is necessary in order to fully assess the effect of treatment. These children in particular will get the most out of growth hormone therapy if it is commenced early, which means intervening as soon as growth velocity falls.

The appreciation of the normal pulsatile pattern of the secretion of growth hormone has led to modification in the administration of replacement therapy. It appears that the same overall weekly dose is more effective when given daily than when given as a three-times-a-week schedule (Hindmarsh and Brooke, 1988).

The possibility that increasing the frequency of injection further – for example, to three times a day – may be even more effective, is currently being investigated. Once established, the daily administration of growth hormone is usually straightforward and without side effects. The possibility of using growth hormone-releasing hormone (GHRH) for replacement therapy is under investigation and appears to be effective although as yet there is no depot preparation (Brain *et al.*, 1990). There is no good evidence that exogenous growth hormone promotes tumour recurrence (Arslanian *et al.*, 1985), although the obvious high chance of coincidental recurrence whilst on growth hormone therapy has promoted anecdotal reports.

Growth hormone is usually continued until either the child is contented with the achieved height, bone fusion is detected or growth has ceased. In girls, only a very little further growth can be expected following the start of menstruation.

(b) Thyroid hormone insufficiency

Thyroid insufficiency following treatment of childhood malignancy may be classified as primary, i.e. as a result of the direct effect of radiation on the thyroid gland, or secondary, because of damage to the hypothalamic-pituitary axis. The former mechanism is by far the commonest, most often occurring in children irradiated for treatment of medullo-blastoma or Hodgkin's lymphoma.

Although the thyroid gland is generally considered to be a relatively resistant organ, it may be more vulnerable to the effects of radiation during childhood (Shalet *et al.*, 1977). Certainly, it would appear that doses in the order of 40 Gy, conventionally fractionated, are highly likely to result in thyroid dysfunction (Abusrewil *et al.*, 1989). The interval after treatment to the peak incidence of thyroid dysfunction is not yet known since good prospective studies are not yet available (Shalet, 1983). However, from the accessible data, it would seem that the majority of abnormalities are detected within five years of completing radiotherapy (Livesey and Brook, 1989).

Measurement of serum thyroid-stimulating hormone (TSH) concentration is the most sensitive method for detecting thyroid dysfunction and is the most common abnormality seen in children following radiotherapy, the majority of whom are biochemically euthyroid (Brown *et al.*, 1983). The optimum management of these children with compensated hyothyroidism has not yet been rationally defined, but it has been shown that this group of patients have alterations in the cardiac systolic time interval which can be reversed by thyroxine replacement (Ridgway *et al.*, 1981). Another concern is that there is some evidence that a persistently elevated serum TSH concentration may have a role in the development of subsequent thyroid malignancies (Doniach, 1963). Although it is not known whether suppression of the TSH level with exogenous thyroxin is protective, it is general policy to give thyroxin to those children whose TSH is elevated. Most centres would now therefore recommend that thyroid function be assessed annually, and that because of the risk of thyroid malignancy, patients should be followed up for life with the aim of detecting any suspicion of thyroid carcinoma early.

It seems that if chemotherapy has any effect on thyroid function, then it is probably small. However, the suggestion that chemotherapy may have an independent contribution to thyroid function has recently been made (Livesey and Brook, 1989).

(c) Gonadal dysfunction

The clinical picture of gonadal dysfunction following radiotherapy is complex, mainly because of the strong dependence of outcome both on age and radiation dose. In addition, the situation is often confounded by the concurrent use of chemotherapy which may independently, or synergistically, cause gonadal damage. Despite this complexity, it is clear that the ovary and testis are both radiosensitive organs and that the effects on the germ cell line are greater than those on the Sertoli/Leydig cells. The available clinical dose-response data is somewhat blurred by uncertainty in radiation dose, particularly where the gonads lie outside the high dose volume.

In the few studies of ovarian function which are uncomplicated by the effects of cytotoxic agents, it has been shown that children treated by fractionated, whole abdominal radiotherapy to a dose of 20–30 Gy are highly likely to develop subsequent ovarian failure (Shalet *et al.*, 1976a; Himmelstein-Braw *et al.*, 1977). However, in women over the age of 40, the ovaries are much more sensitive and a dose of only 6 Gy will induce an artificial menopause (Lushbaugh and Casarett, 1976). Unlike the situation with other tissues, the effect on fertility of fractionating the dose is uncertain, making it difficult to compare different clinical treatment schedules (ICRP, 1984). Nevertheless, allowing for this uncertainty, an upper limit for the LD_{50} of the human oocyte has been calculated to be in the order of 4 Gy (Wallace *et al.*, 1989), which is lower than had been previously estimated. This means that children whose ovaries have only received a small dose of radiation need to be followed up with a view to detecting any decline in function. The availability of effective replacement therapy means that these children can successfully be 'guided' through a 'normal' puberty and develop secondary sexual characteristics which are such an important part of body image and self-assurance and therefore, critical in terms of quality of life.

Fortunately, the management of primary gonadal failure is relatively straightforward, and by administering either oestrogen or testosterone it is fairly easy to induce puberty. However, it is important that these pubertal changes are allowed to evolve slowly so that, for girls, there is adequate development of the uterus and the future possibility for *in vitro* fertilization. Unfortunately, testosterone cannot yet be given as an oral preparation and is currently given as a monthly, subcutaneous depot injection. On the other hand, oestrogen can be given orally, although its absorption by this route is very variable; the effectiveness of a trans-dermal preparation is currently being investigated with very encouraging results.

Secondary gonadal failure as a result of radiotherapy to the hypothalamic-pituitary axis is much less common and usually occurs only as part of a general hypopituitary picture. These children retain potential fertility and, using pulsatile administration of gonadotrophin-releasing hormone, it is possible to induce puberty and ovulation (Stanhope *et al.*, 1987).

30.4.4 CATARACT FORMATION

It has long been recognized that, after a prolonged delay, radiation can induce posterior subcapsular cataract formation in the optic lens. It appears that this is due to the effects of ionizing radiation on the germinative zone in the pre-equatorial region of the anterior lens epithelium. The damaged cells,

or their remnants, are gradually pushed to the posterior pole of the lens at which point cataract may be detected. The resultant deterioration in vision is obviously a significant handicap and therefore the dosimetry of treatment set-up and dose-response information has been investigated. Early dosimetry studies suggested that the minimum cataractogenic dose for a single fraction was 2 Gy, and for fractionated treatment given over three weeks to three months it was 4 Gy (Merriam and Focht, 1957). In this study, all patients receiving more than 11.5 Gy developed cataract irrespective of the fractionation schedule used. Furthermore, it became apparent that lower lens doses were associated with a longer latency and with a greater chance of subsequent cataracts being stationary rather than progressive. Since then a number of other studies have looked at the question of cataractogenic dose and shown considerable variation. However, in practice, every effort is made to keep the dose to the lens to a minimum (Harnett *et al.*, 1987), for example, by using the type of lead blocks described earlier, but without compromising disease control. Nevertheless, should cataract develop despite shielding, surgery is now a possibility in all patients and the resultant deficit can be corrected using an intra-ocular lens implant when appropriate. This development has had a major influence on the significance of the opposing risks of cataract formation and tumour recurrence.

30.5 TREATMENT OF THE PSYCHOLOGICAL SEQUELAE OF RADIATION MORBIDITY

30.5.1 NEUROPSYCHOLOGICAL AND INTELLECTUAL DEFICITS

Taking the survivors of childhood malignancy as a whole, the incidence of significant neuropsychological dysfunction appears to be low (Holmes *et al.*, 1975). However, for certain tumour types, namely brain tumours and acute lymphoblastic leukaemia which together constitute more than half the paediatric oncology population, significant deterioration in global IQ and specific cognitive deficits have been described (Meadows *et al.*, 1981; Moss *et al.*, 1981; Danoff *et al.*, 1982). These late effects have been quite extensively studied but it is difficult to attribute blame, at least in a quantitative fashion, because of the many possible contributing factors. This is particularly the case with brain tumours where the tumour itself, raised intra-cranial pressure, hydrocephalus, radiotherapy and other forms of therapy may share joint responsibility for final functional outcome. The inclusion of many different brain tumour types, with the accompanying variation in treatment, makes the interpretation of studies of this group of patients particularly difficult. Children treated for acute lymphoblastic leukaemia are much more uniform as a group, have larger numbers of long-term survivors, and have therefore been the subject of more detailed investigations. However, even here, there are complicating factors such as initial central nervous system disease, central nervous system relapse, type of CNS directed therapy and approach to neuropsychological assessment.

Confining the discussion to acute lymphoblastic leukaemia, the result of studies addressing neuropsychological outcome appear to be discordant. This has recently been systematically examined in an attempt to define the discrepancies and to search for a possible common underlying neuropathological mechanism (Williams and Davis, 1986). Twenty-eight studies, performed over a nine-year period, were reviewed; from the pooled data it was not possible to implicate any particular form of CNS therapy as being more likely to induce cognitive impairment. In other words, the children who received cranial irradiation as part of their CNS therapy fared no worse than those treated with intrathecal methotrexate alone or intrathecal methotrexate combined with high dose intravenous methotrexate. Similar results, from a single centre study looking at children treated on a single protocol with no evidence of CNS disease at diagnosis, failed to show any treatment-related difference when the children were examined with standardized memory measures (Mulhern *et al.*, 1988). Another study, looking at academic achievement as a functional measure of neuropsychological outcome, failed to show any difference between patients who had cranial irradiation and those who did not (Allen *et al.*, 1990).

Recent results looking at neuro-developmental status in young children and infants treated for brain tumours are also interesting (Mulhern *et al.*, 1989). In this study 14 young children were given prolonged pre-irradiation chemotherapy with the aim of delaying cranial irradiation for as long as possible to allow a greater degree of CNS maturation. What was interesting in this study was the finding of a significant degree of deceleration of linear and psychological growth during the chemotherapy phase. This further supports the increasing evidence that factors other than radiotherapy may have an important influence on the final functional status of these children. With the current trend towards replacing radiotherapy with chemotherapy, either for CNS therapy in leukaemia or for treatment of brain tumours in very young children, it is essential that a full evaluation of the toxic effect of these therapeutic manoeuvres is performed.

Irrespective of causal factors, and the overall variation of the treated population from normal controls, it certainly appears that some children develop late problems which translate into educational and learning difficulties and which finally determine their achievements in terms of personal and professional life style. The possibility of reversing, or at least teaching these children to compensate for their disabilities, is being investigated. Although this needs to be done systematically, there is some indication that rehabilitative measures, such as special training or tutoring to sustain attention and concentration, may be of benefit (Peckham *et al.*, 1988). What is encouraging to the further development of this approach is the probability that the learning deficits are specific and not indicative of global mental retardation.

REFERENCES

Abusrewil, S.S., Mott, M.G., Oakhill, A. *et al.* (1989) Thyroid function in survivors of cancer. *Arch. Dis. Child.*, **64**, 709–12.

Allen, A., Malpas, J.S. and Kingston, J.E. (1990) Educational achievements of survivors of childhood cancer. *Paediatrics, Haemetology and Oncology*, **7**, 339–45.

Arslanian, S.A., Becker, D.J., Lee, F.A. *et al.* (1985) *Am. J. Dis. Child.*, **139**, 347–50.

Baram, T.Z., Eys, J. van and Pack B. (1986) Optimal surgery and MOPP chemotherapy in infants with primitive neuroectodermal tumours of the posterior fossa. *Ann. Neurol.*, **20**, 423.

Bedford, M.A., Bedotto, C. and Macfaul, P.A. (1971) Retinoblastoma: study of 139 cases. *Br. J. Ophthalmol.*, **55**, 19–27.

Berry, R. (1980) Effect of timing between drugs and radiation on type of interaction. *Int. J. Radiat, Oncol. Biol.*, **6**, 957–9.

Blatt, J., Lee, P., Suttner, J. and Finegold, D. (1988) Pulsatile growth hormone secretion in children with acute lymphoblastic leukaemia after 1800 cGy cranial radiation. *Int. J. Radiat. Oncol. Biol.*, **15**, 1001–6.

Bleyer, W.A. and Poplack, D.G. (1985) Prophylaxis and treatment of leukaemia in the central nervous system and other sanctuaries. *Sem. Oncol.*, **12**, 131–48.

Brain, C.E., Hindmarsh, P.C. and Brook, C.G.D. (1990) Continuous subcutaneous GHRH (1–29) NH$_2$ promotes growth over one year in short, slowly growing children. *Clin. Endocrinol.*, **32**, 153–63.

Brown, I.H., Lee T.J., Eden, O.B. *et al.* (1983) Growth and endocrine function after treatment for medulloblastoma. *Arch. Dis. Child.*, **58**, 722–7.

Constine, L.S., Cann, D., Woolf, P. *et al.* (1989) Radiation-induced hypothalamic and pituitary injury in children following treatment of CNS malignancies. *Paediatr. Res.*, **25**, 149a.

Constine, L.S., Donaldson, S.S. and McDoughall, I.R. (1984) Thyroid dysfunction after radiotherapy in children with Hodgkin's disease. *Cancer*, **53**, 878–83.

Danoff, B.F., Cowchock, S., Marquette, C. *et al.* (1982) Assessment of long-term effects of primary irradiation for brain tumours in children. *Cancer*, **49**, 1580–6.

Doniach, I. (1963) Effects, including carcinogenesis, of ^{131}I and X-rays on the thyroid of experimental animals. *Health Phys.*, **9**, 1357–62.

Duffner, P.K., Cohen, M.E., Voorhess, M.L. *et al.* (1985) Long-term effects of cranial irradiation on endocrine function of children with brain tumours. *Cancer*, **56**, 2189–93.

Duffner, P.K., Cohen, M.E., Horowitz, M., *et al.* (1986) Post-operative chemotherapy and delayed irradiation in children <36 months of age with malignant brain tumours. *Ann. Neurol.*, **20**, 424 (abstract).

Edwards, M.S.B., Wara, W.M., Urtasun, R.C. *et al.* (1989) Hyperfractionated radiation therapy for brain/stem glioma: a phase I/II trial. *J. Neurosurg.*, **70**, 691–700.

Flamant, F., Rodary, C., Voûte, P.A. and Otten, J. (1985) Primary chemotherapy in the treatment of rhabdomyosarcoma in children: Trial of the International Society of Paediatric Oncology (SIOP) preliminary results. *Radiother. Oncol.*, **3**, 187–292.

Goffinet, D.R., Martinez, A., Pooler D. *et al.* (1983) Paediatric brachytherapy, in *Model Interstitial and Intracavitary Radiation Management* (ed. F.W. George III) Masson, New York, pp. 57–70.

Harnett, A.N., Hungerford, J.L., Lambert, G.D. *et al.* (1987) Improved external beam radiotherapy for the treatment of retinoblastoma. *Br. J. Radiol.*, **60**, 753–60.

Himmelstein-Braw, R., Peters, H. and Faber, M. (1977) Influence of irradiation and chemotherapy on the ovaries of children with abdominal tumours. *Br. J. Cancer*, **36**, 269–75.

Hindmarsh, P.J. and Brook, C.G.D. (1988) Contribution of dose and frequency of administration to the therapeutic effect of growth hormone. *Arch. Dis. Child.*, **63**, 491–4.

Holmes, G.E. and Holmes, F.F. (1975) After ten years, what are the handicaps and life styles of children treated for cancer? *Clin. Paediatr.*, **14**, 819–23.

ICRP (1984) Non-stochastic effects of ionising radiation, ICRP Publication 41 (Pergamon Press, Oxford).

Jacobs, J.S., Walker, R.W., Jennings, M.T. and McElwain, M.C. (1989) Pre-radiation chemotherapy in the treatment of infant brain tumours. *Ann. Neurol.*, **26**, 459.

Jaffe, N., Toth, B.B., Moar, R.E., *et al.* (1984) Dental and maxillofacial abnormalities in long-term survivors of childhood cancer. Effects of treatment with chemotherapy and radiation to the head and neck. *Paediatr.*, **73**, 816–23.

Kirk, J.A., Raghapathy, P. and Stevens, M.M. (1987) Growth failure and growth hormone deficiency after treatment for acute lymphoblastic leukaemia. *Lancet*, **i**, 190–3.

Le Floch, O., Donaldson, S.S. and Kaplan, H.S. (1976) Pregnancy following oophoropexy and total nodal irradiation in women with Hodgkin's disease. *Cancer*, **38**, 2263–8.

Livesey, E.A. and Brook, C.G.D. (1989) Thyroid dysfunction following radiotherapy and chemotherapy of brain tumours. *Arch. Dis. Child.*, **64**, 593–5.

Lushbaugh, C.C. and Casarett, G.W. (1976) The effect of gonadal irradiation in clinical radiation therapy: A review. *Cancer*, **37**, 1111–20.

Malpas, J. (1988) Cancer: the consequences of cure. *Clin. Radiol.*, **39**, 166–72.

Maurer, H.M. (1978) The Intergroup Rhabdomyosarcoma Study: update, November 1978. *Natl. Cancer Inst. Monogr.*, **58**, 61–8.

Maurer, H.M., Beltungady, M., Gehan, E.A. *et al.* (1988) The Intergroup Rhabdomyosarcoma Study 1. A final report. *Cancer*, **61**, 209–20.

Meadows, A.T., Gordon, J., Massari, D.J. *et al.* (1981) Declines in IQ scores and cognitive dysfunctions in children with acute lymphocytic leukaemia treated with cranial irradiation. *Lancet*, **ii**, 1015–8.

Merriam, G.R. and Focht, E.F. (1957) A clinical study of radiation cataracts and the relationship to dose. *Am. J. Roentgenology*, **77**, 759–85.

Moss, H.A., Nannis, E. and Poplack, D. (1981) The effects of prophylactic treatment of central nervous system on the intellectual functioning of children with acute lymphocytic leukaemia. *Am. J. Med.*, **71**, 47–52.

Mulhern, R.K., Horowitz, M.E., Kovnar, E.H. *et al.* (1989) Neurodevelopmental status of infants and young children treated for brain tumours with pre-irradiation chemotherapy. *J. Clin. Oncol.*, **7**, 1660–6.

Mulhern, R.K., Wasserman, A.L., Fairclough, D. and Ochs, J. (1988) Memory function in disease-free survivors of childhood acute lymphocytic leukaemia given CNS prophylaxis with or without 1,800 cGy cranial irradiation. *J. Clin. Oncol.*, **6**, 315–20.

Peckham, V.C., Meadows, A.T., Bartel, N. and Marrero, O. (1988) Educational late effects on long-term survivors of childhood acute lymphocytic leukaemia. *Paediatrics*, **81**, 127–33.

Plowman, P.N., Doughty, D. and Harnett, A.N. (1988) Paediatric brachytherapy. I The role of brachytherapy in the multi-disciplinary therapy of localised cancers. *Br. J. Radiol.*, **62**, 218–22.

Ridgway, E.C., Cooper, D.S., Walker, H. *et al.* (1981) Peripheral responses to thyroid hormone before and after 1-thyroxin therapy in patients with sub-clinical hyothyroidism. *J. Clin. Endocrinol. Metabol.*, **53**, 1238–42.

Riseborough, E.J., Grabias, S.L., Burton, R.I. and Jaffe, N. (1976) Skeletal alterations following irradiation of Wilms' tumour: with particular reference to scoliosis and kyphosis. *J. Bone Joint Surg.*, **58**, 526–36.

Rivera, G.K., Buchanon, G., Boyett, J.M. *et al.* (1986) Intensive retreatment of childhood acute lymphoblastic leukaemia in first bone marrow relapse: a paediatric oncology study. *N. Engl. J. Med.*, **315**, 273–8.

Shalet, S.M., Rosenstock, J.D., Beardwell, C.G. *et al.* (1977) Thyroid dysfunction following external irradiation for Hodgkin's disease in childhood. *Clin. Radiol.*, **28**, 511–15.

Shalet, S.M. (1983) Disorders of the endocrine system due to radiation and cytotoxic chemotherapy. *Clin. Endocrinol.*, **18**, 637–59.

Shalet, S.M., Beardwell, C.G., Morris-Jones, P.H. *et al.* (1976a) Ovarian failure following abdominal irradiation in childhood. *Br. J. Cancer*, **33**, 655–8.

Shalet, S.M., Beardwell, C.G., Pearson, D. *et al.* (1976b) The effects of varying doses of cerebral irradiation on growth hormone production in childhood. *Clin Endocrinol.*, **5**, 287–90.

Stanhope, R., Brook, C.G.D., Pringle, P.J. *et al.* (1987) Induction of puberty by pulsatile gonadotrophin-releasing hormone. *Lancet*, **ii**, 552–5.

Tefft, M. (1977) Radiation related toxicity in National Wilms' Tumour Study Number 1. *Int. J. Radiat. Oncol. Biol. Phys.*, **2**, 455.

Thomas, P.R.M., Thefft, M., D'Angio, G.J. and Norkool, P. (1988) Validation of radiation dose reductions used in the Third National Wilms' Tumour Study (NWTS-3). Proceedings of the American Society of Clinical Oncology, **29**, 227.

Thomas, P.R.M., Theft, M., Farewell, V.T. *et al.* (1984) Abdominal relapses in irradiated Second National Wilms' Tumour Study patients. *J. Clin. Oncol.*, **2**, 1098–101.

Thomson, E.S., Afshar, F. and Plowman, P.N. (1988) Paediatric brachytherapy. II Brain implantation. *Br. J. Radiol.*, **62**, 223–9.

Vaeth, J.M., Levitt, S.H., Jones, M.D., *et al.* (1962) Effects of radiation therapy in survivors of Wilms' tumour. *Radiology*, **79**, 560.

Wallace, W.H.P., Shalet, S.M., Hendry, J.H. *et al.* (1989) Ovarian failure following abdominal irradiation in childhood: The radiosensitivity of the human oocyte. *Br. J. Radiol.*, **62**, 995–8.

Williams, J.M. and Davis, K.S. (1986) Central nervous system prophylactic treatment for childhood leukaemia: neuropsychological outcome studies. *Cancer Treat. Rev.*, **13**, 113–27.

Chapter 31

Philosophy of follow-up methods

E. DOUEK

31.1 INTRODUCTION

Dramatic advances in paediatric oncology have resulted in improved survival rates and careful follow-up on a long-term basis is now mandatory. Overall survival figures of 65–75% have led to 1/1000 of the population now, in their third decade, surviving a childhood malignancy (Young *et al.*, 1986). The nature of follow-up management depends on timing in relation to therapy. Baseline parameters will allow follow-up during therapy to establish (a) the response to therapy, and (b) the timing of achieving a complete response. Subsequent repeated reviews are carried out to detect relapse at an early stage in patients whom it is still possible to cure by the early introduction of salvage therapy.

Follow-up should, however, not be simply concerned with detection of relapse: with prolonged survival, follow-up of early and late complications of treatment is becoming ever more important. The oncologist, who is interested in response rates and survival curves, should work towards giving maximum benefit for the minimum overall toxicity. Follow-up, therefore, is intended to consider the wellbeing of children with cancer to ensure that they achieve normal or maximal growth maturation and psycho-social adaptation despite the setbacks of intensive cancer therapy. The growing child it should be remembered may be more vulnerable to the delayed adverse sequelae of cancer therapy.

The risk factors for relapse and treatment complications should also be considered. Careful history taking, examination, and relevant investigation (with the above thoughts in mind) will lead to optimal follow-up management. This chapter attempts to outline the various risk factors and complications involved and gives suggestions for follow-up of the more common paediatric malignancies. Some guidelines are common irrespective of disease, e.g. children who receive >300 mg/m^2 of anthracycline should have ECG and/or ECHO studies, on treatment and repeated 6 and 12 months off treatment. Similarly renal function and audiometry should be documented after each 200 mg/m^2 of cisplatin and repeated off treatment at 6 and 12 months.

31.2 ACUTE LYMPHATIC LEUKAEMIA (ALL)

Investigations during continuing therapy that include 12-weekly height and weight measurement and full blood count (FBC) every two to four weeks. Once treatment is complete the patient should be seen monthly for a year, and two-monthly for the second year. At each visit a blood count is taken and full clinical examination is performed, including regular auxology. More detailed investigations may be needed if the initial therapy caused untoward toxicity. Relapse is most common in the first year off treatment, and recurrence is rare if the patient is clear of disease after four years. At relapse full clinical examination and investigation of bone marrow, and CSF are mandatory. Extramedullary relapse documentation should also be carried out, with biopsy of testis and lymph nodes, as indicated clinically.

Late neurological dysfunction may occur in children because of the use of neurotoxic treatment modalities (Meadows and Evans, 1976; Copeland *et al.*, 1985). Patients with acute leukaemia as well as central nervous system tumours run a higher risk as radiotherapy has often been used in treatment schedules. If concomitant CNS directed chemotherapy is involved the risks are even greater. As these two groups of malignancies account for some 50% of childhood cancers, neuropsychological dysfunction is a significant problem overall for childhood cancer survivors. The frequency and severity of these problems will be related to radiotherapy volume, dosage and timing of treatment. Simple neuropsychometric tests can be performed during the first few weeks of treatment and thereafter at one, two and three years from diagnosis. Serial scans may be useful in patients who have received cranial irradiation, especially if radiotherapy occurred in early childhood (Riccardi *et al.*, 1985).

Evaluation of neurological dysfunction should involve a multidisciplinary approach, and include input from a paediatric endocrinologist since the hypothalamic/pituitary

volumes may have been in the radiation field. The age of the child is important, with early treatment causing greater deficit. More careful attention should therefore be directed to cognitive and developmental function so that special needs can be picked up early. On the whole, specific tests, e.g. EEG, EMG, should only be performed if there is a deficit: the clinician should also be aware that anomalies were not a pre-existing feature. Subtle abnormalities in an asymptomatic child may presage clinical deficits. Generally, an assessment of 'development' one to two years after treatment cessation and then every two to three years until early adulthood, should be performed.

31.3 WILMS' TUMOUR

Follow-up in these patients will be related to both stage and histopathology; those with mesoblastic nephroma, for example, will rarely have distant spread unless there has been tumour rupture. D'Angio *et al.* (1989) reviewed 1400 patients and established differing sites of secondaries at diagnosis and local/distant relapse sites of primary renal tumours. Follow-up management for Wilms' tumour should include:

1. On treatment
   (a) Stages 1–3: chest radiography (AP/LAT) every six to eight weeks. Abdominal ultrasound every three months.
   (b) Stage 4: monthly chest x-ray to review shrinkage of metastases. Abdominal ultrasound monthly to assess time for surgery. A chest x-ray should be taken every six weeks after surgery until the end of treatment.
2. Follow-up off treatment
   (a) Clinic visits two monthly for first year, with a chest x-ray every eight weeks for one to one-and-a-half years. Then three-monthly for twelve months

(Stages 1–3), or for two years (Stage 4), six-monthly for a third year.

(b) Abdominal ultrasound six-monthly for two years. Patients at particular risk of abdominal relapse may be scanned more frequently (D'Angio *et al.*, 1989);

(c) Relevant bone/liver/brain scans can be performed three-monthly for one year then six-monthly for two years and annually to the fifth year (D'Angio *et al.*, 1989).

Patients with associated features, e.g. Beckwith's syndrome, hemihypertrophy, or aniridia, should be watched carefully with regard to the remaining kidney. If there has been unilateral removal of a tumour, the contralateral side should be ultrasound scanned three-monthly during the first two years post surgery then six-monthly for a further three years and annually for another five years.

Long-term follow-up involves looking for the late effects of radiotherapy on soft tissues, bowel, and bone (Evans *et al.*, 1986). Second tumours can occur in irradiated sites, e.g. thyroid/breast in patients with lung secondaries (D'Angio *et al.*, 1976; Meadows *et al.*, 1985).

Gastrointestinal symptoms may give clues as to whether treatment has left residual problems, e.g. adhesions, strictures, ulceration and malabsorption. There may be problems relating to site of tumour, e.g. liver in field if right-sided, or extent of irradiation (whether whole abdomen or flank irradiation is given). Fibrosis of the gut is worse with radiation following surgery and usually occurs within five years. The onset can be insidious compared to the detection of chronic enteritis, and the input of the gastroenterologist may be helpful. Careful auxology and follow-up of spinal growth is mandatory.

Nephrotoxicity can be acute or chronic. A single check on renal status within several months of treatment is adequate if all the results are normal. Compromising a remaining kidney is hazardous so acute problems such as an infection of the urinary tract must be treated rapidly and followed up to ensure the infection has been eradicated. Blood pressure checks should be carried out at every visit.

31.4 NEUROBLASTOMA

The follow-up programme should include appropriate tissue scans as well as monitoring tumour markers. Urinary VMA, HVA and dopamine are standard. NSE and ferritin levels may be useful markers in Stages 3–4 where the disease load can be followed from initial treatment to remission. The n-*myc* amplification and diploid DNA index are indications for closer follow up, especially in low stage disease. *m*IBG scans are useful for restaging, particularly in detecting residual bone marrow involvement.

1. Off treatment
   (a) Clinic follow-up monthly for three months, two-monthly until one year off treatment, and then three- to four-monthly for the next year;
   (b) Urinary catecholamines should be checked at each visit. Children treated with platinum should have GFR/audiology checked six-monthly for the first eighteen months off treatment.

Children with stage 4 disease who have received aggressive chemotherapy do not need intensive monitoring after treatment as early detection is of relapse not going to alter prognosis. Once three years from diagnosis have lapsed all investigations can be stopped.

31.5 NON-HODGKIN'S LYMPHOMA

Full follow-up includes repeating baseline parameters on treatment and, because of the

605

high salvage rate in this disease, close off treatment surveillance.

1. On treatment
   (a) stages 1–3:
      (i) prior to each pulse of chemo-therapy FBC; UEs; LFTs should be carried out;
      (ii) chest x-ray three-monthly or sooner if disease at presentation;
      (iii) ultrasound or CT scan monthly to CR;
      (iv) height and weight three-monthly.
   (b) stage 4:
      (i) BM if positive, should be repeated at end of each cycle until CR or if there is a prolonged delay in treatment due to poor marrow recovery;
      (ii) CSF: If positive at presentation, it should be repeated at times of thera-peutic LPs for each course;
2. End of treatment
   BM/LP; chest x-ray, CT scan, ultra-sound as appropriate;
3. Off treatment
   Two-monthly visit for one year, then three-monthly for second year. Image primary site(s) each visit.

31.6 HODGKIN'S DISEASE

In Hodgkin's disease, follow-up should include:

1. On treatment
   (a) chest x-ray if primary; monthly to CR, otherwise eight-weekly.
   (b) abdominal ultrasound or CT scan at time of stopping treatment in supra-diaphragmatic cases (Stage 1–2) or monthly to document time of com-plete remission of infradiaphragmatic disease. If the patient had lymphangio-graphy, a plain abdominal film at the times of the chest x-rays. If gallium

scan is positive, a repeat scan at three months into treatment and at the end.
2. Off treatment
   (a) Monthly visits for three months, then two-monthly for the rest of that year. This is followed by three-monthly visits for the next two years and six-monthly for the subsequent three years. Height and weight should be measured at each visit.
   (b) chest x-rays (each visit); abdominal ultrasounds six-monthly for the first two years if positive at diagnosis.

Males, if postpubertal after treatment, should have a check sperm count and testos-terone and FSH/LH levels. Females should be asked about their menstrual history. If amenorrhoea is present, check FSH/LH/oestrogen levels.

Because of the widespread nature of the disease several vital organs may be exposed to toxic therapy. Accurate treatment records are therefore essential when these patients are followed up. Thyroid dysfunction can occur with both direct and indirect irradiation with a risk of hypothyroidism and secondary malignancy. High risk groups should have six-monthly thyroid function tests and be treated appropriately. If on thyroxine, checks need to be made regularly for at least five years. Any signs of thyroid swelling/nodularity demand imaging, thyroid func-tion tests – including TBG levels – and biopsy.

Cardiac function can be compromised by both radio- and chemotherapy, and the com-bination of this treatment can be very cardio-toxic. If the patient is under fifteen years of age and has an anteriorly weighted field, the risks are higher. An underlying cardiac ano-maly or pre-existing hypertension also raise the chances of long-term damage. The sev-erity of dysfunction is related to age, sche-dule and cumulative anthracycline dose. Low risk patients do not benefit from serial non-invasive monitoring. However, if patients are at risk, follow-up should be for life as there may be a long latent period; they should have regular evaluation, e.g. nuclear scans two- to four-yearly and more frequent use of ECGs, echocardiograms and assessment of ejection fractions at points in between.

Patients receiving whole lung irradiation are at risk of chronic respiratory problems especially if irradiation was given in infancy. The use of bleomycin compounds the situation.

31.7 EWING'S SARCOMA/PRIMITIVE NEUROECTODERMAL TUMOURS (PNET)

Follow-up for Ewing's sarcoma/PNET includes the following:

1. On treatment
   X-ray, CT or MRI of primary two-monthly until surgery; chest x-ray every three cycles of chemotherapy; bone scan pre surgery.
2. Off treatment
   X-ray CT/MRI of primary; chest x-ray; CT scan/MRI chest and primary; bone scan.

Once treatment is completed, two-monthly visits in year one, three-monthly in year two, four-monthly in year three and finally six-monthly for two further years are necessary. Initially, chest/primary imaging is performed two- to three-monthly for two years, then four-monthly for two years, then thereafter every six months.

It should be remembered that relapse can occur up to ten years post therapy. Extraosseous tumours are rapid growing so follow-up visits could be more frequent earlier on. More vigilant surveillance should be carried out in the poorer risk groups, e.g. patients with bulky disease, older rather than younger patients, and poor risk primary sites, e.g. pelvis. There may be some hope of salvage if radiotherapy has not already been given. Females do slightly better than males

(Cangir *et al.*, 1990). Second tumours in the radiation portal should be looked out for. If the resection margins were difficult to obtain and >5% viable tumour cells are present post chemotherapy there is a higher chance of relapse (Terrier *et al.*, 1989).

31.8 OSTEOGENIC SARCOMA

Follow-up management for osteogenic sarcoma should include:

1. On treatment
   (a) chest x-ray eight-weekly and CT or MRI of primary site pre surgery.
   (b) LDH level; ploidy of tumour; tumour necrosis levels after chemotherapy – these all affect outcome and are worth documenting.
2. Off treatment
   Chest x-ray (or CT if suspicious). Scan of primary site if there has not been an ablative procedure.
   Note: follow-up usefulness is debatable following radical chemotherapy and ablative surgery with regard to altering prognosis except for small numbers of lung secondaries.

The patient should be reviewed two-monthly for the first year with chest and stump x-ray every four months. If the limb has been preserved, follow-up should be more assiduous as local relapse may be salvageable, e.g. CT scan limb four-monthly off treatment.

Follow-up should continue four-monthly in the second and third years off treatment, six-monthly for two more years.

Orthopaedic advice is invaluable especially if a prosthesis is involved. Fitting and function must be assessed in relation to growth and development. Scoliosis evaluation should be done every six to twelve months with two plane imaging especially during the growth spurt of puberty.

31.9 RHABDOMYOSARCOMA/SOFT TISSUE SARCOMA

Follow-up management for rhabdomyo-sarcoma/soft tissue sarcoma should include:

1. On treatment
   (a) chest x-ray eight-weekly (every third cycle of treatment AP/LAT) and repeat imaging of primary and metastatic sites prior to local therapy. This is repeated at the end of treatment.
2. Off treatment
   (a) two-monthly visits for the first year, three-monthly the next, and four-monthly visits for the third year. For the next two years the visits are six-monthly and, after this, on a yearly basis.
   (b) a chest x-ray is taken at each visit for five years. Repeat imaging of the primary site three-monthly in patients where the site has not been managed with either radical radiotherapy or surgery, as relapse could be salvageable by local radiotherapy or surgery.

For genitourinary rhabdomyosarcomas, repeat cystoscopy at the above time points may be appropriate.

It is important that a maxillofacial surgeon (for jaw tumours) or a urological surgeon (for bladder primaries) become involved so that long-term effects are minimized with retention of maximal possible function. A bladder compromised by radiotherapy and cyclophosphamide needs to be followed up with regular urinalysis/cytology. If symptoms develop, regular cystoscopy may be needed.

31.10 CENTRAL NERVOUS SYSTEM TUMOURS

Follow-up management for CNS tumours should include:

1. During treatment:
   (a) baseline simple neuropsychometry;
   (b) in medulloblastoma, serum non specific enolase (NSE) levels can be measured and used to evaluate response;
   (c) CT scan/MRI scan post surgery and at six and thirteen weeks later; thereafter as clinically indicated to determine progress or relapsed disease.
2. Follow-up imaging is the same as that for diagnosis and is reviewed six-monthly for five years.

Approximately 10% of CNS tumours occur in children under two years of age. In these patients there is a high risk of sequelae if radiotherapy is given. Psychometry and developmental assessment should be performed three-monthly for the next two years and then when necessary in the light of developmental needs.

Visual and auditory dysfunction can occur due to a treatment volume which includes the orbits and inner ear (Kirkbride and Plowman, 1989). Anticipation of damage may reduce the degree of developmental interference. Frequent assessment is important as simple corrective treatment can be very effective, e.g. cataract removal, corrective lens, grommet insertion, and modification of causative chemotherapy.

31.11 GERM CELL TUMOURS

Follow-up management for germ cell tumours should include:

1. On treatment:
   (a) measurement of AFP/β-hCG pre removal of primary then weekly until normal levels are reached. (The half-life of AFP is four to nine days.) These can then be repeated with each course

of treatment. A chest x-ray is taken with every other course.

2. End of treatment
   repeat measurement of AFP/β-hCG levels, and imaging of the chest and primary site as well as the site of any secondaries, e.g. bone scan.

3. Off treatment
   monthly visits for the first year, then two-monthly for the next, with AFP/β-hCG taken each visit. Then three-monthly for a further year, clinical review six-monthly for another and thereafter on an annual basis. A chest x-ray can be taken at each visit. If the β-hCG was normal at diagnosis it does not need to be repeatedly measured.

Imaging of the primary site (ultrasound or CT) is performed three-monthly off treatment. If there is any abnormal renal, audiological or lung function, continued assessment is mandatory.

31.12 HEPATOBLASTOMA

Follow-up management for hepatoblastoma should include:

1. On treatment
   (a) AFP weekly until normal and then with each cycle of therapy.
   (b) a chest x-ray is taken with each course, if there are lung secondaries, until there is complete remission, and every three courses in other cases.
   (c) abdominal ultrasound/CT scan of the liver every three courses and immediately prior to possible surgical resection.

2. Off treatment
   (a) monthly review for a year, then two- and three-monthly for the second and third year respectively. The AFP is measured at each visit for three years and a chest x-ray taken for two years.

The liver is imaged three-monthly off treatment for two years.

31.13 THE CHILD PATIENT IN ADULTHOOD

Increasing numbers of patients are surviving to adulthood. Delayed or poor growth can be psychologically traumatic so careful auxology until growth is complete is vital. During this time weight gain must also be watched carefully. Stress tests for growth hormone responses may be useful although clinical response to growth hormone can sometimes be disappointing. The onset of puberty brings sexual maturation but this also can be delayed or fail to develop. The help of a skilled paediatric endocrinologist will be vital.

Risks will be higher if combined chemotherapy and radiotherapy have been given. Recovery of ovarian failure is unlikely if menstruation has not returned in three months off treatment.

In males, azoospermia may be irreversible (Green *et al.*, 1981). Many patients have abnormal spermatogenesis at diagnosis (Thadil *et al.*, 1981; Vigersky *et al.*, 1982). If given testicular radiotherapy prepubertally, such patients show decreased testosterone despite a rise in LH, with delayed onset of puberty. The use of alkylating agents further impairs fertility.

At some point a patient will have to be informed of the possibilities or otherwise of parenthood. This interview should never be rushed and the facts must be clearly explained. When pregnancy is achieved good antenatal care is essential, especially if the pelvis has been irradiated. Facilities for premature delivery should be available.

Another emerging problem is that of secondary malignancy developing in 3–12% of patients initially treated for Hodgkin's disease within twenty years of initial diagnosis. It is usually a leukaemia and the risk

Table 31.1 Suggested points to be covered at follow-up review

1. History of any intercurrent illness	
2. Systems review	
3. Development of any benign tumours or other cancers	
4. Medication	prophylaxis, compliance, viral status and the need for vaccination, immunoglobulin, administration of *Pneumovax*
5. Educational:	achievements, special needs, areas of weakness
6. Employment:	regular, handicap, discrimination, insurance
7. Mental welfare:	finances, family, peers, friends, domestic harmony, steady sexual relationship, fertility, contraception, libido, pregnancies
8. Future aims:	understanding of disease, treatment and prognosis. Quality of life

may be higher in splenectomized patients. Solid tumours occur later on, often within radiation portals. The risk is of the order of 3–6% and there may be a latency period of ten to fifteen years (Meadows *et al.*, 1989). Life-long surveillance will be necessary to assess the carcinogenicity of newer modalities such as total body irradiation and intensive chemotherapy.

In conclusion, the therapy team must be aware of the survivor's psychosocial needs and welfare. The following Table (31.1) gives a summary of the information that should be obtained from survivors of childhood cancer in order to ensure a continuity of follow-up care.

REFERENCES

Cangir, A., Vietti, T.J., Gehan, E.A. *et al.* (1990) Ewing's sarcoma metastatic at diagnosis: Results and comparisons of two Intergroup Ewing's Sarcoma Studies. *Cancer*, **66**, 887–93.

Copeland, D.R., Fletcher, J.M., Pfefferbaum-Levine, B. *et al.* (1985) Neuropsychological sequelae of childhood cancer in long-term survivors. *Pediatrics*, **75**, 745–53.

D'Angio, G.J., Breslow, N., Beckwith, J.B. *et al.* (1989) Imaging studies for follow up of patients with primary renal tumours of childhood. *Med. Paed. Oncol.*, **17**, 313.

D'Angio, G.J., Meadows, A., Miké, V. *et al.* (1976) Decreased risk of radiation associated malignant neoplasms in actinomycin-D treated patients. *Cancer*, **37** (supp), 1177–85.

Evans, A.E., Breslow, N., Norkool, P. and D'Angio G.J. (1986) Complications in long-term survivors of Wilms' tumour. *Proc. Am. Assoc. Cancer Res.*, **27**, 204.

Green, Brecher, M.L., Lindsey, A.N. *et al.* (1981) Gonadal function in paediatric patients following treatment of Hodgkins' disease. *Paed. Oncol.*, **9**, 235–44.

Kirkbride, P. and Plowman, P. (1989) Platinum chemotherapy and the inner ear: implication for 'standard' radiation portals. *Br. J. Radiol.*, Vol. 62, 457–62.

Meadows, A.T., Baum, E., Fossati-Bellani, F. *et al.* (1985) Second malignant neoplasms in children. Update of the late effects study group. *J. Clin. Oncol.*, **3**, 532–8.

Meadows, A.T., Obringer, A.C., Marrero, O. *et al.* (1989) Long-term follow-up of Hodgkins' disease. *Med. Paed. Oncol.*, **17**, 479–84.

Meadows, A.T. and Evans, A.E. (1976) Effects of chemotherapy on the central nervous system. *Cancer*, **37**, 1079–85.

Riccardi, R., Brouwers, P., Dichiro, G. and Poplack, D.G. (1985) Abnormal computed tomography brain scans in children with acute lymphoblastic leukaemia: serial long-term follow-up. *J. Clin. Oncol.*, **3**, 12–18.

Terrier, P., Terrier-Lacombe, M.J., Contesso, G. *et al.* (1989) Extensive pathological examination of post-chemotherapy surgical specimens of Ewing's Sarcomas: prognostic value. *Med. Ped. Oncol.*, **17**, 282.

Thadil, J.-V., Jewett, M.A., Rider, W.D. *et al.* (1981) Effects of cancer and cancer treatment on male fertility. *J. Urology*, **126**, 141–5.

Vigersky, R.A., Chapman, R.M., Berenberg, J., Glass, A.R. *et al.* (1982) Testicular dysfunction in untreated Hodgkins' disease. *Am. J. Med.*, **73**, 482–6.

Young, J.L., Ries, L.G., Silverberg, E. *et al.* (1986) Cancer incidence, survival and mortality for children younger than fifteen years. *Cancer*, **58**, 598–602.

Chapter 32

The child in the community

N. PATEL

With current treatment regimens, approximately 60% of all children with cancer are now long term survivors. Most respond to initial chemotherapy and will return to their homes and schools often whilst receiving treatment. It is these children who need the early intervention of community support, and it is clear that, overall, community services are inadequate for such patients. Thus a child with cancer, with his or her special needs, is currently unlikely to receive adequate community support. Apart from the immediate and extended family unit, the child with cancer and family find themselves in contact with several professional people within a very short time. From a community point of view, it is worth considering the composition and role of the primary health care team.

32.1 THE ROLE OF THE GP

A GP may encounter perhaps only one child with cancer throughout his or her practising career. Even so, a child with cancer may have been seen by the GP several times prior to referral to a District Hospital or specialist centre. The child's family may have lost confidence in the GP with ensuing feelings of anger or even resentment. To help the family regain their confidence in the GP it is important to explain the rarity of childhood cancer

to family members, and to re-establish early contact. In some cases the GP may not know the actual diagnosis of his or her young patient until confirmation is sent by the specialist centre, which may take several weeks.

The task of early liaison with the GP can be undertaken by either the specialist hospital community paediatrician or the community-based paediatric nurse, who provides the necessary information regarding the child's diagnosis, treatment plan and problems relating to possible side-effects of treatment. This enables the physician to make appropriate arrangements so that the family can have easy access to his or her medical services. This in turn lessens the parents' anxiety and helps to gain or regain their confidence. Regular liaison also encourages the GP to keep in touch with the specialist centre and make occasional visits to the unit.

Outpatient treatment regimens render the child only moderately neutropenic, but always, to some extent, immunocompromized. In this case, the local paediatrician or GP may be involved. A low threshold for contacting the specialist centre is essential, but a number of simple anxieties can be dealt with locally. Infectious disases are a common problem, particularly chickenpox and measles. Contact with other children who are in the infectious period either before or after the appearance of a rash is an indication for prophylactic hyperimmune globulin in the case of measles, or zoster immunoglobulin in the case of chickenpox. There is, however, no point in administering either of these if over 72 hours have elapsed since the time of contact. The morbidity of chickenpox has been dramatically reduced by intravenous acyclovir which should be given at the first sign of any rash. The intravenous route should initially be used, although it may be changed to the oral route if there is a rapid response. Recrudescence of both herpes simplex and zoster lesions should be actively treated with oral or intravenous acyclovir. Although these may seem initially innocuous, they can become rapidly progressive.

Contact with other infectious diseases, such as mumps or rubella, is of little significance and reassurance of the parents is all that is necessary. Keeping a child with cancer away from school for prolonged periods from fear of contacting an infectious disease is a difficult problem. In general, this is undesirable, as these children should be allowed to maintain a lifestyle which is as close to normality as possible.

Septrin prophylaxis is given to children on continuing therapy for acute leukaemia, to prevent *Pneumocystis carinii* pneumonia. Despite this, any child with a dry persistent cough or tachypnoea should be immediately referred back to the specialist centre for assessment and advice.

32.2 THE ROLE OF THE HEALTH VISITOR

Health visitors can play an important role in giving young children (<5 years of age) with cancer and their families continuous psychosocial support throughout the illness. Although adequate support may be given to mentally and physically handicapped children, when the health visitor encounters a child with cancer it may be difficult to face the family because of lack of information about the

diagnosis and treatment. If the child is under the age of five at the time of diagnosis, the health visitor is more likely to know the family than if the child is older. The hospital community liaison nurse can establish early contact with the health visitor, so that a home visit is made soon after the child's discharge from hospital.

In the case of an older child, the health visitor may need to make contact with the family and gain their confidence so that the family identify this interaction as beneficial. There will also be a need to contact the child's school and the school nurse.

Health visitors are expert at monitoring the developmental milestones of children under the age of five, therefore observation and early detection of a child's slowness in any development area would enable referral to the appropriate agencies, for example, portage system assessment for children under five with a brain tumour, where development may be hindered because of the tumour. Overall, health visitors can help the family of a child with cancer by organizing practical help, such as voluntary baby-sitters, home help or Family Aid through social services where necessary, or by just listening and giving them time to express their views and concerns.

32.3 THE ROLE OF THE DISTRICT NURSE

In recent years, district nurses have become involved in the care of the young. In some parts of Britain, paediatric district nursing services are being set up. The district nurse's involvement in the care of the child with cancer may follow surgical mangement, and either the District Hospital or the GP will have requested nursing services for home care. Where such a service is available, early liaison by the hospital community nurse will enable the paediatric district nurse to establish contact with the family. This allows added support for the family and child, i.e. care of central venous lines, home medication, and palliative care if the occasion arises.

32.4 THE ROLE OF SCHOOL NURSE AND COMMUNITY PAEDIATRICIAN

In recent years the school nurse has played an important part in the care of the child with cancer at school. This function is that of 'health educator' and of assessing the child's educational needs. Home tuition may be opted for, if necessary, or the child may be encouraged to settle into a school routine. Psychological help for the child and family can be initiated by the community paediatrician.

The community social worker may have to be involved where family stresses, financial or otherwise, are increased, or the care of siblings is at risk due to the parents' need to spend time with their sick child.

Nurses funded by charitable organizations play a major role in supporting the child and family through the terminal phase of the illness. If the family live some distance from the child's treatment centre, the hospital liaison nurse or community paediatric nurse should establish early contact with the various supporting agencies before the parents take their child home. Early discharge planning in such instances is essential.

32.5 EDUCATION

Education plays an important role in the formative years of all children. The child who is faced with a life-threatening illness may develop changes in self-image and begin to feel 'different' because of the illness and side-effects from the treatment. This may lead to 'opting out' of the educational system, which is in itself traumatic. Separation of an ill child from the parents for playschool, nursery or infants school can be stressful for both child and family.

The community liaison nurse helps the child to overcome this anxiety and adjust into the school environment. Interaction with the school involves giving correct information regarding the child's illness and treatment plan; offering information about the child's physical changes and how to cope with specific situations, for example, regrowth of hair following loss. The issue of infections, especially problems related to chickenpox and measles, must be addressed, giving clear guidelines on what action to take. The school must be flexible while the child is undergoing treatment. Lack of energy is to be expected during this period, and teachers need to understand that this will improve once the child has finished treatment.

32.5.1 THE ROLE OF THE TEACHER

After the specialist nurse has informed the teacher(s) about the child's illness, the teacher will be equipped to explain the child's absence from the class and to remember the child during school activities. Other children will be prepared for the possible physical changes of the ill child, such as loss of hair during treatment and the reasons why, changes in weight, or loss of a limb through surgery or dysfunction due to a tumour. During hospitalization, it is important that the teacher keeps in touch with the child and the family. Following treatment, it is important to welcome back the child as 'normal'.

32.5.2 HOME TUITION

Children undertaking intensive chemotherapy regimes at frequent intervals over a six-month period or longer, or those who have to undergo bone marrow transplantation, miss long periods of schooling. The hospital teacher should liaise with the local education authority to arrange for home tuition once the treatment plan is known. This will enable the child to maintain the school pace and eventually to return to the school routine. In exceptional cases, home tuition may be necessary to give the child time to adjust to the physical and emotional changes, on the understanding that a return to school must take place once the child feels ready for that.

32.6 HOME VISITS

Therapy for childhood cancer has become more aggressive and complex, and at the same time increasingly more successful. The approach to care for the child with cancer can roughly be divided into three stages:

1. time of diagnosis and administration of therapy;
2. time of remission and anticipated good health;
3. if the treatments are unsuccessful, the period leading to the death of the child.

Each of these requires different kinds of support, which cannot always be provided by members of the community, and are usually handled by the multidisciplinary team of the specialist centre. Home visits provide an opportunity for families to continue to seek new information, and to clarify recently acquired information about their child's disease and treatment. The dramatic increase in the number of children surviving cancer has created this need, and specialist nurses help the affected family to adjust to the new circumstances coming to terms with the diagnosis of cancer and its treatment. In the long term, they provide follow-up care for the surviving patient.

32.6.1 OBJECTIVES AND NURSE'S ASSESSMENT OF HOME VISIT

Each family has individual needs, and the specialist nurse must be able to consider social, cultural, religious and language factors. The home nurse provides an assessment of the family and their coping mechanisms, the home environment, teaching of procedures, patient advocacy, health education and supportive counselling.

Discussion of the diagnosis is vital. Clarification of medical terminology may be necessary where perhaps the word 'tumour' is not equated to cancer due to language difficulties. Parents and child should have an understanding of the disease process and treatment protocols. They need to know that, although two children may have a similar diagnosis, the tumour bulk, site and extent at presentation determine the eventual outcome of the child's illness.

Parents need clear instructions on how to look after a Hickman or Broviac line, and, likewise, a guideline to follow if the child shows signs of infection due to a low blood count or has contact with measles or chicken-pox. The ultimate aim of home visits is for parents to be less dependent on the specialist unit and become competent advocates for their child's health needs.

Siblings are encouraged to visit freely in a 'family-centred care' unit. However, experience and studies show that certain stresses are unique to the siblings of a child with cancer. These include feelings of abandonment due to recurring periods of separation; envy, resentment and rivalry in younger children; feelings of guilt, distress and learning difficulties or lack of concentration in older siblings. As the child with cancer becomes an object of natural total concern, parents should be made aware of the 'needs' of healthy children. Occasionally, the services of a child psychologist may be required.

During a home visit it is important to identify the members of the extended family and friends. In many instances, good friends and the church support the family through their difficult periods. The parents need reassurance about not feeling guilty in accepting a 'helping hand'.

32.7 NURSING THE TERMINALLY ILL CHILD AT HOME

32.7.1 HOME CARE RESOURCES

At the terminal phase of the child's illness, parents are confronted with a period of unknown duration and their role as parents is threatened. 'Anticipatory grief' tests the individual, marriage, siblings and other family members. Research and experience shows that most parents opt to care for their dying child at home.

There are important issues to be considered and discussed at this stage. First, whether such home care is feasible, and secondly, whether it is desirable. Furthermore, the issue of the effect of the dying child on healthy siblings must be dealt with. Therefore, the choice of the child and family to return to the hospital must be emphasized. Such a dialogue builds a trusting relationship between the nurse and parents, which in turn leads to open communication. The two fears that are regularly uppermost in parents' minds are:

1. uncontrollable symptoms, especially pain;
2. the fear of the unknown at the time of actual death.

The home care nurse should reassure the family that a support service operating 24-hours a day will be available and will be provided as and when necessary. Psychologically, the parents will have been dependent on the unit staff throughout the child's active treatment period, and unfamiliar outside nursing help will not be easily accepted. From the practical point of view, if the family live some distance from the treatment centre, early intervention from paediatric community nursing services and GP is important. Early liaison with the primary health care team and relevant agencies will facilitate the availability of the team within 24 hours of the

child's discharge from hospital. If within travelling distance, it is important for the home care nurse to meet the team. This enables the child and parents to build up confidence in the services provided by the community.

Nurses in the paediatric setting have to remember certain home care criteria:

1. in the home environment, the parent is the primary care giver;
2. the nurse is a facilitator in achieving the child's peaceful death;
3. the physician needs to be approachable, available and flexible;
4. access to adequate, necessary medication should be easily available;
5. the home care nurse or specialist unit should be easily available to the GP as a resource.

32.7.2 THE ROLE OF THE HOME CARE NURSE

The physical, psychological and emotional support required by families and children who are dying at home falls within the remit of professional nursing. Therefore certain guidelines are necessary which will assist the home care nurse in maximizing the child's and family's comfort.

Pain control is a paramount issue. Oral analgesia is very effective until the child is unable to swallow. Subcutaneous or intravenous pain control will then become necessary. Parents may have to be taught about dosage, frequency and administration of drugs via a syringe driver pump. They soon become proficient at such a task, which gives them a degree of control over the situation.

Other potential symptoms, such as nausea, vomiting, constipation and mouth ulcers, should be assessed regularly and treated accordingly. As far as possible, hospital visits should be minimized for psychological and physical comfort to the child and his family.

Physical comforts must be assessed and provided. Wheelchair, commode, sheep-skin or a special mattress should be readily available. Mobility must be maintained for as long as possible, especially where a pump is used for some time.

Changes in the living accommodation will be necessary, to allow the child to be nursed in the centre of the family for comfort and security. The home care nurse should monitor and evaluate the child's condition and deterioration over a period of time, therefore continuity of care on a daily basis will be of paramount importance. It may be that although parents want to nurse their child at home, they do not wish for their child to die at home. The nurse must remain in close contact with the physician, so that the child can be moved into hospital at the appropriate time. Parents will require clear guidelines as to whom to contact when the child dies, especially at night, if the nurse or doctor is not present.

After the death of a child, the family usually disassociate from members of the hospital staff and try to readjust to family patterns. Grief will be the most important issue at this stage, and bereavement support care must be provided as part of total care for these parents.

Overall, the importance of adequate psychosocial support for children with cancer and their families in the community needs to be recognized and provided, especially in view of long-term survival of these young patients.

REFERENCES

Ferguson, J. and Hobbie, W. (1985) Home visits for the child with cancer. *Nursing Clinics of North America*, **20**(1), 109–15.

Hersh, S.P. and Wiener, L.S. (1989) Psychosocial support for the family of the child with cancer, in *Principles and Practice of Pediatric Oncology*, (eds P.A. Pizzo, D.G. Poplack) J.B. Lippincott, Philadelphia, pp. 897–913.

Hinds, C. (1985) The needs of families who care for patients with cancer at home: are we meeting them? *J. Adv. Nursing*, **10**(6), 575–81.

Houlton, E. (1986) The Jacks of all trades. *Senior Nurse*, **5**(2), 24–5.

Kohler, J.A. and Radford, M. (1985) Terminal care of children dying of cancer – quantity and quality of life. *Br. Med. J.*, **291**, 115–6.

Lansky, S.B., List, M.A. and Ritter-Sterr, C. (1989) Psychiatric and psychological support of the child and adolescent with cancer, in *Principles and Practice of Pediatric Oncology*. (eds P.A. Pizzo, D.G. Poplack) J.B. Lippincott, Philadelphia, pp. 885–96.

Lauer, M.E. and Camitta, B.M. (1980) *J. Paediatr.*, **97**(6), 1032–35.

Lauer, M.E., Mulhern, R.K., Hoffman, R.G. and Camitta, B.M. (1986). Utilisation of hospice/home care in paediatric oncology (in USA). *Cancer Nursing*, **9**(3), 102–7.

Martinson, I.M., Modlow, D.G., Armstrong, G.D. *et al.* (1986) Home care for children dying of cancer. *Research in Nursing and Health*, **9**(1), 11–16.

Norman, R. and Bennett, M. (1986) Care of the dying child at home: a unique co-operative relationship. *Australian Journal of Advanced Nursing*, **3**(4), 3–16.

Price, B.J. (1979) Caring for the child with cancer: the nurse practitioner. *Cancer Nurse*, **75**(11), 48–50.

Ross, A.K. (1985) Supportive care for families of dying children. *Nursing Clinics of North America*, **20**(2), 457–65.

Chapter 33

Care of the dying child

A. GOLDMAN

33.1 INTRODUCTION

The death of a child is one of the most distressing and traumatic events which can happen to any family, leaving a permanent mark on their lives. The prognosis for childhood cancer continues to improve and cure can now be anticipated for about 65% of the children diagnosed. The remainder, however, do die; 396 children in England and Wales in 1988 (Office of Population Censuses and Surveys). The majority of these children die from progression of their malignant disease but some will die from the side effects of treatment.

33.2 CESSATION OF TREATMENT

When a child with a malignant disease suffers a relapse there are no firm criteria about when to stop treatment that is directed against the cancer and focus on palliative care. There appears to be a wide variation of opinion between oncologists; in a recent survey of United Kingdom Children's Cancer Centres the percentage of children dying from progressive disease who were still having chemotherapy varied from 0–30%. Many variables, both conscious and unconscious, may affect the practising oncologist and little has been written about the process involved

in making what are often difficult and stressful decisions (Maher and Jefferis, 1990).

Some of the factors which are clearly relevant include the likelihood of effecting a cure or good remission with further treatment, the availability of good second line drugs, and how well the child has tolerated previous treatment both physically and psychologically. Some areas which are less clearly defined are the oncologist's personal approach: how easy he or she finds it to give up the struggle; how much interest they have invested in new agents; how strongly they feel that parents should share the responsibility for decisions, and at what age and how much they believe children themselves can contribute (Nitschke *et al.*, 1982; Kamps *et al.*, 1987).

At this point in the disease process, the way interviews with families are conducted, as at other critical points in the disease, is important. The manner in which information is imparted and the emotions that information elicits are likely to remain as vivid lifetime memories and may influence the family's manner of coping subsequently (Woolley *et al.*, 1989). It is important to leave the family with a clear message that although the child is not going to be cured of his or her cancer and is going to die they are not being abandoned. They should understand that palliative treatment will be available and have a general picture of how this will be organized. They will need some time to think through the situation and they should know who will be contacting them to explain the details and answer their questions when they have had this time.

33.3 THE PROVISION OF CARE

Traditionally, providing terminal care has been part of the role of the paediatric oncologist; in contrast with the carefully designed and monitored protocols of anti-cancer treatment, however, palliative care has been much more variable, reflecting the skills and personal practice of individuals. With the formation of the hospice movement and the development of palliative medicine as a speciality, standards of practice in palliative care are becoming more clearly defined. Although it remains the responsibility of the paediatric oncologist to assure that optimum care is available for the dying child as well as their family, it is increasingly common for the actual care to be undertaken by staff with expertize in palliative medicine.

The sick child will need somewhere to be cared for with love and security where they can die with as much dignity and peace as possible. They require competent medical and nursing management of any symptoms they develop; both the child and family will also need skilled help and support in facing the physical and emotional problems of the impending death. This chapter will look at these aspects of care in more detail. It is important when planning terminal care to be as flexible as possible so that different families have as much choice and control as possible.

33.3.1 WHERE TO LOOK AFTER THE CHILD

When there is no longer any expectation of cure the family are faced with a choice of where to care for their dying child. At the turn of this century the pattern was for children to die at home; death in hospital later became routine. Currently, after a gradual reintroduction, home care has become acceptable again. The range of possibilities include nursing the child at a cancer centre, at their local hospital, at home, or in a hospice. The aim should be to offer the family a choice and to discuss with them the advantages and disadvantages of each situation so that they can choose which feels right for them.

The cancer centre can provide both a sense of security for the family and continued care by the team with whom they are familiar. There are, however, many disadvantages for both the family and staff. The environment is inevitably institutional and often cramped; in addition, parents lack a sense of control. The contrast between the gentle pace and unintrusive needs of palliative care and the more positive aggressive approach to curative treatment are apparent to families and it is difficult for staff who have to oscillate between the two. The cancer centre is often a long way from the child's home, making visits more difficult so that siblings and members of the wider family may be excluded. A local hospital may be able to provide more conducive surroundings but may know the family less well and lack confidence and experience in palliative care, particularly in the use of strong analgesics.

To be cared for at home, in familiar surroundings, is almost always the preference of the child. This gives parents the opportunity to maintain family life as near to normal as possible and continue to have control of their child's care. There is evidence that long-term problems for bereaved parents and siblings are also reduced (Lauer *et al.*, 1983; Mulhern *et al.*, 1983). Heavy responsibility falls on the parents as well as on the primary health care team who rarely encounter dying children and may feel ill equipped to deal with their

619

medical and emotional needs. For a family to have the confidence and skills to look after their child successfully at home, support is vital. A number of paediatric oncology departments have developed facilities in order to offer home care. These vary depending on local needs and resources and include centrally based teams which travel out to children at home (Goldman *et al.*, 1990), specialist nurses based at hospitals throughout the health region (Chambers *et al.*, 1989) and paediatric community nursing services (Kohler and Radford, 1985).

In adult cancer care many deaths now occur in hospices but although three hospices for children exist in the United Kingdom they have found their developing role has differed from those in adult medicine. Comparatively few children with cancer have been admitted; most of their patients have long-term problems from metabolic or neurodegenerative diseases and many of their admissions are for

respite care (Burne *et al.*, 1984). Families for whom hospices have played a role have been those with children with brain tumours and the prospect of a long slow deterioration, and families in whom complex social circumstances make home care difficult.

In 1986, with the provision of a hospital-based symptom care team in the department of haematology and oncology at Great Ormond Street, families who chose home care symptom management were offered psycho-social support and liaison with their primary health care team, providing a 24-hour on call service for advice by telephone or home visits. The percentage of families whose children died at home changed from 19% between 1978–81 before the team began, to 75% between 1987–89 (Fig. 33.1).

33.4 SYMPTOM MANAGEMENT

A systematic approach is as important to

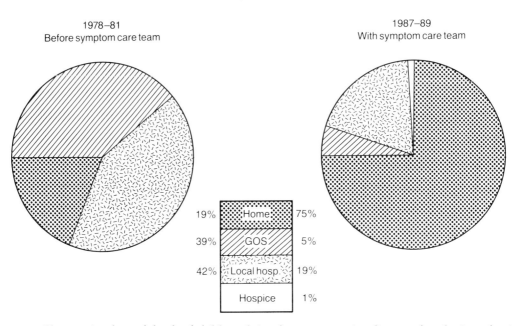

Fig. 33.1 Changes in place of death of children dying from progressive disease after the introduction of the hospital-based symptom care team, in 1986, at the Hospital for Sick Children, Great Ormond Street, UK.

620

symptom management as it is to tackling the diagnostic problem. Many symptoms give rise to complex experiences including both a physical response and an emotional component and both of these must be considered. A knowledge of the child's tumour and its usual metastatic pattern should be combined with a detailed history and assessment of the separate problems. A plan of management can then be devised and instituted. Frequent review and reassessment are vital so that treatment can be modified to provide optimum symptom relief.

Although it is possible to provide good symptom relief for the majority of children, there are some for whom it is not complete and a few who have severe and resistant problems. It is important to set realistic goals in management and work towards improvement gradually. If parents are given over-optimistic reassurances that all symptoms can be relieved completely they may be disappointed, distressed, and lose their trust in medical staff.

33.4.1 PAIN

One of the worst fears for parents of a child with progressive malignant disease is that they will suffer pain. This is a realistic concern. In a study of a group of 76 children from the Hospital for Sick Children, Great Ormond Street who died from progressive malignant disease over a period of two years, opioid analgesics were required by 87% during their terminal illness. Although a number of the children (17%) needed these for less than 24 hours, 70% required opioids for between two and 370 days (median 21 days). (Goldman and Bowman, 1990). Effective pain control is an important part of the management of the dying child.

(a) Assessment

It is valuable to build up as clear a picture of

a child's pain problem as possible, within the limitations imposed by their age and level of understanding. Aspects of the pain to consider are its site, nature, frequency, intensity, and the factors that relieve or exacerbate it.

There are many problems inherent in the measurement of pain because it is subjective and influenced by many variables. This is complicated further in children by their range of cognitive development, their limited means of expression, their lack of experience of pain, and our lack of understanding of the physiology of pain in children. Recently interest and research into children's pain and its assessment has increased and a number of reliable and useful tools are available (McGrath and Unruh, 1987; Bayer and Wells, 1989; McGrath, 1990). Many of the measurement techniques have been used primarily in a research context but they are also applicable in clinical practice. The approach chosen needs to reflect the child's age and level of understanding as well as the information requested.

For babies, scales and coding systems have been developed and validated; these depend on observation of facial expression, body movement, and cry. In pre-school and older children, various self-report systems have been developed. Variations of linear analogue scales can be understood by children as young as six years and for younger children techniques using more concrete ideas have been developed such as pain thermometers, ladders, 'smiley charts' of ranked facial scales (both photographs and drawings) and poker chips (which correspond to 'pieces of hurt'). These measures can be completed at regular intervals and can provide a guide to the severity of the pain and the effects of treatment over a period of time.

In terminally ill children we still tend to depend primarily on clinical observations and parents' understanding of their own children. These apparently 'unscientific' approaches should not be scorned; McGrath *et al.* (1985) has shown that estimates of a child's pain made at the time – by several independent observers using a visual analogue scale – correlate well both with each other and with detailed behavioural techniques. However, more caution may be needed with retrospective reports of pain. Both children and parents appeared to overestimate pain frequency, intensity and duration (of headaches) over the previous month compared with actual diary-kept records (Andrasik *et al.*, 1985).

(b) Management

When a child's pain has been assessed and its nature and cause elucidated as far as possible, a plan of management can be made. This may include choices from a number of approaches (Table 33.1). The choice will depend not only on what is most likely to be effective but also on what is acceptable to the child and family. In particular, numerous oral medications may not be tolerated, especially by younger children, and so it may not be possible to use theoretically useful drug combinations.

Table 33.1 Approaches to pain management

Pharmacological		
Analgesics	mild	paracetamol
	moderate	dihydrocodeine
	strong	morphine
Non steroidal anti-inflammatory agents (NSAIDS)		
Antidepressants and anticonvulsants		
Steroids		
Palliative chemotherapy		
Palliative radiotherapy		
Anaesthetic blocks		
Psychological approaches		

(i) Analgesics

Analgesics still form the backbone to most pain management plans for terminally ill children. The analgesic chosen will depend on the severity of the child's pain. Most children, after their disease has relapsed, develop pain gradually and so can be treated with mild analgesics initially progressing to moderate and then strong ones as the pain increases. A wide range of analgesics is available but there are a few which are well tried and whose side effects are well known and these form the basic analgesic ladder. Important general principles relating to analgesic use are to prescribe them regularly according to their length of action (and not on an 'as required' basis) and also to regularly reassess the patient so that treatment can be modified to provide optimal pain relief. When changing drugs because pain relief is inadequate then a drug from the next rung of the analgesic ladder should be chosen rather than an alternative of similar strength.

For mild pain in children, the drug of choice is paracetamol, a mild non-narcotic analgesic. Although aspirin is an effective analgesic, its use as a routine in children has decreased since the recognition of its association with Reye's syndrome. Also, because of its adverse effect on platelet function, it is avoided in oncology and haematology patients. Additionally, there is the possibility of gastritis.

When pain is no longer relieved by regular paracetamol a mild opioid such as codeine or dihydrocodeine can be prescribed. These have the same potential side effects as stronger opioids and these are described in more detail below. In practise, these drugs are usually well tolerated. The only side effect likely to be troublesome is constipation and initial drowsiness which may be noticed by some children. Codeine is a useful stepping stone from mild to strong pain analgesics for the child's pain and also for the parent who is coming to terms with a need for increasingly potent analgesia.

For severe pain, strong opioid analgesics are essential. Many myths and fears still prevail about their use, both among the lay public and among professionals, many of whom are unfamiliar with the use of strong analgesics, especially in children. Successful introduction of the drugs and management of the child's pain often depends on tackling these concerns.

For parents there is often a large emotional hurdle to be overcome in admitting that their child's disease has progressed to an extent that they need opioids. It may signal to them a final acknowledgement that the disease is incurable and their child is going to die. If this is so, it must be explored before they will tolerate allowing the drugs to be given to their child. They may feel that opioids will hasten their child's death but can be re-assured that this has not proved to be the case in adults. They may be afraid that by starting too soon 'nothing will be left' if the child's pain becomes more severe; again they can be reassured. They may have inappropriate fears of addiction or worries about side effects. It is important to try to get to the root of their particular concern so that appropriate explanations can be given.

Health care professionals are often nervous of using strong opioids in children and worry particularly about respiratory depression. Although opioids decrease the respiratory response to hypoxia and hypercapnia there appears to be a wide margin between the doses required for analgesia and those causing respiratory failure. Respiratory depression is uncommon in patients receiving opioids for pain due to cancer and appears to be no more common in children above the age of three months than in adults receiving comparable plasma opioid levels (Shannon and Berde, 1989). Confusion still arises between physical dependence and psychological addiction to opioids. Physiological dependence will develop following regular administration of opioids over one to two weeks but this rarely presents a clinical problem. If a child's pain and therefore their analgesic needs decreased, for example, after radiotherapy to a bony metastasis, then symptoms of withdrawal can be avoided by gradually decreasing the dose of opioids over a number of days. There is no evidence that appropriate administration of opioids for pain produces psychological addiction.

In the UK, the strong opioids used most widely and those recommended are the morphine preparations. These are pure agonists and have no ceiling effects, providing increasing analgesia with increasing doses. There are no established indications for the partial agonists or mixed agonists/antagonists.

Morphine is available in preparations that are active over 3–4 hours and also in slow release form, active over 12 hours (MST). In children, the advantage of the less frequent medication is considerable. The theoretical disadvantage is lack of flexibility in dose variation but this can be overcome by providing patients with a short-acting morphine preparation to use for breakthrough pain while the MST dose is gradually increased to give full analgesia. Patients vary in the dose of opioids required to produce analgesia and the dose should be titrated to produce the required clinical effect. The initial recommended dose of MST for children who have pain unresponsive to codeine are 1 mg/kg/dose twice daily (Goldman and Bowman, 1990). For four-hourly oral preparations, 0.3 mg/kg/dose is suggested.

In addition to providing analgesia, opioids have a range of other physiological effects which include sedation, dysphoria, respiratory depression, cough suppression, decreased gut motility, nausea, urinary retention, biliary spasm and pruritis. Although these may produce some clinically evident side effects, they rarely limit the use of the drugs. Sedation is common in children, particularly over the first two days of using a strong opioid, but gradually wears off. It is very important to warn parents about this as otherwise they may attribute the child's drowsiness to rapid disease progression and may fear the child's imminent death. Constipation is also common and can be troublesome if adequate laxatives are not given routinely. The administration of regular lactulose is often sufficient and is well tolerated by children but if not oral stimulant laxatives or rectal preparations should be introduced. Nausea attributable to opioids appears to be rare. Overt dysphoria is also rare in children although some report having vivid nightmares. Pruritis is uncommon and may respond to antihistamines. Occasionally this particular side effect can be intolerable and alternative opioid preparations may be better tolerated. The active metabolite of morphine is excreted renally and in patients with renal impairment care must be taken with the dose and frequency of administration of strong opioids to avoid overdose.

The route of choice for analgesics is oral. Nausea and vomiting, decreased level of consciousness, inability to swallow or occasionally flat refusal to take oral medication, may make it necessary to find an alternative. Rectal preparations of morphine and the longer-acting oxycodone are available. It has also been suggested that controlled release morphine tablets can be used rectally in end stage patients (Maloney *et al.*, 1989). For some patients and staff this is not an attractive choice but can be useful, particularly in children who are no longer conscious and within the last hours before death. The most convenient alternative to the oral route is a continuous subcutaneous infusion. Drugs can be delivered by a small portable syringe driver attached to a narrow gauge needle, sited on the abdomen, upper arm, or leg. The syringe containing the drugs can be replaced every 24 hours and parents can be taught how to do this themselves. If the child has a permanent in-dwelling intravenous catheter such as a Hickman, then this can be used conveniently for a continuous infusion, but the disadvantage of the intravenous route is

that tolerance builds up rapidly and escalation to very high doses occurs.

(ii) Non steroidal anti-inflammatory agents

These drugs are thought to produce analgesia through acting peripherally to inhibit prostaglandin synthetase. They have a particular role in the management of bone pain from metastatic tumour and can be used effectively in combination with opioids. Response to one NSAID does not predict response to others so it may be worth trying several preparations; choice for children may be influenced by the availability of suspensions and slow release once-daily preparations. The gastric irritation these drugs can cause may be of concern, particularly for those who have low platelet counts. This can be helped by giving H_2/receptor blockers such as ranitidine. The potential benefits must be weighed against the unacceptability, to many children, of multiple medications.

(iii) Anti-depressants and anti-convulsants

Neuropathic pain, from tumour invasion or compression, characteristically has a burning or tingling quality and may be shooting and stabbing in nature. It is relatively unresponsive to opioid drugs and may be severe and difficult to relieve. Tricyclic anti-depressants such as amitriptyline can diminish this type of pain. The action appears to be distinct from its anti-depressant effect as it occurs with much lower doses (0.5–1/5 mg/kg at bedtime) and within a couple of days. Carbamazepine and phenytoin may also be helpful for nerve pain. They appear to act through reduction in spontaneous neuronal firing. Doses should be built up to the tolerated maximum before the trial of that drug is abandoned.

(iv) Steroids

Steroids have been widely used in adult palliative care. However, the problems may be greater than the benefits unless life expectancy is very short. Dexamethasone is usually the drug of choice and although advantages may be apparent at first as the disease progresses, a time comes when increasing the dose no longer helps. It is then difficult to reduce the dose because symptoms recur and meanwhile the problems from side effects continue.

Steroids reduce pain caused by compression and distension due to intracerebral tumours, peripheral nerve involvement, bony metastases, and stretching of the liver capsule. They may also improve appetite and general well being. Side effects include unpleasant changes in mood and behaviour (which are common), gastritis, and the rapid alteration of physical appearance. These side effects are often distressing to both children and their parents. Marked weight gain can make nursing care difficult and as mobility decreases in children with central nervous system tumours skin problems can be exacerbated.

(v) Palliative chemotherapy

The use of chemotherapy may be considered to provide pain relief. A situation in which it can be particularly helpful is that of central nervous system leukaemia where regular intrathecal drugs can dramatically relieve symptoms.

(vi) Radiotherapy

Radiation can alleviate many symptoms and should be considered in the case of a radiosensitive tumour with a clearly defined site. Pain due to bony metastases, symptoms from obstruction by mediastinal or pelvic masses, spinal cord compression and local recur-

rences in skin and soft tissue are particular situations where it may be helpful. The use of very short courses, preferably single fraction, in palliative medicine have been explored and recommended; unfortunately this is still not common practice in the United Kingdom (Price *et al.*, 1986; Crellin, 1989).

(vii) Anaesthetic blocks

These are not very often used in paediatrics. Most children have widespread disease at the time of relapse and their tumours progress rapidly. Occasionally they may be helpful and the skills of an anaesthetist familiar with the techniques should be sought.

(viii) Psychological help for pain

Explanations of the causes of pain, exploration of fears of the disease and its outcome, and reassurance have a vital role in management and help resolve the psychological component of pain. Hypnosis, distraction, and the relaxation techniques developed to help with painful procedures during treatment, also have a role in the pain of progressive disease (Zeltzer and LeBaron, 1986). Children are susceptible subjects, enjoy these procedures and there are no unpleasant side effects. Both children and parents can rapidly learn the process themselves and benefit from this increased sense of control. The techniques can be particularly useful for the child who has intermittent episodes of increased pain where raising the overall level of their analgesics causes unacceptable drowsiness, and in order to help with insomnia and anxiety.

33.4.2 BLOOD AND PLATELET TRANSFUSIONS

The nature of childhood tumours is such that many terminally ill children have bone marrow infiltration, resulting in low platelet counts and anaemia. It is possible to provide both platelet and red cell transfusions over many months and often there is a dilemma of whether to do so, how often, and for how long.

(a) Platelets

For a child who is terminally ill from leukaemia a massive cerebral bleed may mean a relatively easy death. On the other hand, for a child to choke from massive haemoptysis is frightening for the patient, distressing for the carers, and will leave the family with unforgettably painful memories of the time of death. During chemotherapy it is routine to give a child platelets when the blood level falls below 20×10^9 per litre as there is a significant risk of spontaneous bleeding. However, there are few guidelines in the literature for this situation in terminal care and practice tends to depend on personal judgement. Routine platelet transfusion according to the level of the platelet count has not been our regular practice. We have given platelets only when bleeding problems which interfere with the quality of life have occurred; for example, persistent nose bloods or haematemesis, but not petechiae. However, children with a past history of significant bleeding problems, such as those with myeloid and acute promyelocytic leukaemia, have had regular platelet transfusions. There have been suggestions that haemostatics such as tranexamic acid may help to reduce spontaneous bleeding even when platelets are low (Avvisati *et al.*, 1989; Chambers *et al.*, 1989).

(b) Blood

Red cell transfusions may offer a child marked improvement in the quality of life when no other symptoms than those of anaemia are present. Each situation must be judged at the time it occurs and in consultation with the family. It is important to be clear, before beginning red cell transfusions, of their value and purpose at this particular point in the illness. Emphasis should be placed on the symptoms of anaemia and on the fact that the purpose of the transfusion is to relieve these symptoms so that the child can continue an otherwise good quality of life. It should be clear from the start that there will come a point when his quality of life has declined to an extent that blood transfusions may no longer be appropriate.

If a child has a central line, *in situ* transfusions can be given easily and atraumatically. Platelets, which take only a short time to infuse, can be given readily at home either by a specialist nurse, the local family doctor, or the district nurse. Routine cover or immediate access to hydrocortisone and antihistamines should be available. Transfusion of blood requires more time and is usually more conveniently done in the hospital as a day or overnight admission.

33.4.3 GASTROINTESTINAL PROBLEMS

Nausea and vomiting are the most prominent gastrointestinal symptoms in palliative care. They are often multifactorial in origin but the predominant cause should be sought so that anti-emetic treatment can be planned rationally, using the appropriate drugs according to the site of the emetic stimulus (below and Chapter 28).

Drugs such as the phenothiazines and haloperidol are believed to act via the chemoreceptor trigger zone and are therefore appropriate for the nausea of endogenous or iatrogenic chemical stimuli. The nausea due to raised intracranial pressure responds best to cyclizine. Metoclopramide, which is contra-indicated in the vomiting caused by intestinal obstruction, may be helpful in the overflow vomiting which occurs when the stomach is compressed by an external mass.

The role of the newer 5HT antagonists is being addressed in the treatment of nausea and vomiting of chemotherapy (Pinkerton *et al.*, 1990), but has not yet been explored in terminal care. A combination of anti-emetics working synergistically may be more helpful than a single drug.

For a mild gastrointestinal problem, oral drugs may help but rectal or parenteral routes are often needed. Drugs such as cyclizine and haloperidol, which are compatible with opioids, can be given in combination with them via a subcutaneous syringe pump. Both chlorpromazine and prochlorperazine are skin irritants. The drug methotrimeprazine can be given subcutaneously and is markedly sedating as well as anti-emetic – something which may be useful in an anxious or agitated patient.

Constipation, usually a side-effect of opioids, should be anticipated and treated vigorously. Oral drugs are preferable and combinations of stool softeners such as lactulose or docusate with stimulants like biscodyl and danthron can be used. Rectal measures may be needed if prophylaxis is unsuccessful. Poor oral hygiene is common in debilitated patients and good mouth care should be encouraged with appropriate use of anti-fungal agents if necessary.

33.4.4 OTHER SYMPTOMS

A variety of other symptoms may occur, depending on the site of the tumours. Information specific to children is scarce but useful advice for a range of problems common in adult palliative care can be adapted (Twycross and Lack, 984; Regnard and Davies, 1986).

33.5 PSYCHOLOGICAL SUPPORT

The need for and importance of psychological support for the dying child and the family is generally acknowledged. However, psychological support can be difficult to define precisely and to provide effectively. The aim is to relieve psychological distress and approaches to achieving this are through establishing a dialogue, identifying the patient's real concerns, listening, acknowledging feelings, and opening possible avenues of thought and action (Lansdown and Goldman, 1988). The provision of psychological support in paediatrics involves considering the needs of the parent and siblings as well as the patient. Care of the bereaved family is a separate issue that will not be considered in this chapter.

A major area of concern for parents is the need for information. Questions about the illness, its past treatment, terminal course, symptoms and their relief, length of time, the death itself, and funeral plans, may all be asked or be the unspoken cause of anxiety. Honest and full answers covering the factual content of the questions is necessary and should be followed by exploration of the feelings which are associated. Parents may need to talk of their sadness, confusion, anger, guilt or any of the multitude of feelings which are involved in trying to make sense of and come to terms with the death of a loved child.

Marital counselling is not part of the brief of the terminal care team but it is appropriate to acknowledge the stress of a child's illness on a marriage, give both partners opportunities to talk of how the child's impending death is affecting them – separately, if appropriate – and if necessary to offer referral to a marriage counselling organization.

Parents will often ask for advice in dealing both with the sick child's questions and those of the siblings. Adults are often at a loss when they try to communicate openly with children. Help can be offered on age-appropriate approaches.

Children's concepts of death and of their illness develop gradually. (Kane, 1979; Lansdown and Benjamin, 1985). Their level of understanding will influence their concerns and the ways in which to work with them in order to help. Children tend to appreciate more than adults expect (Bluebond-Langner, 1978) and are aware of death at as young as three years of age. At first they think of death as an ill-defined reversible state, associated with separation and loss of movement; a fuller awareness, including the permanence and universality of death, develops with time. Most seven-year-olds have a complete or almost complete understanding.

Parents can be helped to communicate with their children, not only through direct conversation, but by being alert to their indirect approaches: 'I don't need any more new toys now'. Some children can express themselves more readily through play or drawing or may respond to an opening provided by reading a story involving illness or death (Wass, 1984; Lamers, 1986). Parents are often grateful for the opportunity of anticipating awkward situations and of rehearsing their response.

Most parents find they are able, with encouragement and support, to be open with siblings. However, even for the most open, the idea of facing a child's own death with the child him or herself is immensely difficult. Mutual pretence between parents and the sick child is a common phenomenon (Bluebond-Langner, 1978) which can result in the child being denied an opportunity to express his own fears.

It is not always possible to break the pretence but parents may be helped to recognize that it exists and allow the child a chance to talk to a third person. Anxiety in children – which may also be manifest as nightmares, withdrawn behaviour, or aggression – is commonly reduced if they can understand and anticipate events as much as possible. Discussing their death may precipitate feelings of distress and anger in the child but if these can be acknowledged and expressed openly stress can be reduced. The child will also have the opportunity of fulfilling any plans and of saying goodbye.

Talking to patients about bad news and death is rarely easy. The doctor or nurse may themselves be affected by many fears, some overt and some hidden, which can interfere with the effectiveness of their conversation (Buckman, 1984). It appears that even staff committed to care of the dying consistently use distancing tactics and avoid getting too close to their patients' suffering (Maguire, 1985). Provision of teaching in communication skills and adequate support for staff involved in terminal care is important. It will help them to provide optimum care for their patients while at the same time maintaining their own job satisfaction and equilibrium.

REFERENCES

Andrasik, F., Burke, E.J., Attanasio, V. and Rosenblum, E.L. (1985) Child, parent and physician reports of a child's headache pain: Relationships prior to and following treatment. *Headache*, **25**, 421–5.

Avvisati, G., Buller, H., Wouter ten Cate, J. and Mandelli, F. (1989) Tranexamic acid for control of haemorrhage. *Lancet*, **2**, 122–4.

Bayer, J. and Wells, N. (1989) The assessment of pain in children. *Pediatr. Clin. N. Am.*, **36**, 837–54.

Bluebond-Langner, M. (1978) The private worlds of dying children. Princeton University Press, Princeton, NJ.

Buckman, R. (1984) Breaking bad news: why is it still so difficult? *Br. Med. J.*, **288**, 1597–9.

Burne, S.R., Dominica, F. and Baum, J.D. (1984) Helen House – a hospice for children: analysis of the first year. *Br. Med. J.*, **289**, 1665–8.

Chambers, E.J., Oakhill, A., Cornish, J.M. and Curnick, S. (1989) Terminal care at home for children with cancer. *Br. Med. J.*, **298**, 937–40.

Crellin, A.M., Marks, A. and Maher, E.J. (1989) Why don't British radiotherapists give single fractions of radiotherapy for bone metastases. *Clin. Oncol.*, **1**, 63–6.

Goldman, A., Beardsmore, S. and Hunt, J. (1990)

Palliative care for children with cancer – home, hospital or hospice. *Arch. Dis. Child.*, **65**, 641–43.

Goldman, A. and Bowman, A. (1990) The role of oral controlled release morphine for pain relief in children with cancer. *Palliative Medicine*, **4**, 279–85.

Kamps, W.A., Akkerboom, J.C., Kingma, A. and Bennett Humphrey, G. (1987) Experimental chemotherapy in children with cancer – a parent's view. *Pediatr. Hematol. Oncol.*, **4**, 117–24.

Kane, B. (1979) Children's concepts of death. *J. Genet. Psychology*, **134**, 141–53.

Kohler, J.A. and Radford, M. (1985) Terminal care for children dying of cancer: quantity and quality of life. *Br. Med. J.*, **91**, 115–6.

Lamers, E. (1986) Books for adolescents, in *Adolescence and Death* (eds C.A Corr and J.N. McNeill), Springer-Verlag, New York.

Lansdown, R. and Benjamin, G. (1985) The development of the concept of death in children aged 5–9 years. *Child Care Health Dev.*, **11**, 13–20.

Lansdown, R. and Goldman, A.G. (1988) The psychological care of children with malignant disease. *J. Child. Psychol. Psychiatr.*, **29**, 555–67.

Lauer, M.E., Mulhern, R.K., Wallskog, J.M. and Camitta, B.M. (1983) A comparison study of parental adaptation following a child's death at home or in the hospital. *Pediatrics*, **71**, 107–11.

McGrath, P.A. (1990) *Pain in Children: Nature, Assessment and Treatment.* Guilford Press, London.

McGrath, P.A., DeVeber, L.L. and Hearn, M.T. (1985) Multidimensional pain assessment in children, in *Advances in Pain Research and Therapy* (eds H.L. Fields, R. Dubner and F. Cervero) Raven Press, New York, pp. 387–393.

McGrath, P.J. and Unruh, A. (1987) *Pain in Children.* Elsevier, Amsterdam.

Maguire, P. (1985) Barriers to psychological care of the dying. *Br. Med. J.*, **291**, 1711–13.

Maher, E.J. and Jefferis, A.F. (1990) Decision making in advanced cancer of the head and neck: variation in the views of medical specialists. *J. Roy. Soc. Med.*, **83**, 356–9.

Maloney, C., Kaye Kesner, R. Klein, G. and Bockenstette, J. (1989) Rectal administration of MS Contin: Clinical implications of use in end stage cancer. *Am. J. Hospice Care*, **6**, 34–5.

Mulhern, R.K., Lauer, M.E. and Hoffman, R.G. (1983) Death of a child at home or in the hospital: subsequent psychological adjustment of the family. *Pediatrics*, **71**, 743–7.

Nitschke, R., Bennett Humphrey, G., Sexauer, C.L. *et al.* (1982) Therapeutic choices made by patients with end-stage cancer. *J. Pediatrics*, **101**, 471–6.

Office of Population Censuses and Surveys. Mortality statistics in childhood. 1988 Mortality Statistics. DH2 No. 15. HMSO.

Pinkerton, C.R., Williams, D., Wooton, C., Meller, S.T. and McElwain, T.J. (1990) 5HT3 antagonist, ondansetron – an effective outpatient antiemetic in cancer treatment. *Arch. Dis. Child.*, **65**, 822–55.

Price, P., Hoskin, P.J., Austin, A., Palmer, S.G. and Yarnold, J.R. (1986) Prospective randomised trial of single and multifraction radiotherapy schedules in the treatment of painful bony metastases. *Radiotherapy and Oncology*, **6**, 247–55.

Regnard, C.F.B. and Davies, A. (1986) *A guide to symptom relief in advanced cancer.* Distributed by Haigh & Hochland, Manchester, UK.

Shannon, M. and Berde, C. (1989) Pharmacologic management of pain in children and adolescents. *Pediatr. Clin. N. Am.*, **36**, 855–72.

Twycross, R.G. and Lack, S.A. (1984) *Therapeutics in Terminal Cancer.* Churchill Livingstone.

Waas, H. (1984) Books for Children, in *Childhood death.* (eds H. Wass and C.A. Corr). Hemisphere, London.

Woolley, H., Stein, A., Forrest, G.C. and Baum, J.D. (1989) Imparting the diagnosis of life threatening illness in children. *Br. Med. J.*, **298**, 1623–6.

Zeltzer, L. and LeBaron, S. (1986) The hypnotic treatment of children in pain. *Adv. Dev. Behav. Pediatr.*, **7**, 197–234.

Index

Page numbers in italics refer to figures, those in bold refer to tables.

630

639

trilateral 283
triple-freeze cryotherapy 277
Retinoids 372
Retinomas 273
Reverse genetics 35
Rhabdomyosarcoma (RMS)
  aetiology and genetics 291–2
  alveolar, genetic
    abnormalities **62**
  alveolar (ARMS) *294*–5, 297
  botryoid 293
  chemotherapy **305–9**
  classification 292–6
  clinical manifestation 296–*7*
  congenital anomaly
    association 292
  development 54
  diagnostic biopsy 300–1
  embryonal (ERMS) 293, 295
  follow-up studies 608
  high grade 294–5
  histogenesis 55–6
  incidence **3**, 5, 291
  International Study
    Committee on
    classification 292–3
  IRS clinical grouping
    classification **138**
  leiomyomatous 294
  liver 424
  low grade 293–4
  megatherapy 472, 474
  multidrug resistance 105–6,
    318
  pattern of spread 296
  primary excision 301–2
  primary sites 295–6
    distribution **295**
  prognostic factors 299–300
  radiation sensitivity **79**
  radiotherapy 303–5
    trials 590
  second tumours 316–17
  secondary surgery 302
  spindle cell 293–4
  staging investigation 297–8
  staging systems 298–9
    clinical categories **299**
  surgical management 300
  survival
    by disease extent **310**
    by primary sites **310**
  treatment
    modalities 300–10
  ultrastructural features **60**

see also Soft tissue sarcomas
Ribosome inactivating proteins
  (RIP) 522
Ricin 463, 496–7, 522
Ridgeway sarcoma model 461
RNA analysis, enzyme
  degradation 67
RNA diagnostics 65–7
RNAse protection assay *66*–7
Rye histopathological
  classification 217

Sacrococcygeal tumour 397–8
Salivary gland tumours 451–3
Sarcomas, *see* Soft tissue
  sarcomas
School nurse, role of 614
Schwannoma 244, 315–16
Scleral plaque therapy for
  retinoblastoma 277–8
Scoliosis after Wilms'
  tumour 386
Screening for
  neuroblastoma 126–30
Seascale
  birth risk study 18
  school risk study 18
Selective bowel
  decontamination
  (SBD) 584–5
Sellafield, paternal radiation
  risk 19
Seminoma 392
Septrin prophylaxis in acute
  leukaemia 613
Serotonin, in carcinoid
  tumour 120
Shanghai, paternal radiation
  risk 19
Shimada histopathological
  classification 466
SIOP 138, 139, 234, 317
  brain tumour trial 259
  liver tumour
    grouping system *417*
    study 417
  MMT-89 317
  radiotherapy trial 590
  RMS primary
    distribution **295**
  Study Group 221
  study MMT-89 304, 317
  Study on soft tissue
    sarcomas 307–*8*

TMN staging system for soft-
  tissue sarcomas 299
Wilms' tumour
  classification **382**–3
  management *383–4*
  pathology 380
SIOP–Intergroup European
  Study on soft tissue
  sarcomas 309
Slot blots 65
Small cell lung carcinoma
  (SCLC), mutations 38
Smoking and childhood
  cancer 7
Societe Internationale
  d'Oncologie Pediatrique
  (SIOP), *see* SIOP
Soft tissue sarcomas
  bladder–prostate,
    therapy 309
  differential diagnosis **313**
  follow-up studies 608
  incidence 291
  late sequelae 316–17
  megatherapy **472**
  non rhabdo (NRSTS) 311–
    19
    chemotherapy 311–13
    chemotherapy
      response 318–19
    clinical features **312**
  orbit, therapy 309
  parameningeal head-neck,
    therapy 309
  paratesticular, therapy
    309–10
  prognostic factors 317
Somnolence syndrome 191
Southern analysis *63*–4
Southern blotting 410
Southwest Oncology Group
  (SWOG), hepatoblastoma
  study 413
Spheroid model systems 496
Spinal cord tumours 244
Spinal irradiation and
  growth 532
Spironolactone 167
Stereotactic multiple arc
  rotational technique
  (SMART) 256
Stereotactic radiotherapy 592
Sternberger's PAP method 59
Strawberry naevus 456
Streptavidin 502

Stress
  cardiac damage
    recurrence 558
  and catecholamine metabolite
    secretion 117
Sublingual gland tumours 452
Suramin 512
Survival
  definition 158
  disease-free, definition 158
  event-free, definition 158
Surviving fraction equation 74
Sympathogonia 359
Synaptophysin 314
Synovial sarcoma 311, 315
  genetic abnormalities **62**

T-cell
  antigen receptor 31
  depletion (TCD) 170–2
  function in Langerhans cell
    histiocytosis 434
  lymphoblastic lymphoma 53
  proliferation in NHL 200
  receptor gene 31
Tadpole cells 293
Tamoxifen 456
Tanner growth charts 554
Targeting therapy 495–505
Teacher, role of 614
Teeth, radiation damage 316
Teicoplanin 166–**8**
Teilum's classification of germ
  cell tumours *112*
Teniposide,
  pharmacokinetics **92**
Teratoma **393–4**
  abdominal 399
  head and neck 399
  histology 396
  mature 249, 251
  mediastinal 398–9
  see also Germ cell tumour
Testis
  function after
    chemotherapy 543–5,
    550–2, 553
  irradiation 546, 549–50, 551
  tumours 401–2
    differential diagnosis **399**,
    401
    UKCCSG staging
      system **402**
Tetrahydrocannabinol
  (THC) 573

Thalassaemia, mutations 35
Therapeutic drug monitoring
  (TDM) 525
Therapeutic index 87
Thioguanine 168
6-Thioguanine (6-TG),
  pharmacokinetics **90**
Thiopurine methyltransferase
  (TPMT) 105
Thiotepa, for brain
  tumours 478–**9**
Thymidylate synthase (TS) 95
Thyroid carcinoma *446–8*
  iodine uptake 495
Thyroid dysfunction, after
  irradiation 542
Thyroid hormone
  insufficiency 596–7
Thyroid nodules, benign 541
Thyroid tumours, after
  radiation 541
Ticarcillin 577
Toluidine dye (MTT) assay 105
Topoisomerase II, action
  98–100
Total body irradiation (TBI)
  84–5, 464–5
  role 467–71
Totally protected environment
  (RPE) 584
Transcobalamin I, marker 123
  in fibrolamellar hepatocellular
    carcinoma 423
Transient myeloproliferative
  disorder (TMD) 180–1
Translocation breakpoints 30
Treatment evaluation
  difference in response
    149–50
  no difference in
    response 148–9
  variability of response *147–8*
Trichrome stain 57
Tuberous sclerosis, childhood
  cancer risk 12
Tubular fertility index
  (TFI) *543–5*
Tubulin, binding to vinca
  alkaloids 99
Tumour
  antibody penetration
    failure 499
  benign 54–5
  borderline 54–5
  chromosome analysis 42

diagnostic methods 56–61
DNA evaluation 63–4
histogenesis 55–6
model systems 523
mutations 38–9
radiosensitivity 74
second primary 564
survival relationship to gross
  tumour response 75
targeting therapy 495–505
Tumour growth factor
  (TGF) 512
Tumour growth fraction 87
Tumour lysis syndrome 164,
  203
Tumour markers 356–9
  biological 109–12
  clinical use 108
  enzymes *356*
  hormonal 126
  as prognostic factors 125–6
Tumour necrosis factor
  (TNF) 171, 343, 372
Tumour node metastases (TNM)
  classification 136, 138
  general principles **137**
  for neuroblastoma **354**
  relevance to paediatrics
    137–8
  for soft-tissue sarcomas **299**
  staging system outline 137
  for Wilms' tumour **383**
Tumour staging, purpose 136
Tumour suppressor gene 31,
  34
  in 11p13 41
Tumour-associated
  antigens 520
Turcot's syndrome 11
Twins
  and childhood cancer 11
  leukaemia risk 181
  Wilms' tumour in 379
Tyrosine protein kinases
  513–14

Ultrasound, safety 5
US National Cancer Institute
  drug screening
    programme 523
  infection control studies 577
  SEER Programme 52–3
  small cell lung tumour
    studies 512